THE BASIC PHYSICS OF RADIATION THERAPY

THE BASIC PHYSICS
of
RADIATION THERAPY

(*Second Edition*)

By

JOSEPH SELMAN, M.D., F.A.C.R., F.A.C.P.

Clinical Assistant Professor of Radiology, The Southwestern Medical School
University of Texas
Director, School of Radiologic Technology, Tyler Junior College
Attending Radiologist, Medical Center Hospital
Attending Radiologist, Mother Frances Hospital
Consultant in Radiology, East Texas Chest Hospital
Tyler, Texas

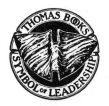

CHARLES C THOMAS • PUBLISHER
Springfield • Illinois • U. S. A.

Published and Distributed Throughout the World by

CHARLES C THOMAS • PUBLISHER
Bannerstone House
301-327 East Lawrence Avenue, Springfield, Illinois, U.S.A.

ISBN 0-398-03247-5

Library of Congress Catalog Card Number 74 9589

First Edition, 1960
First Edition, Second Printing, 1973
Second Edition, 1976

*With THOMAS BOOKS careful attention is given to all details of
manufacturing and design. It is the Publisher's desire to present books that
are satisfactory as to their physical qualities and artistic possibilities and
appropriate for their particular use. THOMAS BOOKS will be true to
those laws of quality that assure a good name and good will.*

Library of Congress Cataloging in Publication Data

Selman, Joseph.
    The basic physics of radiation therapy.

    Bibliography: p.
    1. Radiotherapy.   2. Radiation.   I. Title.
[DNLM: 1. Food. 2. Nutrition. QU145 H178f]
RM859.S4   1974   615'.842   74-9589
ISBN 0:398-03247-5

Printed in the United States of America
BB-14

Preface to the Second Edition

AS would be expected, a number of advances have taken place in the physics of radiotherapy during the thirteen-year time span between the First and Second Editions. However, none of these may be considered monumental.

One significant change has been in units and terminology—the further clarification of the concepts of radiation exposure and dosage. While this seems to have been stabilized for the time being, there is on the horizon the threat of a more scientific, but at the same time a vastly more complex International System of Units (S.I.). This has already been accepted by the Soviet Union as well as the member countries of the European Economic Community. The S.I. will be touched upon, although there is still considerable resistance to its adoption in the United States.

In this edition, emphasis has been shifted to megavoltage radiation, and rightly so. Whereas formerly kilovoltage radiation (200 to 300 kV) had been the "backbone" of irradiation therapy the advent of cobalt 60 teletherapy, followed by the linac, has all but made kilovoltage radiation obsolete except for certain limited indications. A separate section has been added to cover electron beam therapy.

Because of growing interest in radiotherapy with heavy particles (high-LET radiation), a new chapter has been introduced to deal with this modality. Special emphasis in this regard has been placed on neutron and negative pion beams. This new chapter has been deliberately placed after that on radiobiology to provide the rationale for the use of high-LET radiation.

In general, the text has been almost completely rewritten, obsolete material eliminated, some sections combined, and some chapters rearranged. Although illustrations and tables from the First Edition have been retained wherever applicable, a number have been updated and new ones added.

v

The chapters covering radionuclides have been reworked and made more comprehensive. The diagnostic use of radionuclides has been minimized and major attention directed to their therapeutic application.

Radiation protection in therapy, including radionuclides, has been expanded. An example of the computation of wall protective barriers has been included, for the author feels that the radiotherapist should have at least a basic understanding of how this is done, despite the fact that it is the ultimate responsibility of the radiation physicist.

In addition to the appreciative acknowledgement of the data furnished by the manufacturers of therapy equipment cited in the First Edition, the author wishes to thank Varian for kindly providing important material on their linac units through John C. Ford, Ph.D.; and to Atomic Energy of Canada, Ltd. Revision of earlier illustrations and preparation of new ones have again been admirably executed by A. Howard Marlin, for which the author is most appreciative.

Finally, many thanks are due Charles C Thomas, Publisher, in the person of Payne Thomas, for providing the opportunity and encouragement toward the realization of this Second Edition.

JOSEPH SELMAN, M.D.

Preface to the First Edition

PHYSICS has played a dominant role not only in the birth and development of Therapeutic Radiology, but also in the charting of its future course. Every major advance in the technical aspects of radiation therapy has been predicated on new information in physics and engineering. This is evidenced particularly by the advent and popularization of supervoltage therapy and medical radioisotopes.

To the resident in radiology, physics often looms as a major obstacle in a varied and intensive program. So often, the newcomer to radiology is keenly aware of his deficient background in the physical sciences, making his task even more difficult. Yet, a secure foundation in radiologic physics is necessary both as a part of any successful training program and as a basis upon which to build future knowledge. The chore of keeping abreast of new developments in therapy methods and apparatus, and of appraising their value, is facilitated when the radiologist is adequately trained in physics. However, there is no consensus among teachers of radiology as to the amount of time that should be devoted to physics in the average residency training program. While some believe that there is already too much emphasis on the physical basis of radiotherapy, others are of the opinion that in many cases this is being grossly neglected. Despite this difference of opinion, there can be no question that the better the radiologist's training in physics, the more intelligently he can plan his therapy and the more satisfactory will be his relationship with his consulting physicist.

The purpose of this book is to explain the fundamental physical principles underlying radiation therapy in as comprehensive and comprehensible a manner as possible, without sacrificing accuracy for simplicity. Wherever possible, the material is presented from the standpoint of the radiologist who, from his own experience,

vii

is aware of the problems confronting the resident in radiology. It is hoped that such a presentation will be of benefit not only to the resident but also as a refresher course for the practicing radiologist. Furthermore, in view of the present trend toward two-year courses in schools of X-ray technology, this book may serve to direct more attention to the physics of radiation therapy in the X-ray technician's training program. To facilitate adaptation to various curricula, the chapters and sections are so arranged that certain material can be excluded without jeopardizing the continuity of the text. For this reason, a minimum of cross references has been used; each section has been made as complete as possible in its own right.

Since experienced teachers are well aware of the shortcomings of most neophytes where mathematics is concerned, the first chapter is devoted to the mathematical concepts pertinent to Therapeutic Radiology. Matter, energy, and radiations are then covered in survey fashion in order to acquaint the student with modern "pure" physics in preparation for the more specific aspects of radiation therapy physics. The production and properties of orthovoltage X rays are reviewed briefly, since most students will have had a certain amount of instruction along these lines. The greatest emphasis is placed on the interactions of radiation with matter, radiation dosage and quality, therapy planning, supervoltage and telecurietherapy, radioactivity and nuclear physics, and radium and radioisotope therapy. Finally, detailed consideration is given to radiobiology and health physics since these are assuming a position of ever-increasing importance not only in medicine, but in the world at large.

The Bibliography has been assembled at the end of the book in order to facilitate the location of references. A supplementary list of textbooks and other books for collateral reading has been added to broaden the scope of the student's background.

The kindness and interest of the following physicists, who reviewed portions of the manuscript and offered valuable suggestions, is acknowledged with sincere appreciation, although the author assumes full responsibility for any errors of commission or omission: Kenneth E. Corrigan, Ph.D.; Gerald E. Swindell, M.S.; Jack S. Krohmer, M.A.; and Lawrence Brown, Ph.D.

Several commercial organizations have been most cooperative in furnishing data on various types of equipment and devices: Picker X-ray Corporation; High Voltage Engineering Corporation; General Electric X-ray Corporation; Tracerlab, Inc.; Victoreen Instrument Company; Nuclear-Chicago Corporation; Machlett Laboratories, Inc.; Gilbert X-ray Company of Texas; and North American Philips Company, Inc. Thanks are also due those authors and publishers who so generously permitted the use of their published data, as well as those whose original ideas and works bear the mark of anonymity.

Special recognition must be given the artist, Howard Marlin, for his admirable execution of the illustrations from the sketches provided by the author. The author's secretary, Mrs. Charlene Lane, should also be mentioned with gratitude for her diligence in typing the major part of the manuscript, including the tables.

Finally, the interest and encouragement of Charles C Thomas, Publisher, and their most competent staff are greatly appreciated, as have been their invaluable suggestions during the preparation of the manuscript.

JOSEPH SELMAN, M.D.

Contents

THE BASIC PHYSICS OF
RADIATION THERAPY

CHAPTER 1

Simple Mathematics of Radiation Therapy

FROM its earliest days physics has evolved hand-in-hand with mathematics to reach its present advanced position. Moreover, mathematics continues to serve the physicist in a number of ways. Not only does it facilitate the comprehension of physical principles, but it also aids in the correlation of experimental and observational data. Furthermore, it makes possible the development of new concepts.

For the student of radiologic physics in particular, mathematics is essential both as an aid to learning and as a means or handling the data pertinent to radiation therapy. Since an insight into the physics of radiation therapy may be gained without resorting to higher mathematics, only those mathematical processes that are applicable to this field will be presented here.

PROPORTION

One of the more fundamental mathematical concepts is *proportion,* which simply expresses the equality of two *ratios* or *fractions.* Three main types of proportion are used in radiologic physics: (1) simple direct proportion, (2) simple inverse proportion, and (3) inverse square proportion.

Simple Direct Proportion. We may represent simple direct proportion in three ways: *algebraic* or *arithmetic, geometric,* and *graphic.*

1. *Algebraic or Arithmetic Proportion.* At a half price sale the ratio $\frac{1}{2}$ indicates the fraction by which the list price would be reduced on any given article. Thus, if an item were marked $2.00, its sale price would be $1.00. To represent such a simple situation in algebraic terms immediately establishes the basic concept of

1

proportion. If x is to be the sale price, and the list price happens to be $6.00, a proportion can be set up as follows:

$$\frac{x}{6} = \frac{1}{2}$$

Solving this equation by cross multiplication, we obtain

$$2x = 6$$
$$x = 3 \text{ dollars, the sale price}$$

Simple direct proportion can be stated algebraically as follows:

$$\frac{y}{x} = \frac{b}{a} \tag{1}$$

This means that y is as many times greater than x, as b is greater than a. y/x is a ratio that is equal to the ratio b/a. If any three of these factors are known, the fourth can easily be determined by equation (1).

Note that in any given proportion, the ratio is constant. Thus, in equation (1), b/a is a constant. Substituting the constant k for b/a in equation (1),

$$\frac{y}{x} = k$$

$$y = kx \tag{2}$$

k is called the **constant of proportionality.** Whenever a variable such as y (known as the *dependent variable*) is proportional to another variable such as x (known as the *independent variable*), then it is equal to a constant times the variable, as noted in equation (2). y is said to be a function of x often expressed as $y = f(x)$. Only if the constant is known can the dependent variable corresponding to any given independent variable be found.

2. *Geometric Proportion.* When two triangles are of the same shape, though of different size, they are said to be **similar triangles.** In plane geometry, such similar triangles have the property of proportionality of their corresponding sides (i.e. the sides

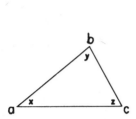
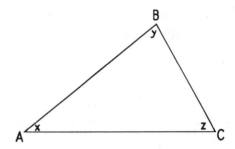

FIGURE 1.01. Similar triangles. $AB/ab = BC/bc = CD/cd$ because the corresponding sides are directly proportional when the corresponding angles are equal.

opposite the equal angles). In Figure 1.01 the corresponding sides are proportional:

$$AB/ab = AC/ac$$

$$AB/ab = BC/bc$$

$$BC/bc = AC/ac$$

In other words, the ratio of any two corresponding sides is the same as that of any other two corresponding sides. Or, a side is just as many times greater than its corresponding side, as any other side is greater than its corresponding side.

3. *Graphic Proportion.* A simple proportion may be expressed in the form of a *graph.* For example, the diameter of an X-ray beam is directly proportional to the target-skin distance. If a series of actual measurements is made and tabulated, it might appear as shown in Table 1.01. Note that the ratio of any field

TABLE 1.01
DATA ILLUSTRATING SIMPLE DIRECT PROPORTION; THE RELATIONSHIP
OF TARGET-SKIN DISTANCE TO DIAMETER OF A BEAM

Target-Skin Distance	Diameter	Ratio of Diameter to Distance
cm	*cm*	
10	8	$8/10 = 4/5$
20	16	$16/20 = 4/5$
30	24	$24/30 = 4/5$
40	32	$32/40 = 4/5$
50	40	$40/50 = 4/5$

diameter to its corresponding distance, 8/10, is the same as that of any other, such as 24/30. In each case, the ratio can be reduced to 4/5.

This information has been plotted in graphic form in Figure 1.02. The graph (curve) is represented by a straight line with its origin at 0. The **slope** of the curve is the ratio of the **vertical distance** of any given point to its **horizontal distance** from the origin (i.e. the ratio of the y to the x coordinate). For example, the vertical dotted line intersects the curve at twenty-four units above the origin, and it also intersects the horizontal line at thirty units from the origin. The slope is therefore 24/30 = 4/5. Stated algebraically, if y is the field diameter and x is the target-skin distance,

$$y = \frac{4}{5}x$$

Note that the constant of proportionality and the slope of the curve are exactly the same, in this case 4/5. Thus, for any distance x, the field diameter y can readily be determined either from the graph or from its algebraic counterpart.

Simple direct proportion has wide application in radiology. For example, we know that the output X of an X-ray machine is proportional to the exposure time t. Therefore, the equation for exposure as a function of time is

$$X = kt \tag{3}$$

where k is the constant of proportionality. If the exposure in 1 min is 50 roentgens (R), then according to equation (3) k is 50 (since $t = 1$). Now with an exposure time of 4 min ($t = 4$)

$$X = 50 \times 4 = 200 \text{ R}$$

Thus, the exposure with a particular set of operating factors can be found, for time t, only if the constant of proportionality is known.

Simple Inverse Proportion. In this type of proportion, the dependent variable changes in the opposite direction from the independent variable. For example, if the independent variable is doubled, the dependent variable is halved.

1. *Algebraic Inverse Proportion.* In simple inverse proportion,

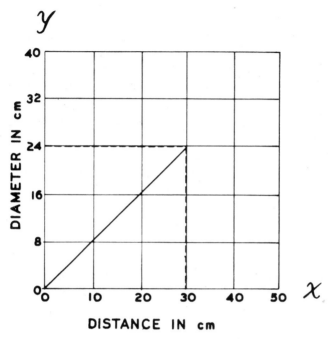

FIGURE 1.02. Graphic representation of simple direct proportion. The diameter of an X-ray beam is directly proportional to the distance from the source. The dotted lines indicate that at a distance of 30 cm, the diameter of the beam is 24 cm. At ⅓ the distance, or 10 cm, the diameter of the beam is also decreased to ⅓, or 8 cm. The slope of the curve is determined by the ratio of the vertical coordinate (such as 24) to the horizontal coordinate (such as 30) of a given point. In this case, the slope is 24/30 = 4/5.

the variables are represented by inverted ratios. For example if x is inversely proportional to y, and if the value of x is x_1 when y is y_1, what will the value of x be when y is y_2? Inverse proportion can be represented as follows:

$$\frac{x_1}{x_2} = \frac{y_2}{y_1} \tag{4}$$

An actual example will clarify this. It is well known that the time needed to deliver a given dose of radiation with radium is inversely proportional to the number of milligrams in the source. If 10 mg Ra provides a certain dose in 2 hr, 20 mg would give the same dose in 1 hr, and 40 mg would give it in ½ hr. Representing this algebraically, if N is the amount of Ra and T is the exposure time,

$$\frac{N_1}{N_2} = \frac{T_2}{T_1} \tag{5}$$

Suppose $N_1 = 25$ mg and $T_1 = 4$ hr to deliver a given dose. What would the treatment time T_2 be with 50 mg Ra? Here $N_2 = 50$ mg. Substituting these values in equation (5),

$$\frac{25}{50} = \frac{T_2}{4}$$

$$T_2 = \frac{100}{50}$$

$$T_2 = 2 \text{ hr}$$

Error in setting up an inverse proportion is minimized if each ratio is made up of the same units. In the above example, note that the left side of the equation consists of mg in the numerator and denominator, while in the right side, time appears in both the numerator and denominator, although inverted.

2. *Graphic Inverse Proportion.* A simple inverse proportion may be expressed in graphic form. Suppose the data in Table 1.02 were obtained under actual conditions. When plotted graphically, they would generate the curve in Figure 1.03. It can be shown that the product of each pair of variables equals a constant. Starting with the equation for inverse proportion,

$$\frac{N_1}{N_2} = \frac{T_2}{T_1}$$

and crossmultiplying,

$$N_1 T_1 = N_2 T_2 = \text{constant}$$

Thus, in any inverse proportion,

$$xy = k, \quad \text{or} \quad y = k/x \tag{6}$$

This can be verified by referring to Table 1.02.

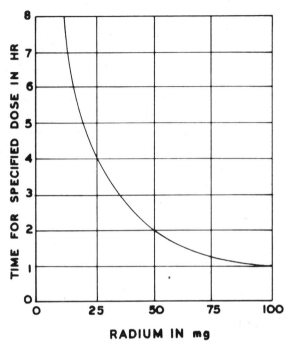

FIGURE 1.03. Graphic representation of simple inverse proportion. The time for a specified dose is inversely proportional to the quantity of radium. For example, 50 mg Ra gives a certain dose in 2 hr. Doubling the amount of Ra to 100 mg reduces the treatment time to 1 hr for the same dose.

Inverse Square Proportion. Of fundamental importance in radiation physics is an understanding of the relationship between the radiation intensity or exposure rate at a point and its distance from the source—the *inverse square law*. Radiation intensity

TABLE 1.02
DATA ILLUSTRATING INVERSE PROPORTION—RELATION BETWEEN
THE QUANTITY OF RADIUM AND THE REQUIRED TREATMENT
TIME TO GIVE THE SAME TOTAL DOSE

Radium	Time for Specified Dose	mg-hr
mg	hr	
100	1	100
50	2	100
25	4	100
12.5	8	100

means the amount of radiation striking a unit area in unit time, such as photons/cm^2/sec. Exposure rate in radiology may be expressed in roentgens per min (R/min). The mathematical basis of the inverse square law is fairly straightforward and can be demonstrated in algebraic, geometric, and graphic forms.

1. *Algebraic Inverse Square Proportion.* If intensities or exposure rates of radiation such as i and I are measured at corresponding distances d and D, and if i is inversely proportional to d^2, then when D is twice d, I will be $\frac{1}{4}i$. This relationship can be expressed as follows:

$$\frac{i}{I} = \frac{D^2}{d^2} \tag{7}$$

For example, if $i = 100$ R/min when $d = 20$ cm, what will the value I be when D is 40 cm? Substituting in equation (7):

$$\frac{100}{I} = \frac{(40)^2}{(20)^2} = \frac{1,600}{400} = \frac{4}{1}$$

$$4I = 100$$

$$I = 25 \text{ R/min}$$

Note that as the distance was doubled, from d_1 to d_2, the resulting exposure rate I_2 became $\frac{1}{4}$ the initial exposure rate I_1.

2. *Geometric Inverse Square Proportion.* Inverse square proportion can also be expressed and solved geometrically. If a beam of radiation emerges from a *point source* and passes through a *square* diaphragm, the area covered by the radiation at any distance can be represented as in Figure 1.04. At distance D the radiation will cover a square area X^2; at distance d it will cover a square area x^2. According to simple geometry (similar triangles), the lengths of the sides of these squares are proportional to their respective distances from the source:

$$\frac{X}{x} = \frac{D}{d} \tag{8}$$

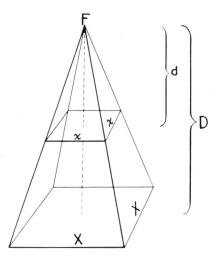

FIGURE 1.04. Inverse square law of radiation. The lower plane X is at a distance twice that of the upper plane x from the focal spot F. Since side X is equal to $2x$, the area of the lower plane is $X^2 = 4x^2$. Thus, at twice the distance, the same amount of radiation is spread over an area 4 times as great and therefore the intensity or exposure rate must be $\frac{1}{4}$ as great.

Squaring both sides of equation (8), we find that the areas are proportional to the squares of their respective distances:

$$\frac{X^2}{x^2} = \frac{D^2}{d^2} \tag{9}$$

But the exposure rate of a beam of radiation is ***inversely*** proportional to the area which it covers, and this is in turn proportional to the square of the distance according to equation (9). Therefore,

$$i \text{ is proportional to } \frac{1}{d^2}$$

or

$$i = \frac{k}{d^2}$$

and

$$I = \frac{k}{D^2}$$

Dividing these two equations,

$$\frac{i}{I} = \frac{D^2}{d^2} \tag{10}$$

3. *Graphic Inverse Square Proportion.* The same concept of inverse square proportionality may be expressed graphically. Actual experimental data are presented in Table 1.03. When plotted graphically, the curve in Figure 1.05 is obtained. Since exposure rate is inversely proportional to distance squared,

$$I = \frac{k}{D^2}$$

$$ID^2 = k \tag{11}$$

This can be verified by referring back to the tabulated data (Table 1.03) for the graph in Figure 1.05. If the values in the distance column are squared and multiplied by the corresponding exposure rate, the product is a constant, as shown in Table 1.03. This provides a means of greatly simplifying the use of the inverse square law. In actual practice, first determine the constant of proportionality for the given situation, and use this to find the exposure rate at any other distance. For example, suppose that under specified conditions the output of a therapy machine is 100 R/min at 100 cm. Since

TABLE 1.03
DATA ILLUSTRATING INVERSE SQUARE PROPORTION—RELATION
BETWEEN THE RADIATION EXPOSURE RATE AND
THE DISTANCE FROM THE SOURCE

Exposure Rate	*Distance*	$Id^2 = k$
R/min	*cm*	
160	10	$160 \times 10^2 = 16{,}000$
40	20	$40 \times 20^2 = 16{,}000$
10	40	$10 \times 40^2 = 16{,}000$
2.5	80	$2.5 \times 80^2 = 16{,}000$

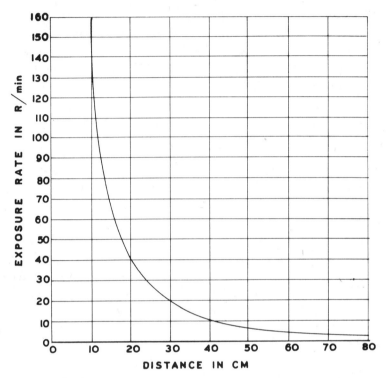

FIGURE 1.05. Graphic representation of inverse square proportion. At a distance of 20 cm, for example, the exposure rate is 40 R/min. Doubling the distance to 40 cm reduces the exposure rate to ¼ the initial value, or 10 R/min.

$$ID^2 = k$$

$$100 \times (100)^2 = k$$

If one needs to know the output i at some other distance d, such as 50 cm, assuming that the radiation is coming from a point source,

$$id^2 = 100 \times (100)^2$$

$$i \times 50^2 = 100 \times (100)^2$$

$$i = \frac{100 \times 100 \times 100}{50 \times 50} = 400 \text{ R/min}$$

The same result can be obtained by use of equation (7).

Since the inverse square law may not apply exactly in actual practice, radiotherapy equipment should be calibrated at various distances by careful measurement. However, application of the inverse square law serves as an approximate check on the accuracy of such measurements.

MATHEMATICAL LAW OF DECAY

Whenever the dependent variable decreases by the same fraction, for equal increments of the independent variable, a **decay** or "die-away" **curve** is obtained. Strictly speaking, however, it is really a **survival curve**, as will be demonstrated below. In simpler terms, if y decreases by the same fractional amount, such as $1/10$, whenever x increases by a fixed amount, such as 1 sec, the value of y will decrease along a curve known as an **exponential decay curve.** This type of mathematical relationship applies especially to radioactive decay, absorption of monochromatic radiation by filters, and survival of cell cultures exposed to increasing doses of radiation.

Without going into mathematical details, the general form of the exponential equation for the decay curve may be stated as follows:

$$A = A_o e^{-\lambda d} \tag{12}$$

where A is the quantity **remaining** after the original quantity A_0 has been influenced by a change in variable d, λ is the decay constant for a given material, and e is a constant (natural logarithmic base). The exponent $-\lambda d$ is negative because A is decreasing.

When applied to radioactive decay, equation (12) may be represented as follows:

$$N = N_o e^{-\lambda t} \tag{13}$$

where N is the number of atoms remaining at the end of time t, N_o is the initial number, and λ is the decay constant. From this equation it can be seen that a radioactive substance gradually decreases in quantity with the passing of time.

When a narrow beam of monoenergetic (same energy) X rays passes through a sufficiently thin filter, the resulting decrease in radiation exposure rate as the filter thickness is increased, can be represented by an equation in the same form as equation (12):

$$I = I_o e^{-\mu d} \tag{14}$$

where I is the **remaining** intensity of the beam after passing through a filter of thickness d, and μ is the linear attention coefficient characteristic of the given material.

While the actual use of this form of equation requires a knowledge of logarithms, it is possible to develop a simple graphic concept without logarithms.

$$N = N_o e^{-\lambda t}$$

where N is the number of radioactive atoms remaining at the end of time t, N_o is the initial number, and λ is the decay constant for a given radioactive nuclide. Since e is also a constant, the equation may be written in the form

$$N = N_o k^{-t} \tag{15}$$

or,

$$N = \frac{N_o}{k^t}$$

(because $k^{-t} = 1/k^t$)

If equation (15) is allowed to take on different values of t in seconds, and if k were to equal 2, and if there are 1280 radioactive atoms initially (N_o), then the different values of N may be found by means of the equation and tabulating the results as in Table 1.04.

Note that this is exactly as stated at the beginning: as time t increases by the same interval, the number of atoms remaining is reduced by the same fraction ($\frac{1}{2}$ in this case). Again note that it is **not** reduced by the same amount; but, **by the same fraction.** Thus, as time increases from zero to 1 sec, the number of atoms

TABLE 1.04
DATA ILLUSTRATING RADIOACTIVE DECAY; THE FRACTIONAL
DECREASE IN THE NUMBER OF ATOMS OF A RADIOACTIVE NUCLIDE
WITH THE PASSING OF TIME WHEN K EQUALS 2

Time (t)	$N = N_0/k^t$	No. of Atoms Remaining at End of Time t
sec		
0	$1280/2^0 = 1280/1$	1280
1	$1280/2^1 = 1280/2$	640
2	$1280/2^2 = 1280/4$	320
3	$1280/2^3 = 1280/8$	160
4	$1280/2^4 = 1280/16$	80
5	$1280/2^5 = 1280/32$	40
6	$1280/2^6 = 1280/64$	20

is changed from 1,280 to 640, or by a factor of ½. With each increment of time of 1 sec, the number of atoms is decreased by ½. Thus, at the end of the next second, the number of atoms decreases from 640 to 320. At the end of the third second, the number decreases to 160, etc. This is shown also in graphic form in Figure 1.06A. The plot is represented by a decay curve which is concave upward when ordinary graph paper is used.

If we plot the same data on *semilog* paper we obtain a straight line curve (see Fig. 1.06B). The reason for this is that the vertical scale is not uniform, the actual measured distances along it representing *ratios.* Thus, the distance measured along the vertical scale between 200 and 400 is the same as the distance between 100 and 200, a factor of 2 in both instances, even though in the first case the interval represents $400 - 200 = 200$ atoms, and in the second case the same interval represents $200 - 100 = 100$ atoms. The vertical scale is, therefore, said to be *logarithmic.*

On the other hand the horizontal scale is laid off in uniform intervals, each division actually representing a *difference* between two values instead of a ratio. It is a *linear* or *nonlogarithmic* scale. Therefore, the plot is called semilogarithmic or semilog because only one scale, in this case the vertical one, is logarithmic.

Other vertical scales could be selected in which the factor would have some value other than 2, but the result would still be a straight line curve, although it would have a different slope.

Because derived data can be obtained more easily and with greater accuracy from a semilog plot (for example, half-life, half

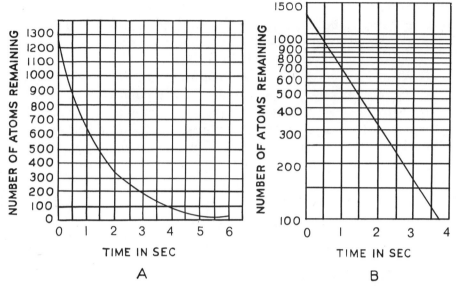

FIGURE 1.06. Radioactive decay curves. A. Plotted on ordinary graph paper. B. Plotted on semilogarithmic paper.

value layer), this is the customary method of graphic representation of radioactive decay and X-ray absorption data.

SIGNIFICANT FIGURES

A set of numerical data obtained by measurement will have a degree of reliability that depends on the precision of the measuring instrument. For example, if a ruler is calibrated in divisions of 0.1 cm we can estimate a measured length to the nearest 0.05 cm, especially with the aid of a magnifying lens. But it must be borne in mind that this is no more than an estimate. Obviously, no greater reliability is possible with this particular ruler. The digit representing the limit of reliability is called the *last significant figure or digit.*

The rules for determining the number of significant figures in a given number are as follows:

1. *When there are no digits after the decimal point,* the first significant figure is the first nonzero digit, and the last significant figure is the last nonzero digit. For example, 256 has three significant figures, as does 2560.

2. *When there are digits after the decimal point*, the first significant figure is the first nonzero digit, and the last significant figure is the last digit even if it is 0. Thus, 0.61 and 0.061 each has two significant figures, whereas 0.0610 has three.

When numbers are *added or subtracted*, the answer can have no more significant figures after the decimal point than the number with the smallest number of significant figures after its decimal point. For example, in weighing three samples with weights reliable to 0.1 g and 0.01 g, respectively, and adding the results, we obtain a sum that is no more reliable than the measurements made with the 0.1 cm ruler. Thus,

$$
\begin{array}{lr}
\text{item 1} & 1.42 \text{ g} \\
\text{item 2} & 21.2 \\
\text{item 3} & \underline{4.71} \\
& 27.3
\end{array}
$$

Note that there is one digit to the right of the decimal point in the answer because there is one measurement, item 2, that has only one digit to the right of the decimal point.

If at least one of the added numbers has no digits after the decimal point, the sum contains the same number of significant figures as that number. Thus,

$$
\begin{array}{r}
7640. \\
7.56 \\
\underline{5.1} \\
7650.
\end{array}
$$

In subtraction the answer may actually have fewer significant figures than either of the original numbers, as in the following

$$
\begin{array}{r}
365.78 \\
-364.47 \\
\hline
1.31
\end{array}
$$

In *multiplication and division* the number of significant figures in the answer will be the same as that in the number having the least number of significant figures:

$$25.23$$
$$\times 1.21$$
$$\overline{30.5}$$

The discussion of significant figures is incomplete without considering the process of **rounding off** (approximation) of the last significant figure. A good rule is as follows: if the digit *following* the last significant figure is larger than five, the last significant figure is increased by one; if less than five, it is unchanged; if equal to five, the last significant figure is approximated to an even number. Of course, the digits beyond the last significant figure are then dropped. The rule applies as follows:

46.238 is rounded off to 46.24
46.234 is rounded off to 46.23
46.235 is rounded up to 46.24
46.225 is rounded down to 46.22

where the answer is to be stated in four significant figures.

It is important in the rounding off process, to do so after the answer has been obtained. However, when a slide rule or logarithms are used, each number must first be rounded off according to the number of significant figures of the slide rule or log table before being entered into the computation. The answers will have the proper number of significant figures.

In summary, then, the concept of significant figures permits the approximation, to a reasonable degree of reliability, of the last digit in a number representing any kind of measured quantity. This tends to minimize the likelihood of conferring spurious accuracy on a measurement or computation.

DECIMAL SYSTEM AND SCIENTIFIC NOTATION

Ordinary scientific calculations rely on the decimal system which is based on the position of digits relative to a point called the **decimal point.** Fractional values in terms of tenths, hundredths,

TABLE 1.05

ten thousands	thousands	hundreds	tens	units	decimal	tenths	hundredths	thousandths	ten thousandths
5	4	3	2	1	.	1	2	3	4

thousandths, etc. are assigned to each of these positions, as shown in Table 1.05.

To convert ordinary fractions to decimals, we divide the numerator by the denominator and carry the answer to as many figures as are significant. For example,

$$2/3 = 0.667$$

which is read as "six hundred sixty-seven thousandths." If it were carried to 2 places,

$$2/3 = 0.67$$

it would read as "sixty-seven hundredths."

Although the decimal system is admirably suited to ordinary problems, it becomes exceedingly cumbersome when applied to very large or very small numbers. This applies especially to radiation physics wherein quantities are so often extremely large or small, requiring modification of the decimal system.

Suppose we take the quantity 2^3. In this instance, 2 is called the **base** and 3 the **exponent.** The indicated operation is that 2 be multiplied by itself 3 times, that is, $2^3 = 2 \times 2 \times 2 = 8$. We may state this also as "2 raised to the third power."

Another example is 10 to the fourth power, or $10^4 = 10 \times 10 \times 10 \times 10 = 10,000$. When 10 is raised to a power, the resulting number is 1 followed by the number of zeros indicated by the exponent, the so-called **powers-of-ten system.**

$$10^0 = 1$$
$$10^1 = 10$$
$$10^2 = 100$$
$$10^3 = 1,000$$
$$10^4 = 10,000$$

This information can be used to simplify the expression of very large quantities. For example, we know that 100,000,000 atoms of a light element, when lined up in a row, will measure approximately 1 cm in length. To express this in the powers-of-ten system, we simply count the zeros to the right of 1 and place this number as an exponent of 10,

$$100,000,000 = 10^8$$

Another application of this principle is as follows: take the number 56,100,000,000,000,000,000,000. It is obvious that such a number cannot be stated simply, nor can it readily be used in calculations, without resorting to the powers-of-ten system. First, we place a decimal point after the 5, and then we count the number of places to the right of this decimal point, which turns out to be 22. The number then becomes 5.61×10^{22}. It can easily be stated as "five point six one times 10 to the twenty-second." Furthermore, it is recognized much more promptly than the original long form with numerous zeros strung out after the significant figures.

Now let us consider the expression of *very small numbers* in simple form. This involves the use of *negative exponents*. For example, $10^{-1} = 1/10$. Similarly, $10^{-2} = 1/10^2 = 1/100$. In other words, a number raised to a negative power equals the reciprocal of the number raised to the same positive exponent. This is shown in the following list:

$$
\begin{aligned}
10^0 & && = 1.0 \\
10^{-1} &= 1/10^1 && = 0.1 \\
10^{-2} &= 1/10^2 = 1/100 && = 0.01 \\
10^{-3} &= 1/10^3 = 1/1,000 && = 0.001 \\
10^{-4} &= 1/10^4 = 1/10,000 && = 0.0001
\end{aligned}
$$

With the conventional method of expressing small numbers, such as 4.0×10^{-3}, we can see that the negative exponent indicates the number of decimal places to the left of a digit, *including the digit*. Thus, $4.0 \times 10^{-3} = 0.004$.

Let us look at a more complicated number, such as the mass of an electron at rest, 0.00000000000000000000000000009107 gram, and convert it to a power of ten by reversing the above procedure. At first sight, the verbal expression of this number and its use in computation would seem almost hopeless. However, according to the rule of negative powers of 10, we shift the decimal point 28 places to the right, placing it after the 9. The number may then be stated as 9.107×10^{-28}, which may be read as "nine point one oh seven times ten to the minus 28."

Finally, it is important to indicate the rules for this system of notation in mathematical operations. If we are to **multiply** two large numbers, such as $10^{21} \times 10^{16}$, the exponents are added to make a new exponent for the base 10. Thus,

$$10^{21} \times 10^{16} = 10^{(21+16)} = 10^{37}$$

If these numbers are to be **divided,** the exponent of the divisor is subtracted from the exponent of the dividend, the difference then representing the new exponent of the base 10:

$$10^{21} \div 10^{16} = 10^{(21-16)} = 10^{5}$$

If negative exponents are involved, the rules of algebraic addition must be used. Thus,

$$10^{25} \times 10^{-14} = 10^{[25+(-14)]} = 10^{11}$$

$$10^{25} \div 10^{-14} = 10^{[25-(-14)]} = 10^{(25+14)} = 10^{39}$$

A final example will serve to summarize these rules for the simplification of very large and very small numbers.

$$\frac{4.2 \times 10^{7} \times 5 \times 10^{-3}}{2 \times 10^{4} \times 2.5 \times 10^{-2}} = \frac{21.0 \times 10^{4}}{5 \times 10^{2}} = \frac{21.0 \times 10^{2}}{5} = 4.2 \times 10^{2}$$

$$(4.2 \times 10^{2} \text{ is the same as } 420)$$

It should be emphasized at this point that numbers expressed as powers of 10 **cannot be simply added or subtracted,** unless the powers of 10 are the same and of the same sign:

$$10^{5} + 10^{5} = 2 \times 10^{5}$$

$$4 \times 10^{-5} - 3 \times 10^{-5} = 10^{-5}$$

To add or subtract numbers expressed as powers of 10 where

the exponents are different, they must first be converted to ordinary notation:

$$10^4 + 10^3$$

$$10,000 + 1,000 = 11,000 = 1.1 \times 10^4$$

A simpler method is to convert to the *same* power of ten:

$$10^4 + 10^3 = (10^3)(10^1) + 10^3$$

Factoring, we obtain

$$10^3(10 + 1) = 11 \times 10^3 = 1.1 \times 10^4$$

THE SLIDE RULE

One of the most useful aids to computation in physics is the *slide rule.* It is a simple mechanical device which facilitates certain mathematical operations. The precision of this instrument is approximately 0.1 percent, considered to be adequate for problems encountered in radiation therapy. (More advanced types of slide rules permit the handling of complex functions, but these will not be discussed.)

The description of the use of the slide rule will be based on the 10-inch simplex model and it is essential that the reader have one before him so that the discussion may be closely followed. Inexpensive slide rules are available at most school supply stores.

A slide rule consists of a grooved *body* and a central sliding part called the *slide.* Attached to it is a movable glass runner called the *cursor,* in the center of which is a vertical *hairline* (see Fig. 1.07).

Only the operations of multiplication and division will be described. More intricate details in the use of the slide rule may be obtained from suitable manuals.

Scales *C* and *D* are used in both multiplication and division. The scale divisions become smaller by the same fractional amount (logarithmic) along the scale toward the right. (Logarithms are necessary only in *making* the scale divisions, but this is beyond the scope of the discussion.)

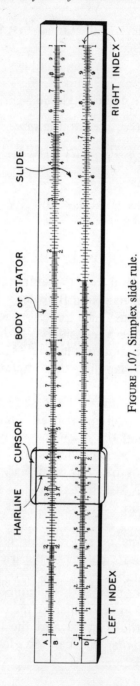

Figure 1.07. Simplex slide rule.

First the scale must be read accurately. Note in Figure 1.07 that each scale is divided by ten numbered *primary* marks, the last mark on the right being the number 1 instead of 10. The number 1 on the extreme left end of the slide is the *left index;* the 1 at the extreme right end of the slide is the *right index.* Between primary marks 1 and 2 there are 9 *secondary marks,* each of which

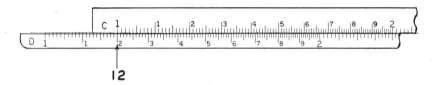

FIGURE 1.08.

represents a digit in the second place in the number. Thus, in Figure 1.08 the reading would be 12.

Between these secondary marks are *tertiary* marks, each of which has a value of 1 in the third place, in the same range of

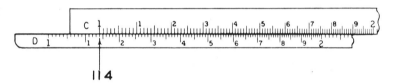

FIGURE 1.09.

the scale. In Figure 1.09 the arrow points to a scale reading of 114. Positions between these tertiary divisions are estimated and appear in the fourth place. In Figure 1.10 the arrow points to

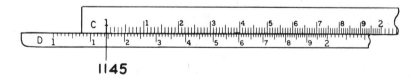

FIGURE 1.10.

1145. In Figure 1.11 the arrow points to a scale reading of 1041. Between primary marks 2 and 4, the divisions are reduced in

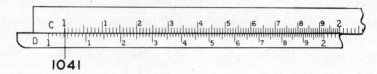

1041

FIGURE 1.11.

number. The secondary divisions have the value 1 in the second place, and the tertiary divisions 2 in the third place. In Figure 1.12 the arrow indicates a reading of 212. If the scale reads half-

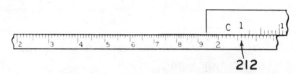

212

FIGURE 1.12.

way between the tertiary divisions, as in Figure 1.13, the reading as indicated by the arrow is 213.

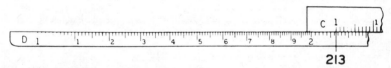

213

FIGURE 1.13.

Beyond primary mark 4, each secondary mark again has the value of 1 in the second place, but the tertiary marks now indicate a value of 5 in the third place (see Fig. 1.14). Values for positions between the tertiary marks must be estimated.

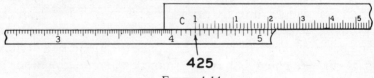

425

FIGURE 1.14.

The number of significant figures depends on the portion of the scale being read. Between primary marks 1 and 2, the answer appears in four significant figures of which the first three are read directly and the last one is estimated. Beyond primary mark 2, the answer contains three significant figures, the last one being approximated. We must emphasize again that the discussion in this paragraph and in those which follow can be understood only if a slide rule is at hand to verify each description or instruction.

The rules for ***multiplication*** with a slide rule are simple, being based on the addition of the chosen scale numbers; the answer appears as though the numbers had been multiplied. For example, suppose a position of the slide and body is selected as in Figure 1.15. The distance $x_3 = x_1 + x_2$ when the lengths of these seg-

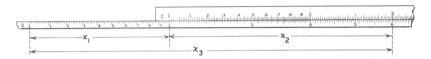

FIGURE 1.15. The left index of the C scale has been placed over 2 on the D scale. The total distance up to a given number on the D scale, such as 6, represented by x_3, is equal to the actual lengths of the two segments x_1 plus x_2; but since the scales are logarithmic, this sum represents multiplication of the two segments. Thus, segment x_1 denotes 2 on the D scale and segment x_2 denotes 3 on the C scale, the product being 6, represented by total segment x_3.

ments are actually measured (disregarding the numerical values indicated on the slide rule). But because of the logarithmic nature of the scale divisions, in which the actual distance between primary marks 1 and 2 is equal to that between 2 and 4, and between 4 and 8, the answer as it appears on the slide rule represents multiplication. In Figure 1.15 the left index of the slide is placed exactly above 2 on the body (scale D). If you now look at 3 on the slide (scale C) you will see directly below this the answer 6 on scale D. Obviously, 2 has been multiplied by 3 and the answer appears below the multiplier. It must be emphasized that the decimal point is not indicated but is determined by approximation, as described below.

The general rule for multiplication by use of scales C and D on the slide rule can now be stated. To multiply two numbers:

1. Disregard the decimal point.
2. Place the index of the C scale opposite either of the numbers (which are to be multiplied) on the D scale.
3. Move the cursor until the hairline coincides with the other number on the C scale.
4. The answer will appear under the hairline on the D scale.
5. The decimal point is then located by rough calculation.

An example of the application of these rules follows. Suppose the numbers 2.5 and 24.2 are to be multiplied. The left index of C is placed opposite 25 on the D scale. The hairline is now set over 242 on the C scale and the answer appears under the hairline on the D scale, as in Figure 1.16. The answer will read 605. To find the position of decimal point, inspect the two numbers.

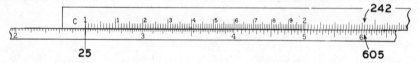

FIGURE 1.16. Multiplication by means of a slide rule. The left index of C has been placed over 25 on the D scale. The hairline (not shown) is moved to coincide with 242 on the C scale, and the product, 605, appears directly below on the D scale.

It is obvious that $2 \times 25 = 50$ is a rough approximation to the numbers actually being multiplied. Therefore, the answer with the correctly placed decimal point is 60.5.

If the answer cannot be read on the D scale because the second of the numbers to be multiplied is on a part of the slide projecting beyond the body, use the right index. In this case, the right index of scale C is placed over the larger number on scale D, and the cursor is moved until its hairline is over the other number on scale C; the answer will then appear directly below on scale D.

The rules for *division* are just as simple. If x is to be divided by y, x is the numerator and y is the denominator.

1. Disregard the decimal point.
2. Place the denominator on scale C exactly above the numerator on scale D.

3. Slide the cursor to bring the hairline over the index on *C* within the body.
4. The quotient will appear on *D* scale under the hairline.
5. The decimal point is located by approximation, as before.

Suppose we wish to divide 26 by 13. Place the line corresponding to number 13 on scale *C*, directly over 26 on scale *D*. The answer appears on the *D* scale exactly below the left index of scale *C*, as shown in Figure 1.17.

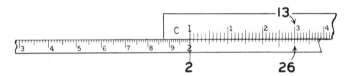

FIGURE 1.17. Division by means of a slide rule. Twenty-six is to be divided by 13. The hairline (not shown) is placed over 26 on the *D* scale and the slide bearing the *C* scale is moved until 13 also coincides with the hairline. The quotient, 2, appears directly under the left index of *C* on the *D* scale.

In solving a problem in which a series of numbers appears, requiring multiplication and division, such as

$$\frac{a \times b \times c}{x \times y \times z}$$

we divide *a* by *x*, multiply by *b*, divide by *y*, multiply by *c*, and finally divide by *z*. This will save a great deal of unnecessary shifting of the indicator with its attendant errors.

The slide rule may also be used as a simple means of solving proportion, which, as we know, is the equality between two ratios. Suppose we have the proportion

$$x/6 = 1/3$$

Place 1 on the *C* scale over 3 on the *D* scale. Now move the slide until the hairline is over 6 on the *D* scale, the value of $x = 2$ appearing on the *C* scale directly above 6.

Although the slide rule has long served as an indispensable tool for simplifying many kinds of computations, it is rapidly being supplanted by the new family of ***electronic calculators.***

Ranging from very simple and inexpensive pocket models, to quite elaborate units, they make possible a great variety of computations with remarkable speed and accuracy. Furthermore, not only do the smaller models locate the decimal point, but some will even round off the answer to the desired number of significant figures.

CHAPTER 2

Matter and Energy

HISTORICAL BACKGROUND

ONE of the most fascinating aspects of science is its historical development. This applies particularly to the evolution of the modern concept of the structure of matter and its relationship to energy.

Ancient Theories. More than 2,000 years ago the Greek philosopher Democritus taught that matter is composed of perpetually moving tiny invisible and indivisible particles called *atoms* (*a* = not, + *temnein* = to cut). Based solely on speculation, this ancient atomic theory proposed that if a piece of matter were repeatedly subdivided, there would ultimately remain tiny particles that could not be further subdivided. These ultimate particles were called *atoms*. Aristotle (384 to 322 B.C.) opposed this concept by advancing his own theory that all matter was composed of one or more elements: air, earth, fire, and water. This absurd theory held sway throughout the Middle Ages.

Dalton's Theory. The beginning of the nineteenth century saw the revival of the atomic theory in a new and scientific form. On the basis of careful quantitative study, John Dalton, an English Quaker schoolmaster, published *A New System of Chemical Philosophy* (1808) in which he stated that all matter is "constituted of a vast number of extremely small particles or atoms of matter bound together by a force of attraction."

Dalton's work established several facts about the structure of matter that had a profound impact on the development of the modern view of atomic structure:

1. Ultimate particles of a substance (element or compound) are alike for that particular substance.
2. Chemical analysis and synthesis may separate and combine these ultimate particles, but can neither create nor destroy them (*Law of Conservation of Matter*).

3. Chemical elements combine in simple proportions.
4. Relative weights of the ultimate particles (atoms) of a given element can be determined by comparison with other elements, and are constant. (Periodic chart)

Avodagro's Law. Dalton did not differentiate atoms from molecules. This remained to be done in 1811 by his Italian contemporary, Avogadro, whose observations led to this modern concept: *a molecule is the smallest particle of a substance that can exist and have the properties of larger masses of that substance.* Ordinary gases such as hydrogen, oxygen, and nitrogen are made up of molecules that consist of two atoms joined together. A molecule is also the smallest particle of a compound; thus, a molecule of sodium chloride consists of an atom of sodium combined with an atom of chlorine. Sodium and chlorine are examples of *elements.* *An atom is the smallest particle of an element that still has the identifying properties of that element.* An atom cannot be subdivided by ordinary chemical means, but as we shall see later, it can be subdivided by special physical methods.

Avogadro also advanced the theory that equal volumes of all gases have the same number of molecules under the same conditions of temperature and pressure. This has come to be called *Avogadro's Law.* The present application of this law is of utmost importance in atomic physics.

Prout's Hypothesis. In 1816 the English physicist William Prout advanced the hypothesis that the weights of various elements relative to hydrogen, which was taken arbitrarily as 1, should be whole numbers. For instance, if a hydrogen atom is assumed to be 1 unit, an atom of oxygen would be 16, an atom of nitrogen would be 14, and so on. But the more accurately these weights were determined, the more certain it became that these were *nearly* but not quite whole numbers, so for a time Prout's hypothesis fell into disfavor. Only with the advent of modern physics has the essential correctness of his theory been confirmed.

Mendeleev's Law. In 1896 the great Russian chemist Dmitri Mendeleev published his observations on the relationship between the properties of elements and their atomic weights. Upon arranging all the known elements in order of increasing atomic weight, he discovered a periodic or repetitive similarity in their properties. For example, he found that the eighth element after fluorine is chlorine, both of these having similar chemical properties. The eighth element beyond chlorine is bromine, which also has properties similar to chlorine and fluorine. The eighth element beyond bromine is iodine, and this, too, resembles fluorine, chlorine, and bromine chemically. In fact, this family of elements is called the *halogens.* Inspection of Table 2.01, known as the *Periodic Table of the Elements,* reveals the other families of elements appearing in vertical groups. Mendeleev's theory, modified by certain exceptions and revisions, contributed greatly to the establishment of atomic theory on a firm scientific basis. Its early popularity was in no small measure due to Mendeleev's correct prediction of the discovery of certain elements such as germanium and gallium. (The periodicity of the properties of elements was also discovered independently by J. L. Meyer.)

Arrhenius's Theory. Finally, the existence of atoms was further supported by the theory of electrolytic dissociation advanced by the Swedish chemist Svante Arrhenius. According to his concept, when a salt such as sodium chloride (NaCl) is dissolved in water, each molecule divides into 2 charged atoms, Na^+ and Cl^-. These are called *ions* (from the Greek verb *ienai* = to go) because they migrate in an electric field.

Avogadro's Number. It has already been pointed out that according to Avogadro's Law, equal volumes of all gases have the same number of molecules under standard conditions. It has also been indicated that the atoms of all elements can be assigned certain characteristic numbers which represent the average weight of that atom relative to some atom taken as a standard. Originally the standard element was oxygen, but the modern standard is carbon 12. The *atomic mass* is the mass of an atom of any element relative to that of carbon 12 taken as 12.000. On this basis the *atomic mass unit* is $1/12$ the mass of a carbon 12 atom. For example, the sulfur 32 atom has a mass $32/12 = 2.67$ times that of the carbon 12 atom. (The term atomic weight is used in chemistry to express the average weight of an element relative to the carbon atom taken as 12.)

Avogadro suggested that ordinary gases consist of molecules, each containing two atoms joined together. For example, a mole-

TABLE 2.01

THE PERIODIC TABLE OF ELEMENTS
(MODERN VERSION)

	I A	II A	III A	IV A	V A	VI A	VII A		GROUPS		I B	II B	III B	IV B	V B	VI B	VII B	O
Period 1	H 1.008 *Hydrogen* 1																	He 4.003 *Helium* 2
Period 2	Li 6.94 *Lithium* 3	Be 9.01 *Beryllium* 4											B 10.81 *Boron* 5	C 12.01 *Carbon* 6	N 14.007 *Nitrogen* 7	O 15.999 *Oxygen* 8	F 19.0 *Fluorine* 9	Ne 20.18 *Neon* 10
Period 3	Na 22.99 *Sodium* 11	Mg 24.31 *Magnesium* 12											Al 26.98 *Aluminum* 13	Si 28.09 *Silicon* 14	P 30.97 *Phosphorus* 15	S 32.06 *Sulfur* 16	Cl 35.45 *Chlorine* 17	Ar 39.95 *Argon* 18
Period 4	K 39.10 *Potassium* 19	Ca 40.08 *Calcium* 20	Sc 44.96 *Scandium* 21	Ti 47.90 *Titanium* 22	V 50.94 *Vanadium* 23	Cr 52.0 *Chromium* 24	Mn 54.94 *Manganese* 25	Fe 55.85 *Iron* 26	Co 58.931 *Cobalt* 27	Ni 58.71 *Nickel* 28	Cu 63.55 *Copper* 29	Zn 65.30 *Zinc* 30	Ga 69.72 *Gallium* 31	Ge 72.59 *Germanium* 32	As 74.92 *Arsenic* 33	Se 78.96 *Selenium* 34	Br 79.90 *Bromine* 35	Kr 83.80 *Krypton* 36
Period 5	Rb 85.47 *Rubidium* 37	Sr 87.62 *Strontium* 38	Y 88.91 *Yttrium* 39	Zr 91.22 *Zirconium* 40	Cb 92.91 *Columbium* 41	Mo 95.94 *Molybdenum* 42	Tc (99) *Technetium* 43	Ru 101.07 *Ruthenium* 44	Rh 102.91 *Rhodium* 45	Pd 106.4 *Palladium* 46	Ag 107.87 *Silver* 47	Cd 112.40 *Cadmium* 48	In 114.82 *Indium* 49	Sn 118.69 *Tin* 50	Sb 121.75 *Antimony* 51	Te 127.60 *Tellurium* 52	I 126.90 *Iodine* 53	Xe 131.30 *Xenon* 54
Period 6	Cs 132.90 *Cesium* 55	Ba 137.34 *Barium* 56	Lanthanides 57–71	Hf 178.49 *Hafnium* 72	Ta 180.95 *Tantalum* 73	W 183.85 *Tungsten* 74	Re 186.2 *Rhenium* 75	Os 190.2 *Osmium* 76	Ir 192.2 *Iridium* 77	Pt 195.09 *Platinum* 78	Au 196.97 *Gold* 79	Hg 204.59 *Mercury* 80	Tl 204.37 *Thallium* 81	Pb 207.19 *Lead* 82	Bi 208.98 *Bismuth* 83	Po (210) *Polonium* 84	At (210) *Astatine* 85	Rn (222) *Radon* 86
Period 7	Fr (223) *Francium* 87	Ra (226) *Radium* 88	Actinides 89–102															

Lanthanide Series	La 138.91 *Lanthanum* 57	Ce 140.12 *Cerium* 58	Pr 140.91 *Praseodymium* 59	Nd 144.24 *Neodymium* 60	Pm (145) *Promethium* 61	Sm 150.4 *Samarium* 62	Eu 152.0 *Europium* 63	Gd 157.25 *Gadolinium* 64	Tb 158.92 *Terbium* 65	Dy 162.5 *Dysprosium* 66	Ho 162.5 *Holmium* 67	Er 167.26 *Erbium* 68	Tm 168.93 *Thulium* 69	Yb 173.04 *Ytterbium* 70	Lu 175.0 *Lutetium* 71

Actinide Series	Ac (227) *Actinium* 89	Th 232.04 *Thorium* 90	Pa (231) *Protoactinium* 91	U 238.03 *Uranium* 92	Np (237) *Neptunium* 93	Pu (244) *Plutonium* 94	Am (243) *Americium* 95	Cm (247) *Curium* 96	Bk (247) *Berkelium* 97	Cf (251) *Californium* 98	Er (254) *Einsteinium* 99	Fm (257) *Fermium* 100	Md (256) *Mendeleium* 101	No (254) *Nobelium* 102	Lw (257) *Lawrencium* 103

* Elements that are of special interest are in **bold face** type.
Mass number of most stable isotope is in parenthesis.

cule of oxygen contains two atoms of oxygen having an atomic weight of 16. Therefore the molecular weight of oxygen is $2 \times 16 = 32$. If we take a mass of oxygen in grams equal numerically to its molecular weight, that is, 32 grams, it is called a **mole** or **gram molecular weight** of oxygen. Similarly, a mole of nitrogen would contain 28 grams ($2 \times$ atomic wt 14).

It has been found experimentally that a mole of any gas, under standard conditions of temperature and pressure, occupies a volume of 22.4 liters. According to Avogadro's Law, this volume should contain the same number of molecules of any gas, a number that has actually been determined since Avogadro's time: 1 mole or 1 gram molecular weight of a substance contains 6.023×10^{23} individual molecules, called **Avogadro's number.**

Since 6.023×10^{23} molecules of an element or compound equal 1 gram molecular weight, we can actually determine the weight of 1 molecule as follows:

$$6.023 \times 10^{23} \times \text{weight of 1 molecule} = 1 \text{ gram molecular weight or mole}$$

$$\text{weight of 1 molecule} = \frac{1 \text{ mole}}{6.023 \times 10^{23}}$$

For example, in the case of oxygen:

$$\text{weight of 1 molecule of oxygen} = \frac{32}{6.023 \times 10^{23}} = 5.31 \times 10^{-23} \text{ g}$$

An extension of this principle allows us to find the weight of an **atom:**

$$6.023 \times 10^{23} \times \text{weight of 1 atom} = 1 \text{ gram atomic weight}$$

$$\text{weight of 1 atom} = \frac{1 \text{ gram atomic weight}}{6.023 \times 10^{23}}$$

In the case of oxygen, having atomic weight 16,

$$\text{weight of 1 atom of oxygen} = \frac{16}{6.023 \times 10^{23}} = 2.66 \times 10^{-23} \text{ g}$$

Using Avogadro's number, we can find the **number of atoms** in a given weight of any element. For example, how many atoms are there in 1 gram of copper? The atomic weight of copper is 63.55, so its gram atomic weight is 63.55 g. Therefore, 1 gram represents 1/63.55 of a gram atomic weight. Since 1 gram atomic weight contains 6.023×10^{23} atoms, 1/63.55 of a gram atomic weight, or 1 gram of copper contains:

$$(1/63.55) \times 6.023 \times 10^{23} = 0.0948 \times 10^{23} = 9.48 \times 10^{21} \quad \text{atoms.}$$

States of Matter. Daily experience teaches us that matter can occur in three states: *solid, liquid,* and *gaseous.* The explanation for this is apparent from the preceding discussion on the discontinuity of matter; that is, the existence of atoms and molecules.

A *gas* has neither constant shape nor constant volume, and presents no surface. The molecules of a gas fill a container because they are in continual random motion. This accounts for the phenomenon of gas pressure, which is caused by the collision of the agitated molecules with the walls of the container. Not only are gases readily compressible, but they also diffuse or spread through empty space, through other gases, and even through solids and liquids.

A *liquid* has constant volume but indefinite shape, assuming the form of the container, but having a flat upper surface. The molecules of a liquid tend to glide over each other, but do not separate completely as do the molecules of a gas. Liquids are incompressible.

A *solid* has constant form and volume, its entire surface being free. The atoms of a solid are relatively fixed in position by attractive forces, thereby forming crystals.

Any substance can be made to exist in any of the three states, depending on the temperature and pressure. Water is a liquid under ordinary conditions. Upon being heated, its molecules move more and more rapidly until a critical temperature is reached —the boiling point. At this temperature, the water is converted to the gaseous state, known as steam. If water is cooled sufficiently, its molecular motion decreases until another critical temperature—the freezing point—is reached. At this point the water crystalizes to the solid state as ice.

ATOMIC AND MOLECULAR SIZE

Application of the foregoing principles allows indirectly the determination of molecular and atomic diameters. This is remarkable, considering the unbelievably small dimensions of these particles. An approximation can be reached quite readily. Water is H_2O—each molecule contains 2 atoms of hydrogen and 1 atom of oxygen. Therefore, the molecular weight of water is $1 + 1 + 16 = 18$. One mole of water weighs 18 g and occupies a volume of 18 cc under standard conditions (temperature 0 C, and pressure 760 mm mercury). Assuming that the molecules fill the entire space,

$$\frac{18}{6.023 \times 10^{23}} = 3 \times 10^{-23} \text{ cc} = \text{volume of 1 molecule}$$

If the molecules are assumed to approximate a spherical shape, the volume is less, that is, about 2×10^{-23} cc. The radius of a sphere can easily be determined from its volume, since $V = \frac{4}{3}\pi r^3$. In this case the *radius* is 1.7×10^{-8} cm, a value agreeing reasonably well with the experimentally determined radius of the lighter atoms. The accepted *diameter* of the lighter atoms is about 3×10^{-8} cm (1 angstrom = 10^{-8} cm).

STRUCTURE OF THE ATOM

Historical Background. As late as the latter part of the last century, atoms were considered to be the smallest existing material particles. However, the experiments of Franklin, Faraday, Stoney, J.J. Thomson, and others had begun to cast serious doubt on the belief that the atom could not be subdivided into smaller particles. Thus, in 1897 a British Physicist, Sir J.J. Thomson, proved that the cathode rays in a Crookes tube consist of a stream of negatively charged particles that are identical to the *electron,* proposed earlier by Stoney as the unit of electric charge. Thomson advanced the idea that the electrons in the Crookes tube originate in the atoms of the cathode metal. He visualized the atom as consisting of a positively charged medium within which the negatively charged electrons are in constant motion. Since the atom is ordinarily neutral, he supposed the positive charge to be exactly equal to the number of negative charges represented by the electrons. Thus, electrons are the first subatomic particles to have been discovered.

As the result of inconsistencies in Thomson's concept of atomic structure, the Japanese physicist, Nagaoka (1904), proposed in rough outline our present picture of the interior of the atom. He visualized it as consisting of a central positive charge surrounded by electrons, much as the sun is encircled by its planets.

It remained for Ernest Rutherford in 1914, working in Thomson's laboratory, to discover the positively charged particle which we now know as the *proton.* Rutherford found its charge to be equal and opposite to that of the electron, and its mass nearly equal to that of the hydrogen atom. Moreover, he proved that these positively charged particles exist in all matter. Upon bombarding thin metals with α particles of radium, he found that the α particles were deflected at angles too large to be accounted for by collision with the much lighter atomic electrons. He reasoned, therefore, that the α particles must have collided with heavy particles, which he decided were positively charged *nuclei.* In other words, Thomson's concept of electrons imbedded in a sea of positive electricity had to be abandoned and replaced by Rutherford's model, that of a *positively charged nucleus surrounded by rapidly revolving electrons.* The positive charge of the nucleus was due to the presence of one or more protons, the second subatomic particle to be discovered.

In this country, Langmuir and Lewis suggested that the electrons in various atoms occupied definite positions around the nucleus, called *shells.* The electrons were either stationary or vibrating. Although this was an attractive theory, it raised a number of objections which were finally resolved by the Danish physicist Niels Bohr. In 1913, working in Rutherford's laboratory, Bohr proposed an atomic model in which the electrons revolve about the nucleus in definite orbits. As long as an electron remains in its particular path, no radiation of energy occurs. But whenever an electron jumps from an orbit of higher energy level to one of lower energy level, energy is radiated.

In 1932 James Chadwick, an assistant to Rutherford, discovered the third subatomic particle, the **neutron.** This particle has very nearly the same mass as the proton, but carries no electrical charge. Furthermore, although it may be stable while inside the nucleus, it is unstable (radioactive) when free.

Present Concept of Atomic Structure. On the basis of the preceding review, we can now delineate a simple model of atomic structure. The same basic plan applies to the atoms of all elements, but the number and arrangement of the component parts are different. Because the modern wave-mechanical and relativistic model of atomic structure is much too complex for our consideration, we shall adhere to a simpler version which, nevertheless, answers our purpose.

1. *The Nucleus.* In the center of any atom is found a *positively charged nucleus* around which swarm the negatively charged *electrons.* The number of electrons in a neutral atom exactly equals the number of positive charges in the nucleus (see Fig. 2.01).

Within the nucleus of all atoms (except hydrogen 1) there are two main types of particles. One is the *proton,* which carries a positive charge equal and opposite to that of the electron. The other is the *neutron,* which is uncharged and has about the same mass as a proton.

The positive charge on the nucleus is due entirely to the *number of protons* it contains. Furthermore, the number of protons in the nucleus of an atom characterizes that particular element and none other. All atoms of a given element have the same

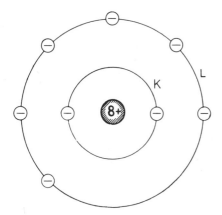

FIGURE 2.01. General atomic model according to the Bohr Theory. The nucleus is at the center, in this case bearing 8 positive charges (protons). An equal number of electrons is present in the surrounding shells. Actually, each electron moves in its own elliptical or circular zone called an *orbital.*

number of positive nuclear charges—the neutrons add mass to the nucleus but no charge.

Because the proton and neutron have very nearly the same mass (proton mass about 1836 and neutron mass about 1839 times the resting mass of the electron), it is obvious that the mass of an atom is concentrated in its nucleus. The term *nucleon* refers to the proton or the neutron.

Since all protons are similarly charged and are closely packed in the nucleus, what keeps them from flying apart and disrupting the nucleus? There is evidence that several factors tend to prevent this and thereby contribute to nuclear stability. These include: (1) *short range forces*—all nucleons have a strong mutual attraction at distances less than the nuclear diameter; (2) *geometric arrangement*—certain spatial configurations of nucleons favor nuclear stability; (3) *neutrons* act as a sort of nuclear "glue," although in excess they reduce nuclear stability; (4) *pions* contribute in some way to the attractive forces between nucleons. These factors will be discussed in greater detail on pages 333 to 336.

It is important to know that nuclear energy is *quantized*. The nucleons are arranged in particular energy levels, so that a shift of particles from a higher to a lower energy level results in the emission of energy in the form of γ rays. Quantization means that these emitted rays can have only certain discrete energies; that is, they do not exhibit a continuous spectrum.

In addition to protons and neutrons, the nucleus contains a variety of particles, the nature and function of which are, as yet, imperfectly understood. Of interest in this connection are the *mesons*. Several types of mesons have been identified, but at present the most abundant are the π mesons, or *pions*, with a mass 273 times that of the electron, and the μ mesons, or *muons*, with a mass 207 times that of the electron. Both types may have either positive or negative charges, or they may be neutral. Free pions are unstable, decaying to muons and neutrinos.

2. *The Orbital Electrons.* According to our simple model, the electrons are the *only* particles swarming in orbitals around the nucleus. The total number of such orbital electrons is equal to the number of positive charges—protons—in the nucleus of a *neutral* atom. According to Bohr's theory, there are two opposing and

equal forces which keep the electrons in orbit. One is *centrifugal force*, tending to pull the electron away from the nucleus. The other is the *electrostatic force* which tends to pull the negative electron toward the positive nucleus. Since these forces are normally equal, the electron remains in its orbit unless some extraneous force upsets the equilibrium, resulting in displacement of the electron from its orbit. It would be anticipated that the orbital electrons, moving at terrific velocities, would radiate energy. However, the revolutionary aspect of Bohr's theory requires the assumption that so long as an electron remains in an orbit, it does not radiate energy. As well be shown later, energy is radiated only during the transition of an electron from outer to inner orbits. It should be pointed out that according to the modern quantum-mechanical concept, the orbit is no longer regarded as a fixed line in space but rather a *zone* of electron activity around the nucleus. Hence, the concept of an orbit has been replaced by the *orbital* which is the zone around the nucleus in which a particular electron has the greatest probability of being located.

The shapes of the orbitals are *circular* or *elliptical.* Their distance from the nucleus determines their so-called *energy level.* By convention, it is stated that all the electrons in orbitals having nearly the same energy level occupy the same *shell.* It should be mentioned that the terms *shell* and *orbit* are often loosely used interchangeably, but if it is borne in mind that these really represent *electronic energy levels,* no confusion should result. For simplicity, an atom is often represented with electrons in circular rings, each ring representing an energy level shell. Each shell may contain a limited maximum number of electrons, according to the *Pauli Exclusion Principle.* The shells are identified by letters of the alphabet, the innermost being the K shell, the second L, the third M, and so on. The *maximum number* of electrons permitted in the various shells are 2 in the K shell, 8 in the L shell, 18 in the M shell, etc. A number called the *principle quantum number* and symbolized by the letter n has been assigned to each shell. Thus, for the K shell $n = 1$, for the L shell $n = 2$, etc.

Each element in the Periodic Table (see Table 2.01) has one more orbital electron than the one preceding it. When a given element such as neon has its outermost shell filled to capacity (in this case,

8 electrons), the next element, sodium, has an additional shell
with one electron in it (see Fig. 2.02A). On the other hand, according to the Bury-Bohr Principle, the **outermost** shell of any
element can never contain more than 8 electrons, even though
this shell has a greater maximum number assigned to it. For
example, argon has 8 electrons in its outermost or *M* shell. Although the *M* shell can hold a maximum of 18 electrons, the next
element, potassium, instead of adding a ninth electron in the *M*
shell, starts the *N* shell with one electron (see Fig. 2.02B), and
calcium adds another electron to the *N* shell. Only then does the
following element, scandium, begin to fill the previously incom-
pleted *M* shell. In other words, in shells such as *M*, *N*, and *O*
which may contain more than 8 electrons, only 8 electrons enter
and then a new shell is started for the additional electron in the
next element, the incomplete shell being filled later in the atomic
series. However, when finally completed, no shell can hold more
than the maximum number of electrons assigned to it by the exclusion principle. It should be mentioned that the shells beyond
K are made up of **subshells,** but their consideration is beyond our
scope.

As stated, shells represent *energy levels,* a very important concept
in radiation physics. An electron in the *L* shell is at a higher energy
level than one in the *K* shell; if an *L* electron jumps to a vacancy

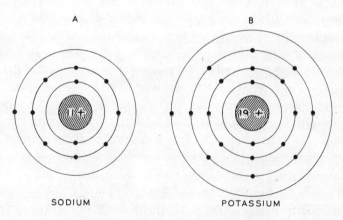

A   B

SODIUM   POTASSIUM

FIGURE 2.02. Examples of elements with a single electron in the outermost shell
(valence +1).

in the K shell, or K energy level, the atom loses energy which is radiated as an X-ray photon. On the other hand, energy must be supplied to move an electron from a lower to a higher energy level (e.g. from the K to the L shell) in accordance with the Law of Conservation of Energy. This is analogous to the increase in potential energy of mass when it is raised. The energy needed to displace an electron from a particular shell to a point remote from the nucleus is called the *electronic binding* energy, or simply the *binding energy*, of that shell for the atom in question. Since energy must be supplied, the binding energies are negative. For example, in Figure 4.10 the binding energy for the K shell of tungsten is -69.5 keV, and that of the L shell is -11.0 keV. Since a change in energy equals the initial energy state minus the final energy state, the displacement of an electron from the K to the L shell of *tungsten* would require

$$-69.5\,\mathrm{keV} - (-11.0\,\mathrm{keV}) = -58.5\,\mathrm{keV}$$

Note the negative sign in the answer, indicating that energy must be supplied to the atom. On the other hand, when an electron transition occurs between the L and the K shells, the characteristic X-ray photon has an energy of

$$-11.0\,\mathrm{keV} - (-69.5\,\mathrm{keV}) = +58.5\,\mathrm{keV}$$

Here the sign in the answer is positive because energy is emitted.

We may conclude that energy absorbed or emitted by an atom is *quantized* just as it is in the nucleus. Thus energy is absorbed or emitted in definite, discrete quantities—*quanta*—rather than in a continuous spectrum.

Penetrating and ionizing radiations of high energy (short wavelength) originate in the nucleus and in the *inner* and *intermediate* electron orbits. On the other hand, the emission of low energy (long wavelength) radiation such as ordinary light involves electron transitions in the *outermost* orbits.

In general, chemical compounds are formed by the exchange or sharing of electrons in the outermost shells of atoms. Figure 2.03 shows the formation of sodium chloride from its elements by means of an *ionic bond.* Another type of chemical union involves

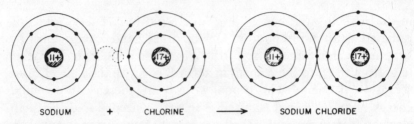

SODIUM   +   CHLORINE   ⟶   SODIUM CHLORIDE

FIGURE 2.03. The chemical combination of sodium and chlorine to form the compound sodium chloride, by sharing the valence electron.

a **covalent bond,** the sharing of a common electron as in the formation of water.

One of the remarkable facts about the atom is the incredible vastness of the empty space it contains as compared with the dimensions of the nucleus and electrons. The diameter of the lighter elements is about 3×10^{-8} cm (or 3 Å), whereas the diameter of the electron is about 10^{-13} cm. In other words, the electron is 10^{-5} or one one-hundred-thousandth the size of an atom. The average nucleus measures about 10^{-12} cm in diameter. Thus, while matter may seem to be continuous as it is perceived by the senses, it actually consists mainly of empty space within which are located widely separated nuclei and orbital electrons. If an atomic nucleus were magnified to a diameter of 1 meter (m) the atom would measure about 10,000 m across, and on this scale, an electron would measure less than 0.1 m.

Atomic structure may be summarized as follows: the atoms of all elements consist mainly of empty space, in which are found the same fundamental building blocks—protons, neutrons, and electrons. These building blocks are arranged as follows:

1. **Nucleus**—contains one or more **nucleons:**
   a. *Protons*—elementary particles having a single positive charge of 1.6×10^{-19} coulomb and a mass of 1.67×10^{-24} gram. They may exist free in nature, but soon annex an electron to form a hydrogen atom. Physical symbol of proton, $_{1}^{1}\text{H}$.
   b. *Neutrons*—fundamental particles carrying no charge and having a mass very slightly greater than that of a proton. They are unstable when free in nature, giving rise to a proton, an electron, and an antineutrino ($\tilde{\nu}$). Physical symbol of neutron, $_{0}^{1}\text{n}$.

(In addition, the nucleus contains a great multiplicity of particles, the nature and function of which are not yet clear. One of these, the π meson or pion, is thought to be concerned with nuclear stability.)

2. **Orbits**—circular or elliptical—containing:

    a. *Electrons*—elementary particles with a unit negative charge of 1.6×10^{-19} coulomb (equal and opposite to that of a proton) but with a mass at rest equivalent to about $1/1,836$ that of a proton, that is, about 9×10^{-28} gram. Electrons may be readily stripped from atomic orbits by various means and can exist free in nature for long periods of time. Physical symbol of electron, $_{-1}^{0}e$.

Thus, the smallest integral units of matter are the atoms, but they have a definite internal structure and are made up of still smaller particles. As will be seen in the next section, the nuclei of all atoms of the same element contain the same number of protons, whereas the nuclei of different elements contain different numbers of protons. Atoms of different elements may, under suitable conditions, combine in definite proportions to form compounds.

ATOMIC NUMBER

You will recall that Mendeleev arranged the elements in the order of increasing atomic weights, the result being embodied in the Periodic Table. Neither he nor his contemporaries understood the true significance of this sequence.

With the advent of the *Bohr Theory*, new light was shed on the meaning of the Periodic Table. The orderly position of each element in the table was found to have deep physical significance. For example, hydrogen occupies position 1, helium 2, lithium 3, beryllium 4, boron 5, and so on. These numbers are now known to represent much more than the artificial placement of each element in a schematic table; they actually state the number of positive charges (protons) in the nucleus of that particular atom. Accordingly, hydrogen has one positive charge, helium 2, lithium 3, beryllium 4, and boron 5.

The number of positive charges in the nucleus of an atom is called its atomic number. All atoms of the same element have the same atomic number. Conversely, atoms of different elements must have different atomic numbers. The atomic number is a fixed characteristic of any given element. If the number of nuclear protons is changed, the atomic number is changed and the element is thereby converted to some other element corresponding to the new positive charge on the nucleus.

Thus, the individuality of the different elements depends primarily on the number of protons in the nucleus. The symbol for atomic number is Z.

MASS NUMBER

Referring again to the Periodic Table (see Table 2.01), we see that each element has a designated atomic weight. We found earlier that the atomic weight represents the mass of an element relative to carbon 12 which is assumed to have 12 atomic mass units. Previously, this was the sole significance attached to atomic weights. Modern theory has exposed the much deeper meaning of the relative weights of atoms. Since the nuclear particles— protons and neutrons—weigh nearly 2,000 times as much as the electron, virtually all of the mass of the atom is concentrated in the nucleus. If each nucleon (proton or neutron) is assigned the arbitrary value of 1 atomic mass unit (amu), and all the mass units of a given nucleus are added, the total is called the *mass number*. In other words, *the mass number of an atom is equal to the total number of nucleons (protons and neutrons) in the nucleus.* It turns out that the mass numbers are *nearly* the same as the atomic weights recorded in the Periodic Table. The physical symbol for mass number is A. The atomic mass unit is 1/12 of the atomic mass of carbon 12, or 1.66×10^{-27} kg.

The mass number, unlike the atomic number, is *not* characteristic of a given element. Thus, most elements occur in nature as a mixture of atoms of slightly different mass numbers. *Atoms of the same element which differ in mass number are called isotopes.* The occurrence of isotopes is explained by the presence of different numbers of neutrons in the nucleus, changing the mass number but not the atomic number since the neutrons do not contribute to the nuclear charge. In other words, *isotopes of the same element differ only in the number of neutrons in the nucleus;* the number of protons remains the same. As will be seen

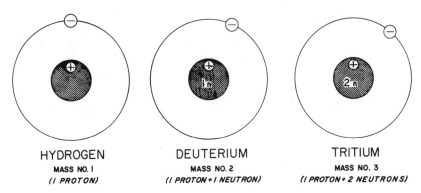

HYDROGEN
MASS NO. I
(I PROTON)

DEUTERIUM
MASS NO. 2
(I PROTON + I NEUTRON)

TRITIUM
MASS NO. 3
(I PROTON + 2 NEUTRONS)

FIGURE 2.04. The isotopes of hydrogen. All three have the same atomic number, but differ in mass number. Ordinary hydrogen (A = 1) is known as *protium*. Tritium does not occur naturally and is radioactive. (From J. Selman, *The Fundamentals of X-ray and Radium Physics,* 5th ed. [Springfield, Charles C Thomas, 1973].

later, isotopes can be made artificially by subjecting stable atoms to irradiation by subatomic particles such as neutrons. Some of these isotopes are stable, whereas others are radioactive. It must be emphasized that all the isotopes of a given element have the same chemical properties because they have the same number of orbital electrons distributed in identical shells. For example, ordinary hydrogen or **protium** has 1 proton. If a neutron is added the mass number increases by 1, but the atomic number does not change; we then have an isotope of hydrogen called **heavy hydrogen** or **deuterium.** If a second neutron is introduced into the nucleus, the resulting isotope has a mass number of 3, but it has all the chemical characteristics of protium and deuterium; however, this isotope, called **tritium,** is radioactive (see Fig. 2.04). All three isotopes of hydrogen contain one orbital electron, hence the similarity in their chemical properties. The term **nuclide** is preferred over *isotope* to designate a nucleus having a particular number of protons and neutrons in a particular energy state.

EQUIVALENCE OF MASS AND ENERGY

According to classical physics, the mass of a body is a measure of a property of matter called **inertia**—the resistance which the mass offers to a change in motion. Thus, a body which is at rest tends to remain at rest, whereas a body moving with constant speed in a straight line (i.e. constant velocity) tends to remain in motion in a straight line, unless acted upon by an outside *force.* A simple definition of force is a push or a pull; it is always required to overcome inertia, that is, to put a resting body in motion or to change the motion of a moving body.

Weight is not the same thing as mass; weight is simply the force with which the earth attracts a given mass, and may vary with geographic location. However, the weight of a body is proportional to its mass.

Energy is defined as the *ability to do work,* and work equals the product of a *force* acting upon a body, by the *distance* through which it moves,

$$W = fs \tag{1}$$

where W is work, f is force, and s is distance in the direction in which the force acts. Energy and work may be expressed in the same units, for example, ergs or joules.

There are two types of mechanical energy, *potential* and *kinetic.* *Potential* or *stored* energy is the energy a body has because of its position or deformation. For example, a ball situated on a hill has more potential energy than at the bottom of the hill; the ball will therefore roll down the hill to a lower energy level. On the other hand, a coiled spring represents energy stored by its deformation as it is wound.

Kinetic energy is the energy a body possesses by virtue of its motion, and exists only while the body is moving. If a ball is located on a hill and is allowed to roll down, its potential energy is gradually converted to kinetic energy. The classical equation for kinetic energy is

$$E = \tfrac{1}{2}mv^2 \tag{2}$$

where E is kinetic energy, m is mass, and v is velocity. The correct units must be used; thus, E is in ergs if m is in grams and v is in cm per sec.

There are several *forms of energy,* including heat, electrical, magnetic, mechanical, chemical, electromagnetic, and atomic. Most forms of energy can be converted to other forms. Thus, a steam engine converts heat into mechanical energy. An electric generator changes the kinetic energy of a waterfall into electrical energy. Chemical energy is released or absorbed during the interaction of atoms, with resulting rearrangement of the atoms. In all these conversions, the process is not 100 percent efficient; a variable amount of energy is always lost in the form of heat.

Atomic energy is produced by certain changes occurring within atomic nuclei. If this energy arises in the nucleus and is released in an extremely short interval of time, the effect may be explosive, as in the atom bomb.

In classical physics there are two conservation laws. The *Law of Conservation of Matter* states that *matter* can neither be created nor destroyed. The *Law of Conservation of Energy* states that *energy* can neither be created nor destroyed. It remained for Einstein to tie these two laws together by showing that mass and energy are equivalent, so both conservation laws really state the same principle. According to his concept, and one now generally accepted, mass and energy are mutually interconvertible—when matter is made to "disappear" an equivalent amount of energy "appears," and conversely. Einstein's equation for the equivalence of mass and energy is as follows:

$$E = mc^2 \qquad (3)$$

where E is energy in ergs; m is mass in grams; and c is velocity of light, 3×10^{10} cm/sec in air, and is constant.

The unit of energy most often used in radiologic physics is the *electron volt* (eV), defined as the kinetic energy an electron acquires when it is acted upon by 1 volt. One electron volt equals 1.6×10^{-12} erg. In radiation physics, the useful energies range from a few thousand electron volts up to the millions and even billions of electron volts. The abbreviations for these units are as follows:

1 electron volt = 1 eV
1 thousand electron volts = 1 kiloelectron volt = 1 keV
1 million electron volts = 1 MeV
1 billion electron volts = 1 BeV

According to Einstein's equation, the amount of energy that would be liberated by complete conversion of a mass of 1 gram may be calculated as follows:

$$E = mc^2$$

$$= 1 \times (3 \times 10^{10})^2$$

$$E = 9 \times 10^{20} \text{ ergs}$$

This tremendous amount of energy, sufficient to raise the temperature of almost 240,000 tons of water from the freezing point to the boiling point, may be expressed in electron volts in the following manner:

Since 1 eV = 1.6×10^{-12} erg, 9×10^{20} ergs represent:

$$\frac{9 \times 10^{20}}{1.6 \times 10^{-12}} = 5.6 \times 10^{32} \text{ eV or } 5.6 \times 10^{26} \text{ MeV}$$

Returning now to the discussion of mass number, we may investigate more closely the meaning of the mass units in their relationship to atomic energy. The mass of the nucleon is only approximately equal to 1 atomic mass unit, this degree of precision being adequate for ordinary chemical problems. But in nuclear physics, where a higher order of precision is essential, it is found that the actual atomic mass of many elements is in some cases more, in others less, than the mass that would be expected from simple addition of the constituent nucleons.

The bearing of this observation on nuclear physics may be indicated by what is to follow. The mass of a proton is 1.00727 atomic mass units (amu), that of a neutron 1.00866. The helium nucleus is known to contain 2 protons and 2 neutrons. Therefore,

$$2n = 2 \times 1.00866 = 2.01732 \text{ amu}$$

$$2p = 2 \times 1.00727 = \underline{2.01454} \text{ amu}$$
$$\text{Total} \quad 4.03186 \text{ amu}$$

The total 4.03186 is the anticipated mass of a helium nucleus. But its actual mass is 4.00151. Therefore, the combination of 2 protons and 2 neutrons in a helium atom has resulted in a loss of 4.03186 —

4.00151 = 0.03035 amu. This deficit is called the **nuclear mass defect** or **binding energy**. If the nucleus were to be disrupted into its individual nucleons, this amount of energy would have to be added to the nucleus. Since 1 amu = 931 MeV, the binding energy of the helium nucleus is

$$0.03035 \times 931 = 28.3 \text{ MeV}$$

The **formation** of one helium nucleus by the combination of 2 neutrons and 2 protons would therefore liberate about 28.3 MeV of energy!

From the foregoing discussion, we may conclude that a definite mass was transformed to energy during the union of 2 protons and 2 neutrons in the production of a helium nucleus. This conversion of mass to an equivalent amount of energy is in accord with Einstein's equation set forth above, and is a process which is believed to be going on continuously in the sun and other stars. In order to free the 4 nucleons from the helium nucleus, the same amount of energy must be introduced, being reconverted to mass and distributed among the 4 nucleons as follows:

Formation of Helium Nucleus:

$$2p + 2n \longrightarrow 1 \text{ helium nucleus} + 28.3 \text{ MeV (binding energy)}$$

Destruction of Helium Nucleus:

$$1 \text{ helium nucleus} + 28.3 \text{ MeV} \longrightarrow 2p + 2n$$

where p represents proton and n neutron.

If the binding energy is divided by the number of nucleons, the result is the **binding energy per nucleon.** In the preceding example,

$$28.3/4 = 7.08 \text{ MeV per nucleon}$$

for the helium nucleus (α particle) whose mass number is 4. Interestingly enough, the average binding energy per nucleon of all the stable nuclei with mass numbers of 10 or more ranges from about 7.5 to 9 MeV. However, there is a sharp decrease in the average binding energy per nucleon for atoms with mass number less than 10.

CHAPTER 3

The Nature of Radiation

DEFINITION

RADIATION *is the process of emission of energy by atoms, and the transmission of this energy through space.*

TYPES OF RADIATION

Energy may be transmitted through space in two forms: *particles* and *waves.* As described on pages 53 to 54, these are not completely distinct entities. Particle radiation consists of minute bits of matter traveling with a certain velocity, and therefore possessing kinetic energy similar to larger bodies of matter in motion. It may be recalled that the classical equation for kinetic energy of bodies moving at ordinary speeds (i.e. much less than that of light) is:

$$E = \tfrac{1}{2}mv^2 \tag{1}$$

where E is the kinetic energy in ergs, m is the mass in grams, and v is the velocity in cm/sec. Thus, a particle with a given mass moving through space with ordinary velocity would have a kinetic energy derived according to equation (1).

Radiation in the form of *waves* is somewhat more difficult to understand. Everyone is familiar with the waves passing outward from a pebble falling upon the surface of a pond. Such waves represent cyclic deformity of a medium—water—from stresses set up by the pebble. Energy is transmitted by this wave *form* passing across the water, although the water itself does not pass outward. It actually moves up and down, as is evident from the rise and fall of a cork on its surface.

In the case of wavelike radiation, energy is propagated through space by *electromagnetic waves.* However, there is no transmitting medium. Wave radiation includes all the familiar types of radiant

50

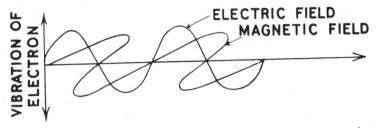

FIGURE 3.01. The electrical and magnetic components of an electromagnetic wave oscillate (vibrate) in mutually perpendicular planes.

energy: radio, infrared, visible light, ultraviolet, X rays, and γ rays.

The two general forms of radiation include a number of specific types. Those which are of greatest interest in radiation therapy will be discussed under separate headings.

ELECTROMAGNETIC RADIATION

Electromagnetic waves are generated by oscillations (vibrations) of electric charges. It is well known that moving free electrons always have an associated magnetic field (electromagnetism). A *field* is a region in which a particular kind of force is exerted. When a free electron oscillates, it sets up a changing magnetic field which in turn gives rise to an oscillating electric field. These two fields pass outward in a straight line (in limited space), vibrating at right angles to each other, and to the direction in which they move (see Fig. 3.01). The combination of these two oscillating fields resulting from electron vibration constitutes the *electromagnetic wave*. To simplify the discussion, we represent an electromagnetic wave as a single transverse wave, as in Figure 3.02.

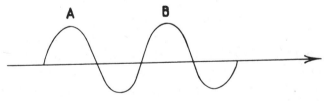

FIGURE 3.02. Ordinary representation of an electromagnetic wave. The spatial distance between two successive peaks, such as A and B, is the wavelength λ. The number of cycles per second is the frequency ν.

The speed of all waves of this type, regardless of their origin, is the same as the speed of light *in a vacuum:* about 3×10^{10} cm per second, or 186,000 miles per second. This is a universal constant. Figure 3.02 shows two of the attributes of an electromagnetic wave—*frequency* and **wavelength.** Frequency, symbolized by v (Greek letter "nu"), is the number of waves passing a given point each second, or the number of vibrations occurring per second, usually termed cycles per sec or hertz (Hz). The distance AB, between two successive crests, is the wavelength, symbolized by λ (Greek letter "lambda"). The wavelength and frequency are very simply related to the speed of the wave. If v waves pass a given point in space in one second, and if each wave is λ cm in length, then it is obvious that at the end of one second, the waves will have moved a distance equal to the length of each wave multiplied by the number of waves during one second. Since the distance the waves move per second represents their velocity,

$$c = v\lambda \tag{2}$$

where c is the velocity of light, v is the frequency of the electromagnetic wave, and λ is its wavelength. It is obvious from equation (2) that if v is doubled, λ is halved; if v is tripled, λ is divided by 3, etc., since their product must always be equal to the constant $c = 3 \times 10^{10}$ cm per second.

Because of the extremely short wavelengths of the radiations used in therapy, a unit that is much smaller than the cm has been introduced for the sake of convenience. This is the angstrom, usually abbreviated Å.

$$1 \text{ Å} = \frac{1}{100,000,000} \text{ cm}$$

or

$$1 \text{ Å} = 10^{-8} \text{ cm}$$

(Note that the angstrom is of the same order of magnitude as the diameter of an atom of low atomic number.) The wavelength of red light is 7600 Å; that of blue light is 4000 Å. X rays have a range of wavelengths extending from about 0.0005 Å to 120 Å, while γ rays range from less than 0.001 Å to 1.5 Å (see Fig. 3.03). In general, it may be stated that X rays arise from the oscillation

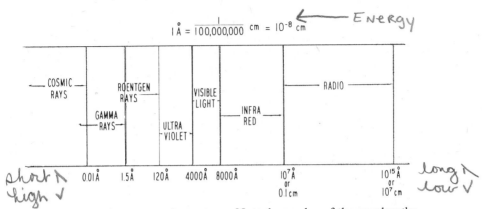

FIGURE 3.03. The electromagnetic spectrum. Note the overlap of the wavelengths of X and γ rays. (From J. Selman, *The Fundamentals of X-ray and Radium Physics,* 5th ed. [Springfield, Charles C Thomas, Publisher, 1973].)

of orbital electrons or in transitions of orbital electrons from higher to lower energy levels corresponding to shells nearer the nucleus. On the other hand, γ rays are emitted during the transition of particles within atomic *nuclei* or by reactions between fundamental particles. However, one must never lose sight of the fact that X rays and γ rays are essentially similar in nature— highly energetic electromagnetic waves. The properties of electromagnetic waves depend only on their frequency or wavelength, and not on their site of origin.

ELEMENTARY QUANTUM THEORY

Scientists have discovered that particle and wave radiations are not entirely distinct entities. Certain phenomena associated with electromagnetic waves cannot be adequately explained on the basis of wave motion alone. For example, in the photoelectric effect, an orbital electron can be dislodged only by a photon possessing a certain minimum energy. The atom becomes excited and an electron immediately drops into the vacant space or *hole* in the shell, with emission of radiation having a characteristic frequency known as *characteristic radiation* (see Fig. 3.04). The shift of an electron between shells is called a *transition.* Such behavior can be explained only if the radiation acts as though it also has the characteristics of particles. In other words, electro-

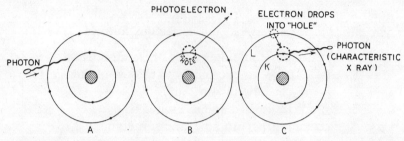

FIGURE 3.04. The production of characteristic X rays. *A.* An incident photon is absorbed by an atom, an orbital electron being ejected as a *photoelectron.* All the energy of the photon is used up in this process of *true absorption. B.* The atom is now in an *excited state;* and it is also *ionized*, since an electron has been completely removed from the atom. *C.* An electron from some higher energy level fills the "hole" in the *K* shell, with resulting emission of a characteristic X-ray photon. (Actually, a series of electrons cascade from outer to inner shells to fill successive holes.)

magnetic radiation behaves as though it consists of **both** waves and energy particles. The term **quantum** or **photon** has been applied to these tiny packets of energy.

In 1900 the corpuscular aspect of electromagnetic radiation was embodied in the quantum theory by Max Planck, a renowned German physicist. Stated mathematically,

$$E = h\nu \tag{3}$$

where E is the quantum energy in ergs, h is a constant called Planck's constant (6.625×10^{-27} erg-sec), and ν is the frequency of the electromagnetic wave in cycles per sec or hertz. This equation indicates that the energy of a quantum or photon is directly proportional to the frequency of the wave; the higher the frequency, the more energy propagated by the wave. Note that we usually express energy in keV or MeV.

Figure 3.04 shows how, in the photoelectric process, an atom absorbs and emits X and γ rays (i.e. photons) in limited, discrete energy units: quanta, as just described. Thus, a particular species of atom (i.e. element) can absorb and emit only certain quanta and no others. An atom, on absorbing an appropriate quantum $h\nu$, ejects an orbital electron as a photoelectron. Immediate electron transition occurs, accompanied by the emission of discrete quanta in the form of X rays characteristic of the atomic species. The entire process may be summarized as follows:

photoelectric effect

1. *hv* photon = binding energy of electron orbit
   + kinetic energy of ejected photoelectron
2. vacancy or hole in shell, and
3. atom now ionized and in excited state
4. electron drops into hole, and simultaneously,
5. atom radiates energy quanta = characteristic X rays.

X RAYS

Production of X Rays. As already indicated, X rays are one variety of electromagnetic radiation, ordinarily having a wavelength shorter than 120 Å. Their average wavelength in superficial therapy is about 0.5 Å, in deep therapy about 0.15 Å, and in million volt therapy about 0.01 Å. X rays are generally produced in one of two ways:

1. *Sudden slowing or stopping of high speed electrons* occurs as they strike the target of an X-ray tube. Upon approaching the positively charged nuclei of the target atoms, the energetic negative electrons are deflected from their initial path, undergoing acceleration, that is, a change in direction. In accordance with electromagnetic theory, an accelerating electron emits electromagnetic radiation—a *photon.* Since the photon's energy must come from the electron's kinetic energy, the electron moves away from the atom with reduced energy (and speed), thereby satisfying the Law of Conservation of Energy. The electron may lose all its energy in one encounter, or may do so in multiple encounters, so that the resulting radiation appears in a continuous spectrum of energies ranging from zero to the maximum kinetic energy of the electrons entering the atomic nuclear fields. This process is called *bremsstrahlung* or *brems radiation,* a German word meaning braking radiation, because it is associated with a slowing of the electrons; the greater the initial velocity of the electron and the closer the electron approaches the nucleus, the more energetic the brems radiation (i.e. the higher the keV or MeV). But the quantity of radiation per unit time (i.e. intensity) is proportional to the atomic number of the target.

2. **When electrons jump from outer to inner orbitals** radiation in the form of **characteristic X rays** is emitted as just described on page 54 to 55. The initial removal of the inner orbital electron may be accomplished by various means, such as interactions with X rays, γ rays, or electrons. In one type of **nuclear reaction,** a K electron may be captured by the nucleus with resulting conversion of a nuclear proton to a neutron, a process known as **K capture.** The resulting hole in the K shell is promptly filled by another electron with emission of characteristic X rays. Characteristic radiation does not exhibit a continuous spectrum.

The subject of X-ray production will be discussed at length in Chapter 5, but a summary should aid in understanding X-ray spectra. In the modern X-ray tube, introduced in 1913 by William D. Coolidge, two electrodes are inclosed in an evacuated glass tube. The **cathode** or **filament** is heated by a low voltage current, with liberation of electrons by **thermionic emission.** A large positive potential then applied to the anode drives the electrons across a gap toward the anode (target). The energy of these electrons depends on the applied potential difference, and is measured in electron volts. (An electron volt is the energy acquired by an electron when it is accelerated through a potential difference of 1 volt.)

Upon entering the tube target, usually **tungsten,** the high speed electrons interact with the atoms and produce X rays by the two processes described above. In the low and orthovoltage regions the resulting X-ray beam consists of a continuous spectrum of brems radiation (about 80%), upon which is superimposed a discontinuous spectrum of characteristic radiation (about 20%).

X-ray Spectra. An X-ray beam is **heterogeneous** or **polyenergetic,** consisting of photons ranging in energy from a minimum to a maximum. The reasons for this are as follows: (1) multiple encounters of the electrons with the target atoms in the X-ray tube, with conversion of various amounts of electron energy to X rays; (2) production of characteristic radiation; and (3) in certain types of X-ray units, fluctuation of the applied potential imparting a variety of energies to the electrons, manifested by a range in energy of the resulting X-ray photons.

A particular X-ray beam can be specified very adequately by sorting out its rays according to wavelength, or its photons according to energy. This may be clarified by an analogy.

TABLE 3.01
HEIGHT DISTRIBUTION OF A CLASS OF
SENIOR HIGH SCHOOL BOYS

Height	Number of Boys
in.	
63	1
64	2
65	4
66	7
67	13
68	14
69	15
70	15
71	14
72	10
73	7
74	1

Suppose we wish to classify a population of high school senior boys on the basis of height. We would first measure all the boys in the designated population and group them according to height. These data would then be set down as in Table 3.01 and plotted graphically as in Figure 3.05, the number of boys in each group being the dependent variable, and the height the independent variable.

Similarly, we can sort out the rays or photons in a given X-ray beam by means of a special instrument known as an X-ray spectrometer, determining the **spectrum** (that is, relative intensities,

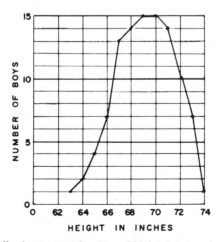

FIGURE 3.05. Distribution curve of a class of high school senior boys according to height. Note the peak incidence at 68 to 70 inches.

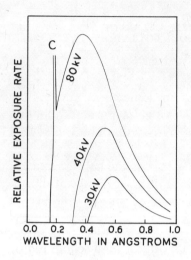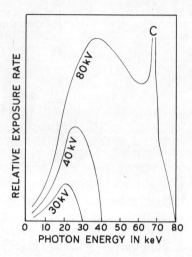

FIGURE 3.06. Spectral distribution curves of X radiation at 30, 40, and 80 kV. *K-characteristic radiation* appears as a peak at *C* (actually, a group of closely spaced peaks). The binding energy for the *K* shell is 69.5 kV. The remaining curves represent *general radiation*. Note that the curves in the left figure are based on the wavelength of the X rays, whereas those in the right figure are based on photon energy.

a measure of relative numbers) of X rays of various wavelengths. When these data are plotted as in Figure 3.06, a **spectral distribution curve** is obtained, in this case representing X-ray beams produced in a tungsten target by three different applied potentials—30, 40, and 80 kV. A curve is also included for spectral distribution according to photon energies, now the preferred method. The peak of the 30 kV curve occurs at about 0.55 Å, the wavelength of most of the rays in this particular beam. The curve crosses the horizontal axis at 0.41 Å, which is the minimum wavelength (or highest energy) ray occurring in the beam. **The minimum wavelength depends only on the peak kilovoltage** and is obtained from the equation:

$$\lambda_{min} = \frac{12.4}{kV} \qquad (4)$$

where λ_{min} = minimum wavelength in Å

kV = peak kilovoltage applied to tube

If kV = 30, then from equation (3),

$$\lambda_{min} = \frac{12.4}{30} = 0.41 \text{ Å}$$

The curve crosses the horizontal again somewhere above 1 Å, which is the limitation imposed by the glass port and cooling oil of the X-ray tube; longer wavelength radiation is absorbed by these materials.

A comparison of these curves shows that as the kV is increased, not only is there a relative increase in the number of rays of shorter wavelengths, but also an absolute increase in the number of rays of all wavelengths.

If a sufficiently high kV is applied (at least 69.5 kV), the curves are modified by the appearance of a *sharp peak* at about 0.2 Å, because of the addition of K-characteristic radiation from the tungsten target.

The same principle may be used in plotting relative intensity as a function of *photon energy,* a more modern way of representing the spectral distribution of an X-ray beam (see Fig. 3.06, right). The conversion from wavelength to photon energy is easily made by use of equation (4). For example, the energy of a photon with a wavelength of 0.2 Å is obtained as follows:

$$\lambda = \frac{12.4}{\text{photon energy in keV}}$$

$$\text{photon energy} = \frac{12.4}{\lambda}$$

$$\text{photon energy} = \frac{12.4}{0.2} = 62 \text{ keV}$$

A closer look at the spectral distribution curves in Figure 3.06 reveals that those obtained with an applied potential of 30 or 40 kV with a tungsten target are smoothly curved lines without irregularities. A portion of the curve obtained at 80 kV has a similar appearance. These smooth curves represent the *continuous spectrum* of brems radiation mentioned above. Sometimes this is called white radiation because of the analogy with white light which, upon passage through a prism, separates into its spectrum of the familiar rainbow wavelengths or colors.

The curve obtained at 80 kV exhibits a peak C superimposed on the continuous spectrum. This peak represents the **characteristic radiation** produced by the transition of orbital electrons to holes in the K shell of excited target atoms, in this case, tungsten. Let us look a little more closely at how characteristic radiation is produced. A high speed electron in the X-ray tube may interact with an inner shell electron in one of the target atoms. Ejection of the electron leaves a hole in the shell, the atom now being excited. Immediately an electron from some more distant shell drops into the hole with emission of an X-ray photon whose energy will depend on the difference in energy levels of the two shells involved in the electron transition. Thus, if an electron drops from the L to the K shell, the difference in energy may be represented by $W_L - W_K$ where W_L is the energy level of the L shell and W_K is the energy level of the K shell. Therefore,

$$W_L - W_K = h\nu$$

where $h\nu$ is the energy of the characteristic photon.

It should be pointed out that the spectrum of a beam scattered by passage through matter differs from that of the primary beam and must be measured in a suitable phantom. In general, the peak of the spectral distribution curve occurs at a lower photon energy than that of the primary beam.

We may summarize the types of X rays found in an ordinary X-ray beam as follows:

1. **White Radiation**—continuous spectrum due to:
    a. Some electrons striking target nucleus and being stopped in one collision (brems rays).
    b. Most of the electrons being stopped only after multiple decelerations (brems rays).
    c. Variation in energy imparted to electrons by fluctuations of applied potential (e.g. alternating current).
2. **Characteristic Radiation**—sharp peaks in continuous spectrum due to:
    a. Transitions of electrons between orbits deep within the target atoms.

Properties of X Rays. As already noted, X rays are a form of electromagnetic radiation and therefore have the same general properties. However, X rays also possess certain peculiarities which set them apart. As far as radiotherapy is concerned, their two most important characteristics are (1) their marked penetrating ability, and (2) their ability to interact in various ways with matter through which they pass. The penetrating ability of X rays makes it possible to apply them in the treatment of deeply situated tumors. Their interaction with matter, causing ionization and excitation of atoms in the tissues leads to biologic changes which may be controlled, within limits, to destroy selectively certain malignant tumors. More specific effects of X rays will be discussed in detail in the appropriate sections. (See especially Chapter 4.)

GAMMA RAYS

Sources. Gamma rays originate from two main sources: (1) excited atomic nuclei and (2) annihilation reaction.

1. *Nuclear Excitation.* Whenever a radioactive nucleus decays by emission of an α or a β particle, the daughter nucleus has a different atomic number than the parent. In most instances the daughter nucleus is left in an *excited state* (surplus of energy called *excitation energy*). Note that there are nuclear energy states analogous to orbital electronic energy states. Usually the excited daughter nucleus de-excites or decays immediately (half-life less than 10^{-13} sec) by γ-ray emission, to the lowest energy state, called the *ground state.* However, in some cases the excited daughter lingers in this condition for a significant period of time; if it decays with a half-life greater than 10^{-6} sec, it is said to have been in the *metastable state,* and its decay is designated as an *isomeric transition.* In either case, the emission of γ photons is the means whereby excited nuclei may decay to ground state when they cannot get rid of their surplus energy by particle emission alone. It must be stressed that the energy of the γ photon is characteristic of the excited *daughter nucleus,* and not the parent. An example of isomeric transition is technetium 99m (m indicates

metastable state) to ground state technetium 99 by γ-ray emission with a half-life of six hours.

Certain radioactive nuclei undergo particle decay to daughters which are immediately in the ground state. Under these circumstances no γ radiation occurs.

As will be described more completely in Chapter 11, nuclear excitation can also be induced by a process called ***radiative capture.*** When atoms are irradiated with slow neutrons, any nucleus which happens to capture a neutron enters an excited state. In returning to ground state, the excited nucleus emits a γ ray as described above. Radiative capture is also possible, though less likely, with certain other types of bombarding particles.

Nuclear excitation can be caused by still another process—***electron capture.*** In neutron-poor nuclei in which the neutron-proton (n/p) ratio is too small for maximum nuclear stability, an electron from the K shell or, more rarely, from the L shell, may fall into the nucleus and combine with a proton to form a neutron (see Fig. 3.07). Because of the disappearance of one nuclear positive charge, the atomic number of the daughter is one less than that of the parent. The daughter is usually excited as the result of electron capture, whereupon it decays to ground state by γ emission. Auger electrons are also ejected by interaction of characteristic X rays with orbital electrons.

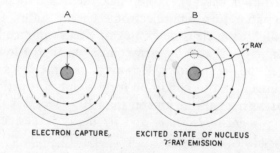

FIGURE 3.07. Emission of γ radiation as the result of electron capture. This is followed immediately by orbital electron transition and emission of a characteristic X-ray photon, not shown. (Radioactive chromium 51 decays to vanadium 51 by this process.)

Finally, certain excited nuclei can dissipate their excitation energy not only by direct γ-ray emission, but also by an alternate route—*internal conversion.* Here an interaction occurs between the nucleus and an inner shell electron, usually a K electron. In the process, the energy that would otherwise be emitted as a γ ray is transferred to the electron, now an *internal conversion electron.* It is ejected from the atom with the following energy

$$E_{ie} = h\nu - E_K$$

where E_{ie} is the kinetic energy of the internal conversion electron, $h\nu$ is the energy of the internally converted γ photon, and E_K is the binding energy of the K shell. The *internal conversion coefficient* for a particular shell, such as α_K for the K shell, is defined as follows:

$$\alpha_K = \frac{\text{number of } K \text{ conversion electrons}}{\text{number of unconverted } \gamma \text{ rays}}$$

An example is as follows: if the internal conversion ratio is 0.3, how many conversion electrons and γ rays would appear for 1000 nuclear transformations? Let e_c be the number of electrons and γ_u the number of unconverted photons. Then,

$$\gamma_u = 1000 - e_c$$

$$\frac{e_c}{\gamma_u} = \frac{e_c}{1000 - e_c} = 0.3$$

$$e_c = 300 - 0.3e_c$$

$$e_c \simeq 230$$

$$\gamma_u \simeq 770$$

The internal conversion coefficient increases with increasing atomic number and with decreasing γ energy.

The origin of γ rays and the fate of those which happen to be internally converted may be conveniently summarized by a diagram, shown in Figure 3.08. This reveals that the γ radiation (as well as the characteristic radiation) arises in the daughter atom, after the parent has lost a nuclear α or β particle.

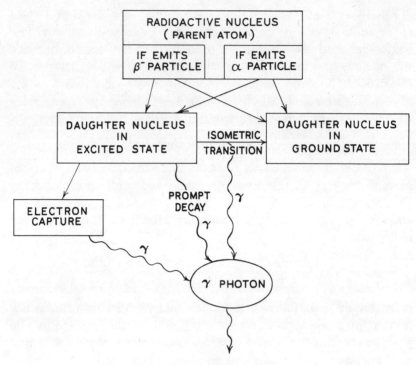

FIGURE 3.08. Schematic diagram showing sources of γ rays.

2. *Annihilation Reaction.* The origin of positrons (positive electrons) is discussed later in this chapter. When a positron that is at rest combines with a negatron (negative electron), their total mass is "annihilated" and converted to an equivalent amount of energy in accordance with $E = mc^2$, where E is the energy in ergs, m is the mass in grams, and c is the velocity of light in a vacuum (about 3×10^{10} cm/sec). The energy is radiated in the form of two γ rays, each with an energy of 0.51 MeV, moving in opposite directions.

Properties of Gamma Rays. There is no fundamental difference between γ rays and X rays, as they are both highly energetic photons belonging to the general category of electromagnetic radiation. Gamma rays are characterized by their wavelength and energy, and travel with the same speed as light in air or a vacuum. They display marked penetrating ability which depends on their extremely high energy and short wavelength. The quantum theory applies just as it does with other types of electromagnetic radiation. As described before, γ rays differ from X rays only in their site of origin; that is, γ rays arise in atomic nuclei and in the annihilation process. Depending on their energy, they interact with matter in the same way as X rays.

Energy of Gamma Rays. There are several methods available for determining the energy of γ rays.

1. *Crystal Diffraction.* When γ rays pass through certain crystals, they are scattered to form a diffraction pattern. Spectrographic analysis serves to measure the wavelength of the photons and, from this, their frequency and energy can be computed by equations (2) and (3). This method is suitable for γ rays with energies up to about 0.75 MeV.

2. *Photoelectric Interaction* (see page 87). When γ photons pass through a layer of matter, in this instance a pure element, a fraction of the photons will interact with inner orbital electrons and eject them as photoelectrons. The photon disappears, its energy being partitioned between W_K the binding energy of the K shell, and E_e the kinetic energy of the photoelectron:

$$hv_\gamma = W_K + E_e$$

Since E_e can be measured by spectrography, and W_K is already known for pure elements, hv_γ can easily be computed. In a similar manner, Compton recoil electrons (see page 91) resulting from the interaction of γ rays with light elements such as carbon can be used to determine the energy of the incident γ rays.

3. *Internal Conversion.* In the case of elements decaying by internal conversion (see above), the energy of the γ ray undergoing conversion can be readily determined. If the energy of the internal conversion electrons is measured by spectrometry, and to this energy is added the binding energy of the electron shell, the sum represents the energy of the converted γ photon:

$$hv_i = E_{ic} + W_K$$

where hv_i is the energy of the internally converted γ ray, E_{ic} is the energy of the internal conversion electron, and W_K is the binding energy of a K shell electron for this particular atom.

4. *Pair Spectrometry.* This method is applicable only to γ rays with energies greater than 1.02 MeV. When such highly energetic photons pass close to the nuclei of heavy elements (lead is most often used in this device), the photons disappear, each giving birth to a positron-negatron pair. (A positron is a positively charged electron.) The positrons and negatrons are separated by means of a magnetic spectrograph and their energy is measured. The energy of a pair, plus 1.02 MeV, equals the energy of the original γ photon.

5. *Scintillation Spectrography.* A specially designed scintillation detector with a pulse height analyzer can be calibrated against γ rays of known energy. The calibrated scintillation spectrograph can then be used to determine the energies of γ rays from various sources.

RADIATION OF PARTICLES

The transmission of energy by moving *particles* has already been mentioned, and will now be described. In general, this is called *corpuscular radiation.* It includes the following:

1. Alpha (α) particles
2. Beta$^-$ (β^-) particles or negatrons
3. Beta$^+$ (β^+) particles or positrons
4. Protons (p)
5. Neutrons (n)
6. Neutrinos (v)
7. Antineutrinos ($\tilde{v}$)
8. Mesons (μ, π, etc.)

Wilson Cloud Chamber. One of the most valuable instruments for the detection and identification of corpuscular radiation is the *Wilson cloud chamber.* It operates on the principle that under certain conditions water or alcohol vapor will condense in the form of tiny droplets upon ions. The chamber is a cylindrical container fitted with a piston (see Fig. 3.09). Water placed in the container will normally evaporate until a state of equilibrium is reached between those molecules of water that are escaping into the air within the chamber, and those that are re-entering

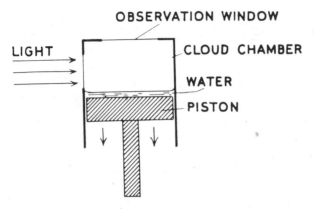

FIGURE 3.09. Wilson cloud chamber.

the water. When an ionizing particle enters the vapor in the chamber, it produces ions by collision with gas molecules in the air. If, at the same instant, the piston is suddenly pulled out, the vapor equilibrium is upset and vapor molecules will condense on the ions, thereby tracing the path of the entering particle. In other words, the ion tracks formed by an ionizing particle are traced by the condensed water droplets. These tracks can be photographed through a window at the top of the chamber. Although the cloud chamber is extremely simple in principle, it has been indispensable not only in the study of the properties of known corpuscular radiations, but also in the discovery of new ones. (See page 82 for a description of the Glaser bubble chamber.)

ALPHA PARTICLES

In the radioactive decay of certain heavy elements such as radium, thorium, and uranium, α particles are ejected from the atomic nuclei. *Alpha particles are identical with helium nuclei,* consisting of two protons and two neutrons in close association (see Fig. 3.10). They therefore bear two positive charges. Furthermore, because of their large mass, they move relatively slowly for a given energy ($\frac{1}{2}mv^2$). Hence, they readily *ionize* and *excite* atoms lying in their path. Recall that *ionization* is the complete removal of one or more electrons from an atom, whereas *excitation* is the raising of an electron to a higher energy level within the

ionization → is the complete removal of one or more electrons from an atom.

excitation → rasing of electron to higer energy level with in the atom.

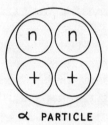

α PARTICLE

FIGURE 3.10. Diagram of an α particle. This is the same as the nucleus of a helium atom. The diagram shows the constituents of the α particle, and not necessarily their arrangement.

atom. These two processes are caused by the interaction of the strongly positive field of the α particle with the orbital electron's field. An atom which has lost one or more of its orbital electrons in this manner is said to be *ionized* and is called a positive ion because it is left with excess positive charge.

On combining with two electrons, an α particle becomes a neutral helium atom (see Fig. 3.11).

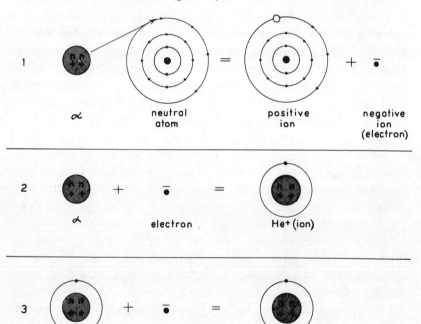

FIGURE 3.11. The steps in the acquisition of electrons by an α particle to form a neutral helium atom.

Thus, the double positive charge on the massive α particle renders it an extremely powerful ionizing particle. When α particles pass through a Wilson cloud chamber (see Fig. 3.09) they ionize the air within, and water vapor condenses on the ions, revealing their paths. Upon photographing these α tracks, one can determine the distance that the particular α particle has traveled in air. The α track is relatively thick and straight.

The distance traveled by the α particles from a given source in a particular medium is called their *range.* Ordinarily, range is specified in air under standard conditions of temperature and atmospheric pressure. For example, the range of radium alphas is 3.3 cm in air or 0.05 mm in soft tissue, which means that over this distance all the α particles have lost their energy through excitation and ionization. They are almost completely stopped by a sheet of paper, by the outer layer of the skin, or by 0.06 mm aluminum (Al). It has been found that the α particles from a given radionuclide such as radium (see page 394) all have nearly the same range in a given material. The range depends on the initial velocity of the α particle as it leaves the nucleus and on the medium through which it passes. The Geiger formula originally gave the range in air for radium-C (radiobismuth) α particles and may be expressed approximately as follows:

$$R \approx kv^3 \tag{7}$$

where R is the range in cm of air, k is a constant, and v is the initial velocity in cm/sec. Furthermore, for α particles from other radioactive nuclides, the constant k has the same value as for those from radium-C, namely 9.7×10^{-28}. The initial velocity of α particles depends on the decay rate of a particular radionuclide; the higher the decay rate, the greater the initial velocity.

Despite the fact that most α particles emitted by a given radionuclide have the same initial velocities, they do not have exactly the same range. The reason for this is that they do not all lose precisely the same amount of energy in their interactions with atoms along their paths. Therefore, there is a *slight* variation in their individual ranges, or lengths of path, a phenomenon called *straggling.*

Since the initial velocities of the α particles emitted by a particular radionuclide are virtually alike (or may occur in mono-energetic groups) and since all α particles have the same mass, they must all have nearly the same kinetic energy, that is, $\frac{1}{2}mv^2$. It is this energy which is used up in the process of ionization and excitation by α particles. Each time an α particle raises an electron to a higher energy level, or dislodges an orbital electron from an atom with formation of ion pairs, it loses a fraction of its kinetic energy. For example, a radium α particle has an initial energy of 4.66 MeV = 4.66 × 10⁶ eV. Since an average energy of 33.7 eV in air, called the W-quantity or W, is required to liberate one ion pair,

$$\frac{4.66 \times 10^6}{33.7} = 1.38 \times 10^5 \text{ ion pairs}$$

or approximately 140,000 ion pairs are liberated by a single α particle with this energy.

If the initial velocity of an α particle is known, its energy can be determined by simple arithmetic. The initial velocities from various sources have a minimum value of about 1.4 × 10⁹ cm per sec, and a maximum of about 2 × 10⁹ cm per sec (about 1/20 to 1/15 the speed of light). Since the mass of an α particle is 6.65 × 10⁻²⁴ g, the kinetic energy of the slowest ones is calculated as follows:

$$E = \frac{1}{2}mv^2$$

$$E = 1/2 \times 6.65 \times 10^{-24} \times (1.4 \times 10^9)^2$$

$$E = 6.5 \times 10^{-6} \text{ erg}$$

Since 1 MeV is equivalent to 1.6 × 10⁻⁶ erg,

$$E = \frac{6.5 \times 10^{-6}}{1.6 \times 10^{-6}} = 4.1 \text{ MeV}$$

In a similar manner, the energy of the fastest α particles is calculated to be 10 MeV.

The ability of a rapidly moving particle to produce ionization is designated by the term *specific ionization,* defined as the number of ion pairs liberated per cm of path in a given medium, usually air. It must be emphasized that the number of ions liberated per cm is entirely different from the total number of ions produced over the full range of the α particle. The total number of ions produced increases with the velocity (or energy) of the α particle. But in the case of ions per cm—specific ionization—a curious situation exists: the specific ionization increases as the velocity of the ionizing particles decreases! This is shown in Figure 3.12. It is noted that as the distance of the α particles from their source increases, the curve rises to a maximum known as the **Bragg peak**. This is explained by the observation that as the α particle slows down along its path (due to interactions with atoms) it remains in the vicinity of atoms longer, with a greater probability of ionizing them by interaction of its strongly positive field with the atomic orbital electrons. As a result, there is an increased density of ionization at the end of an α-particle track (as well as that of other charged particle tracks), an observation that can easily be made in a Wilson cloud chamber. The small tail at the end of the curve in Figure 3.12 represents straggling of the range which has been described above.

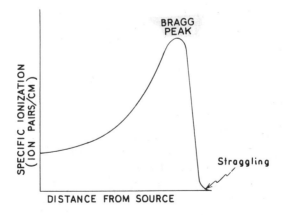

FIGURE 3.12. The relationship of specific ionization of α particles to the distance from the source. Note the marked increase in specific ionization toward the end of the path, as shown by the sharp peak in the curve (i.e. the Bragg peak).

BETA⁻ PARTICLES (NEGATRONS)

All available evidence indicates that β^- particles are identical with electrons, having the same mass and carrying a unit negative charge. The term β^- particle is customarily reserved for high speed negative electrons emitted by unstable atomic nuclei whose n/p ratio is too large for nuclear stability. But in the preceding chapter no mention was made of the existence of electrons within nuclei. Furthermore, careful studies rule out the possibility of electrons existing in a free state within the nucleus. How, then, can their origin in the nucleus be explained?

The first plausible theory of the origin of β^- particles postulated the conversion of a nuclear neutron to a proton and an electron (Fermi), the latter being ejected immediately from the nucleus as a β^- particle. However, this theory, although correct as far as it went, later proved to be incomplete (see below).

The *emission* of β^- particles differs fundamentally from that of α particles. It may be recalled that the latter all leave the atomic nuclei of a given element, endowed with nearly the same energy—that is, α particles are virtually monoenergetic. Gamma rays, too, are emitted in distinct energy ranges, corresponding to intranuclear energy levels. On the other hand, β^- particles are emitted in a continuous range of energies (corresponding to various speeds) varying from zero to a maximum. For example, radium-C β^- particles have energies from zero up to a maximum of 3.15 MeV. If the intensities of the β^- particles are plotted against their corresponding energies, an asymmetrical bell-shaped spectral distribution curve is obtained with a peak intensity corresponding to about one-third the maximum energy. The continuous spectrum of β^- particle energy has been explained by Pauli as follows: each particle leaving the nucleus with less than the maximum energy is accompanied by a neutral particle with an extremely small mass (several hundredths of that of an electron) and fantastic penetrating ability, called a *neutrino*. Actually, there are two kinds of neutrinos, the one accompanying the β^- particle being an *antineutrino* ($\bar{v}$). The energy of any given β^- particle plus its antineutrino is equal to the energy of the fastest β^- particle emitted by the atoms of a given nuclide and is a constant for that nuclide. In other words, there is a partition of energy between the β^- particle and its antineutrino:

$$\begin{array}{c} \text{energy of} \\ \beta^- \text{ particle} \end{array} + \begin{array}{c} \text{energy of} \\ \text{antineutrino} \end{array} = \begin{array}{c} \text{energy of} \\ \text{fastest } \beta^- \text{ particle} \end{array} = \begin{array}{c} \text{energy difference between} \\ \text{initial and final states} \end{array}$$

Thus, a fast (high energy) β^- particle is accompanied by a small antineutrino, whereas a slow (low energy) β^- particle is accompanied by a high energy antineutrino. The existence of the neutrino, an extremely difficult task, was proved in 1953 by Reines and Cowan.

The following equation summarizes β^- decay or de-excitation of certain radionuclides, a process that is more likely to occur with those that are neutron rich:

$$\underset{\text{neutron}}{{}^{1}_{0}n} \longrightarrow \underset{\text{proton}}{{}^{1}_{1}H} + \underset{\substack{\beta^- \text{ particle} \\ \text{or negatron}}}{{}^{0}_{-1}e} + \underset{\text{antineutrino}}{\tilde{\nu}}$$

In this reaction, the proton remains in the nucleus, while the β^- particle and antineutrino are emitted.

Although the β^- particles emitted by a given type of atom have a continuous range of energies as noted above, there is an exception in that some of them occur in **monoenergetic groups.** This phenomenon, manifested by sharp peaks in the otherwise smooth spectral distribution curve, is explained by the presence of **internal conversion electrons.** All are negative electrons, of course, but they differ in origin; the β^- particles arise in the nucleus and their energies lie on a smooth spectral distribution curve. The internal conversion electrons, on the other hand, originate usually in the K shell (much less often the L or M shell) and carry **discrete** nuclear de-excitation energies; they are responsible for the appearance of discontinuity peaks in the spectral distribution curve.

The **energy** of β^- particles refers to their kinetic energy, which depends on their velocity and mass (mass must be corrected for relativity effect as described below). Electron energy may be simply expressed in electron volts, 1 eV being the amount of energy an electron acquires when accelerated by 1 volt. The maximum energy (E_{max}) of β^- particles from various radionuclides ranges from about 0.01 to 5 MeV. In general, the average energy E_{av} of a β^--particle beam is equal to about one-third the maximum energy: $E_{av} \simeq \frac{1}{3} E_{max}.$

An interesting phenomenon is the increase in the mass of an electron as its velocity approaches that of light, as originally predicted by Einstein. This is called the **relativistic increase in mass**. Table 3.02 indicates the mass of an electron at various speeds relative to its mass at rest. These values were obtained from

$$m = \frac{m_0}{\sqrt{1 - \dfrac{v^2}{c^2}}} \tag{8}$$

where m is electron mass at velocity v, m_0 is electron mass at rest, and c is the velocity of light. Note that as v becomes vanishingly small compared to c (true of bodies traveling at ordinary speeds), v^2/c^2 becomes so small it can be neglected; m then equals m_0 in equation (8). As v approaches the speed of light, the entire denominator becomes vanishingly small and the value of m increases without limit (see Table 3.02).

TABLE 3.02
RELATIVITY EFFECT—THE INCREASE IN MASS OF AN ELECTRON
AS ITS VELOCITY APPROACHES THE VELOCITY OF LIGHT

Velocity of Electron Relative to Velocity of Light	Mass of Electron Relative to Its Resting Mass
v/c	m/m_0
0	1.0
0.1	1.00005
0.5	1.16
0.999	22

The **range** of β^- particles in air is difficult to determine because their small mass allows them to be deflected into a zig-zag course by the atoms with which they interact. This is in contradistinction to α particles which have a straight course in air, allowing their range to be determined more easily. The range of β^- particles is usually measured in solid material, this being expressed in grams per square centimeter (g/cm^2). The reason for the choice of this unit is that β^- particles are slowed down mainly by interaction with orbital electrons and, to a much smaller degree, with

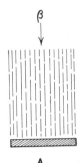
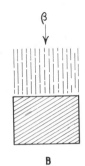

FIGURE 3.13. The absorption of β particles. The block in *A* is denser material than in *B*. However, if each presents the same number of mg per cm² to the incident beam, absorption will occur equally in both blocks.

A   B

atomic nuclei. In general, all elements (other than hydrogen) have nearly the same number of electrons per gram. Obviously, for the same number of orbital electrons to be available, a larger thickness of a less dense than of a denser material will be required to stop the β^- particles of a given energy range. This is illustrated in Figure 3.13 where blocks of material of different densities are placed in the path of a stream of β^- particles. In both cases, the same cross-sectional area, 1 cm², has been selected. The absorber in *A* is denser than in *B*. Therefore a greater thickness of *B* is required to absorb the β^- particles per unit cross-sectional area. Thus, if 10 g/cm² of *B* is required to absorb all the β^- particles, it means that a slab 1 cm² in area and of sufficient thickness to weigh 10 g must be used. In the case of absorber *A*, 10 g/cm² will also be needed, but since *A* is denser, a slab 1 cm² in area will not have to be so thick as *B* in order to weigh 10 g. As a practical application of this principle, the mica window of a Geiger tube will absorb the same fraction of a stream of β^- particles as an aluminum window having the same number of g/cm².

The range of the β^- particles of radium is 1 cm in soft tissue. They are almost completely stopped by 0.5 mm platinum (Pt), 1 mm silver (Ag), 1 mm lead (Pb), or 2 mm brass.

Since β^- particles are charged, their electric fields facilitate the removal of orbital electrons from atoms in their path, with resultant ionization of these atoms. The energy given up in this process (33.7 eV per ion pair formed) reduces the energy (and velocity) of the β^- particles, and after a sufficient number of collisions, their energy decreases to zero. At this point, the particle has reached the end of its range. The number of ion pairs produced per cm

TABLE 3.03
COMPARISON BETWEEN α AND β PARTICLES, WITH ENERGY OF 2 MeV.
VALUES ARE APPROXIMATE

	Average Range in Air	Specific Ionization
	cm	*ion pairs/cm*
α particles	1	60,000
β⁻ particles	1,000	50

of path is called *specific ionization*. Since a β^- particle has a smaller mass and a smaller charge than an α particle, it has a smaller specific ionization. Thus, 2-MeV β^- particles liberate about 50 ion pairs/cm of air, in contrast to 60,000 ion pairs/cm for 2-MeV α particles.

At the same time, β^- particles have an extremely long range in air as compared with α particles; β^- tracks in a cloud chamber are long, thin, and zig-zag so that the range must be determined by summation of these irregular tracks. The maximum range of 2-MeV β^- particles is found to be about 1,000 cm in air, as compared with about 1 cm for 2-MeV α particles (see Table 3.03).

BETA⁺ PARTICLES (POSITRONS)

A *positron* is a subatomic particle which has the same mass as an electron, but carries a positive charge. The positive charge on the positron exactly equals the negative charge on the electron. The symbol for positron is $_{+1}^{0}e$ or β^+ (contrasted with negatron or negative electron $_{-1}^{0}e$).

First discovered by Anderson in cosmic rays, positrons are emitted by certain unstable nuclei in the process of arriving at a stable form. However, this requires a large excess of energy which is not available in most unstable elements, so that positron emission is not a common occurrence.

In general, neutron-deficient nuclei, that is, those having an n/p (neutron/proton) ratio too low for stability, may de-excite and achieve stability by emitting a β^+ particle. This requires an available nuclear energy of *at least 1.02 MeV* (equivalent to the mass defect represented by two electron rest masses). A nuclear proton disappears and a neutron appears in its place, a β^+ particle being emitted together with a neutrino:

$$^1\text{H} \longrightarrow \ _0^1\text{n} \ + \ _{+1}^{\ 0}\text{e} \ + \ \nu$$

proton   *neutron*   *positron*   *neutrino*

remains in nucleus

emitted

The 1.02 MeV is needed because the emission of a positron re-duces the nuclear positive charge by 1 unit, and therefore an orb-ital electron must be lost to maintain the electrical neutrality of the atom. Thus, the daughter atom has two less electrons than the parent, and the rest mass of these two electrons is equivalent to 2×0.51 MeV = 1.02 MeV. (Note that in **negatron** emission the atom gains one unit of positive charge and an orbital elec-tron, that is, the atom both loses and gains an electron.) Any energy in excess of 1.02 MeV is shared between the positron and the neutrino in a manner analogous to that of the negatron and its antineutrino.

If a neutron-poor nucleus has an excitation energy **less than 1.02 MeV** it can still gain a neutron by the process of **electron cap-ture.** Here an orbital electron, usually from the K shell but less likely from shells farther out, is captured by the nucleus. A nu-clear proton disappears and a neutron appears in its place ac-cording to the following equation:

$$_1^1\text{H} \ + \ _{-1}^{\ 0}\text{e} \ \longrightarrow \ _0^1\text{n} \ + \ \nu$$

proton   *electron*   *neutron*   *neutrino*

capture   *remains in nucleus*   *emitted*

The nuclear excitation energy must be at least equivalent to the binding energy of the captured electron in its shell, plus the energy of the neutrino. Since the binding energy of the electron has a definite value, the neutrino does, too (instead of a range of anti-neutrino energies with negatron emission). Obviously, character-istic X rays are also produced because electron capture leaves a hole in the corresponding shell. In addition, **Auger** (pronounced o'zhay) electrons are emitted as the result of interaction between some of the characteristic X rays and orbital electrons of the same atom.

In a neutron-poor radionuclide whose nuclear excitation energy is greater than 1.02 MeV, some atoms may de-excite by positron emission, whereas others may do so by electron capture. In other words, these two processes are in competition in the same nuclide. The term *branching* designates a type of decay in which certain radionuclides can de-excite by alternate processes. The ratio of the number of atoms de-exciting by capture to those by positron emission is the *branching ratio* for electron capture. For example, sodium 22 has a branching ratio for electron capture of 10 percent.

Finally, some radionuclides that are neutron-poor and have excitation energy in excess of 1.02 MeV can de-excite by either of the three processes: negatron emission, positron emission, or electron capture. An example of this is arsenic 74 (negatron 32%, positron 30%, and electron capture 38%).

Another source of positrons is *pair production*. Whenever high energy photons containing more than 1.02 MeV pass close to a nucleus, they may disappear, at the same time giving rise to a pair of oppositely charge electrons; in other words, a positron and a negative electron.

Regardless of the origin of a positron, it soon loses energy and in about 1 billionth of a second unites with a negative electron. Together they disappear and give rise to two photons of 0.51 MeV each, moving in opposite directions (see Fig. 4.07). Conversion of the positron-electron pair to a pair of photons is known as the *annihilation reaction* (see page 64).

NEUTRONS

The discovery of the *neutron* forms a most interesting chapter in the history of atomic physics. In 1920 Rutherford postulated the existence of a neutral subatomic particle. Shortly afterward, Harkins in the United States made the same suggestion and is believed to have coined the term "neutron" in 1921. Subsequently, a number of physicists observed a type of radiation which was electrically neutral, but which they could not explain. The first of these were the German physicists Bothe and Becker who, in 1930, found that the bombardment of beryllium with polonium α particles caused the emission of extremely penetrating, electrically neutral radiation which they misinterpreted as γ radiation. Two years later, Joliot and Curie in France repeated this error. In 1932, twelve years after Rutherford's original prediction, one of his assistants, James Chadwick, definitely established the existence of the neutron, thereby ushering in the Atomic Age and, with it, the new field of Nuclear Medicine.

Neutrons are particles of about the same mass as a hydrogen atom but carrying *no charge*. Thus, they are not deflected by an electrical or magnetic field (as are α and β particles). Furthermore, neutrons are not directly ionizing because there is no associated electrical field to interact with atomic orbital electrons. Instead, they may collide directly with atomic nuclei, and it is the *recoil* of these nuclei, especially of the lighter elements, which causes ionization. Thus, *neutrons may be said to ionize indirectly,* liberating about 1 ion pair per 100 cm of path in air.

The symbol for the neutron is $_0^1 n$, indicating mass number 1 and atomic number zero. A neutron does not exist in the free state except for very short intervals of time. There are two reasons for this phenomenon. First, the neutron is radioactive, disintegrating to a proton, an electron, and an antineutrino, as described above, with a half-life of about 12.8 min:

$$_0^1 n \quad \rightarrow \quad _1^1 H \quad + \quad _{-1}^0 e \quad + \quad \tilde{v}$$

neutron   proton   electron   antineutrino

In the second place, because they are uncharged, neutrons enter atomic nuclei very easily, unopposed by a nuclear electrostatic field. In other words, an atom in the path of a neutron does not offer an electrical barrier to its penetration of the nucleus. Therefore, neutrons which fail to disintegrate lose their free state by entering atomic nuclei.

Because neutrons are not emitted by any of the naturally occurring radioactive nuclides, they must be obtained artificially. Several sources of neutrons will be indicated briefly, but first the notation of elements in nuclear physics will be presented. The number above and to the left of the chemical symbol is called the **superscript** and represents the mass number. The number below and to the left of the symbol is the **subscript** and represents the atomic number. Thus, $^{16}_{8}O$ refers to the oxygen atom with mass number 16 and atomic number 8. Examples of neutron sources are as follows:

Classic example

1. *Alpha particle interaction with beryllium ($^{9}_{4}Be$).*

$$^{9}_{4}\text{Be} \quad + \quad ^{4}_{2}\text{He} \quad \longrightarrow \quad ^{12}_{6}\text{C} \quad + \quad ^{1}_{0}\text{n}$$

  beryllium   *α particle*   *carbon*   *neutron*

2. *Deuteron interaction with deuterium ($^{2}_{1}H$).*

$$^{2}_{1}\text{H} \quad + \quad ^{2}_{1}\text{H} \quad \longrightarrow \quad ^{3}_{2}\text{He} \quad + \quad ^{1}_{0}\text{n} \quad + \text{ 3.2 MeV}$$

 deuterium   *deuteron*   *helium*   *neutron*

          (rare isotope)

3. *Photodisintegration—irradiation of certain nuclides with energetic γ rays.* Notice that energy must be absorbed (i.e. supplied) for this reaction to take place.

$$^{2}_{1}\text{H} \quad + \quad h\nu \quad \longrightarrow \quad ^{1}_{1}\text{H} \quad + \quad ^{1}_{0}\text{n}$$

 deuteron   *γ photon*   *·proton*   *neutron*

      (2.2 MeV)

4. *Stripping process.* When a high energy deuteron collides with the edge of an atomic nucleus, the proton portion of the deuteron may be stripped off while the neutron portion goes on alone (Oppenheimer-Phillips Mechanism):

$$^{2}_{1}\text{H} \quad \longrightarrow \quad ^{1}_{1}\text{H} \quad + \quad ^{1}_{0}\text{n}$$

 deuteron   *proton*   *neutron*

5. *Nuclear reactor or atomic pile.* This is the most prolific and important source of neutrons and will be taken up in detail on pages 375 to 386.

Neutrons are usually classified as *fast, intermediate, slow,* and *thermal.* The fast neutrons impart their kinetic energy to nuclei with which they collide, and the recoil of such nuclei, carrying as they do positive charges, results in ionization of other atoms. The slowest or ***thermal*** neutrons have about the same kinetic energy as molecules at ordinary temperature. Because they move slowly and have no electrical barrier to overcome, they easily enter atomic nuclei, thereby producing stable, or radioactive, isotopes.

Fast neutrons must be slowed down before they can participate in certain nuclear reactions. Since they lose more energy by ***nuclear recoil*** when they encounter nuclei whose mass is similar to their own, the ***lighter*** atoms are most efficient in slowing them to thermal levels. Water and paraffin, containing a relatively high percentage of hydrogen, are best suited for slowing down neutrons and are widely used for this purpose. A 1-MeV neutron requires about 18 collisions with hydrogen nuclei, or 150 collisions with the heavier oxygen nuclei, to be reduced to thermal range which averages about 0.025 eV.

Since neutrons ionize indirectly through recoil of the atomic nuclei with which they collide, they cannot readily be detected by ordinary methods such as the Wilson cloud chamber or the Geiger counter. One method utilizes a proportional type of ionization chamber either lined with boron (isotope ^{10}B) or containing it as a part of the gas filling. The neutrons interact with the ^{10}B producing lithium recoil nuclei and α particles, both of which ionize the gas in the chamber and are thereby detected. Another type of counter uses the fission principle (see page 377); such a fission chamber has one electrode coated with uranium 235 mixed with a phosphor that scintillates when it is struck by fission particles. The latter can be counted by means of a photomultiplier tube (see pages 486 to 488). A third method is photographic; recoil nuclei produced by the interaction of neutrons with low atomic number elements are detected by their tracks in photographic film.

ORBITAL ELECTRONS

The electrons emitted by certain nuclei and ordinarily called β particles have already been described. Before leaving the subject of particles, we must consider briefly the corpuscular radiation consisting of *orbital electrons.*

Whenever photons of sufficient energy (such as X rays and γ rays) or charged particles (such as α and β particles) interact with orbital electrons of atoms in their path, the electrons may be dislodged and fly off into space. Consisting of two types, *photoelectrons* and *recoil electrons,* they will be considered in greater detail in Chapter 4. Suffice it to say, these primary electrons cause ionization by collision with other atomic orbital electrons and may also produce secondary X rays and characteristic X rays as the result of these interactions. Such reactions continue until all the energy of the primary electrons has been dissipated. It is principally the ionization and excitation by electrons that is responsible for the therapeutic effect of X and γ rays.

COSMIC RAYS

Although they are of no practical concern in therapy, *cosmic rays* are of general interest in radiation physics. It was known early in this century that ordinary air is ionized, as shown by the leakage of a charge from an insulated electroscope. Furthermore, the rate of leakage increases at high altitudes. This has been found to be due to the entrance of extraterrestrial *cosmic rays* into the earth's atmosphere. Cosmic rays are of two types. The *primary cosmic rays,* arising in outer space, consist mainly of high energy protons (more than 2.5 billion electron volts), but also include α particles, atomic nuclei, and high energy electrons and photons. *Secondary cosmic rays* are produced by interaction of primary cosmic rays with nuclei in the earth's atmosphere and consist mainly of mesons (most are π mesons, but μ, τ, and κ are also present), electrons, and γ rays. Most cosmic rays observed in the laboratory are of the secondary type. They are so penetrating that they can pass through lead many feet thick.

Glaser Bubble Chamber. Because of the low density of the gas in a Wilson Cloud Chamber, interactions with high energy radiations are sparse and may be impossible to detect. A more efficient type of chamber, one that has become indispensible in the investigation of nuclear radiation of all types, was devised in

1952 by D. A. Glaser. In this instrument, called a **bubble chamber**, a superheated liquid serves as the medium in which ionization tracks are manifested as bubbles that are more closely spaced than the droplets in a cloud chamber.

When a liquid is heated to the boiling point under ordinary conditions, bubbles of vapor are released into the liquid as it boils. However, if the liquid is carefully heated in a vessel with exceptionally smooth walls its temperature may be raised above the boiling point without bubble formation—it is now a **superheated liquid.** Passage of ionizing radiation through such a superheated liquid results in bubble formation about the released ions to produce bubble tracks. The spacing of the bubbles depends on the specific ionization of the radiation being observed, and may approach 0.025 cm.

Various liquids have been used in bubble chambers including liquid hydrogen, liquid nitrogen, ordinary ether, and others. Because the density of such liquids greatly exceeds that of the gas in a cloud chamber, the tracks produced by extremely high energy radiation are short enough to be detected, especially if the chamber dimensions are adequate.

In actual use, compression of the liquid in a smooth walled chamber permits heating above the boiling point. Upon sudden release of the pressure the liquid becomes superheated and sensitive to the passage of ionizing radiation. However, the period of sensitivity is fairly short, bubbles soon appearing even without the passage of radiation, although in no specific pattern. The compression and superheating process then has to be repeated. In more advanced equipment, the sensitization of the bubble chamber can be synchronized with the entry of the radiation being studied.

The bubble chamber has greatly extended the possibility of detecting and observing the properties of a host of nuclear radiations that are beyond the capacity of the cloud chamber.

SUMMARY

Radiation is the process of emission of energy by atoms, and the passage of this energy through space.

There are two *types* of radiation:
1. *Wave*—electromagnetic—X rays and γ rays. Transverse waves associated with vibrating electric charges.
2. *Corpuscular*—streams of particles including α particles, negatrons (β^-), positrons (β^+), neutrons, neutrinos, antineutrinos, orbital electrons, and others. (Certain aspects of wave radiation require the assumption that waves are companied by discrete energy corpuscles: photons or quanta.)

The *sources* of radiation are:
1. *Atomic Nuclei*
   a. Alpha particles (helium nuclei)
   b. Beta particles (fast negatrons and positrons)
   c. Gamma rays
   d. Neutrinos
2. *Atomic Orbits*
   a. Electrons
   b. X rays
3. *Brems Rays*—arise during deceleration of energetic electrons, as in X-ray tube.
4. *Annihilation Radiation*—combination of positron and negatron which immediately disappear and give rise to 2 γ photons.
5. *Cosmic Rays*—outer space.
   a. *Primary*—high energy protons, electrons, and γ rays; α particles; atomic nuclei.
   b. *Secondary*—mesons; electrons; γ rays.

CHAPTER 4

Reactions Between Radiation and Matter

PHOTON INTERACTIONS WITH MATTER

IN order to comprehend the mode of action of electromagnetic radiation on living tissues, we must first understand the various types of interactions of radiation with matter in general. These interactions occur between the incident radiation and the atoms lying in its path, the type of reaction depending on the energy and nature of the radiation, and the atomic number of the substance being irradiated.

We have already seen that X and γ rays are physically *identical,* occupying the same region of the electromagnetic spectrum and behaving at the same time both as waves and as energy quanta (photons). Because of their essential similarity, one may consider X and γ photons together in discussing their interaction with matter.

In general, X and γ photons liberate primary electrons from orbits of atoms by various types of interactions. But this is, at best, an inefficient process, relatively few such electrons being freed directly. However, the released primary electrons display significantly greater efficiency in exciting and ionizing atoms in their path. Thus, *it is the energy and spatial distribution of the primary electrons freed by X and γ rays that are mainly responsible for the resulting radiobiologic effects.* We therefore regard X and γ rays as *indirectly ionizing radiation.*

The liberation of primary electrons, as we shall soon discover, involves energy absorption; it is axiomatic that *only absorbed energy contributes to radiobiologic effects.* For this reason, detailed consideration will be given to the processes by which X and γ rays dislodge orbital electrons.

Five different interactions may occur when matter, regardless of its state, is irradiated by high energy photons: (1) transmission

85

of photons unchanged; (2) unmodified (classical or coherent) scattering; (3) photoelectric absorption; (4) modified scattering; and (5) pair production. As will be pointed out later, the predominant type of reaction depends on the energy of the incident photon and the atomic number of the material being irradiated. Since nuclear reactions are not involved in ordinary X- and γ-ray therapy, the discussion will be limited to the interaction of photons with orbital electrons. Each class of interaction will be discussed separately.

1) **Transmission of Photons.** It has already been indicated that the atom consists largely of empty space, only a minute fraction of its volume being occupied by the nucleus and the orbital electrons. Thus, the actual particles in the atom (protons, neutrons, electrons) constitute about 10^{-12} or one one-million-millionth of its volume. Because of this, a large fraction of the photons in any given beam passes directly through the atom without encountering an electron. Furthermore, the absence of a charge on the photon prevents the usual interaction of electrical fields, thereby increasing the likelihood that a photon may pass through an atom unhindered (see Fig. 4.01). However, such an event is not really an interaction because the transmitted photons do not lose energy and are therefore entirely ineffective in therapy, unless they later succeed in interacting with an orbital electron.

2) **Unmodified (Classical, Coherent, or Rayleigh) Scattering.** Orbital electrons that are bound, relative to incident *very low energy* photons, are made to oscillate with the same frequency as the photons. The oscillating electrons radiate photons having the same frequency, these photons constituting the scattered radi-

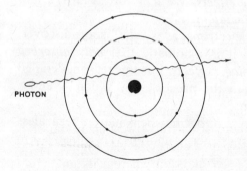

PHOTON

FIGURE 4.01. Simple transmission of a photon.

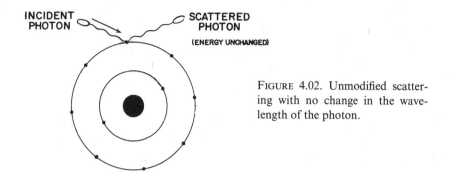

FIGURE 4.02. Unmodified scattering with no change in the wavelength of the photon.

ation. The incident photons, in effect, have "rebounded" from the firmly bound electrons with a change in direction but with no change in energy (see Fig. 4.02). This type of reaction occurs only if the incident photon does not have sufficient energy to dislodge the electron and is of minor significance in irradiation therapy, although it may impair the resolution of scintiscans with low energy radionuclides.

3) **Photoelectric Interaction with True Absorption.** According to the modern view of atomic structure, the orbital electrons occupy certain energy levels with respect to the nucleus. How is this explained? Since the nucleus carries a net positive charge, and the electrons in the shells are negative, there is an electrical force of attraction exerted between the nucleus and the electrons. This force is greatest between the electrons in the innermost (K) shell and the nucleus; and least between the electrons in the outermost shell and the nucleus, simply because of the effect of the greater distance. Much more work would therefore have to be done to lift an electron from the K shell away from the nucleus and out of the atom than would be required to remove an electron from an outer one, such as the N shell.

On this basis, the energy level of a given electron shell specifies the amount of work required to remove an electron from that energy level to such a distance from the nucleus that the force of attraction between them would approach zero. The electrons nearest the nucleus are therefore at the lowest energy level, while those farther out are at higher energy levels. Figure 4.03 represents a simplified energy level diagram wherein its analogy

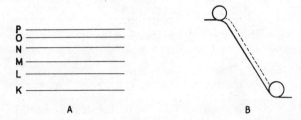

FIGURE 4.03. Energy level diagram of electronic shells (*A*) compared with a ball at various positions on a hill (*B*).

to a ball on a hill is demonstrated. The energy level of a shell is the **_binding energy_** of an electron in that shell.

Suppose that a block of matter is irradiated by a beam of X or γ rays. Photons whose energy approximates the energy level of a particular shell have a high probability of giving up their energy to the atom which then ejects an electron from that shell. In a naive sense, the photon "collides" with the orbital electron, freeing it. As shown in Figure 4.04A, if the *hv* of the incident photon is at least equal to, but does not greatly exceed, the *K* energy level, a *K* electron may be freed. Any of the photon's energy in excess of the electron's binding energy will be transferred to the electron in the form of kinetic energy (energy of motion), and the electron will escape from the atom. Such an interaction

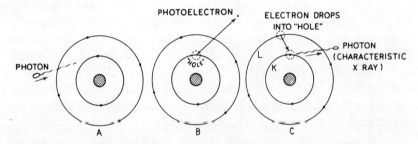

FIGURE 4.04. Photoelectric interaction. *A*. An incoming photon gives up *all* its energy to the atom which ejects a bound orbital electron as a *photoelectron*. *B*. The atom is now *excited* and *ionized*, since an electron has escaped from the atom. *C*. An electron from some higher energy level fills the "hole" in the *K* shell, with resulting emission of a characteristic X-ray photon. (Actually, there is a *series* or *cascade* of electrons to fill successive holes, giving rise to a series of characteristic photons).

in which all of the energy of the photon is used up in (1) dislodging the electron and (2) giving it kinetic energy, is called the *photoelectric effect*. The electron so liberated is called a *photoelectron*.

The term *K-absorption edge* refers to the peak absorption occurring as the energy of the incoming photons approximates the binding energy of the K shell.

The energy exchange occurring in a photoelectric interaction may be further clarified by a simple equation (Einstein):

$$h\nu_{photon} = W_K + E_e \qquad (1)$$

where $h\nu_{photon}$ is the energy of the incident photon, W_K is the energy associated with the K energy level (sometimes called the binding energy or escape energy of the electron in the K shell), and E_e is the kinetic energy of the photoelectron. A similar equation applies to photoelectric interaction with electrons in other energy levels.

If the incoming photon has less energy than the binding energy associated with the K shell, but nearly that of the L shell, then it is likely to release a photoelectron from the L shell. The same principle applies to shells farther out.

It should be emphasized that in the photoelectric process the *entire energy* of the photon is dissipated in releasing a photoelectron and giving it kinetic energy. The photon actually disappears in this process. Therefore, photoelectric interaction results in *true absorption* of the incident photon. This is followed promptly by the emission of *characteristic radiation* (see pages 97 to 103).

Photoelectrons are ejected at progressively smaller angles relative to the direction of the incoming photons as the energy of the latter increases; that is, ejection occurs more and more forward. For example, photoelectron ejection angles range from 90° for incident photon energy of a few keV, to about 10° for 1.5-MeV photons. Accompanying the decrease in the angle is an increase in the energy of the photoelectron.

In summary, photoelectric interaction consists of:

a. *Absorption of* a photon by an atom, wherein the energy of the photon exceeds the shell binding energy of the electron, with increasing probability of interaction as these energies approach equality.

   b. _**Emission**_ of the electron with kinetic energy equal to the difference between the energy of the photon and the binding energy of the electron for the involved shell. The atom is now ionized and excited.

   c. _**Excited atom**_ regains its normal state by emitting **characteristic photons** (X rays) whose energy equals the difference in energy levels between which orbital electron transition has occurred.

   d. _**Characteristic photons**_ may in turn cause excitation and ionization of the same or other atoms by the same process.

   The probability of a photoelectric interaction varies directly with the third power of the atomic number (Z^3) of the absorber, and inversely as the third power of the energy ($1/hv)^3$ of the incident photon. It is the principal type of interaction of photons with energies up to about 50 keV (accelerating potential about 100 kV) and with atoms of high atomic number (bone minerals *vs* soft tissue).

4) **Modified** (**Compton**, **incoherent**, **or** **inelastic**) **Scattering**. This produces *scattering absorption* of incoming photons, and

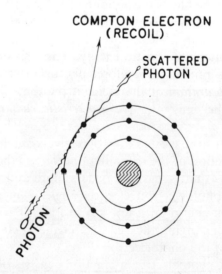

FIGURE 4.05. Compton interaction. The scattered photon has less energy and a longer wavelength than the incident photon.

occurs mainly between *high energy photons* (higher than those in-volved in photoelectric collision) and *loosely bound (outer shell) electrons.* The incident high energy photon interacts with a remote orbital electron which requires an insignificant amount of energy for its removal. Therefore the incident photon gives up only a part of its energy to the electron which is ejected as a *recoil electron* or *Compton electron* with kinetic energy equivalent to the loss of energy of the incident photon.

$$E_r = \Delta(hv) \qquad (2)$$

where E_r is the kinetic energy of the recoil electron, and $\Delta(hv)$ represents the decrease in energy of the incident photon during the encounter. The photon, now with reduced energy (and there-fore longer wavelength), proceeds in a direction at some angle to its original path. After the collision, the photon is a *scattered photon* because of this change in direction. The energy inter-change may be expressed simply as follows:

$$hv = hv_s + E_r \qquad (3)$$

where hv is the energy of the incident photon, hv_s is the energy of the scattered photon, and E_r is the kinetic energy of the recoil electron. The binding energy of the outer electrons, being almost nil, is disregarded in the Compton Effect.

Note that only that fraction of the incident photon's energy which imparts kinetic energy to the recoil electron is truly ab-sorbed in the Compton interaction. The energy remaining in the

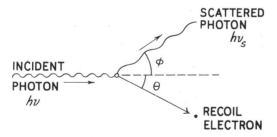

FIGURE 4.06. Angular relations in the Compton interaction: the smaller the angle of scatter, ϕ, of the photon, the less energy imparted to the recoil electron, and therefore the less energy lost by the original photon. The incident photon loses max-imum energy in a head-on collision, reversing its direction ($\phi = 180°$).

scattered photon is available for further interactions with other electrons by either the photoelectric or the Compton process. In a Compton interaction the scattered photon differs from the incident photon in two important respects: (1) its direction may be altered, and (2) its energy may be decreased (wavelength increased).

The *angle* at which the incident photon is scattered determines the increase in wavelength of the scattered photon (or its decrease in energy). The crucial factor is the angle ϕ which the path of the scattered photon makes with the initial direction of the incident photon (see Fig. 4.06). This relationship is expressed by the following equation:

$$\Delta\lambda = 0.024(1 - \cos\phi) \text{ Å} \tag{4}$$

where $\Delta\lambda$ is the increase in wavelength of the scattered photon as compared with the incident photon, and $\cos \phi$ is the cosine of the scattering angle. If ϕ is known, its cosine may be found in published trigonometric tables. Equation (4) shows that *in the Compton Effect, the increase in wavelength of the scattered photon depends only on the angle of scatter;* it has nothing whatever to do with the wavelength of the incident photon. It is interesting to note that if the incident photon collides head-on with the electron, the photon is scattered directly backward, the angle of scatter being 180°. Since cosine 180° is − 1, equation (4) becomes:

$$\Delta\lambda = 0.024[1 - (-1)]$$

$$\Delta\lambda = 0.024 \times 2 = 0.048 \text{ Å}$$

Thus, if the incident photon has a wavelength of 0.1 Å, the scattered photon in a head-on collision will have a wavelength of 0.1 + 0.048 = 0.148 Å. The loss of energy represented by this increase in wavelength will be carried off by the recoil electron. For example, a 1-MeV photon striking an electron headon "bounces back" with an energy of about 200 keV, while the electron shoots forward with an energy of about 800 keV.

If a photon undergoes a glancing interaction with an electron, the photon is not scattered, but proceeds in its original direction. In this case, the recoil electron is projected at an angle of 90°,

ϕ is 0°, and cos ϕ is 1. Substituting in equation (4), the change in wavelength is

$$\Delta\lambda = 0.024(1 - 1)$$

$$\Delta\lambda = 0.024 \times 0 = 0$$

Thus, the change in wavelength of the scattered photon varies from 0 when collision is such that photon continues directly forward, to a maximum of +0.048 Å when scattering of the photon is directly backward.

As far as the recoil electron is concerned, the more nearly the incident photon makes a direct hit, the more nearly the recoil electron is projected in a forward direction and the more kinetic energy it acquires.

The Compton Effect assumes major importance with X and γ rays having an energy of at least 100 keV; with this energy, about 99 percent of the primary electrons are recoil electrons while only 1 percent are photoelectrons (in water). Under these conditions, about 91 percent of the liberated energy is carried by the recoil electrons. It should be emphasized that 100 keV is equivalent to an accelerating voltage of about 200 kVp.

The probability of a Compton interaction varies in approximately inverse ratio to the energy of the incident photon ($1/h\nu$) and is virtually independent of the atomic number of the medium. However, it varies directly with the number of electrons per gram of the medium, so that more such interactions occur in fat than in an equal mass of bone.

5) **Pair Production.** When a photon with an energy of at least 1.02 MeV (equivalent to the rest mass of two electrons) passes near an atomic nucleus, it may interact with the strong nuclear electrical field and disappear, giving rise to two oppositely charged particles of equal mass—a negative electron or *negatron*, and a positive electron or *positron*. This process is called *pair production*. Any photon energy in excess of 1.02 MeV is shared almost equally between the particles in the form of kinetic energy. The negatron behaves in the same manner as any other negative electron. The positron, too, slows down by interacting with atoms; however, when it reaches thermal velocity (average velocity of molecules

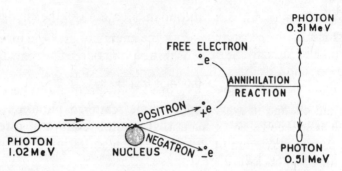

FIGURE 4.07. Pair production and annihilation. The incident photon (1.02 MeV or greater) forms a negatron-positron pair in the vicinity of an atomic nucleus. The positron, upon coming to rest, combines with a free electron to form two 0.51 MeV photons by the *annihilation reaction*.

at ordinary temperatures), it combines with an electron to form a *positronium* which disappears in 10^{-10} sec to produce two photons each with an energy of 0.51 MeV moving in opposite directions. The conversion of particles to photons is termed the *annihilation reaction* (see Fig. 4.07). The probability of pair production per atom increases rapidly with an increase in the energy of the incident photon. In contrast to this, the probability of annihilation increases with a decrease in the energy of the positron, reaching a maximum when the positron is almost at rest.

In summary, we have first a conversion of energy to matter, and then reconversion of matter to energy in strict accord with Einstein's equation, $E = mc^2$:

1. *Pair Production.*

$$h\nu \longrightarrow {}_{-1}^{0}e + {}_{+1}^{0}e$$

1.02 MeV   negatron positron
photon

2. *Annihilation Reaction.*

$${}_{-1}^{0}e + {}_{+1}^{0}e \longrightarrow h\nu + h\nu$$

0.51 MeV   0.51 MeV
photon   photon

The probability of pair production varies approximately in direct ratio to the second power of the energy $(hv)^2$ of the incident photon, and directly with the atomic number of the medium. Pair production exceeds the Compton Effect above 20 MeV. At very high energies, above 50 MeV, pair production becomes almost the sole form of interaction of photon radiation and matter. This is particularly true when the irradiated material has a high atomic number.

INTERACTIONS OF CHARGED PARTICULATE RADIATION WITH MATTER

TEST

The interactions of α and β particles with matter have already been considered in detail in the preceding chapter. However, a summary of these reactions may be instructive.

It should be pointed out that such interactions are of two main types—elastic and inelastic. An *elastic interaction* is one in which the total kinetic energy of the interacting particles is the same before and after the interaction; that is, there is no change in the kinetic energy of the system. On the other hand, an *inelastic interaction* is one in which the total kinetic energy changes as the result of the interaction.

Alpha Particles. When an α particle, which carries two positive charges, collides with an orbital electron, that is, comes close enough to it for their *electrical fields to interact*, the electron may be kicked out of its orbital. The atom is now *ionized*, becoming a positive ion; the ejected electron is the negative ion. This process is analogous to the expulsion of orbital electrons by X- or γ-ray photons. With every such collision the α particle loses an amount of energy equal to the binding energy of the electron plus the kinetic energy of the electron. This is an *inelastic interaction* because some of the energy of the α particle was used to raise the electron to a higher energy level. After a certain number of such collisions, the kinetic energy of the incident α particle is reduced to zero. Eventually, the α particle takes on two electrons, becoming a neutral helium atom. The ionized absorbing atom, now in an *excited state*, returns to its normal energy state by transition of an electron from an outer orbit to fill the hole left by the liberated electron, radiating a characteristic X-ray photon in the process. Thus, the sequence of events is analogous to that during certain photon interactions with atoms.

The α-particle track in a Wilson cloud chamber, which resembles its track in tissues, is straight and thick because of its strong ionizing ability. Its distance or *range* in tissues before being stopped is about 0.05 mm.

Beta⁻ Particles. The interaction of β^- particles with matter occurs in a manner similar to that of α particles: interaction with orbital electrons which may be ejected from the atom, resulting in ionization of the atom; or only raising electrons to higher energy levels, resulting in excitation. These are *inelastic interactions.* After a number of such interactions the incident β^- particles are slowed to the point where they lack sufficient kinetic energy to cause further ionization. The paths of β^- particles in the cloud chamber are zig-zag because of their small mass and charge, as contrasted with α particles which possess a mass about 7,000 times as great and a double charge. For the same reasons, the ionization tracks of β^- particles of equivalent energy are not so dense as those of α particles. However, there is one important difference in the interaction of α and β particles with matter. Beta particles can also lose energy by a process called *bremsstrahlung* (see pages 55 to 56). This is another example of an *inelastic* interaction.

The process of bremsstrahlung depends on (1) the *atomic number (Z) of the absorber,* and (2) on the *energy of the β^- particles.* Thus, the probability of bremsstrahlung radiation is directly proportional to Z^2. This explains why low atomic number materials such as plastics are more efficient protective shields for β^--particle emitters such as phosphorus 32 and strontium 90. As the energy of the β^- particles increases, the associated bremsstrahlung photons are radiated at progressively smaller angles, approaching the direction of motion of the particles. For example, with 1-MeV β particles this angle is about 10° to 20°. Conversely, bremsstrahlung for 100-keV electrons is radiated mainly at large angles, approaching 30° to 60°.

It is possible for β^- particles to interact *elastically* by removing outer shell or free electrons; as their binding energy is virtually nil, there is no change in the total energy of the reacting particles.

An interesting phenomenon is associated with the passage of high speed charged particles, such as betas, through transparent media such as water or glass. The speed of light in these media is less than that of the charged particles and their passage is associated with the emission of a weak bluish-white light called *Cerenkov radiation.* This has been explained as a sort of electromagnetic shock wave. A special counter has been designed to utilize Cerenkov radiation to detect high energy particles.

Beta$^+$ Particles. As we have already seen, positrons have an extremely short, independent existence. They dissipate their energy in the same manner as negative β particles. But when a positron comes to rest, it unites with a negatron; immediately both particles disappear, giving rise to two 0.51 MeV photons which proceed in opposite directions (see Fig. 4.07). The interaction of these photons with matter is the same as that of any other photons of the same energy.

CHARACTERISTIC OR FLUORESCENT RADIATION

We have already mentioned the characteristic radiation associated with X-ray production and photoelectric interaction. It will be instructive to consider the subject of characteristic X rays in more detail.

As described above, the electron shells about the nucleus of an atom represent energy levels within the atom, the shell nearest the nucleus (that is, the K shell) being at the lowest energy level, and the shells farther and farther from the nucleus (L, M, N, etc.) at progressively higher energy levels. The energy holding an electron in its shell may be called the *binding energy*, which may be defined as the energy required to lift an electron from its particular shell to a point just outside the atom. Since more work is needed to remove an electron from an inner shell than from a more distant one, it follows that the binding energies become progressively smaller in successive shells farther and farther from the nucleus. When an electron is raised from an inner to an outer shell, the atom absorbs energy. Conversely, when an electron jumps from an outer shell to a hole in an inner one, the work must be returned in the form of energy radiated by the atom, thereby satisfying the Law of Conservation of Energy. No energy is absorbed or emitted by a stable atom so long as its electrons remain in their respective orbitals.

How are such *electron transitions* brought into play? *Any form of radiation,* regardless of whether it is electromagnetic (X or γ rays) or corpuscular (α or β particles), can cause the ejection of a firmly bound orbital electron if it can bring enough energy to the atom. Thus, the incident radiation must have an amount of energy at least equal to that associated with the energy level of the electronic shell. During the ejection of the orbital electron, energy is absorbed by the atom equal to the binding energy of the electron in its shell. (Any additional energy imparted to the escaping electron in the form of kinetic energy is abviously not absorbed by the atom.)

Because the nucleus of an atom of high atomic number carries a large positive charge, there is a strong force of attraction between the nucleus and the orbital electrons. Therefore, more work is required to pull an electron out of its shell in such an atom than in an atom of low atomic number. Thus, 1.56 keV is required to release an aluminum ($^{27}_{13}$Al) K electron, whereas 87.5 keV is needed to dislodge a lead ($^{207}_{82}$Pb) K electron.

When an orbital electron is moved to an outer shell, or entirely out of the atom, the atom absorbs energy and is then in an *excited state;* it is now said to be in a higher energy state. If the electron is removed completely, not only is the atom excited, but is said to be *ionized* as well because there is now a deficit of one electron leaving one excess positive charge on the nucleus. Thus, in the process of excitation an *ion pair* may be formed, consisting of the positively charged atom and the ejected negative electron. This is shown in Figure 4.08.

Immediately after excitation, that is, in about 10^{-8} sec, an electron jumps from some higher energy level, or perhaps from outside the atom, into the vacated space in the shell. Since the

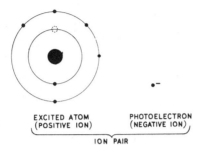

EXCITED ATOM
(POSITIVE ION)

PHOTOELECTRON
(NEGATIVE ION)

ION PAIR

FIGURE 4.08. Diagram of an ion pair. The electron soon attaches itself to an atom or molecule to form a negative ion.

transition of an electron leaves a hole in its shell of origin which must then be filled by transition of an electron from a still higher shell, there is usually a *cascade* of electrons as holes in successive shells are filled. The excited atom thereby returns to *ground* (most stable) level, radiating a series of characteristic photons with total energy equal to the binding energy of the original ejected electron (see Fig. 4.09).

In order to demonstrate the transition of electrons between energy levels, the physicist makes use of an *energy level diagram* (see Fig. 4.10). This, incidentally, indicates the nomenclature

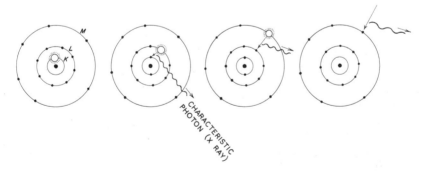

FIGURE 4.09. Characteristic radiation. An electron drops from a higher energy level, such as *L*, to a hole in a lower energy level such as *K*, the difference in these energy states being represented by the energy of the characteristic photon. The resulting hole in the *L* shell is promptly filled by an electron transition from a still higher energy level, etc. Thus, we have cascading electrons associated with a family of characteristic photons.

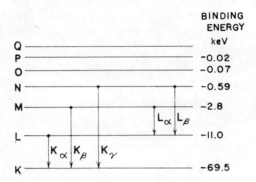

FIGURE 4.10. Electronic energy levels of tungsten. Note that these binding energies become progressively smaller as the corresponding shells become more remote from the nucleus. Terminology has been simplified.

applied to the characteristic radiation arising from such transitions. Note that whenever an electron drops into a vacancy in the *K* shell (*K* energy level), a *K* characteristic photon for that particular atom is emitted. The energy of the characteristic photon equals the difference in the energy levels between which the electron has jumped. For example, if electron transition has occurred from the *L* shell to a hole in the *K* shell, then

$$hv_X = W_L - W_K$$

where hv_X is the energy of the characteristic X ray, and W_L and W_K are the binding energies of the respective shells. Actually, because electron transitions occur in a cascade, a series of characteristic X rays is emitted. The emitted photons are designed as ***characteristic*** or ***fluorescent X rays*** because their wavelength and energy are typical of the stated shell of the atom concerned. Thus, characteristic X rays associated with the *K* shell of copper (Cu) have the same wavelength for all atoms of copper, but are different from those of other elements such as tin (Sn) or iron (Fe). Characteristic X-ray photons emitted by the atom proceed to interact with other atoms and liberate electrons in the same way as the original incident photon, provided it has sufficient residual energy.

Actually, there is a family of *K* characteristic photons, constituting the ***K series***. If the electron jumps from the *L* shell to the *K* shell, it is designated K_α; if it drops from the *M* shell to the K shell it is called K_β. The characteristic photons emitted when electron transition occurs between outer orbits and the L shell constitute the L series. The K and L series are shown in Table 4.01.

TABLE 4.01
SIMPLIFIED TERMINOLOGY DENOTING THE CHARACTERISTIC SPECTRAL LINES IN THE K AND L SERIES

	Shells From Which Electron Transitions Occur			
Series	*L*	*M*	*N*	*O*
K	K_α	K_β	K_γ	K_δ
L		L_α	L_β	L_γ

It must be emphasized that the wavelengths of the photons in the K, L, etc. series are characteristic of a given element so that an unknown element can be identified if its K or L series is measured. This characteristic radiation arising from the interaction of penetrating radiation with atoms may be measured by X-ray spectrometry. When a narrow beam of monoenergetic X rays (i.e. consisting essentially of a single energy or wavelength) passes through matter, the emerging beam of X rays will no longer be monoenergetic, but will consist of a mixture of photons of various wavelengths and energies, resulting from photon interactions with orbital electrons of the specimen. If this emergent beam is now studied by means of an X-ray spectrometer, the intensities of the various wavelengths of X rays in the beam can be determined. The spectrometer is illustrated in Figure 4.11. This emerging beam

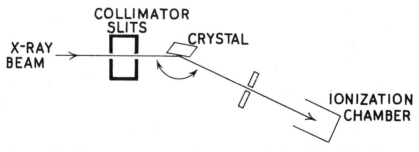

FIGURE 4.11. X-ray spectrometer used to measure the intensities of the photons representing various wavelengths in a *polyenergetic* (heterogeneous) beam. By turning the crystal together with the ionization chamber, the observer can obtain readings for the intensities corresponding to various wavelengths.

which is to be analyzed for its component wavelengths is then passed through a pair of slits in a lead collimator and allowed to strike the crystal face at various angles, the ionization chamber and crystal being lined up correctly for each angle. An ionization reading is taken for each position. Since the photons of a given wavelength are reflected at a particular angle, the series of ionization readings will obviously reveal the intensities of the various wavelengths in the beam being analyzed.

If the various intensities are now plotted against their corresponding wavelengths, **discontinuous peaks** of intensity will be found at certain wavelengths, as shown in Figure 4.12. These peaks are due to characteristic radiation emitted by the irradiated sample. They are called **spectral lines** or **line spectra** (that is, lines of X-ray spectrum), being analogous to the spectrum of visible light produced in a rainbow. The X-ray spectral lines represent the K, L, M, etc. characteristic radiation of the particular element irradiated. The frequency can then be found by the equation discussed earlier, $c = v\lambda$, and from this the energy computed by $E = hv$. A more practical method of measuring X- and γ-ray spectra involves the use of a scintillation or semiconductor detector and a pulse height analyzer. Since the height of the voltage pulses in this system depends on the energy of the entering photons, we have a means of sorting the radiation into its energy components which are then counted by a scaler. A spectral distribution curve is obtained by plotting the counting rate as a function of the individual photon energy.

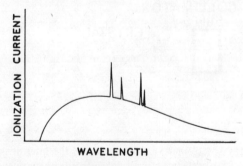

FIGURE 4.12. The type of curve obtained with an X-ray spectrometer. Peaks are caused by characteristic radiation present in the beam.

As the periodic table of elements is ascended (toward higher atomic numbers), the line spectra representing the *K*, *L*, etc. energy levels shift toward the shorter wavelength region because the binding energies of the corresponding energy levels increase with increasing atomic number. For example, aluminum has atomic number 13; its *K* series begins at wavelength 8.320 Å. On the other hand, copper has atomic number 29, and its *K* series begins at wavelength 1.541 Å.

The *fluorescent yield*, that is, the number of characteristic photons per shell hole, may be less than anticipated, a discrepancy explained by the production of *Auger* (pronounced ozhay) *electrons*. These are electrons liberated from shells by energy that would otherwise be emitted as characteristic photons.

ATTENUATION OF PHOTON RADIATION

When a beam of X or γ rays passes through a body of matter, it emerges with less intensity (e.g. R/min) than it had on entering the body. The loss of intensity, or *attenuation* of the beam as it is called, is due to three distinct processes:

1. True absorption
2. Scattering
3. Inverse square law

These will now be taken up in some detail.

True Absorption. We have already discussed this process at length in the preceding sections. In the photoelectric type of interaction of radiation with atoms, the entire energy of a photon is used up in ionizing an atom by ejection of an inner shell electron. If a part of a photon's energy is expended in initiating atomic ionization, only that part is said to be truly absorbed by the ionized atom; consequently, in the Compton process, only a portion of the energy of a given photon is absorbed and that is the portion which gives kinetic energy to a loosely bound orbital electron.

During photoelectric interaction, characteristic radiation is emitted, the wavelength of which is longer than that of the incident photon because the latter had to possess enough energy both to dislodge the electron and to give it kinetic energy. The total energy of the characteristic radiation equals the energy needed to dislodge the electron from a particular shell. In the case of soft tissues we are dealing with atoms of low atomic number in which the binding energies of even the inner shells are very small —about 0.5 keV. Therefore virtually all the energy (hv) of the incident photon is transferred to the photoelectron as kinetic energy.

It is the primary electrons (photoelectrons and recoil electrons) *which carry the truly absorbed energy,* and they in turn expend it in interaction with other atoms to produce secondary electrons, which in turn expend their energy in further interaction. The characteristic radiation may also be absorbed by interaction with atoms in the same manner as the incident photons, or may emerge as part of the exit beam. It must be emphasized that *only the energy that is truly absorbed in releasing primary electrons is effective in producing biological and chemical changes,* and hence is therapeutically useful. True absorption also occurs in pair production as the moving negatrons and positrons expend their kinetic energy in interactions with orbital electrons; the 1.02 MeV required to form each pair is re-radiated and is not absorbed unless the resulting 0.51 MeV photons interact with orbital electrons, mainly by the Compton process.

Scattering. Measurement of a *small field* X-ray beam upon emergence from a body which it has traversed shows loss of energy over and above that lost by true absorption. This is due to change in direction of some photons so they fail to reach the measuring instrument in the center of the beam. Such a change in direction of X or γ photons is called *scattering.* There are three varieties of scattering. First, there is *unmodified* scattering which results when a photon interacts with a nucleus or an inner orbital electron which it cannot dislodge because its energy is less than the binding energy of the electron. During this process, the photon undergoes a change in direction, but retains its original wavelength and energy. This is usually not an important interaction for us.

Another type of scattering reaction occurs in the Compton Effect (see page 90); the interacting high energy photon retains some energy after liberating a recoil electron, this residual energy being less than the photon originally possessed. It therefore undergoes a lengthening of its wavelength, but due to the type of collision, it also suffers a change in direction. This is called *modified scattering* because the photon experiences a modification or change in energy as well as direction.

Finally, an extremely high energy photon may undergo metamorphosis to a positron-negatron pair. The positron, upon slowing almost to rest, combines with an electron to produce two photons, each with an energy of 0.51 MeV, moving in opposite directions. This is really another form of modified scattering, although it must be borne in mind that the scattered photons, each having an energy of 0.51 MeV, may engage in other types of interaction with atoms and be partly or wholly absorbed.

Inverse Square Law. This will be mentioned only for the sake of completeness, as it has already been fully discussed in Chapter 1. Suffice it to say, the X- or γ-ray beam is attenuated by the very circumstance that in passing through a body of matter, its distance from the source becomes progressively greater. Obviously, the greater the thickness of tissue penetrated, the greater will be the distance from the source and the resulting attenuation of the beam on account of the inverse square law.

THE MEANING OF ATTENUATION CURVES

Let us first consider the relatively simple case of a *narrowly collimated* beam of *monoenergetic photons* passing through a *thin* slab of *homogeneous* absorbing material. The attenuation of the beam will depend on the thickness and the atomic number of the absorber and on the energy of the radiation, provided the distance is maintained constant. In Figure 4.13 is shown a narrow beam of X or γ rays incident on a *thin* sheet of homogeneous matter. If the radiation intensity (e.g. exposure rate in R/min)

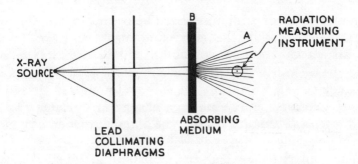

FIGURE 4.13. Diagram of an experimental arrangement for studying the attenuation of x or γ rays. *A* is the radiation transmitted by the absorber (filter). *B* represents various thicknesses of the absorber. Good geometry is achieved by having a narrow beam and thin filters.

is measured at point *A* without the absorber *B*, the recorded value will represent the incident radiation intensity I_0. If, now, a stated thickness of the absorber is placed at *B*, the intensity *I* that is recorded by the detecting instrument will be less than I_0 because of attenuation of the beam. Then,

$$I = I_0 - a \tag{5}$$

where *I* is the transmitted intensity, I_0 is the incident intensity, and *a* is the intensity lost by attenuation. Now let μ (Greek letter "mu") represent the fraction of the radiation intensity lost per cm thickness of the absorber, and *d* the thickness of the absorber. Then $\mu \times d \times I_0$ or $\mu d I_0$ will be equal to the actual loss of intensity *a* in equation (5). The value $a = \mu d I_0$ may now be substituted in equation (5):

$$I = I_0 - \mu d I_0 \tag{6}$$

This equation is an approximation which may be used where μd is less than 0.2. The quantity μ is called the *linear attenuation coefficient* and is defined as *the fraction of the incident radiation lost per unit thickness of absorbing material.* For example, it may be expressed in cm^{-1} or *"per cm."* The value of μ depends on the atomic number and physical state of the absorber, and the energy of the photons but, as will be shown later, this is not a simple relationship.

this refers to material's state such as; liquid, solid, gas

A more precise equation, derived by the use of simple calculus, is as follows:

$$I = I_0 e^{-\mu d} \tag{7}$$

The symbols have the same meaning as before, and e is a constant (base of natural logarithms). This equation has already been discussed in Chapter 1. Its practical application depends on the fact that with a monoenergetic beam (i.e. component photons all have essentially the same energy) each successive thickness d absorbs the same fraction of the incident radiation reaching it. Thus, if a narrow beam with an initial intensity of 10 units passes through a thickness d of a given substance having a linear attenuation coefficient of 0.1, then $10 - (0.1 \times 10) = 9$ units will get through thickness d. These 9 units now represent the incident radiation for the next layer of thickness d. Again, $0.1 \times 9 = 0.9$ units will be lost and $9 - 0.9 = 8.1$ units will be left as the incident radiation for the next layer. This process will continue until the radiation has passed through the entire thickness of the absorber. Since the loss of intensity is always fractional, the intensity of the beam theoretically never reaches zero, but may become extremely small if a large thickness of high atomic number material is used.

One need not use logarithms to apply equation (7). The values of $e^{-\mu d}$ for various values of μd can be found in published tables. Table 4.02 shows some of these values for the purpose of our discussion. Thus, if μ and d are known, let $x = \mu d$, and therefore $-x = -\mu d$. Then look in the column headed e^{-x} in Table 4.02 and read opposite the value of x the corresponding value of e^{-x}. For example, if μ is 0.1 per cm and d is 2 cm,

$$-x = -\mu d$$

$$-x = -0.1 \times 2 = -0.2$$

$$e^{-x} = e^{-0.2}$$

Corresponding to 0.2 in the x column, the value of $e^{-0.2}$ is 0.82.

Knowing $e^{-\mu d}$ in a given set of circumstances, and also knowing the intensity of the incident radiation, we can easily compute the intensity of the transmitted radiation. For example, we just found

TABLE 4.02
EXPONENTIAL FUNCTIONS FOR VALUES OF THE EXPONENT
HAVING TWO SIGNIFICANT FIGURES

x	e^x	e^{-x}	x	e^x	e^{-x}
0.00	1.0	1.0	4.1	60	0.017
0.10	1.1	0.90	4.2	67	0.015
0.20	1.2	0.82	4.3	74	0.014
0.30	1.3	0.74	4.4	81	0.012
0.40	1.5	0.67	4.5	90	0.011
0.50	1.6	0.60	4.6	99	0.010
0.60	1.8	0.55	4.7	110	0.0090
0.70 (0.693)	2.0	0.50	4.8	120	0.0082
0.80	2.2	0.45	4.9	130	0.0074
0.90	2.4	0.40	5.0	150	0.0067
1.0	2.7	0.37	5.1	160	0.0061
1.1	3.0	0.33	5.2	180	0.0055
1.2	3.3	0.30	5.3	200	0.0050
1.3	3.7	0.27	5.4	220	0.0045
1.4	4.1	0.25	5.5	240	0.0041
1.5	4.5	0.22	5.6	270	0.0037
1.6	4.9	0.20	5.7	300	0.0033
1.7	5.5	0.18	5.8	330	0.0030
1.8	6.0	0.16	5.9	360	0.0027
1.9	6.7	0.15	6.0	400	0.0025
2.0	7.4	0.14	6.1	450	0.0022
2.1	8.2	0.12	6.2	490	0.0020
2.2	9.0	0.11	6.3	550	0.0018
2.3	10	0.10	6.4	600	0.0017
2.4	11	0.090	6.5	670	0.0015
2.5	12	0.082	6.6	740	0.0014
2.6	13	0.074	6.7	810	0.0012
2.7	15	0.067	6.8	900	0.0011
2.8	16	0.060	6.9	990	0.0010
2.9	18	0.055	7.0	1100	0.00091
3.0	20	0.049	7.1	1200	0.00083
3.1	22	0.05	7.2	1300	0.00075
3.2	25	0.04	7.3	1500	0.00068
3.3	27	0.04	7.4	1600	0.00061
3.4	30	0.033	7.5	1800	0.00055
3.5	33	0.030	7.6	2000	0.00050
3.6	37	0.027	7.7	2200	0.00045
3.7	40	0.025	7.8	2400	0.00041
3.8	45	0.022	7.9	2700	0.00037
3.9	49	0.020	8.0	3000	0.00034
4.0	55	0.018			

the value of $e^{-\mu d}$ to be 0.82. If I_0 is 100 units (such as R/min) then the transmitted radiation is:

$$I = 100 \times 0.82 = 82 \text{ units}$$

As we have seen in Chapter 1, the graph representing this equation belongs to the family of *exponential* or *logarithmic* curves. This type of graph is shown in Figure 4.14 plotted on conventional graph paper. The vertical axis represents the per-

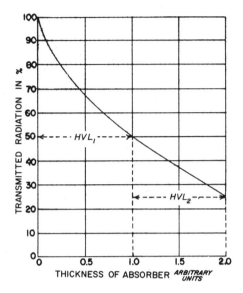

FIGURE 4.14. Transmission curve obtained with a hypothetical *monochromatic* X- or γ-ray beam. The caption on the vertical axis refers to the intensity (e.g. R/min or photons/cm²/sec) transmitted by various thicknesses of a particular absorber, relative to the unfiltered intensity taken as 100 per cent.

cent of the initial radiation intensity passing through various thicknesses of absorbing medium shown along the horizontal axis. A very useful quantity, to be discussed in more detail later, is derived from the curve. This is the **half value layer (HVL)**— that thickness of any given absorber which reduces the intensity of the incident beam 50 percent. In the graph in Figure 4.14 the half value layer is 1.0 mm Cu. It is obvious that if an absorber having a greater attenuation coefficient were substituted, the curve would fall off more rapidly and the half value layer would be less. On the other hand, the more energetic the photons the greater the thickness of absorber needed to reduce the intensity by 50 percent and therefore the less steep the curve would be.

The same data have been plotted on semilog paper in Figure 4.15. Whenever an exponential function is plotted in this manner, the resulting curve is a straight line.

As indicated in the preceding paragraph, there is a definite relationship between the half value layer of a given beam of monoenergetic radiation and its linear attenuation coefficient.

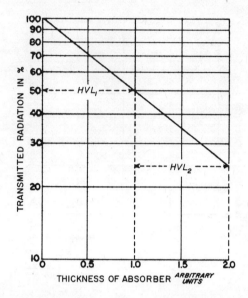

FIGURE 4.15. Same data as in Figure 4.14, semilogarithmic plot, *monoenergetic* beam. Note that the curve is a straight line typical of an exponential function. The linear attenuation coefficient μ_1 is constant and is the slope of the curve. Similarly, the HVL is constant — 3 thickness units for both the first and the second HVL.

This relationship may be readily derived from equation (7). Since the value of I_0 is reduced to 50 percent by one half value layer, I in equation (7) becomes $\frac{1}{2}I_0$. Substituting this value in the equation,

$$\frac{1}{2}I_0 = I_0 e^{-\mu d_{1/2}}$$

$$\frac{1}{2} = e^{-\mu d_{1/2}} = \frac{1}{e^{\mu d_{1/2}}}$$

$$2 = e^{\mu d_{1/2}}$$

$$\log 2 = \mu d_{1/2} \times \log e$$

$$0.3010 = \mu d_{1/2} \times 0.4343$$

$$\mu d_{1/2} = 0.3010/0.4343 = 0.693$$

$$\mu = \frac{0.693}{d_{1/2}}$$

or conversely,

$$d_{1/2} = \frac{0.693}{\mu}$$

Since $d_{1/2}$ is one half value layer,

$$HVL = \frac{0.693}{\mu} \qquad (8)$$

The linear attenuation coefficient μ neglects the physical state of the absorbing medium. Obviously, a given material in the solid state is a more efficient absorber per unit thickness than the same material in the gaseous state because the atoms are more closely spaced in solids. A correction factor, the **density** (g/cm^3) of the material, must be introduced to obtain a modified coefficient which would be independent of the physical state of the absorber. Dividing the linear attenuation coefficient by the density yields a coefficient that is constant for a given absorber regardless of its state; for example, if a certain liquid has a linear absorption coefficient of 0.2 cm^{-1} and a density of 1, and it is then vaporized and the resulting gas has a density of 0.1, the linear attenuation coefficient will be 0.02. In both cases μ divided by the density gives the same result:

$$0.2/1 = 0.02/0.1 = \mu/\rho$$

This modified coefficient is termed ***mass attenuation coefficient***, symbolized by μ/ρ where μ is the linear attenuation coefficient and ρ (Greek letter "rho") is the density. The units needed to express it are derived very simply:

$$\text{units of } \mu = \text{cm}^{-1} = 1/\text{cm}$$

$$\text{units of } \rho = \text{grams/cm}^3$$

Therefore,

$$\mu/\rho = \frac{1/\text{cm}}{\text{g/cm}^3}$$

$$\mu/\rho \text{ or } \mu_m = \text{cm}^2/\text{g}$$

Thus, the mass attenuation coefficient is expressed in cm^2/g, and it may be defined as the fractional attenuation of an X-ray or γ-ray beam per gram of absorber having a unit cross-sectional area. Its symbol in physics is μ_m to differentiate it from the linear attenuation coefficient μ_l.

The mass attenuation coefficient merits further discussion. As already mentioned in the preceding section, the attenuation of an X- or γ-ray beam in its passage through matter is due to three factors: absorption, scattering, and inverse square law. If the distance factor is maintained constant, then only the first two need be considered. Since absorption and scattering are due to three processes—photoelectric effect, Compton Effect, and pair production—the *total mass attenuation coefficient* is the sum of specific attenuation coefficients for each of these processes:

$$\mu_m = \tau_m + \sigma_m + \pi_m \qquad (9)$$

where τ_m ("tau") is the mass attenuation coefficient for the photoelectric effect, σ_m ("sigma") is the mass attenuation coefficient for the Compton Effect, and π_m ("pi") is the mass attenuation coefficient for pair production. The values of these coefficients may be found in published tables for specific conditions. Additional attenuation coefficients are ω for coherent scattering, and π for photodisintegration, but these are not important for us.

The attenuation coefficients vary with the energy of the incident photons and the atomic number of the absorber, but this dependence is different for the various coefficients. The following summary shows these relationships:

1. *Photoelectric Absorption.* The mass attenuation coefficient for the photoelectric effect, τ_m, is nearly proportional to Z^3, where Z is the atomic number of the absorber. Thus, there is a rapid increase in photoelectric absorption with increasing atomic number of the absorber; for example, τ_m is much greater for copper ($Z = 29$) than for aluminum ($Z = 13$), in the ratio of about $29^3/13^3 = 11$ times. The value of τ_m is also approximately proportional to $1/(h\nu)^3$, where $h\nu$ is the energy of the incident radiation. Hence, τ_m increases rapidly as the photon energy decreases;

for example, if photon energy is halved, τ_m increases by a factor of $2^3 = 8$. Furthermore, the probability of a photoelectric interaction increases as the energy of the incident photon approaches that of the energy associated with one of the inner shells; that is, at the absorption edge of a particular shell.

2. *Compton Effect.* The mass attenuation coefficient for Compton scattering, σ_m, is nearly independent of the atomic number of the absorber because this coefficient depends on the number of orbital electrons per gram, which is nearly constant for all elements except hydrogen. The effect of photon energy is more complicated. Since the Compton Effect involves two simultaneous processes: (1) scattering of photons, at various angles, with less energy than the incident photons, and (2) true absorption of energy by recoil electrons, the mass attenuation coefficient for the Compton Effect may be separated into two fractions:

$$\sigma_m = \sigma_{m_s} + \sigma_{m_a} \qquad (10)$$

where σ_{m_s} is the mass scattering coefficient and σ_{m_a} is the mass absorption coefficient for the Compton Effect. It is σ_{m_a} which is important in therapy because it is determined by the energy that is actually absorbed from the beam in the Compton Effect. Therefore, this is the portion of the mass attenuation coefficient that must be correlated with the energy of the incident photons. Since the energy given to the recoil electrons represents the energy lost by the interacting photons, it can be related to the increase in wavelength of the scattered photons. We have already seen that according to equation (4) the change in wavelength of the scattered photon in the Compton reaction is independent of the wavelength of the incident radiation, but depends on the angle of scatter only. In other words, the increase in wavelength of the photon is the same for long wavelength (low energy) and short wavelength (high energy) photons when the angle of scatter is the same. Therefore, a long wavelength photon will undergo *less* change on a percentage basis than will a short wavelength photon under similar conditions. For example, let us consider the change in wavelength of two different photons, one having an energy of

100 keV and the other 1 MeV, when the angle of photon scatter ϕ is 90°, by applying equation (4):

$$\Delta\lambda = 0.024 \, (1 - \cos \phi)$$

$$\Delta\lambda = 0.024 \text{ Å for 90° scatter, since } \cos 90° = 0$$

Therefore, the two photons to be considered will each undergo an increase in wavelength of 0.024 Å. Recall that $\lambda = 12.4/\text{keV}$.

> *100 keV photon* has wavelength of 12.4/100 = 0.124 Å. Scattered photon has wavelength 0.124 + 0.024 = 0.148 Å, which is equivalent to 12.4/0.148 = 84 keV. Energy absorbed is 100 keV − 84 keV = 16 keV. Thus, the percentage of energy absorbed from the 100 keV photon is 16/100 or *16 per cent*, when scatter angle is 90°. *1 MeV photon* has wavelength of 12.4/1000 keV = 0.0124 Å. Scattered photon has wavelength of 0.0124 + 0.024 = 0.0364 Å which is equivalent to 12.4/0.0364 = 340 keV. Energy absorbed, 1000 keV − 340 keV = 660 keV. Thus, the percentage of energy absorbed from 1 MeV (1000 keV) photon is 660/1000 or *66 per cent*. From the preceding calculations, it is evident that the Compton process, with right angle scattering component, results in absorption of 66 per cent of the high energy 1 MeV photons, as contrasted with 16 per cent for the lower energy 100 keV photons.

In summary, we may state that in the Compton Effect a high energy photon transfers a part of its energy to a loosely bound orbital electron which is ejected as a recoil electron. The photon, now with less energy and longer wavelength, is scattered at an angle away from its original path. Only the energy which is imparted to the recoil electron is truly absorbed, the recoil electron constituting one type of primary electron that is capable of producing ionization and excitation, with resulting biologic effects in tissues. The truly absorbed energy is therefore represented by the difference in energy of the incident and scattered photon. The quantity of energy absorbed from the photon is independent of the initial energy of the photon and the atomic number of the absorber. The energy absorbed depends only on the angle of scatter of the photon. However, a higher **percentage** of an energetic photon is absorbed than of a low energy photon. Energy absorption by the Compton interaction predominates over photoelectric interaction and pair formation in soft tissues in the photon energy range of about 60 keV to 15 MeV.

3. *Pair Production.* This process of interaction occurs between extremely high energy photons, exceeding 1.02 MeV, and the strong nuclear electrical fields of atoms in the absorber. It will be recalled that such a photon may disappear and give rise to a negatron-positron pair (see pages 93 to 95). If the incident photon has significantly more energy than 1.02 MeV, the negatron-positron pair will receive the energy in excess of 1.02 MeV in the form of kinetic energy almost equally divided between them. After this energy has been dissipated by interactions with atomic orbital electrons, the positron unites with a negative electron, annihilation takes place, and 1.02 MeV of energy is reradiated. The difference between the total energy of the incident photon and 1.02 MeV therefore represents the energy truly absorbed. In other words, the fraction of the initial energy E that is truly absorbed is:

$$\frac{hv - 1.02}{hv}$$

where hv is the energy of the incident photon. Just as in the case of Compton absorption, the mass attenuation coefficient for pair production consists of two fractions:

$$\pi_m = \pi_{m_a} + \pi_{m_s} \tag{11}$$

where π_m is the mass attenuation coefficient for pair production, π_{m_a} is the mass attenuation coefficient for pair production based on the absorbed energy, and π_{m_s} is the mass attenuation coefficient for that portion of the energy reappearing as annihilation radiation and therefore not really absorbed. π_{m_a} is of utmost importance because it depends on the fraction of the energy of the incident photon per gram of absorber that imparts kinetic energy to the negatron and positron, and hence causes ionization and excitation with attendant biologic effects.

Pair production increases with increasing energy of the incident photons above 1.02 MeV. *The mass absorption coefficient for pair production is proportional to the atomic number of the absorber.* Thus, with photons having sufficient energy to cause pair production at all, the probability of this process is greater in heavy elements such as lead, than in light elements such as carbon, when the incident photons are of similar energy.

Summary. It would be of interest to summarize now the relationship of the three types of absorption of penetrating electromagnetic radiation in tissue. Up to about 50 keV, photoelectric absorption predominates, accounting for about ⅔ of the absorbed energy at 50 keV. At about 60 keV the absorbed energy is about equally divided between photoelectrons and recoil electrons. At 100 keV 91 percent of the absorbed energy is carried by recoil electrons, and at 400 keV this reaches 100 percent, remaining at this level up to 1 MeV. Above 1.02 MeV pair production increases in importance until it becomes equal to the Compton absorption process at about 20 MeV. At 50 MeV the energy carried by electrons resulting from pair production well exceeds that in the Compton process, accounting for about ¾ of the absorbed energy. The above data are based on Table 4.03 and concern absorption in water, which is similar to that in soft tissues. The keV values quoted are usually about one-half the generating the peak voltage of X rays used in therapy.

TABLE 4.03
RELATIVE IMPORTANCE OF THE DIFFERENT TYPES OF
ABSORPTION IN WATER *

| | Relative No. of Processes (%) | | | % Energy Carried by Electrons | | |
Energy of Photons	Photo-electric	Compton	Pair	Photo-electrons	Recoil Electrons (Compton)	Electron-Positron Pairs
10 keV	95	5	0	100	0	0
60	7	93	0	43	57	0
100	1	99	0	9	91	0
400	0	100	0	0	100	0
1 MeV	0	100	0	0	100	0
4	0	94	6	0	93	7
20	0	56	44	0	50	50
24	0	50	50	0	43	57
50	0	29	71	0	24	76

* Johns and Cunningham: *The Physics of Radiation Therapy.* Springfield, Thomas, 1969.

ATTENUATION OF A POLYENERGETIC OR
HETEROGENEOUS X-RAY BEAM

It should be emphasized that the preceding discussion has been concerned primarily with monoenergetic radiation which, in a narrow beam, is characterized by a nearly constant half value layer as it traverses an absorbing medium. The attenuation of a *heterogeneous beam* such as is used in orthovoltage (200 to 300 kV) therapy is more complicated because of the gradual removal of more and more of the soft components of the beam by increasing thicknesses of the absorber (filter). Certain differences from the behavior of a monochromatic beam may be pointed out:

1. A heterogeneous or polyenergetic beam passing through a slab of absorbing material does not undergo a constant fractional reduction of intensity in successive identical layers of the material. Therefore there is *no* constant linear attenuation coefficient for a polyenergetic beam, especially when it has been unfiltered at the outset (see Fig. 4.16).

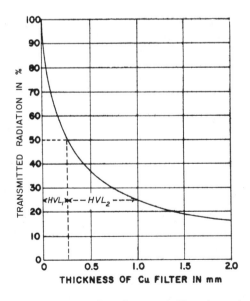

FIGURE 4.16. Transmission curve of a *polyenergetic* X-ray beam (e.g. 220-kV ortho-voltage).

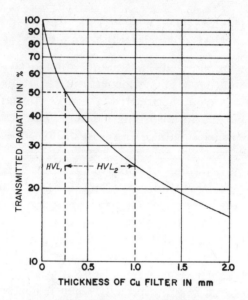

FIGURE 4.17. Same data as in Figure 4.16, semilogarithmic plot, *polyenergetic* beam. Note that this curve is not a straight line as with monoenergetic radiation, but becomes nearly so with increasing filtration. The linear attenuation coefficient μ_1 is not constant here, and neither is the HVL. Thus, the first HVL is 0.25 mm Cu, and the second HVL is 1.0 mm − 0.25 mm = 0.75 mm Cu. In this manner the HVL increases with increasing filtration, approaching a constant after the addition of about 2 HVL's with orthovoltage X rays.

2. As the polyenergetic beam penetrates the absorber (filter) each successive layer of the filter material attenuates the beam a little less than the layer ahead of it (see Fig. 4.16 and 4.17). Thus, the attenuation coefficients (mass and linear) decrease progressively from layer to layer.

3. The half value layer (HVL) of a polyenergetic beam increases progressively as the beam traverses the absorber (see Figs. 4.16 and 4.17). This is to be anticipated from the relation **HVL = 0.693 ÷ (linear attenuation coefficient).** In other words, as the attenuation coefficient decreases, the HVL increases (see Figs. 4.16 and 4.17).

4. For practical purposes, after a polyenergetic beam has passed through a filter thickness equivalent to about 2 HVL's,

the residual radiation that is transmitted behaves almost as though it were monoenergetic, as illustrated in Figure 4.17 where the attenuation curve under actual operating conditions is represented in a semilog plot. Note that the curve approaches a straight line after the first 2 HVL's, that is, it becomes more homogeneous. The energy uniformity of a beam is specified by its ***homogeneity coefficient***—the ratio of the first HVL to the second HVL (see page 210). As the beam hardens, its homogeneity coefficient increases and approaches unity, resembling more and more a monoenergetic beam.

5. In practice a polyenergetic beam approaches homogeneity because, in orthovoltage therapy at 200 to 250 kV, we often use 2 HVL's of copper filtration.

6. The progressive increase in HVL of a polyenergetic beam with increasing filtration results from the relatively greater absorption of the "soft" or low energy photons (except for the absorption edge effect) than of the "hard" or high energy photons, although the latter are also absorbed to some degree. In fact, after the first few HVL's there is greater attenuation of the beam than there is gain in hardness. Therefore there is a practical limit to the amount of filtration of an orthovoltage X-ray beam. The relation of filters to percentage depth dose will be taken up later.

CHAPTER 5

X-ray Production and Control

HISTORICAL INTRODUCTION

IN 1895, during a series of experiments with a highly evacuated Crookes-Hittorf tube, Wilhelm Konrad Roentgen accidentally discovered a new type of radiation which he called *X rays.* The tube consisted of a pear-shaped glass bulb in which were sealed two electrodes: a *cathode* or negative electrode at the small end, and an *anode,* or positive electrode at one side, as shown in Figure 5.01. When a high voltage was applied across the electrodes and the air pressure in the tube was reduced by a vacuum pump, a stream of *cathode rays* passed through the tube from the cathode toward the anode. If the glass at the end of the tube opposite the cathode was thin enough, cathode rays emerged through it into the air beyond. As we have indicated in Chapter 2, these cathode rays were later found to consist of a stream of rapidly moving *electrons.*

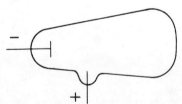

FIGURE 5.01. Crookes-Hittorf tube, forerunner of the X-ray tube.

Roentgen discovered that barium platinocyanide *fluoresces,* emitting visible light when brought near the tube. He then observed that if heavy paper was placed between the end of the tube and the barium platinocyanide screen to absorb the cathode rays, the screen did not stop its fluorescence. This indicated to Roentgen that some phenomenon in addition to cathode rays was responsible for the fluorescence. His scientific genius prompted him to ascribe this effect to a new kind of ray, which he named

X ray, because the letter *x* in algebra indicates an unknown quantity.

In a further series of brilliant experiments, Roentgen soon discovered most of the important properties of X rays. His observations may be summarized as follows:

1. *Penetrating Ability.* Roentgen's most remarkable observation was the *unique ability of X rays to penetrate most solid matter,* a property not ordinarily possessed by ultraviolet or visible light.

2. *Fluorescent Effect.* The rays cause certain crystals such as barium platinocyanide to glow in the dark, a phenomenon called *fluorescence.*

3. *Photographic Effect.* X rays blacken a photographic emulsion in the same manner as visible light.

4. *Rectilinear Propagation.* This property is common to both X rays and light. Both types of radiation *travel in straight lines* in limited space.

5. *Absorption.* Not only do X rays penetrate matter, but they also undergo *absorption* by matter in varying degrees: the thicker and denser the matter placed between the tube and fluorescent screen, the weaker the fluorescence. Thus, lead is an efficient absorber of orthovoltage X rays.

6. *Scattering.* When material is placed behind a fluorescent screen or photographic emulsion it appears to send rays back to the screen or emulsion as though reflecting them. (We now recognize this as actually a scattering of X rays rather than reflection.)

7. *Electrical Neutrality.* X rays cannot be deflected by a magnet, proving that they differ from cathode rays.

8. *Inverse Square Law.* Roentgen demonstrated, by measuring the brightness of the screen's fluorescence at various distances from the tube, that the intensity of the radiation is *inversely proportional to the square of the distance between the tube and the screen.* This principle also governs light and other kinds of electromagnetic radiation.

It is remarkable that so early in the history of this new branch of physics, Roentgen had already observed most of the phenomena associated with X rays. Within a relatively short time after the appearance of his publication, other scientists discovered two more extremely important properties of X rays: ***refraction*** by crystals and ***ionization*** of gases.

Roentgen's outstanding scientific contributions revolutionized classical physics, laying the groundwork for the development of modern physics. He was awarded the Nobel Prize in Physics in 1903, being its first recipient in this field.

PRINCIPLE OF PRODUCTION OF X RAYS

Since the discovery of X rays there has been progressive improvement in the equipment used to generate them. In 1883 Edison sealed a metal plate inside an electric light bulb near the filament, but not touching it. Outside the bulb, he connected the filament to a battery and joined the positive side of the same battery to the metal plate as shown in Figure 5.02. Upon heating the filament, he was amazed to find a current flowing in the plate wire, despite the fact that there was no apparent contact between the plate and filament inside the tube. This was later named the ***Edison Effect.*** It was not adequately explained at the time, but eventually was proved to be due to the evaporation of electrons from the heated filament, a process now called ***thermionic emission.*** The impregnation of such filaments with thorium lowers the temperature of emission and thereby prolongs the life of the

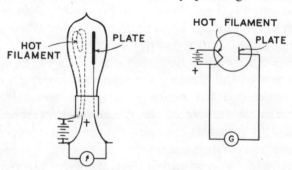

FIGURE 5.02. Edison Effect. When the filament is heated, electrons are emitted from its surface and cross the gap to the plate (anode). This flow of electrons constitutes the plate current and is measured by meter *G* in the plate circuit.

filament. Thoriated filaments are now being used in thermionic rectifiers (valve tubes) and are under investigation for radiographic tubes.

In 1904, Ambrose Fleming in England went a step farther and made the first *diode tube* in which the plate was given a positive charge by a separate "B" battery, with the result that a larger current flowed between the plate and the filament, as shown in Figure 5.03. The term *diode* obviously refers to the presence of two electrodes, a positive plate and a negative filament.

William Coolidge, in 1913, applied this principle in designing the *hot cathode* X-ray tube and thereupon introduced a new method of generating X rays. The following discussion is based on the *Coolidge tube* which, despite important modifications, remains in essence the foundation stone of the modern X-ray tube.

The *principle* of X-ray production may be stated simply as follows: *whenever a stream of high speed electrons strikes matter, X rays are produced.* Several processes are involved:

1. *Bremsstrahlung (brems radiation).* Electrons passing near the positively charged nuclei of the target atoms are accelerated. In doing so they radiate X rays and slow down. The kinetic energy lost by the electrons is equivalent to the energy of these X rays which are called *bremsstrahlung* or "braking" radiation (see pages 55 to 56).

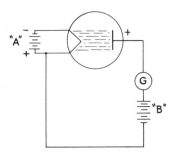

FIGURE 5.03. Diagram of a Fleming diode. The "A" battery supplies the filament current, while the "B" battery places a positive charge on the plate. Note the similarity in principle to the hot filament X-ray tube in Figure 5.04. However, the plate potential (voltage) in the Fleming diode is not large enough to produce X rays.

2. *Characteristic Radiation.* Some of the high speed electrons interact with and dislodge inner orbital electrons from the target atoms, with the result that the atoms become *"excited."* This is followed immediately by the transition of other electrons to replace holes left by the ejected electrons, with attendant emission of *characteristic X-ray photons.* (Note: we saw earlier that atoms can also be excited by interaction with X or γ photons.)

3. *Preliminary Slowing.* Some high speed electrons collide with firmly bound orbital electrons of the target with insufficient energy to dislodge them, merely raising them to a higher energy (or excitation) level. The electrons then proceed with less energy than before and may participate in other interactions such as (1) and (2).

4. *Electrons* ejected from the target atoms may produce bremsstrahlen, or may, in turn, eject secondary electrons.

It is obvious, from a consideration of the intricate processes of interaction between fast electrons and a target, that there is a wide range of energy distribution (therefore, a range of wavelengths) of the emerging X rays. This constitutes the *continuous spectrum.* Superimposed upon this are the discrete *lines of characteristic radiation.* The energy composition of X-ray beams has been described in detail in Chapter 3.

The efficiency of production of X rays, even in advanced modern equipment, is extremely low. For example, *at 100 kV only 0.2 percent of the electrons' energy is converted to X rays,* the remainder appearing as heat. At 200 kV X-ray efficiency is only about 1 percent. However, in the megavoltage range there is considerable improvement with efficiency reaching nearly 100 percent at 20 MeV.

CONDITIONS NECESSARY FOR THE PRODUCTION OF X RAYS

As we have just indicated, X rays are produced whenever fast electrons collide with matter. How can this be accomplished in a practical way? All of the conditions necessary for the production of X rays are admirably fulfilled by the Coolidge tube (see Fig. 5.04) as will be evident in the following discussion:

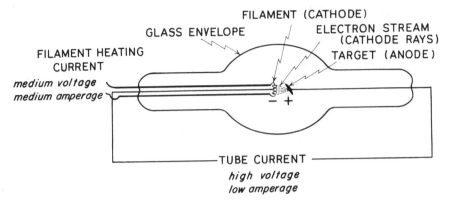

FILAMENT (CATHODE)

GLASS ENVELOPE

ELECTRON STREAM
(CATHODE RAYS)

FILAMENT HEATING
CURRENT

TARGET (ANODE)

medium voltage
medium amperage

− +

TUBE CURRENT
high voltage
low amperage

FIGURE 5.04. X-ray tube (Coolidge type). Compare with the earlier Fleming diode tube in Figure 5.03.

1. *Source of Electrons.* A tungsten wire *filament* or *cathode* serves as the source of electrons. When the filament is heated to incandescence through its own electric circuit it liberates electrons by the process of *thermionic emission.* These electrons remain near the filament as a cloud or *space charge* until a high potential difference is applied across the X-ray tube.

2. *Production of High Speed Electrons.* In order to impart a high speed to the electrons liberated from the filament, two conditions are necessary. First a *large potential difference* (high voltage) must be applied between the tube electrodes in such a way that the filament is charged negatively (cathode) and the target positively (anode). The high potential difference between these electrodes accelerates the electrons toward the anode with velocities ranging from 50 to 98 percent of the speed of light. Second, the tube must be highly *evacuated* in order to eliminate collisions between the electron stream and gas molecules which would slow down the electrons. To maintain the vacuum, a *glass envelope* or *tube* is required.

3. *Sudden Deceleration of Electrons.* The fast electrons must be quickly decelerated for efficient conversion of a part of their kinetic energy to X rays (see pages 55 to 56). The anode of the X-ray tube serves this purpose, acting also as the *target* for the electrons. It usually consists of a high atomic number, high

melting point metal—*tungsten.* Thus, the target fulfills two purposes: (a) to complete the high voltage circuit and accelerate the electrons and (b) to stop these fast electrons. In addition, characteristic X rays are emitted by the target atoms.

By way of summary, then, we can state that the filament current heats the filament to the point of electron emission, forming a space charge. Application of a large potential difference between the electrodes (filament negative, target positive) drives the space charge electrons at high velocity toward the anode (target). When the fast electrons strike the target, their kinetic energy is converted to heat and X rays.

The similarity in the design of X-ray tubes and Fleming's diode in Figure 5.03 is readily apparent. The principal difference between them is the *low* driving voltage used in Fleming's tube, which does not provide the electrons with sufficient kinetic energy to produce X rays

ESSENTIAL FEATURES OF A THERAPY X-RAY TUBE
(200 TO 250 kV)

We may now summarize the construction and operation of a typical therapy tube operated in the conventional 200 to 250 kV region.

1. *Glass Envelope*—constituting the glass tube or enclosure. It serves to insulate the electrodes from each other, and to contain the high vacuum which is required for three reasons. First, the evacuation of the tube removes gas molecules, thereby minimizing collisions between the fast electrons and the molecules. Such collisions would slow down the electrons and cause production of low energy (soft) X-ray photons. In the second place, the evacuation of oxygen from the tube prevents oxidation of the filament. Finally, ionization of any residual gas would result in bombardment and damage of the filament by positive ions.

2. *Cathode* or *filament*—in a circuit supplied with about 6 volts and 4 amps. Electron emission of the filament is very sensitive to filament temperature which depends on the filament current, a small change in the latter causing a large change in electron emission. An increase in the number of electrons liberated at the cath-

ode increases the number available to be driven to the anode; thus, there is a large increase in tube current (milliamperes) resulting from a small change in filament current. Figure 5.05 shows the relation between tube current and filament current in a radiographic tube. Since filament current depends on the filament voltage, a voltage stabilizer must be included in the circuit.

3. *Anode* or *target*—in an orthovoltage tube, usually consists of a tungsten button imbedded in a copper block. Tungsten is used because its high melting point (3370 C) is needed to withstand the heat produced in the anode and to minimize evaporation of the target and consequent coating of the glass aperture of the tube by this metal. A typical anode angle is 30° which, together with the 8 mm focal spot, provides a wide beam of reasonably uniform radiation intensity over its cross section. Furthermore, the large focal spot increases the heating capacity of the anode.

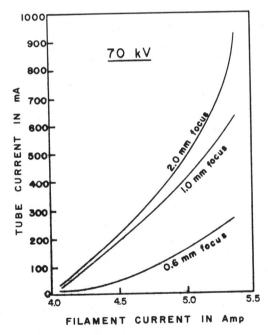

FIGURE 5.05. Relation of tube current (mA) to filament current in a *radiographic* tube. A small increase in filament current causes a large increase in mA.

Because therapy exposures may be as long as ten minutes or more, tube operation is nearly continuous in contrast to intermittent operation of a radiographic tube in short bursts of energy. Therefore, provision must be made for the dissipation of heat produced in the anode. A typical rate of heat production would be 200 kV × 20 mA = 4,000 watts, approximately that in an ordinary electric heater. The simplest method of heat dissipation, applicable to 100-kV equipment, is the use of a large anode with a massive stem to conduct the heat away as rapidly as possible. However, at higher kV elaborate cooling systems are needed, most of which pump the oil into a tank where it is in turn cooled by water circulating in coils immersed in the oil tank. The X-ray tube itself is incased in a metal housing which contains an efficient insulating oil identical with the oil that serves to cool the anode. The high degree of electrical insulation provided by the oil permits the design of smaller and more maneuverable tube housings than would otherwise be feasible.

4. *Large Potential Difference.* To drive the electrons at high velocity from cathode to anode, we must apply a large potential difference as described above. In the process, the electrons acquire a large kinetic energy. If the applied potential difference engenders a velocity of no more than one-half that of light, the following equation holds to a fair approximation:

$$Ee \approx \tfrac{1}{2}m_0v^2 \tag{1}$$

where E is the applied potential difference in electrostatic units (esu), e is the charge on the electron (4.8×10^{-10} esu), m_0 is the mass of an electron at rest (9.11×10^{-28} g), and v is the velocity of a particular electron in cm/sec. Equation (1) may be converted to practical units as follows:

$$\frac{Ve}{300} = \tfrac{1}{2}m_0v^2 \tag{2}$$

where V is the potential difference in volts. Note that as V increases so does v, although not in a simple direct proportion.

At very large values of potential difference the relativistic increase in electron mass has to be taken into account. Under this condition, the appropriate equation for mass stated on page must be substituted for m_o in equation (2).

An electron accelerated through a potential difference of 1 volt acquires an energy of 1 electron volt. Table 5.01 shows the ter-

TABLE 5.01

Potential Difference	Energy of Electron	Abbreviation
1 volt	1 electron volt	1 eV
1,000 volts	1 kiloelectron volt	1 keV
1,000,000 volts	1 million electron volts	1 MeV
1,000,000,000 volts	1 billion electron volts	1 BeV

minology applicable to electrons of various energies. Examples of electron energy as related to the speed of light are as follows:

100 keV   50% of speed of light

200 keV   80% ”   ”   ”   ”

2 MeV   98% ”   ”   ”   ”

Tube current is rated in **milliamperes** (mA) because the current is reduced, by the transformer, to thousandths of an ampere (milliamperes) at the same time that the voltage is stepped up to thousands of volts (kilovolts). We know that under certain conditions, the emitted electrons form a large space charge near the filament and hinder further emission, a phenomenon called **space charge effect.** When a tube operates in this way, the tube current (mA) increases as the kV is increased, as shown in Figure 5.06, because more and more electrons are driven to the anode. The operation of the tube is then said to be **space charge limited.** Orthovoltage tubes of the conventional type usually operate in the space charge limited region.

If the kilovoltage is increased above a certain critical value, **all of the emitted electrons are driven to the anode immediately upon being freed,** and the space charge effect becomes negligible. The tube is then said to be **emission limited** and is operating under **saturation conditions.** Now the milliamperage can be increased only by increasing the filament current to provide additional electrons. The maximum current flowing in the tube, regardless

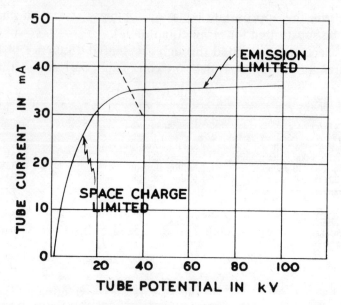

FIGURE 5.06. Relation between tube current (mA) and tube potential (kV). For a given value of filament current, the tube current increases with an increase in the applied potential; in this region, tube operation is *space charge limited*. Beyond the "knee" of the characteristic curve of the tube, nearly all the electrons are driven to the target as soon as they are released from the filament; operation is now *emission limited*. A further increase in kV does not significantly increase the mA. However, to make the mA really independent of the kV at high mA requires the use of a space charge compensator.

of the applied potential, is known as the **saturation current.** With the high mA used in modern radiography, saturation is not reached; therefore, the tube current is made independent of the applied potential by means of a space charge compensator.

RECTIFIER (VALVE) TUBES

As will be shown later, efficiency is improved by conversion of alternating current to **direct current** to energize an X ray tube. Since diode tubes, under ordinary conditions, permit the passage of an electric current only from cathode to anode, they can be used as valves to rectify alternating current, that is, change it to direct current.

Construction. A valve tube has the same general design as an X-ray tube, but certain features set it apart for its own particular function. The cathode of a valve tube consists of a larger filament than that of an X-ray tube. It has its own low voltage circuit to liberate electrons by thermionic emission, and is in series with a high voltage circuit to drive the electrons to the anode. However, as will be shown presently, there is only a *small voltage drop* across the valve tube. The filament of a modern valve tube is *thoriated* to increase emissivity and prolong its life. The anode of the valve tube consists of a large tungsten cylinder surrounding the cathode. Figure 5.07 presents a schematic diagram of a diode valve tube.

Principle of Valve Tube Operation. Unlike a radiographic tube, a valve tube is space charge limited, operating below saturation. There is an abundance of electrons liberated from the large cathode and driven to the massive anode. An increase in the applied kV increases the number of electrons/sec driven to the anode (i.e. the tube current), and conversely. A large stream of electrons is favored by the massive cathode and anode. As a result, the electrical resistance of a valve tube is small and there is only a small kilovoltage drop, 3 kV or less, across its terminals. Such a small drop in kV is insufficient to accelerate the electrons to velocities high enough for the production of X rays. Emission of X rays by a valve tube would obviously be undesirable. Further-

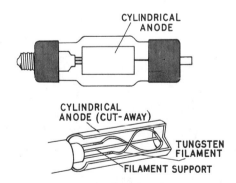

FIGURE 5.07. Type of diode rectifier used in kilovoltage therapy units. The cylindrical anode surrounds the large filament to provide operation below saturation (i.e. in space charge limited region). (Courtesy of Machlett Laboratories, Inc.)

more, any loss of kV across a valve would reduce the available kV applied to the X-ray tube.

Ordinarily, valve tubes are mounted in the transformer casing, immersed in the same insulating oil as the transformer. Such an arrangement permits the design of more compact equipment. Besides, the casing protects against chance production of X rays that might result from a defective valve tube.

GENERATING AND CONTROL EQUIPMENT

Because a large potential difference is needed to accelerate the electrons in an X-ray tube, we must discuss the generation of the required high voltage. However, we shall also describe the devices for varying the high voltage for different therapy technics, and the rectification of alternating current.

High Voltage Transformer. Incoming line voltage is necessarily limited to a level far below that required to operate an X-ray tube. Thus, the usual *maximum* is 230 volts, whereas that needed to operate a conventional X-ray therapy tube ranges from 50 to 250 *kV*. How can the relatively moderate main line voltage be converted to the desired high voltage? This is accomplished by the *transformer,* an electromagnetic device which changes the magnitude of a voltage. As shown in Figure 5.08, a *closed core* transformer consists of two coils of wire insulated from each other and wound around an iron core, the entire assembly being im-

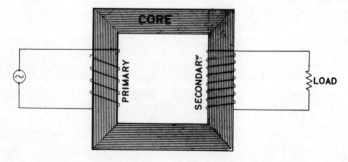

FIGURE 5.08. Closed core ("donut") X-ray transformer.

mersed in a tank of insulating oil. The ***primary voltage*** is applied to one coil (primary coil), inducing the ***secondary voltage*** in the other coil (secondary coil). It must be emphasized that a transformer will operate efficiently only on ***alternating current***. According to the ***Transformer Law,*** the secondary voltage has the same ratio to the primary voltage as the number of turns in the secondary coil has to the number of turns in the primary coil:

$$\frac{V_s}{V_p} = \frac{N_s}{N_p} \tag{3}$$

where V_s is the secondary voltage, V_p is the primary voltage, N_s is the number of turns in the secondary coil, and N_p is the number of turns in the primary coil.

Equation (3) shows that a transformer can either ***increase*** or ***decrease*** the primary voltage, depending on the ratio of the secondary to the primary turns. Thus, if there are fewer turns in the secondary than in the primary, the secondary voltage is less than the primary, and we have a ***step-down transformer.*** On the other hand, if the secondary turns are more numerous than the primary, the secondary voltage is greater than the primary, and we have a ***step-up transformer,*** the type used to change the incoming voltage to the high level needed for sufficient acceleration of electrons in the X-ray tube.

Voltage Control Devices. The X-ray transformer is a stationary device which steps up the input voltage at a *fixed ratio.* For example, if the primary potential is 220 volts, and the ratio of the secondary to the primary turns is 1,000, then the output of the transformer will be 220 × 1,000 = 220,000 volts or 220 kV. But how might we obtain some other voltage such as 100 kV when the line voltage is 220? The answer lies in the use of voltage control equipment which is of two main types: (1) autotransformer, and (2) rheostat.

1. ***Autotransformer.*** Actually, this is a ***variable transformer*** or ***variac,*** placed in the circuit between the main line and the X-ray transformer. Operating on the principle of ***self-induction,*** it consists of a ***single coil*** of wire so arranged that the coil is tapped at regularly spaced intervals. The fractional number of turns de-

limited by any one tap determines the voltage fed to the transformer. The autotransformer law resembles the transformer law:

$$\frac{V_{out}}{V_{in}} = \frac{\textit{number of tapped turns}}{\textit{total number of turns}}$$

where V_{out} is the voltage output and V_{in} is the voltage input. Figure 5.09 shows the principle of the autotransformer and its position in the circuit relative to the transformer. The autotransformer, like the transformer, **operates on alternating current.** Note that the autotransformer so modifies the line voltage that when the resulting voltage is stepped up by the transformer according to its fixed ratio, the desired kilovoltage is induced in the secondary coil of the transformer. For example, suppose we require 100 kV for superficial therapy when the line voltage is 220 and the transformer ratio is 1,000:1. The line voltage is reduced to 100 volts by means of the autotransformer, and this is fed to the primary of the transformer, which multiplies 100 × 1,000, giving the desired 100,000 volts or 100 kV.

2. **Rheostat.** Another device used to control the voltage applied to the transformer is a **variable resistor** called a **rheostat** (see Fig. 5.10). It operates on the basis of **Ohm's Law,** $I = V/R$, which is easily converted to the form

$$V = IR \qquad (4)$$

where V is the potential difference (voltage drop) across the circuit, I is the current in amperes, and R is the resistance of the circuit in ohms.

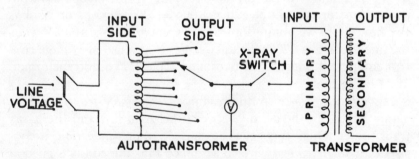

FIGURE 5.09. Relation between autotransformer and X-ray transformer in X-ray circuit.

Thus, if the resistance in a circuit is increased, the voltage drop increases and there is less voltage available to operate the equipment. By use of a rheostat, the resistance and hence the voltage drop can be varied as desired, thereby changing the voltage applied to the transformer. In therapy equipment, a rheostat is placed in series with the primary side of the autotransformer for the purpose of protecting the X-ray tube and cables from the sudden application of high voltage. When the therapy unit (200 to 250 kV) is first turned on, the maximum resistance of the rheostat is in the circuit, allowing only the lowest voltage to be applied to the transformer. As the X-ray tube warms up, the operator manually adjusts the rheostat to progressively smaller values of resistance, thereby increasing the voltage to the desired level. Note that this is done while the equipment is in full operation and X rays are being generated. The autotransformer setting, on the other hand, must be selected *before* the X-ray switch is closed and cannot be changed during tube operation because of the danger of sparking and charring the contacts. Therefore, an autotransformer cannot be used to warm up the X-ray tube, only the rheostat being employed for this purpose. Figure 5.10 shows the connection of the rheostat in the primary circuit. A rheostat can operate on either direct or alternating current.

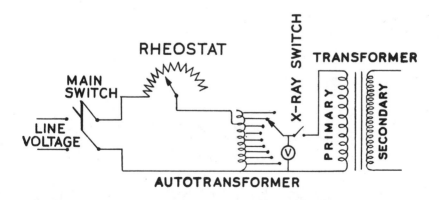

FIGURE 5.10. A rheostat has been added to the primary circuit to permit gradual increase in the potential (up to maximum kV) applied to the X-ray tube.

CURRENT CONTROL IN X-RAY TUBE

In addition to the regulation of tube voltage, provision must be made for the control of **tube current** or **milliamperage.** The tube current consists of a stream of electrons arising at the cathode, and then sent toward the anode by the applied high voltage. The magnitude of the tube current depends on the number of available electrons. This depends on the temperature of the filament which, in turn, is governed by the current in the filament circuit. Here, then, is the key to the control of tube current. By varying the **filament current** we can alter the number of available electrons and hence the tube current (mA).

Two devices are used to modify the current in the filament circuit. First, the **step-down transformer** serves to reduce the line voltage to the proper filament value of about 6 volts. However, this voltage level is fixed. To provide variable control of filament voltage and current, a second device is placed ahead of, and in series with, the filament step-down transformer—a **rheostat** or variable resistor. In accordance with Ohm's Law, as the rheostat is adjusted to increased resistance, there is less voltage and current available to the filament. On the other hand, a decrease in resistance makes more voltage and current available to the filament. In this way the electron emission of the filament is adjusted to obtain the desired tube current (see Fig. 5.11).

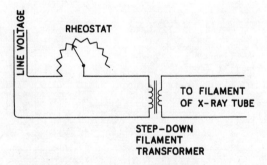

FIGURE 5.11. A rheostat (variable resistor) in the filament circuit serves to vary the filament current and the resulting tube current (mA).

RECTIFICATION

The current in the primary circuit of the X-ray machine, just as in the mains, is an ***alternating*** current (AC). Such a current flows back and forth in the circuit, starting at zero, reaching a maximum in one direction, then declining to zero again. It then reverses its direction, proceeding to a maximum and again returning to zero. The relation of current or voltage to time is shown in Figure 5.12. Note that one cycle is the distance between two successive corresponding points on the curve. The usual alternating current contains 60 such cycles in each second (i.e. 60 Hz) equivalent to 120 alternations of direction in one second. A transformer will operate efficiently only with this type of current. It is completely useless with an unvarying direct current such as one obtains from an electric battery.

On the other hand, an X-ray tube operates most efficiently when it is supplied by a ***direct current,*** flowing always in the same direction from cathode to anode. This is obvious because the cathode is the source of electrons which must be driven toward the anode or target.

It is possible to modify an alternating current to a direct current by ***rectification.*** The simplest method is to supply the stepped-up

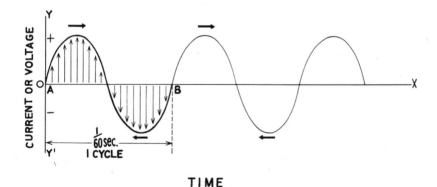

TIME

FIGURE 5.12. Sine curve of 60-cycle alternating current. The thick horizontal arrows show the direction of the current during various parts of the AC cycle. Note that the current reverses its direction every 1/120 sec. The thin lines indicate the variation in voltage or amperage from instant to instant.

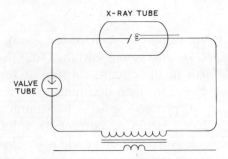

FIGURE 5.13. Half wave rectification with a single valve tube.

alternating current directly to the X-ray tube, a process called *self-rectification*. Since the X-ray tube, under ordinary conditions, allows the passage of current only from the cathode to the anode, it can also rectify an alternating current. The previously available General Electric Maximar® 200 utilized self-rectification. The tube and transformer were mounted in the same case filled with insulating oil, the whole unit being suspended over the patient during therapy. When the alternating potential is in such a direction that the electrons flow from cathode to anode, the tube is conducting. But during the half cycle when the potential reverses, being directed from the anode to the cathode, the tube does not conduct current. The capacity of a self-rectified circuit is limited by the fact that the anode must be prevented from becoming so hot that is emits electrons which could be driven by the inverse voltage toward the cathode, damaging or destroying it.

The cathode can be protected by the addition of a *diode* tube in the secondary circuit. Such a tube, called a *valve tube* or *rectifier,* has both a very large anode and filament to produce a large stream of electrons. Like an X-ray tube, it allows the current to flow in one direction only. During the inverse half of the AC cycle, the total voltage is divided between the valve tube and the X-ray tube, thereby protecting the X ray tube from *inverse voltage.* This type of single valve tube rectification is shown in Figure 5.13. The rectified current is intermittent, resembling that obtained with self-rectification.

The most commonly used types of rectification in 200 to 250 kV equipment are the *Villard Circuit,* and the *constant potential* or

Greinacher Circuit. These are modifications of valve tube rectification, each having certain distinct advantages.

Villard Circuit. An advantage of the Villard circuit is that one
obtains 200 kV from a 100 kV transformer by an ingenious arrangement of valve tubes and capacitors (condensers). Reference to Figure 5.14A will aid in clarifying the description of this
circuit. The current from the transformer is in the correct direction to pass through the valve tubes and capacitors which are
charged as shown; the plates nearest the transformer assume the
same charge as that end of the transformer. Each capacitor is
charged to *one-half* the maximum voltage in the secondary coil
of the transformer. During this half of the AC cycle, no current
flows in the tube because the voltage is inverse.

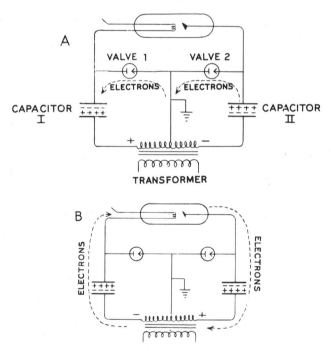

FIGURE 5.14. Villard type of voltage doubling circuit. In *A* the capacitors are each
being charged to one half the total secondary voltage by the transformer. In *B*,
when the transformer reverses polarity, the capacitors discharge simultaneously
through the X-ray tube, adding their total voltage to that supplied by the transformer.

In the next half cycle the transformer changes polarity, as shown in Figure 5.14B. The transformer and the two capacitors are now in series with the X-ray tube. The voltage of the transformer is added to that from both capacitors, each of which now has one-half the transformer secondary voltage, so that the resultant voltage applied to the tube is double that in the transformer secondary:

$$
\begin{array}{ll}
\textit{Voltage on transformer secondary} = & V_t \\
\textit{Voltage on capacitor A} & = \frac{1}{2}V_t \\
\underline{\textit{Voltage on capacitor B} \qquad\quad = \frac{1}{2}V_t} \\
\textit{Total voltage to x-ray tube} \qquad = 2V_t
\end{array}
$$

The voltage on the tube circuit is, then, **intermittent** and **double** that produced by the transformer, as seen in Figure 5.15. Thus, the transformer is rated at 100 kVp, but the machine develops 200 kVp during each cycle, returning to zero between the peaks. A number of such circuits may be connected in series to produce even greater magnification of the voltage, a process called **cascading**.

Although the Villard circuit provides an economical system of rectification, it has certain disadvantages. One of its main deficiencies is the intermittent drop in kV to zero level, with attendant production of low voltage (soft) X rays. These must be minimized by filtration of the X-ray beam to improve its quality, but there is a corresponding loss of X-ray output. Although

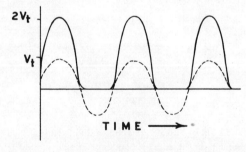

FIGURE 5.15. Voltage curve in Villard circuit. The dotted line represents the voltage developed by the transformer. The solid line represents the doubled voltage (transformer plus capacitor) applied to the X-ray tube.

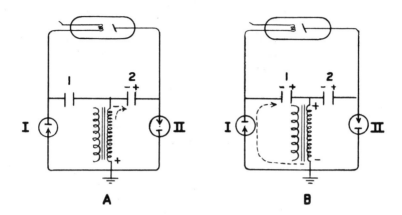

FIGURE 5.16. Greinacher or constant potential type of voltage doubling circuit. With this arrangement of capacitors and valve tubes, the transformer alternately charges capacitor 1 during the first half cycle, and capacitor 2 during the second half cycle. The total voltage of both capacitors, continuously applied to the X-ray tube, undergoes slight fluctuation or *ripple*. (Compare with Fig. 5.14, Villard circuit).

beam attenuation by filters up to 0.5 mm Cu is not too serious, heavier filtration than this so decreases radiation output that treatment time may be excessively prolonged. Therefore, to obtain a penetrating beam of higher output, another, more suitable plan of rectification—the Greinacher Circuit—is necessary.

Constant Potential or Greinacher Circuit. Since low voltage X rays are readily absorbed in the skin and are of no value in the therapy of deep-seated lesions, they must be curtailed by filtration. As a result, the radiation output is less than would be obtained if the kV could be kept at a high level throughout the AC cycle. This problem is solved by the *Greinacher Circuit* which consists of the arrangement of valve tubes and capacitors shown in Figure 5.16.

When the lower end of the transformer is positive as in A, the current flows through capacitor 2 and valve tube II as in Figure 5.16A, the capacitor being charged to the full capacity of the transformer—125 kV. In the next half of the AC cycle, shown in Figure 5.15B, the current flows through valve tube I charging capacitor 1 to a peak 125 kV.

Now the capacitors are fully charged and, being in series with the X-ray tube, their total potential of 250 kV is applied to the X-ray tube. Thus, the constant potential circuit is at the same time a ***voltage doubling circuit.***

During the flow of current through the tube there is only a small drop in kV. This requires explanation. The time it takes for a capacitor to discharge down to 37 percent of its initial charge is called the ***time constant*** of the circuit. The time constant is determined by the product of the resistance *R* and the capacitance *C:*

$$RC = time \quad constant$$

If the capacitance is high, the time constant is long and the capacitor discharges slowly. In the constant potential circuit, the capacitance of the two capacitors is so chosen that there is a ***long time constant.*** Furthermore, the capacitors are kept almost fully charged by the transformer. Consequently, the drop in potential during the operation of the equipment is no greater than 2 or 3 kV and is called ***ripple*** because of the slight fluctuation in voltage as shown in Figure 5.17.

In summary, the capacitors in the constant potential circuit serve as a reservoir of electrical potential maintained at peak level by the transformer. With this type of rectification, the final kV is (1) double the rated voltage of the transformer and (2) main-

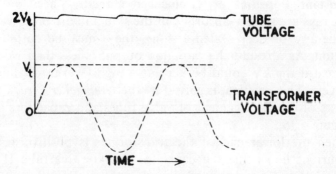

FIGURE 5.17. Voltage curve in a constant potential circuit. The dotted line represents the voltage developed by the transformer. The solid line indicates the doubled voltage supplied to the X-ray tube by the fully charged capacitors in series. Note the relatively slight ripple, twice per cycle, in the latter curve.

TABLE 5.02
COMPARISON IN R/MIN OUTPUT OF A VILLARD AND A GREINACHER
(CONSTANT POTENTIAL) GENERATOR OPERATING AT 200 kVp,
15 mA, AND TARGET-SKIN DISTANCE OF 50 cm

Filter	Villard	Greinacher
	R/min	R/min
0.5 mm Cu	28	75
1.0 mm Cu	16	50
2.0 mm Cu	10	30
3.0 mm Cu	—	20

tained nearly constant. Therefore, the radiation output is maintained at a higher value. Furthermore, since there is no wide fluctuation in kV, there is a lower percentage of soft radiation produced with the constant potential circuit than with the Villard Circuit. The higher initial radiation output of the constant potential unit permits heavier filtration of the beam without unduly attenuating it to uneconomical levels. Table 5.02 compares the radiation output of Villard and constant potential units under similar operating conditions.

CABLES

In all but self-contained therapy units, external conductors are needed to carry the high voltage in the secondary circuit to the X-ray tube. These conductors are known as *cables*, and they must have the following properties:

1. *Shockproof* for the protection of patients and personnel. This is provided by the heavy insulation and the woven wire sheath within the insulating material. The wire sheath is connected to *ground* so that in the event of a break in the insulation, the current would be conducted immediately to ground, protecting against electric shock.

2. *Wear resistant,* preventing damage to the conductors within.

3. *Low resistance* to avoid excessive line voltage drop.

HIGH FREQUENCY X-RAY GENERATOR

Another type of orthovoltage X-ray therapy equipment is the *high frequency generator,* utilizing a *resonance transformer.*

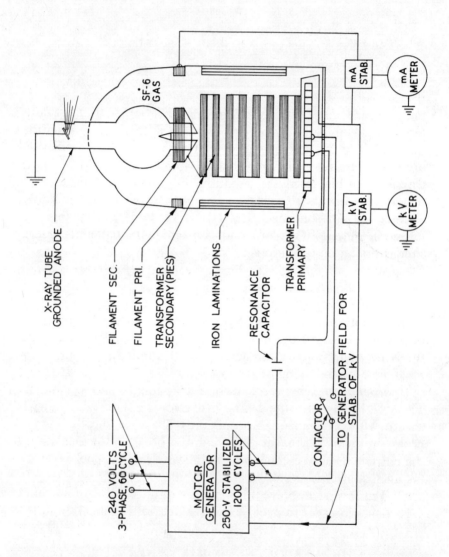

FIGURE 5.18. Schematic diagram of the Picker Vanguard therapy unit. (Courtesy of the Gilbert X-ray Company of Texas.)

Figure 5.18 shows, in schematic form, the construction of the Picker Vanguard. It is supplied by a three-phase 60 cycle alternating current which is converted to a 1,200 cycle alternating current. Since this high frequency current is to supply the primary coil of the transformer, the inductive reactance of the primary circuit would be enormous, resulting in a large voltage drop. To prevent this, a capacitor of suitable size is connected in series with the primary coil so that the circuit will be in *resonance.* Under these conditions, the impedance of the primary circuit is low, and the only hindrance to flow of current is the simple resistance in the circuit. Because of the resonance of the primary circuit supplying the transformer, the latter is called a *resonance transformer.*

The secondary of the transformer differs from a conventional transformer in that it consists of a series of stacked *pancake coils* or *pies.* Furthermore, very little iron core is used to prevent loss of electrical energy in the form of heat within the core. The transformer steps up the secondary voltage to about 280 kV to be applied to a specially designed X-ray tube. A separate filament transformer provides the filament with current appropriate for thermionic emission of electrons.

The X-ray tube differs from conventional tubes in having a *grounded anode.* Furthermore, grounding of the entire tube head eliminates the need for high voltage cables. The tube is self-rectified, operating without an auxiliary rectifying system. The anode is cooled by circulating cold water which is in turn cooled by a separate heat exchanger utilizing tap water. Insulation is accomplished by the highly efficient insulating gas—sulfur hexafluoride—under pressure.

As shown in Figure 5.18, the unit contains both kV and mA stabilizers to avoid excessive variation in radiation output.

This type of equipment generates X rays of high intensity with a wide range of quality, from HVL less than 1 mm Al to 4 mm Cu. Target-skin distance is usually 50 cm for deep therapy, although other distances may be used. It should be mentioned that radiation output with the high frequency generator compares favorably with conventional 250-kV constant potential equipment, for equivalent HVL's.

In general, orthovoltage therapy equipment is now almost obsolete as a result of the introduction of megavoltage devices. However, orthovoltage therapy is still very useful in the management of certain lesions such as carcinoma of the lip and skeletal metastases from carcinoma of the breast.

ULTRA SHORT DISTANCE THERAPY

A novel type of X-ray therapy was first proposed by Chaoul to treat lesions near the surface of the body or within a body cavity. The essential principles of treatment by his method were:

1. Short treatment distance
2. Low filtration
3. Soft radiation
4. Small treatment field

He called this **contact X-ray therapy** because of the short treatment distance, but it is more properly named **ultra short distance therapy**. The Chaoul therapy unit is now obsolete, but the Philips RT 50 is still available for this purpose (see Fig. 5.19).

Philips RT 50. With a minimum target-skin distance of 2 cm there is a steep fall in exposure rate within the first cm below the skin (see Fig. 5.20). Extremely large exposure rates are possible at operating potentials of 10 to 50 kV because of the low inherent filtration of the beryllium window—0.03 mm A1 equivalent. An exposure rate of 10,400 R/min is obtainable even with a tube

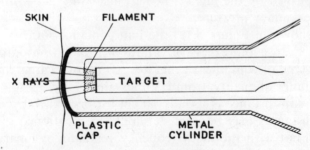

FIGURE 5.19. Schematic diagram of the Philips contact therapy head. Note that the X-ray beam is emitted in the direction of the filament and leaves the end window of the tube. (Courtesy of the North American Philips Company, Inc.)

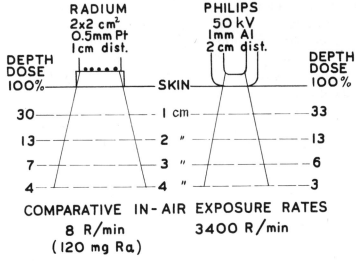

FIGURE 5.20. Comparison of depth doses from a radium plaque and a Philips RT 50 contact therapy unit. The in-air exposure rates are at the level of the skin. (Modified from B. Proctor, J. E. Lofstrom, and C. E. Nurnberger.[69])

potential of 10 kV when no added filter is used. At 50 kV with a 1 mm A1 filter and a 2 cm target-skin distance the output is 3,400 R/min.

The high output and the rapid attenuation of the beam permit marked reduction in treatment time while delivering a large surface exposure and a small dose beneath the skin. These conditions, as well as the elongated shape of the tube and its housing, make the equipment eminently suitable for certain types of dermatologic and intracavitary treatment. However, it should be pointed out that superficial malignant lesions of the skin, especially basal cell carcinomas, are now being successfully managed with chemotherapy (e.g. 5-fluorouracil).

It is interesting to compare the distribution of radium γ rays and Philips X rays under comparable treatment conditions (see Fig. 5.20). The similarity in distribution is striking, but there is a much greater radiation output by the Philips unit than by the milligrams of radium shown. The saving in treatment time is obvious, to say nothing of the much greater personnel protection with the Philips unit.

The General Electric Maximar-100. This is a self-contained, self-rectified unit. It utilizes an X-ray tube of conventional design, encased with its transformer in the tube housing. The important distinguishing feature of the Maximar-100 is the glass aperture of the tube which is made of beryllium glass 0.5 to 1.5 mm thick, equivalent to about 0.1 mm Al. Because such glass transmits very soft X rays, the 50-kV beam is similar to that obtained with the Philips unit with comparable filtration. When unfiltered, the output at 2 cm distance from the surface of the window is 2,000,000 R/min. Furthermore, absorption in air is significant even in a space of a few centimeters.

CHAPTER 6

High-Energy Therapy Units and Particle Accelerators

IN recent years great strides have been made in the development of apparatus delivering beams of high intensity in the multimillion volt region. These include, first of all, the γ-ray emitting *telecurie beam units* originally containing a radium source, but later replaced by one of the artificial radionuclides, mainly cobalt 60. Less widely used for this purpose is cesium 137.

The second general type of equipment produces *megavoltage X rays.* An example is the *Van de Graaff generator* which, for radiation therapy, is usually available with a constant potential output of 2 MV X rays. For practical purposes, the energy of the radiation produced by the ^{60}Co teletherapy unit (1.25 MeV av.) is roughly equivalent to that generated by 2-MV X-ray equipment, any difference being due to the size of the source and the resulting penumbra. Another variety of megavoltage X-ray equipment that is rapidly gaining favor is the *linear accelerator* or *linac,* with models producing X rays ranging in energy from 4 to 35 MV. Still another type, available in some therapy centers, is the *betatron* which can accelerate electrons to energies of 22 to 300 MV, depending on the model. Upon striking the target, these electrons give up their energy in the form of X rays having energies ranging up to the maximum energy of the exciting electrons. The optimum X-ray range with the betatron is 20 to 50 MV, although the usual energy in therapy is about 25 MV.

Other devices used principally for acceleration of heavy particles have no direct application in therapy but will be described for their general interest; they include the *cyclotron* and *synchrocyclotron.* The *nuclear reactor* will be discussed in Chapter 11.

TELECURIE THERAPY

It was found early in the history of radiotherapy that if a sufficiently large source of radium were applied externally, the emitted γ rays could be used to treat a deep-seated tumor. Thus, in 1917 Janeway prepared a "radium pack" which he placed in contact with the patient's skin for the treatment of an underlying lesion. Obviously, the depth dose was small with this form of high powered contact therapy. Later, when large amounts of radium became available, the source was placed at some distance from the skin with consequent improvement in depth dose. Such γ-ray beam therapy in which a powerful radioactive source is placed at a distance from the skin to treat a deep-lying tumor is called *telecurie therapy*.

The early teletherapy units employed radium as the active source. With the rapid growth of nuclear reactor technology, artificial radionuclides, chiefly ^{60}Co and ^{137}Cs, have replaced radium as the active source in telecurie therapy equipment.

COBALT 60 TELETHERAPY EQUIPMENT

When sufficiently large amounts of ^{60}Co became available commercially, it was natural for radiotherapists to turn to it as a substitute for radium in telecurie therapy. High energy X-ray therapy in the 1 million volt region had been used in a few centers in the early 1930's. Radium units had been in use since the 1920's, but despite the fact that radium γ rays have an average energy of about 0.83 MeV, the low intensity of even the most powerful (10 g) sources required such short treatment distances that the central axis depth doses approximated those obtained with 140-kV X rays.

Most of the properties of ^{60}Co make it eminently suitable for telecurie therapy. It is manufactured in the nuclear reactor by the irradiation of stable ^{59}Co with slow neutrons, according to the following equation:

$$^{59}_{27}\text{Co} + {}^{1}_{0}\text{n} \longrightarrow {}^{60}_{27}\text{Co} + \gamma$$

This is an efficient reaction because cobalt happens to have a strong tendency to capture thermal neutrons, that is, the capture cross section is high (see page 380). The decay scheme of ^{60}Co in Figure 6.01 shows why it is such an excellent telecurie source— two energetic γ rays of 1.17 and 1.33 MeV (av. 1.25 MeV) are emitted, equivalent to about 2-MV X rays. Furthermore, the low energy β particles are readily eliminated by a steel capsule. Additional details about the decay scheme of ^{60}Co are given on page 354.

For radiation therapy, the specific activity of the ^{60}Co source should be of the order of 75 to 200 Ci per gram. This requires exposure of the cobalt to neutrons in the nuclear reactor for many months. The advantage of high specific activity is that it makes possible smaller sources to produce beams of high intensity with resulting large exposure rates at long source-skin distances and improved depth dose.

The ^{60}Co Source Housing. We shall turn now to the design of a ^{60}Co source and its housing. As we have already mentioned, stable cobalt is irradiated by slow neutrons in a nuclear reactor to produce radiocobalt. The ^{60}Co source is available as circular discs or slugs, or as pellets grouped in a cluster. An improved process involves neutron activation (in a nuclear reactor) of the stable cobalt in the form of a wire coil (Neutron Products Corp.)

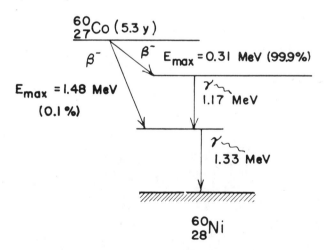

FIGURE 6.01. Decay scheme of cobalt 60. After emitting a β^- particle, nucleus enters an excited state of nickel 60 which immediately decays to ground state by emitting 2 γ rays in succession.

to permit deeper activation of the cobalt. Upon reaching the desired activity, the coil is melted and fabricated into a small cylinder with a diameter of 1.5 or 2 cm, the same diameters in which the other types of ^{60}Co therapy sources are available. The smaller source is preferred because of better geometry, that is, steeper *edge gradient* (smaller "penumbra").

The source is enclosed in a double-layered stainless steel capsule which is sealed by welding to prevent leakage of cobalt particles. It may be mounted in a rotating wheel of tungsten alloy covered with a layer of stainless steel or brass. Rotation of the wheel by a remote control stall-type motor turns the capsule from the "safe" position to the aperture in the housing as shown in Figure 6.02; it is now in the "on" position. At the same time, a spring attached to the wheel is put under tension. Upon completion of the treatment, the stall motor automatically turns off and the spring returns the source to the "off" position. Obviously, no one but the patient should be in the therapy room while the source is in the "on" position.

Another method of controlling the position of the source utilizes a sliding drawer.

It should be pointed out that the protective housing for the source is a massive sphere consisting of an alloy of lead, tungsten, and spent uranium, because this gives excellent shielding per unit mass of material. The highly active sources require a housing about 60 cm (2 ft) in diameter to achieve adequate shielding. If power should fail in the remote control device, a spring promptly returns the source to the "off" position.

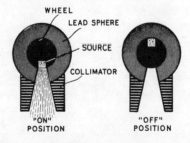

FIGURE 6.02. Wheel type ^{60}Co teletherapy head. In the "on" position, the wheel is rotated to bring the active source to the aperture. In the "off" position, the wheel is rotated away from the aperture.

At a distance of 1 meter in any direction from the source (except the aperture) the maximum exposure rate must not exceed 10 mR/hr, with an average of 2 mR/hr (NCRP *Report No. 33*). The collimating device shall allow no more than 5 percent of the radiation to be transmitted outside the useful beam.

The ^{60}**Co Source.** This is rated either in *curies* or in *rhm units*. A typical installation contains a source rated from about 750 to 9,000 curies and called a *kilocurie* source. However, the output of a ^{60}Co unit depends not only on the number of curies but on the specific activity which is also affected by *self-absorption* of the source. This is absorption of radiation in the source itself, amounting to about 20 to 25 percent per cm of thickness. The output is rated in units of rhm. *One rhm signifies one roentgen per hour at one meter.* Therefore, a 2,000 rhm source would deliver 2,000 R/hr at 1 meter. Because of the problem of protection, the commercial units are often rated on the basis of the maximum rhm which they can safely house. For instance, a 4,000 rhm unit can house a ^{60}Co source up to a maximum output of 4,000 rhm. A stronger source would require a larger protective housing. Figure 14.04 shows a typical ^{60}Co teletherapy unit.

The quality of the radiation emitted by the source does not depend on its curiage, that is, the number of curies. However, to keep treatment time reasonably short, a weak source must be used at a closer distance, producing a more divergent beam and decreasing the depth dose. For example, a 1,000-rhm unit must be used at a distance of 40 to 50 cm to obtain a reasonable treatment time; the 10 cm depth dose through a 100 cm^2 portal is 47 per cent. A 3,000 rhm unit may be operated conveniently at a distance of 80 cm, with a 10 cm depth dose of 56 percent, an increase of nearly 20 percent. The treatment time is approximately the same in both cases. However, the smaller unit may be advantageous in head and neck therapy because of the smaller exit dose.

One of the drawbacks of ^{60}Co in telecurietherapy is its *short half-life,* 5.3 years, requiring adjustment of treatment time according to the decay curve. Furthermore, the ^{60}Co source must be replaced every few years to maintain adequate γ-ray intensity so that treatment time is kept within reasonable limits, still a very expensive procedure. However, maintenance costs and time lost through equipment failure are negligible.

As already mentioned above, the β particles of ^{60}Co are removed by absorption in the stainless steel capsule. Because ^{60}Co γ rays are almost monoenergetic they have a constant HVL— 12 mm lead—so that no filtration is added beyond that required to remove β particles.

At this point we should mention that the housing is equipped with a ***multivaned collimator*** (see Figs. 6.02 and 10.06) originally designed by Johns to delimit the γ-ray beam. Strict collimation is necessary to minimize the significant penumbra associated with the finite area of the source. Further discussion of penumbra and collimation appears on pages 267 to 268.

The protective barriers for the installation of ^{60}Co therapy units will be referred to in Chapter 16. This requires a specially constructed room of adequate wall thickness, based on an HVL of 2.45 in. concrete.

CESIUM 137 TELETHERAPY EQUIPMENT

Because of its relatively long half-life of 30 years, cesium 137 seems to be an attractive source for telecurie therapy. ^{137}Cs is one of the by-products resulting from the fission of uranium in the nuclear reactor. Its decay scheme is shown in Figure 6.03, to be described in more detail later (see page 355). Suffice it to

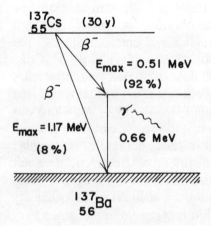

FIGURE 6.03. Decay scheme of cesium 137. Ninety-two percent of the nuclei emit a β⁻ particle, becoming metastable barium 137 (half-life 2.6 min) which decays to stable barium by γ emission (isomeric transition). Eight percent of the nuclei decay directly to stable barium 137 by β⁻ decay.

say here, the main route of decay is via a 0.51-MeV β^- particle and a 0.66-MeV γ ray.

Although the γ rays of ^{137}Cs are less energetic than those of ^{60}Co, they are suitable for certain forms of teletherapy, delivering a better depth dose than orthovoltage X rays (see below, Fig. 10.39). On the other hand, it is questionable whether there is any **biologic** advantage to be gained in teletherapy with radiation in the 1 to 2 MeV range as compared with that of ^{137}Cs at 0.66 MeV, insofar as bone absorption and skin effect are concerned, despite the greater depth dose with the higher energy radiation.

The advantages of ^{137}Cs include, first, its relatively low cost, since it is a waste product of the nuclear reactor. In the second place, because its radiation is less penetrating than that of ^{60}Co, less protection is required. Thus, the **half value layer** of ^{137}Cs γ rays is 6.6 mm of lead in contrast to 12 mm of lead for ^{60}Co. The housing for the ^{137}Cs source can therefore be smaller and more maneuverable, although the protective barriers in the treatment room are only slightly lighter than those required for ^{60}Co. Since ^{137}Cs has a **long half-life** of 30 years, it serves as a more permanent source requiring far less frequent replacement and correction of treatment time than does ^{60}Co. Finally, its smaller exit dose compared to that from ^{60}Co may offer some advantage in certain tumors of the head and neck.

However, there are several noteworthy disadvantages in the use of ^{137}Cs. It has been very difficult to obtain sources with sufficient specific activity to permit a high intensity of γ radiation. The apparent limit of specific activity is now about 80 Ci/g. Furthermore, ^{137}Cs has a high degree of self-absorption, amounting to about 40 percent. Therefore, a large source (about 3 cm in diameter) would be required to provide an activity of 1,500 Ci; but due to **self-absorption,** this would be equivalent to only 900 Ci. Since the Γ factor is about $\frac{1}{4}$ that of ^{60}Co, or 3.2 R/mCi-hr at 1 cm, a simple calculation shows that,

$$3.2 \times 1,500 \times 1,000 \times 0.60 = 2.88 \times (10)^6 \text{ R/hr at 1 cm with a}$$
1,500 Ci unit having 0.40 self-absorption

By the inverse square law (only approximate here because of the large 3 cm source) the exposure rate at 70 cm is:

$$\frac{2.88 \times (10)^6}{(70)^2} = 588 \text{ R/hour at 70 cm SSD}$$

$$\text{or } \frac{588}{60} \cong \text{ about 10 R/min at 70 cm SSD}$$

This is a relatively small output when compared with a 1,500 Ci ^{60}Co source which, under similar conditions, would have a beam output of about 50 R/min. Nevertheless, if short treatment time is not an important economic factor, ^{137}Cs can still be utilized; if the source-to-skin distance is reduced to 50 cm, the output of a 1,500 Ci ^{137}Cs unit would be about 20 R/min, but there would be a significant fall in depth dose.

Another disadvantage of ^{137}Cs is the inherently large penumbra associated with the large source. Although this can be controlled by adequate collimation for stationary therapy, the long distance required between the end of the cone and the skin with rotation therapy interferes with sharp collimation. Therefore, present ^{137}Cs equipment is virtually limited to stationary therapy, but it must be borne in mind that most ^{60}Co sources also have a significant diameter.

In general, it may be stated the ^{137}Cs has many of the desirable features of megavoltage therapy such as skin-sparing and bone-sparing effects, with satisfactory depth dose, and is subject to less complex protection requirements than ^{60}Co. The maximum ionization with ^{137}Cs γ rays is about 1.5 mm below the skin surface, as compared with 5 mm for ^{60}Co, but the difference is of questionable significance as indicated in a report from Oak Ridge in 1955. The absorbed dose per gram in bone from 0.66 MeV photons is the same as in soft tissues. The long half-life of ^{137}Cs is a distinct advantage over ^{60}Co (half-life 5.3 y). However, the high self-absorption of ^{137}Cs together with its low specific activity, limits the radiation output at 50 cm to a value approaching that obtained from a 200 kV Villard X-ray unit. In practice, ^{137}Cs units are usually operated at a distance of 15 to 35 cm.

HIGH ENERGY X-RAY GENERATORS AND
PARTICLE ACCELERATORS

Electrical devices have been designed to produce multimillion volt X rays with properties resembling the γ rays of ^{60}Co. Strictly speaking, all X-ray generators are particle accelerators, since they speed up electrons toward a target where a portion of their energy is converted to X rays. However, in this section we shall describe several of the more important types of particle accelerators used in the generation of megavoltage X rays, and shall also discuss briefly certain devices for the production of short-lived radionuclides.

By way of historic introduction, we should mention that because of the limited usefulness of α particles as projectiles, more efficient methods of obtaining high-speed particles in the megavoltage region had to be devised. In 1930 Cockcroft and Walton used a cascade of capacitors connected in parallel, alternately charging them to a high potential difference and then discharging them in series through a special tube. By this method they succeeded in obtaining a beam of 0.7 MeV protons.

Van de Graaff Generator. The next advance was the *electrostatic generator* designed by Van de Graaff in 1931 and later adapted for radiotherapy. It operates on the principle that a charge applied to a hollow sphere is distributed uniformly over its outer surface, regardless of the initial potential. The construction of a 2-MV Van de Graaff generator is shown schematically in Figure 6.04. A nonconductive fabric belt moves rapidly over the upper and lower pulleys, the latter being motor driven. A 5-kVA generator "sprays" electrons by induction onto the lower end of the belt. The electrons are then carried to the top where a metal screen rubbing against the belt transfers them to the *hemispherical terminal;* here, the electrons are distributed on the external surface in accordance with the laws of electrostatics, resulting in the production of a high negative potential. By means of automatic control of the initial electron spray, the high voltage on the terminal is maintained constant at the desired level. Potentials up to 20 MV can be obtained.

The high voltage on the terminal is then distributed to a series of *cylindrical electrodes* in a multisection X-ray tube by means

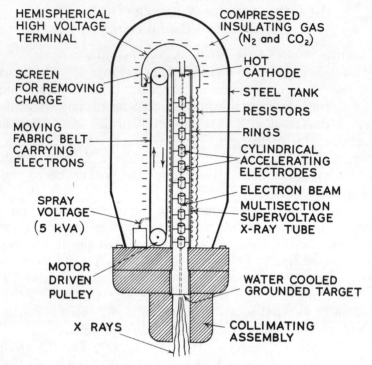

FIGURE 6.04. Schematic diagram of a Van de Graaff generator. (Based on data furnished by courtesy of High Voltage Engineering Corporation.)

of a series of resistors and equipotential rings, the latter surrounding the tube. Because of the progressive fall of potential between successive electrodes, the electrons supplied by the hot cathode at the top of the tube acquire an extremely high velocity. At the same time, as they pass down the tube, they are focused on a fine spot about 5 mm in diameter on the grounded, water cooled transmission type target where megavoltage X rays are produced (2 MV in this case). A heavy lead collimating system provides well delimited beams of various sizes.

The entire unit is placed in a heavy steel tank with insulating gas, either a nitrogen-carbon dioxide mixture or sulfur hexafluoride under a pressure of 6 atmospheres. This provides excellent insulation in a small space, so that the described 2-MV unit measures about 9 feet in height by about 3 feet in diameter.

The Van de Graaff generator also lends itself to the acceleration of positive ions. Positive charges are sprayed onto the belt to produce a high positive potential on the terminal. A source of positive ions is provided at the top of the tube in place of the hot cathode; these ions may be protons or deuterons.

Linear Accelerator. The principle of accelerating ions by a series of cylindrical electrodes was first proposed by Lawrence and Sloan in 1931. Their device, called a *linear accelerator*, consisted of a series of metal electrodes in the form of "cans" open at the ends, enclosed in a vacuum tube. Alternate electrodes (numbered 1, 3, 5, 7, etc.) are connected together to one end of a high frequency electric generator, and the intervening electrodes (numbered 2, 4, 6, 8, etc.) are connected to the opposite end of the generator as shown in Figure 6.05. Thus, at the instant one group of electrodes is charged negatively the other group is charged positively. When a stream of heavy positive ions, such as mercury, is shot into the accelerator, it drifts through the first electrode, or *drift tube.* If the positive ions reach the gap between the first and second drift tube at the instant the latter becomes negative, they will be accelerated toward it. After drifting through tube number 2, if tube number 3 becomes negative at the instant the electrons reach the gap, they will receive another accelerating kick. When conditions are such that the particles always arrive at a gap between electrodes at the instant the alternating current reaches a peak, with an attracting charge on the next electrode,

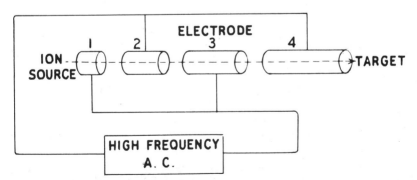

FIGURE 6.05. Diagram of the classical type of linear accelerator for accelerating heavy charged particles such as mercury ions.

TABLE 6.01
COMPARISON OF PARTICLE ACCELERATORS

Type	Particle Accelerated	Applied Voltage	Magnetic Field	Electric Field	Energy of Particles
Van de Graaff Machine	Electrons; protons	5–20 kV	None	—	1 to 20 MeV
Linear Accelerator (Medical)	Electrons; protons	40 kV or more	None	High frequency	up to 35 MeV
Cyclotron	Protons; deuterons; α particles	20 kV or more	Constant	High frequency	up to 40 MeV
Synchrocyclotron	Protons; deuterons; α particles	10 kV or more	Constant	Frequency modulated	up to 400 MeV
Betatron	Electrons	—	Variable	None	up to 500 MeV
Synchrotron	Electrons; protons	—	Variable	Frequency modulated	up to 6 BeV

the machine is said to be in **resonance.** If resonance is maintained for a large series of electrodes, the particles are accelerated to extremely high energies.

The original linear accelerator was 30 feet long and produced a 1.3-MV stream of positively charged mercury ions. This limit could not be exceeded at that time because of nonavailability of ultra high frequency electric generators, and therefore Lawrence devised the cyclotron to obtain particles of higher energy. Furthermore, electrons and positively charged light ions such as protons and deuterons could not be accelerated in this type of device because extremely long drift tubes would be required.

In recent years, with the discovery of radar, extremely high frequency generators have become available for the construction of a different type of linear accelerator or **linac** for X-ray and electron beam therapy. Most **medical** linacs, such as the Clinac®, are of the **standing wave type.** A standing electromagnetic wave is designed to act as an accelerator guide for electrons in a hollow tube 1 to 2 meters long. Electrons are fired by an electron gun, at an energy of about 50 kV, into one end of the tube and are accelerated across a series of resonant cavities, finally striking a transmission type tungsten target to produce X rays. An alternate mode of operation permits extracting the electrons directly for electron beam therapy. However, linacs are much more widely used for megavoltage X-ray than for electron beam therapy, and are available in energies ranging from 4 to 35 MV.

As an example of the features of a linac, the Clinac 4® (see Fig. 6.06) is rated for an electron energy of 4 MeV at the target. This unit has a focal spot size less than 2 mm; hence, there is minimal penumbra. Output at a target-skin distance of 80 cm can be varied continuously from 100 to 350 rads/min, an extremely high value. Fields can be varied from 0×0 to 32×32 cm^2 at 80 cm FSD. The equilibrium depth (maximum ionization) is about 10 mm. Typical isodose curves are shown in Figures 9.19 and 10.42.

The modern linear accelerator can also be applied to protons. Two examples of the proton linear accelerator are the 40-foot 32-MeV unit at the University of California, and the 100-foot 68-MV unit at the University of Minnesota.

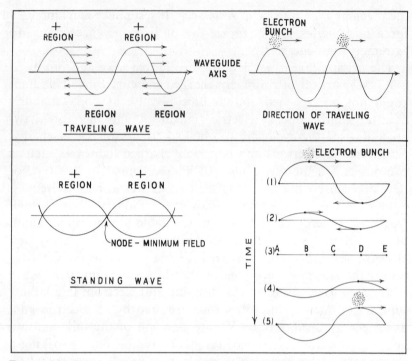

FIGURE 6.06. Principles of traveling and standing wave linear accelerators (linacs). In the traveling wave linac, electron "bunches" introduced by an electron gun are carried by a moving electromagnetic wave, much like a surfboard rider on an ocean wave. In the standing wave linac, the electron "bunches" arrive at the instant the field is maximal in a positive direction as in (1)*B* and (5)*D*. In either type, the electrons attain extremely high energies, but the standing wave linac is a more efficient device. (Courtesy of J. C. Ford and Varian.)

Betatron. In 1941 D. W. Kerst, at the University of Illinois, invented a device with which he accelerated electrons to 2.3 MeV. He named this the ***betatron.*** It consists of a doughnut-shaped glass or ceramic tube placed between the poles of a powerful electromagnet operating at 180 Hz. No electrical field is needed. (Contrast this with the synchrocyclotron in which there is a constant magnetic field and a frequency modulated radio frequency electrical field.) A simplified representation of the betatron is shown in Figure 6.07. An ***electron gun*** introduces electrons at nearly zero velocity into the highly evacuated doughnut. They are accelerated by the rapidly changing magnetic field in the same manner as the electrons in the secondary coil of a transformer. The magnetic field establishes the electrons in an orbit within the doughnut, analogous to a single loop in the secondary coil of a transformer. This so-called **stable** or **equilibrium orbit** has a radius determined by

$$r = \frac{mv}{Bq} \tag{1}$$

where m is the rest mass of an electron, v is its velocity, B is the intensity of the magnetic field, and q is the electron charge. Proper design of the pole pieces insures this relationship, producing the required nonuniform magnetic field.

The electrons are accelerated during the growth phase of the magnetic field, making thousands of revolutions in ¼ cycle of the magnetic alternation (1/720 sec), as shown in Figure 6.08. Note that only the first ¼ cycle of the magnetic flux (flow) is useful in accelerating electrons, the peak velocity being reached at *B*. Now, a special auxiliary coil is used to deflect the electrons out

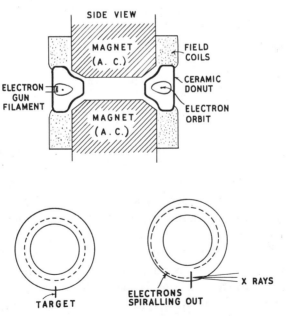

FIGURE 6.07. Diagram of a betatron.

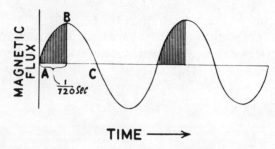

FIGURE 6.08. Electrons spiral out of the betatron in bursts of 1/720 sec, or 1/4 of each cycle; the resulting X rays are also emitted in a 1/720 sec interval during each 1/180 sec.

of their stable orbit, making them spiral outward to strike the target. By this time, the velocity of the electrons may be more than 99 percent that of light. The efficiency of X-ray production is extremely high under these conditions, which means that 24-MeV electrons produce virtually 24-MeV X rays. Obviously, since the electrons are accelerated only during one-fourth cycle, there is a pulsating electron beam striking the target 180 times per second (one pulse for each cycle).

Because the magnetic field strength increases during operation of the betatron, it compensates for the relativistic increase in mass of the electron, accelerating it to very high velocities as already noted. In the large 100-MeV betatron, the electrons reach a velocity 99.99 per cent that of light, undergoing a 200-fold increase in mass! However, beyond a certain acceleration the electron *radiates* energy. For instance, in the 100-MeV betatron about 3 percent of the electron's energy is lost by radiation. Because this radiative loss is proportional to the fourth power of the kinetic energy of the electron, it increases very rapidly as the energy of the electron exceeds 100 MeV. Thus, electron acceleration finally reaches a limiting value because additional imparted energy is radiated. This may be overcome either by increasing the radius of the orbit (larger betatron), or decreasing the number of revolutions the electrons make before striking the target. Both methods are utilized in the largest 340-MeV Kerst betatron equipped with a doughnut 9 feet in diameter, which imparts 3,000 volts per revolution of the electron (as compared with the

100-MeV betatron with a diameter of 5.5 feet and energy increment of 400 volts per revolution of the electron). It is believed
that 500 MeV is probably the maximum energy that can be imparted to electrons by the betatron.

A *beam flattening filter* must be used, thicker in the center
than at the periphery, because the X-ray intensity is much greater
along the beam's central axis than at its edges. In other words,
the beam is sharply peaked in a forward direction. The X-ray beam
produces virtually no side scatter and, with the small target—
about 0.2 mm—the beam edge is sharply defined within the
body. By use of a special device known as an *electron peeler*,
the electrons themselves can be brought out of the betatron as
an electron beam for irradiation therapy (see pages 320 to 322).

The powerful X-ray beam produced by the betatron is being
used in some of the leading medical centers in radiation therapy
of deep-seated tumors, in industry to locate flaws in steel casting,
and in physical research.

Cyclotron. In 1929 E. O. Lawrence proposed a radically
new method of accelerating charged particles to extremely high
velocities, using only a low voltage source. Two years later,
Lawrence and Livingston built the first working model which
they named the *cyclotron.* Its principle is surprisingly simple:
charged particles are gradually speeded up by repeated low
voltage "kicks" provided by a radio frequency low voltage alternating current. Upon being accelerated, the ions travel in a flat
spiral path in which they are kept by a constant magnetic field
directed perpendicular to the plane of the path (see Figs. 6.09
and 6.10). The summation of the repeated low voltage kicks

**CYCLOTRON
"DEES"**

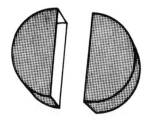

FIGURE 6.09. The accel-
eration chamber of the
cyclotron, called the *dees.*

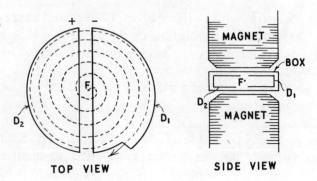

TOP VIEW   SIDE VIEW

FIGURE 6.10. Schematic representation of the position of the dees between the poles of the magnet in a cyclotron.

imparts to the ions an extremely high energy, so the cyclotron generates extraordinarily high voltage using relatively low voltage as its source of energy.

The cyclotron consists of two flat semicircular metal boxes called *dees* because their shape resembles the capital D. The boxes are open only along their straight sides, being arranged so that these open sides face each other with a gap of about 2 to 5 cm as shown in Figure 6.09. The dees are placed in a highly evacuated chamber, but a small amount of gas is introduced to supply the desired charged particles. Thus, for high speed protons, a minute amount of hydrogen gas is chosen. For deuterons, heavy hydrogen is introduced into the chamber. A filament at the center of the chamber emits electrons when heated (thermionic emission), ionizing the surrounding gas. For example, when hydrogen is ionized by the electrons, protons are liberated.

A high frequency alternating current—10^6 Hz (cycles/sec), 20 kV—is now applied to the metal dees which act as electrodes, one being positive and the other negative. The positively charged protons are repelled by the positive D and attracted by the negative D across the gap. Since the charge exists only on the external surface of the dees, there is no electrostatic field within to interfere with the motion of the protons which move in a curved path because of the externally applied constant magnetic field, as shown in Figure 6.10. At the instant the protons reach the opening between the dees, the alternating current reverses its direction, the charges on the dees reverse and the protons receive another push. In other words, the frequency of revolution of the protons must remain in step with the frequency of the AC cycle, for proper function of the cyclotron.

The rapid reversal of charge on the dees, with attendant successive kicks, imparts extremely high velocity and kinetic energy to the protons, causing them to move in a larger and larger circle. Thus, the protons move in a spiral path. Ordinarily, during the operation of the cyclotron, the protons make several thousand revolutions before reaching the side wall of the dees—at this instant the protons pass through the window in one of the dees as shown in Figure 6.10.

For those interested in the mathematical aspects of the cyclotron principle, the radius of the path of an accelerated ion—proton, deuteron, or α particle—depends on the following relationship:

$$r = \frac{mv}{Bq} \tag{2}$$

Note that this is the same as equation (1) for the betatron.

Since m, B, and q are constant for a given high frequency alternating current, it is obvious that the path radius of a given ion depends only on its velocity, becoming greater as the velocity increases and resulting in an increasing spiral path.

Furthermore, as the path becomes longer (spiral), the particle is simultaneously accelerated at the same rate, so the time it spends in each D remains constant and its frequency of rotation therefore remains in step with the current alterations. It is known that

$$s = 2\pi r$$

where s is the length (circumference) of the path in one cycle and r is the radius of the path. But,

$$s = vt$$

where v is the velocity and t is the time for one revolution ("period of revolution"). Therefore, combing these two equations,

$$2\pi r = vt$$

and rearranging,

$$t = \frac{2\pi r}{v} \tag{3}$$

But according to equation (2), $r = mv/Bq$. Substituting this value of r in equation (3),

$$t = \frac{2\pi}{v} \cdot \frac{mv}{Bq}$$

$$t = \frac{2\pi m}{Bq} \tag{4}$$

Note that t is independent of the velocity. Thus, the time for one revolution, t, depends only on the mass of the ion, the field strength, and the charge on the ion. Since these are all constant for a given operational setup, the time for one revolution of the ion in any part of its spiral path is constant and its frequency of rotation therefore remains in step with the frequency of the alternating current. As long as the frequency of the ion rotation equals the frequency of the alternating current, the conditions for correct operation of the cyclotron are fulfilled.

As already indicated, the ion acquires a very high energy. For example, if a proton gains 10 keV with each "kick" or alternation of the current, it would have an energy of 2×10 keV = 20 keV at the end of one complete cycle (2 alternations per cycle), and after 300 revolutions, its energy would be 300×20 keV = 6,000 keV = 6 MeV.

It can be shown that the final kinetic energy of the accelerated ion depends only on the square of the product of the magnetic field strength and the final radius of the path, that is, $(Br)^2$. For this reason, in order to obtain ions with maximum kinetic energy, extremely powerful magnets must be used in the cyclotron, and the dees must be very large to provide the space for a path of large radius. For example, a cyclotron with magnets 15 feet in diameter can produce 200-MeV deuterons.

The question is often asked, "Why cannot electrons be accelerated in a cyclotron?" The answer lies in Einstein's equation for the mass, *m*, of a particle in motion,

$$m = \frac{m_0}{\sqrt{1 - \dfrac{v^2}{c^2}}} \qquad (5)$$

where m_0 is the mass of a particle at rest, v is velocity of the particle, and c is the velocity of light. The equation indicates that when the velocity of the particle is small, the value of v^2/c^2 approaches zero, the denominator is then equal to one, and $m = m_0$. However, as the velocity approaches that of light, the value of v^2/c^2 approaches unity and the denominator becomes vanishingly small so that the mass, *m*, of the particle increases, a phenomenon called ***relativistic increase in mass***. This effect is very large in the case of the electron because of its extremely small rest mass, so that even moderately high velocities increase its mass significantly. For example, a 1-MeV electron has a mass more than twice the rest mass. Now, according to equation (4) the time for one revolution of an ion depends on its mass (in a constant magnetic field). As the electron mass increases, the time of revolution is prolonged, so the electron does not reach the gap between the dees at the instant the alternating current reverses. In other words, the electrons are out of phase with the alternating current and cannot be accelerated. Furthermore, even with heavier ions such as protons and deuterons, relativistic increase in mass prevents acceleration beyond a certain limiting value. In fact, 40 MeV is probably the upper limit for protons.

Although the cyclotron is designed primarily for accelerating protons, deuterons, and α particles, it can be used to obtain other types of subatomic projectiles. For example, if deuterons are accelerated in a cyclotron to an energy of 15 MeV and directed at a beryllium target, a very concentrated beam of neutrons is emitted, containing about one neutron for every 200 colliding deuterons. Such a neutron beam is being tried experimentally in therapy in some centers such as the M.D. Anderson Hospital using the cyclotron at Texas A & M University. Furthermore, a great variety of isotopes can be produced because of the high energy protons and deutrons, as well as neutrons, that can be obtained with the cyclotron. This was the main source of radionuclides for medical and industrial use long before the introduction of the nuclear reactor.

Synchrocyclotron. Because of the relativistic effect of high velocity on mass, we cannot increase the energy of ions simply by building more and more powerful cyclotrons. In 1945, E. M. McMillan in this country and V. Veksler in the Soviet Union independently solved this problem by their discovery of *phase stability*, utilizing the relativistic increase in mass rather than permitting it to hinder further acceleration. If the frequency of the alternating current is slowed down gradually by just the right amount, it will remain in step with ions whose mass is increasing due to the relativity effect of their increasing velocity. Any particles which are moving slower or faster than the main group receive a smaller or larger kick, respectively, so they get into phase with the main group of ions. This tendency for the ions to remain in step as the frequency of the alternating current is modified (frequency modulation) is known as *phase stability.*

The first large scale synchrocyclotron in the United States was the converted giant cyclotron at the University of California. Its magnetic cores contain almost 4,000 tons of iron, wrapped in about 300 tons of copper strips four inches wide. Applied potential across the gap is less than 10 kV. The initial frequency is about 12,500,000 cycles per second, gradually decreasing to 8,500,000 cycles per second during one-half second of operation. The ions travel in a spiral from the center to the window in about 1/1000 second after making about 10,000 revolutions. They emerge in 120 bursts per second, whereas in the conventional cyclotron the particles leave in a nearly continuous stream. The speed of the particles is enormous, approaching one-half the speed of light, as contrasted with 10-MeV α particles from naturally radioactive elements, having a velocity about 1/15 that of light.

The energy which the synchrocyclotron can impart to ions is fabulous. For instance, deuterons can attain an energy of about 200 MeV, protons 680 MeV, and α particles 400 MeV. Particles with such enormous energies can be used to produce, in target atoms, nuclear reactions heretofore impossible. Thus, 200-MeV deuterons can dislodge several neutrons simultaneously from the nuclei of certain heavy atoms. Mesons have also been produced; these are neutral, or negatively or positively charged particles having a mass 200 to 300 times that of an electron.

The extremely energetic particles obtained from this device liberate γ rays and neutrons from atoms with which they collide, thereby representing a source of danger to personnel. Because hydrogen is the best stopping medium for fast neutrons, concrete with its large percentage of water is a very effective shield against the neutrons. The γ rays are absorbed in large part by the calcium in the concrete. A 15-foot thick wall of concrete surrounds the 15-foot synchrocyclotron to provide adequate protection of personnel.

Synchrotron. Machines known as synchrotrons have been designed to accelerate electrons and protons, utilizing a radio frequency alternating current to accelerate the particles, and a modulated magnetic field to take care of the relativistic increase in mass of the accelerated particles. A special ceramic doughnut is used, similar to that in a betatron, but a part is coated with metal to provide the electrical field. The design of the synchrotron, including an electrical field for electron acceleration, allows the use of smaller magnets than does the betatron which depends on its magnet alone for acceleration.

During operation of the *electron synchrotron*, the electrons are first accelerated up to a few MeV as in the betatron. Further energy is then given the electrons by periodic electrical pulses of the *constant* radio frequency electrical field, compensating for the relativistic increase in mass of the revolving electrons. In fact, the increase in energy of the electrons beyond a certain velocity is due to their increase in mass as shown in equation (5). Thus, the synchrotron may be considered as a *ponderator* or "mass-increaser"; the electrons have more energy but no more speed than those in a conventional betatron. As the magnetic field strength increases, the energy of the revolving electrons increases to a maximum, and at this instant the radio frequency oscillating potential is interrupted. The electrons then spiral inward because of the continuing and unopposed increase in the magnetic field strength and strike the target which thereupon emits X rays. The maximum electron energy believed to be feasible with the electron synchrotron is 1 BeV (billion electron volt).

The ***proton synchrotron*** or ***bevatron*** requires variation or modulation of both the radio frequency alternating current which accelerates the protons, and the magnetic field which determines their orbit. This is due to the fact that with a synchrocyclotron, protons would require orbits of large radius to undergo acceleration beyond 450 MeV, necessitating extremely large and heavy magnets. By modulating both the magnetic and electrical fields, a smaller machine can be constructed for the same acceleration of protons. The 6.3-BeV proton synchrotron at the University of California has a magnet weighing 10,000 tons and an orbit diameter of 110 feet. A larger unit, the 33-BeV bevatron, is in use at the Brookhaven National Laboratory, and a 200- to 400-BeV unit with a diameter exceeding 1 mile is under construction for the National Accelerator Laboratory near Chicago.

CHAPTER 7

Quantity of X rays and Gamma Rays

HISTORICAL INTRODUCTION

IN using X and γ rays, the radiotherapist must know the quantity and quality of the radiation in the particular beam. The *quantity* of radiation designates the amount given or absorbed, whereas the *quality* or penetrating ability makes it possible to determine what percentage of the radiation will reach a lesion at a given depth below the body surface. In this chapter, only radiation quantity will be considered, a discussion of quality being reserved for the next chapter.

Very soon after the discovery of X rays, it was found that these rays originate at the target of the X-ray tube and pass out into space in straight lines in a divergent beam. The intensity of the radiation at a given point in the beam may be defined as the quantity of radiant energy passing per unit time through a unit area of the surface perpendicular to the direction of the beam at that point. Thus,

$$I = \frac{Q}{At} \tag{1}$$

where I is the intensity in ergs per cm²-sec when Q is the total quantity of radiant energy in ergs passing through a surface A cm² and t is the time in sec. From this equation is derived the following relation:

$$Q/A = It \text{ ergs/cm}^2 \tag{2}$$

which means that the quantity of radiation per cm² is equal to the intensity times the exposure time.

In radiation physics, according to the ICRU*, the corresponding intensity unit for a polyenergetic beam would be the *energy fluence rate* or *energy flux density* ψ (small Greek psi), defined by

$$\psi = \frac{\Delta N \cdot h\nu}{\Delta a \cdot \Delta t} \tag{3}$$

*International Commission on Radiation Units and Measurements.

Note that the numerator represents the number of photons ΔN times the energy hv of the photons, and the denominator is the area times the time. In other words, equation (3) represents intensity as defined above, that is, the quantity of energy crossing a unit area in unit time. However, these expressions are not useful at present in radiotherapy. Instead, as we shall explain below, we can more conveniently describe the intensity of a beam in terms of the *exposure rate,* based on ionization in air.

When a body is exposed to X or γ radiation, some of the photons pass through unchanged, but a certain fraction is absorbed by interaction with the atoms of the body. The absorbed photons, if sufficiently energetic, liberate photoelectrons, recoil electrons, or negatron-positron pairs. These primary electrons then ionize and excite other atoms nearby. In other words, the absorbed energy causes *ionization* and *excitation* which are primarily responsible for the therapeutic effects of penetrating radiation. Obviously, the direct measurement of the amount of absorbed energy in ergs would be the most precise measure of radiation dosage, but this is too formidable a task in clinical radiotherapy, although we shall see later how this may be determined indirectly.

The early workers in this field attempted to solve the problem in various ways. One method utilized a pastille of barium platinocyanide which changes from green to brown when exposed to ionizing radiation. The degree of color change, compared to a standard, indicates the amount of radiation absorbed. However, this was a crude determination and was not widely accepted. Another method was based on the darkening of a photographic film or plate by the radiation, the degree of darkening being standardized to indicate the quantity of radiation absorbed. This, too, was subject to error, largely because of dependence on the wavelength of the radiation. A third method was based on the production of a standard skin reaction—the so-called *erythema dose.*

In 1908, Villard proposed a unit based on the *ionization of a gas.* This was not accepted until twenty years later when the Second International Congress of Radiology adopted the *roentgen* as the unit of X-ray quantity, defining it in very precise terms as the quantity of radiation producing a definite amount of ionization in a definite, segregated amount of air. The number of ions produced is proportional to the quantity of radiation entering the segregated volume. Furthermore, the amount of energy absorbed in the stated mass of air is proportional to the quantity of radiation, in roentgens (R), incident upon the volume of air. Under carefully specified conditions, so many roentgens will produce so many ions in .air. However, it must be emphasized that only a small fraction of the radiation traversing the selected portion of air actually ionizes atoms. The remainder of the beam passes through unchanged. This becomes even more evident when it is realized that a 1-roentgen exposure of X radiation contains photons having a total energy of about 3,000 ergs. Yet, in passing through 1 cc of air under standard conditions of temperature and pressure (0 C and 760 mm Hg), only 0.11 erg is absorbed in the process of ionization!

It is obvious from the preceding discussion that the roentgen specifies neither the energy in the beam nor the energy absorbed. It merely designates a quantity of radiation, properly called *exposure*, which produces a certain number of ions under strictly limited conditions. The roentgen, as a unit, will now be described.

DEFINITION OF THE ROENTGEN

As defined by the ICRU in 1956 (and omitting the term "dose"), *"one roentgen (R) is an exposure of X or γ radiation such that the associated corpuscular emission per 0.001293 gram of air produces, in air, ions carrying 1 electrostatic unit (esu) of quantity of electricity of either sign."* This definition was not so complicated as it appeared at first sight. Each part was essential and had precise meaning:

1. *"Exposure."* Note that the roentgen is an *amount* of radiation—*exposure*—and not intensity. There is no time factor involved. Nothing is stated about energy absorbed. A roentgen represents a certain amount of radiation, just as a gram is a certain amount of matter.

2. *"X or γ rays."* The definition applies equally to both, up to 3 MeV.

3. *"Associated corpuscular emission."* This refers to the electrons liberated during the interaction of X and γ photons with the atoms present in the air. Most of the ionization in the air is produced secondarily by these photoelectrons and recoil electrons. The measuring device must assure equilibrium conditions (see page 178).

4. *"0.001293 gram of air"* is the mass of 1 cc of air under standard conditions of temperature and atmospheric pressure. A definite amount of air in grams assures that a specific number of atoms will be exposed to the ionizing effect of the radiation. Only a small fraction of these atoms will be ionized.

5. *"Produce in air ions carrying 1 electrostatic unit of quantity of electricity of either sign."* The ions are formed by the interaction of photoelectrons and/or recoil electrons (liberated by the radiation) with atoms of gas in the quantity of air specified. These ions must be separated as soon as they are formed and measured electrometrically before they have had a chance to recombine. If the negative ions are separated from the positive and measured, and the quantity of electricity they carry equals 1 esu, then the initial quantity of photonic radiation responsible for these ions is exactly 1 R. Actually, 1 R produces 2.083×10^9 ion pairs, or that number of ions of either sign, in 1 cc of air at standard temperature and pressure. Thus, 1 esu is equivalent to 2.083×10^9 ions. "In air" is important; if any of the primary electrons or scattered photons strike the walls of the measuring device, they will not interact with atoms in the specified volume of air and an error will thereby be introduced.

Note that this definition specifies the conditions under which the roentgen must be measured. The most recent definition states these conditions in a more general way, although they must nonetheless prevail during measurement. The new definition is as follows:

$$X = \frac{\Delta Q}{\Delta m} \qquad (4)$$

where X is the exposure in R, ΔQ *is the sum of the electric charges on all the ions of one sign produced in air when all the electrons (negatrons and positrons) liberated by photons in a small volume of air of mass Δm are completely stopped in air.* According to this definition *1 R = 2.58 × 10⁻⁴ coulomb/kg air.* We cannot measure the roentgen for photon energies above about 3 MeV for a number of reasons, including the difficulties in achieving electronic equilibrium, uniform electric fields, and efficient collection of ions. Nor can the roentgen be measured for photon energies below a few keV.

From the foregoing definitions, it is obvious that the roentgen is a unit of X- or γ-ray quantity based on the production of a specific number of electric charges in a standard mass of air. When this unit is employed clinically in stating X- or γ-ray exposure, it is the same unit as that derived from ionization in air. It does not indicate the amount of radiation absorbed or the effect the radiation will produce, although we know that the amount of energy absorbed is proportional to the roentgen exposure if all other factors remain constant.

Since its inception, the roentgen has served well as a practical unit of radiation exposure. In radiation therapy, the "intensity" of radiation at a given point in the beam is called the *exposure rate,* and is stated in roentgens per unit time, ordinarily *R/min.* This must be clearly differentiated from *exposure* which is simply stated in *R.* The relationship of dose rate and dose is made clearer by the following equations:

$$exposure\ rate = \frac{exposure}{time}\ R/min \tag{5}$$

$$exposure\ in\ R = exposure\ rate \times time \tag{6}$$

For example, if a certain beam of radiation gives an exposure rate of 100 R/min at a given point, and if this radiation is administered for 2 min, the total exposure is 100 × 2 = 200 R.

MEASUREMENT OF THE ROENTGEN

The adoption of the *roentgen* as a unit of radiation exposure became possible only with the development of a suitable device capable of measuring radiation quantity in terms of ionization in air. Such a device, known as a *free air ionization chamber,* fulfills the requirements specified by the official definition of the roentgen discussed above.

A description of the standard free-air ionization chamber (see Fig. 7.01) will now be presented. The X-ray beam, accurately collimated by a thick lead diaphragm, traverses the chamber, ionizing the air within. Ions are produced throughout the cone of radiation, *PQRS*. But in the volume of air represented by *ABCD*, all the ions are located between the parallel metal plates, P_1 and P_2, the upper one of which is charged to a high negative potential of 1,500–2,000 volts. This repels the negative ions toward P_2. The difference in potential between P_1 and P_2 must be high enough to drive all the negative ions to P_2 before they have had a chance to recombine with positive ions; that is, **saturation conditions** must prevail. Furthermore, the plates must be separated far enough so that they will not be struck directly by photons or by photoelectrons or recoil electrons that have failed to dissipate all their energy in producing ions.

Some of the primary electrons liberated in front of plane *AD* (*X*) will enter the segregated volume *ABCD* to produce ionization, but an equal number of electrons liberated within this volume will pass beyond plane *BC* (*Y*) and produce ions outside this volume, as shown in Figure 7.02. **Electronic equilibrium** is present under these conditions.

Let us refer again to Figure 7.01. The parallel plates labeled "*G*" are grounded **guard plates** whose purpose is to assure a uniform electrical field between plates P_1 and P_2 so that volume *ABCD* is accurately delimited. Without the grounded guard plates, the electrical field would bulge outward at *AD* and *BC*

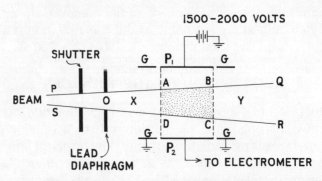

FIGURE 7.01. Standard free-air ionization chamber. For detailed description, see text.

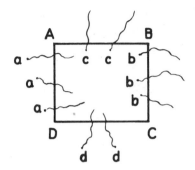

FIGURE 7.02. Electronic equilibrium in the segregated volume of
air—as many electrons enter the
volume from outside as leave the
volume.

instead of having a straight boundary at each end of the segregated volume. The charges collected on plate P_2 are measured by a sensitive electrometer.

Thus far, we have seen that in the free air ionization chamber, a volume of air, *ABCD*, has been segregated and a quantity of X rays has been passed through this volume of air. The liberated ions have been collected, under saturation conditions, and the total charge carried by them has been measured. It remains now to determine accurately volume *ABCD*. Since the beam diverges, and since its edge is not sharply defined due to penumbra, segregated volume *ABCD* cannot be measured accurately. Instead, the **effective volume** is usually employed. If the area of the lead aperture, *O*, is multiplied by the length of the collecting electrodes, the effective volume *A'B'C'D'* is obtained (see Fig. 7.03). But now the exposure given this volume is at *O* rather than at the center of *ABCD*. Because of the inverse square law, the exposure at *O* within the effective volume is the same as the exposure in larger volume *ABCD* at a greater distance from the focal spot, ***provided there is no appreciable attenuation of the beam by absorption between the diaphragm and the segregated volume.*** The expo-

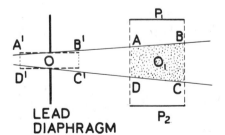

FIGURE 7.03. Volume *A'B'C'D'* is equivalent to volume *ABCD* due to the inverse square law, and can be measured more easily.

**LEAD
DIAPHRAGM**

sure, in roentgens, of the beam entering the chamber is computed by first converting the volume $A'B'C'D'$ to the volume at standard conditions of temperature and pressure (0 C and 760 mm Hg) from appropriate tables. Standard volume is used because the definition of the roentgen specifies 0.001293 g of air, which occupies 1 cc under standard conditions and the volume must therefore be convertible to grams. The charge in esu collected by plate P_2 is obtained from the electrometer reading. If the beam has traversed the chamber for t seconds, the exposure rate at the front of the lead diaphragm may be obtained from the following equation:

$$R/\text{sec} = \frac{Q}{t} \times \frac{1}{A'B'C'D'} \tag{7}$$

where Q is the number of esu collected in time t sec and $A'B'C'D'$ is the area of the aperture times the length of the plate, or the effective volume in cm^3 corrected to 0 C and 760 mm Hg.

The requirements of a standard free-air ionization chamber may be summarized as follows:

1. Primary photons must not hit the plates.
2. Plates must be separated sufficiently so that even the fastest primary electrons can dissipate their energy without first striking one of the plates.
3. Chamber must be far enough from the diaphragm to allow as many primary electrons to enter the segregated volume of air as leave it, in order to have electronic equilibrium.
4. Saturation voltage must be applied to the plates.
5. Segregated volume of air must be measurable to high degree of accuracy.
6. Tiny current carried by ions must be measured with extreme accuracy.
7. It must be assumed that there is no appreciable absorption of photons in air between the diaphragm and the segregated volume of air. When necessary, appropriate correction factors must be applied for absorption in air.
8. The range of the primary electrons must be far less than the mean free path of the photons.

Since the official definition of the roentgen specifies X or γ radiation, let us now see how it actually applies in the case of γ rays. According to the preceding summary the ionization chamber must be of such a size that the fastest primary electrons do not strike the electrode plates, and equilibrium of primary electrons prevails in the segregated volume of air. However, in view of the fact that the fastest electrons liberated by γ rays have a relatively long range in air, the ordinary free air chamber does not meet the dimensional requirement.

The free air ionization chamber used with X rays up to 250 kV has plates measuring about 20 cm long, separated by the same distance. In the case of γ rays, a chamber would have to be equipped with plates about 4 meters long separated by a distance of about 2 meters! Chambers of this size, and even larger, have actually been constructed for the purpose of determining the γ roentgen. However, there is a method utilizing compressed air, up to about 10 atmospheres, in a chamber slightly larger than the one used with 250-kV X rays. Compression of the air forces more molecules into the segregated volume, this being equivalent to a much larger volume of noncompressed air.

According to the most accurate measurements available, the exposure rate of γ radiation at 1 cm from a point source of 1 mg of radium filtered by 0.5 mm Pt is 8.26 $\pm$ 0.5 R/hr (Attix and Ritz,[2] 1956). However, *the most widely used value in clinical radiation therapy is 8.25 R/hr*. This is called the *specific γ-ray constant* (Γ) of radium.

VICTOREEN CONDENSER-R-METER

The standard free-air ionization chamber is not suitable for use in the radiotherapy department, in that it is a delicate precision instrument requiring meticulous technique and, besides, cannot be used in a body cavity. Much more convenient, and sufficiently accurate for the practical calibration of a therapy machine in terms of roentgen output, is the *condenser-R-meter* invented by Fricke and Glasser (see Fig. 7.06). This device should be calibrated periodically against a long-lived radioactive source, or returned to the manufacturer for calibration against a standard free air ionization chamber.

In principle, this practical method of radiation dosimetry is reasonably simple. The device consists of four main parts: (1) a thimble chamber, (2) a stem (capacitor), (3) a measuring system (electrometer), and (4) a battery or other power supply.

Thimble Chamber and Capacitor. Figure 7.04 represents diagramatically a thimble chamber and stem.

The thimble wall is made of bakelite, lined on the inside with a conducting material such as graphite to make contact with the metal stem. A central aluminim wire is the other electrode; it is completely insulated from the thimble and stem. Thus, the central wire and the thimble's conducting surface together make up a capacitor—a device which stores electric charge. The attached stem is also a capacitor, serving to increase the capacitance of the unit.

Why is the thimble chamber a valid device for measuring radiation exposure? The answer lies in the fact that the thimble is designed to be *air equivalent.* To understand air equivalence, let us first refer to Figure 7.05. In *B* is shown the cavity of a hypothetical chamber whose wall consists of ordinary air, the arrows indicating the maximum range of the primary electrons liberated within this "air wall" and causing ionization in the central volume. Evidently, the thickness of the air wall must be at least equal to (or barely greater than) the range of the fastest primary electrons so that even those released in the outermost part of the wall can reach the cavity. At the same time, the photon beam must not undergo excessive attenuation in the wall. Under these

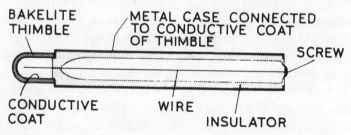

FIGURE 7.04. Thimble chamber and attached stem (capacitor) for Victoreen-R-meter®.

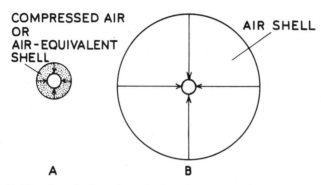

FIGURE 7.05. The air-wall of an air-equivalent shell in *A* undergoes nearly the same degree of ionization as a true air shell in *B* containing the same number of atoms.

conditions, electronic equilibrium will have been achieved. In *A* the air wall has been compressed into a shell (equivalent to the wall of a thimble chamber). The thickness of this shell is such that electronic equilibrium will occur in it just as in the larger thickness of uncompressed air. The mean free path or average distance range of the electrons will be shorter in the compressed air shell than in the uncompressed one, but they will encounter the same number of air molecules. Moreover, the same number of electrons will enter the segregated central air volume in *B* as in *A*, for the same radiation exposure. Such a hypothetical compressed air wall chamber could be used to measure exposure in roentgens since the unit of exposure is based on ionization in air under equilibrium conditions, analogous to the situation in a standard free-air ionization chamber. However, the latter is too cumbersome and too difficult to use in a clinical setting.

Turning now to the thimble ionization chamber, how can it be made air equivalent? This requires that its wall material have the same *effective atomic number* Z_{eff} as air—about 7.64. In other words, the *attenuating properties for X and γ radiation up to 3 MeV should be the same for the thimble wall as for air.* Under these conditions the thimble wall would resemble a shell of compressed air, as described above, in which primary electrons set in motion by X or γ rays would have a reduced distance range relative to that in free air. Note that these electrons are responsible for virtually all the ionization occurring within the small cavity, since the primary electrons released within it produce ionization mainly outside.

Actually, the Z_{eff} of the thimble wall (bakelite, carbon) is more nearly equal to 6. To increase the Z_{eff} to that of air, the central electrode is made of a light metal whose atomic number balances out the Z_{eff} to about 7.6. When the thimble chamber is truly air equivalent the emission of photoelectrons and recoil electrons is similar to that in air and the response of the chamber is proportional to that of the standard free-air ionization chamber. However, wall thickness must be such as to insure electron equilibrium for the energy range of the photons being measured. Since the range of the fastest electrons increases with an increase in the energy of the incoming photons, chamber wall thickness must be increased to coincide with the range of the fastest electrons, thereby achieving *electronic equilibrium* and recording *maximum exposure rates*. In the 100 to 300 kV range, the wall thickness of the thimble is 1 mm, whereas in the case of ^{60}Co γ rays (av. 1.25 MeV) and radium series γ rays (av. 0.83 MeV) the proper wall thickness is 4 mm. Accurate readings require the use of a thimble having a wall thickness appropriate for the particular photon energy range.

The stem to which the thimble is permanently attached is a capacitor, the combination of the two being called the *capacitor chamber*. To the capacitance of this chamber must be added that of the electrometer.

When the thimble is exposed to ionizing radiation after the system (capacitor chamber and electrometer) has been charged to the full voltage, the loss of charge is proportional to the voltage drop, as well as to the exposure in R. The *sensitivity* of the capacitor chamber and electrometer system is the voltage drop per R, and is defined by the following expression:

$$S = k \frac{V}{C} \tag{8}$$

where S is the sensitivity, k is a constant (1000/3), V is the volume of the thimble chamber (cm^3), and C is the capacitance of the system (microfarads). Thus, in measuring a large R exposure we need a chamber of small volume and a system of large capacitance (low sensitivity), and conversely, because sensitivity is directly proportional to the chamber volume and inversely proportional to the capacitance of the system.

Electrometer. The loss of charge resulting from exposure of the thimble to ionizing radiation is measured by an electrometer which gives a readout in R on a calibrated scale. In the Victoreen-R-meter, shown in Figure 7.06, the electrometer portion is of the string type, consisting of a very fine movable platinum wire mounted on a supporting rod and kept under tension by a quartz fiber loop (see Fig. 7.07). The platinum wire, usually called the *string*, is completely insulated from the grounded case. Near the string, and perpendicular to it, is a *deflector electrode.*

In use, the capacitor chamber is inserted into the meter and the entire system charged by a friction wheel or power supply. This places a positive charge on the string, inducing a negative charge on the deflector electrode which then attracts the string, bowing it out of its straight position. The string is now over the zero mark on the scale as seen through the microscope. Next, the capacitor chamber is removed, the protective cap placed on the end away from the thimble, and the chamber placed in the X- or γ-ray beam for exposure during an appropriate time interval

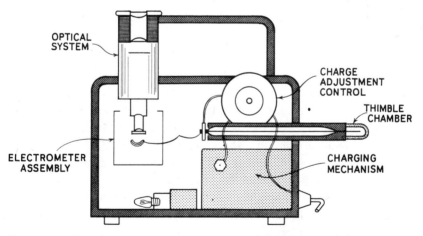

FIGURE 7.06. Diagram of a Victoreen-R-meter®, based on data furnished by the Victoreen Instrument Corporation.

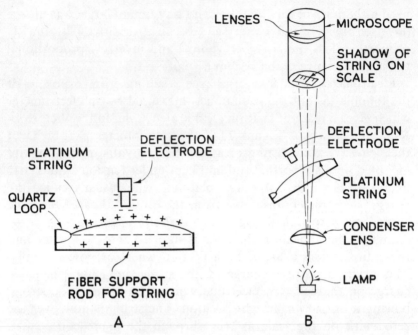

FIGURE 7.07. Details of the components of the Victoreen-R-meter®. In *A* is shown the platinum string supported at one end by a quartz loop to allow motion of the string when acted upon by the oppositely charged deflection electrode. In *B* is shown the arrangement of the microscope, scale, platinum string, and light source.

(i.e. to produce about ½ to ⅔ scale deflection of the string). Because of the protective cap and the design of the chamber, ionization occurs only in the thimble, although with photon energies of 2 MeV or more, significant stem ionization occurs and must be taken into account. The amount of discharge of the capacitor chamber is proportional to the exposure and is measured by reinsertion into the fully charged electrometer, whereupon the deflection of the string decreases, shifting to a new position on the scale. Finally, correction factors must be applied where necessary (see pages 190 to 192). The exposure rate, then, is the corrected R divided by the time during which the chamber was exposed to radiation.

Thimbles of various capacities are available: 25 R, 100 R, and 250 R. There is also a thimble with a capacity of 0.25 R to measure stray radiation.

Calibration of a Victoreen-R-Meter. For maximum accuracy the entire radiation meter requires calibration against a standard free-air ionization chamber, either by the manufacturer, the National Bureau of Standards, or a regional calibration laboratory. This should be done when the instrument is first purchased, and then annually. In addition, local calibration should be performed about every two months against a long-lived radionuclide as a standard, each time under the same geometric setup. Calibration should be carried out for each radiation quality being used. The factor by which the meter reading must be multiplied to obtain the same reading as that at the testing laboratory is called the **calibration factor.** It is of interest that with lower energy radiation in which photoelectric interaction is important, the composition of the thimble wall is critical (probability of photoelectric effect varies directly with Z^3). On the other hand, with higher energy radiation in which Compton interaction predominates, wall composition is not so critical because the probability of this interaction is virtually independent of the atomic number of the absorber; instead, the critical factors are the volume of the chamber or the sensitivity of the electrometer, or both.

OTHER TYPES OF DOSIMETERS

There are several additional types of dosimeters available for radiotherapy. In one way or another, they all measure ionization.

A type of electrometer, not so widely used as the Victoreen-R-meter, is the **Baldwin Farmer Secondary Standard Dosemeter.** In this unit a capacitor chamber is connected by a shielded cable to the grid of an **electrometer tube,** a special type of triode. This device makes it possible to expose the capacitor chamber to the radiation beam while it is attached to the electrometer. Thus, the chamber does not have to be removed and reinserted into the electrometer during the calibration of a therapy machine.

The **integrating dosimeter** is an elaborate device built around a thimble chamber, so designed that it can be set for a given total roentgen exposure. The thimble chamber is placed in the X-ray beam at the center of the treatment field, in contact with the skin.

When the preselected number of roentgens has been delivered, the dosimeter automatically turns off the X-ray machine. Such a dosimeter system is usually employed in administering a daily treatment dose. Because of its complexity, and the resultant danger of error, it should be checked frequently.

Another device used to check radiation output is the *iometer* or *monitor ionization chamber.* It consists of a set of capacitor plates, charged to a known potential. The radiation passes through the capacitor which is placed between the tube and the patient. Ionization of the air in the vicinity of the capacitor results in its discharge approximately in proportion to the radiation exposure. However, since this system is strongly wavelength dependent, it must never be used to determine the exposure in R, nor should it be used for calibration of equipment. It merely indicates the constancy of output under the operating conditions.

The *Failla extrapolation chamber* is exclusively a precision laboratory device. It permits highly accurate determination of exposure in R at the surface and in the depth of a phantom. The air spacing between a pair of extremely thin electrodes is varied by minute degrees, and a curve is plotted showing the relationship of ionization to the electrode spacings. The curve can be extended (extrapolated) to an air space of zero thickness, giving an accurate surface exposure. It can also be used to give precise exposure at any level within a phantom.

CALIBRATION OF AN X-RAY OR GAMMA-RAY BEAM

The exposure in roentgens, as measured by a thimble chamber at a particular distance from an X-ray tube focus or a γ-ray source, with the chamber surrounded by a large thickness of air, is called the *in-air exposure.* No scattering material other than air should be located in the vicinity of the chamber. The determination of the in-air exposure rate is the most satisfactory method of calibrating an X- or γ-ray beam, from the standpoints of both simplicity and reproducibility. When done accurately, this kind of calibration is eminently satisfactory for radiation therapy and should include the following steps:

1. ***Select the Thimble Chamber.*** While this should generally be based on anticipated exposure rate as well as energy of the beam, a 25-R or, at most, a 100-R, chamber is preferred. The capacity of the chamber should be such that about $\frac{1}{2}$ to $\frac{2}{3}$ scale deflection occurs in a convenient time interval of 0.5 to 2 sec. Wall thickness should be adequate for electronic equilibrium; thus, it should be 1 mm for 100- to 250-kV X rays, and 4 mm for cobalt 60 γ rays. However, a 3 mm slip-on cap is available to adapt the 1 mm chamber to the measurement of cobalt 60 γ rays.

2. ***Charge the Capacitor Chamber-Electrometer System.*** Insert the stem or bayonet end of the capacitor chamber into the Victoreen meter and charge until the scale reads "O." The chamber is now fully charged. Recall that during the process, opposite and equal charges are placed on the chamber—central wire positive and wall negative.

3. ***Position the Capacitor Chamber.*** Mount the chamber securely with the thimble portion in the center of the beam at the proposed treatment distance. No objects should be near enough to scatter radiation into the chamber. Avoid having the crosshair shadow of the beam localizer fall on the thimble, and collimate the beam to 10 cm × 10 cm. Readings at the same distance may differ significantly with different size beams because of scattering from within the collimator or cone.

4. ***Make the Exposure.*** Start the exposure, using the timer on the control panel. Be sure to select the correct operating factors. Maximum accuracy is obtained if the exposure is about $\frac{1}{2}$ to $\frac{2}{3}$ the capacity of the chamber. During the actual exposure keep the Victoreen meter outside the therapy room or behind a suitable protective barrier.

5. ***Read the Meter.*** Remove the protective cap and again insert the stem end of the chamber into the meter opening. When the button is depressed, the roentgen exposure (uncorrected) can be read directly on the illuminated scale corresponding to the chamber used. The meter scale is calibrated in R, but the actual deflection of the string shadow on the scale results from the change in potential difference between the central wire and thimble wall due to ionization by the X or γ rays. If the scale were calibrated in volts, a table would have to be used to convert volts

to R. Calibration of the scale in R obviates the need of such a table. Three separate readings should be average for each combination of distance, collimation, and operating factors.

6. **Correct the Exposure Reading.** A number of errors inhere in the calibration of a therapy unit. These will now be summarized.

a. *Stem Ionization or Leakage.* Ionization of air in the stem portion of the capacitor chamber introduces a significant error, especially with high energy radiation and with large capacity chambers (e.g. 100-R and 250-R). This results from the fact that the thimble of such large capacity chambers is **small** and therefore the volume of air in the stem portion is a significantly large fraction of the total volume of the capacitor chamber. Stem ionization or leakage can be determined by placing the chamber first with the thimble alone in the beam, and then turning it to include also the stem. If there is significant leakage, correction should be made, unless this has already been done during the initial calibration of the instrument by the manufacturer or the U.S. Bureau of Standards.

b. *Shutter Time.* Since a finite time is usually required for the shutter mechanism to open and close, the true exposure rate may actually be larger than would be indicated by the measuring instrument. For example, if calibration time is 40 sec and it takes the shutter 4 sec to open and close, the actual "on" time was 36 sec and hence the exposure rate was larger by a factor of 40/36 or 11 percent. A simple way to ascertain shutter time is to make an exposure of the same total duration as that in step 4, but open and close the shutter twice during the exposure. If shutter time is significant, this reading will be less than the one in step 4. The difference is added to the latter to correct for the noninstantaneous opening and closing of the shutter. Let us see how this correction is made in a hypothetical situation:

(1) Scale deflection with 1 opening and closing of shutter is found to be 80 "R" in a total time of 40 sec ("R" is scale deflection uncorrected for shutter time.)

(2) Scale deflection with 2 openings and closings of shutter is 70 "R" in total time of 40 sec.

(3) Loss of R due to shutter time is then 80 "R" − 70 "R" = 10 "R", where "R" is still uncorrected for other factors.

(4) Adding (1) and (3), 80 "R" + 10 "R" = 90 "R" in 40 sec, corrected for shutter time only.

(5) To find actual shutter time we first note that 90 "R"/40 sec = 2.3 "R"/sec. Since we "lost" 10 "R" because of shutter time in step (3),

$$\frac{10 \text{ "R"}}{2.3 \text{ "R"/sec}} = 4.4 \text{ sec, the actual shutter time}$$

(6) In calculating treatment times for the exposure chart, we must include the shutter time, if significant.

c. *Cone Distance Correction.* As shown in Figure 7.08, when a cone is used the thimble cannot be placed at the cone distance because of the diameter of the thimble. The actual distance D of the center of the thimble is the treatment distance d (i.e. focus-skin distance) plus the thimble radius r:

$$D = d + r \tag{9}$$

If the exposure rate measured at the position D of the thimble is I, then the exposure rate i at the true treatment distance d (end of cone) may be obtained with sufficient accuracy by application of the inverse square law as modified on pages 10 and 11. Since id^2 is constant if all operating factors are constant,

$$i = \frac{I(d + r)^2}{d^2} \tag{10}$$

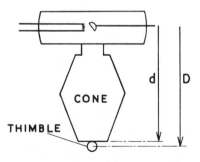

FIGURE 7.08. Inasmuch as the thimble chamber cannot be placed half-way within the cone, its true distance from the target is D, the thimble radius being $D-d$, where d is the target-skin distance.

In general, if the distance of the center of the thimble from the cone end is less than 2 percent of the treatment distance the error is insignificant and may be neglected.

d. *Calibration Factor.* This relates the instrument reading to that of the free-air ionization chamber and is supplied by the manufacturer or calibrating agency.

e. *Temperature and Atmospheric Pressure Correction.* Initial calibration of the capacitor chamber against a free-air ionization chamber is usually carried out under standard conditions of 22 C (295 K or absolute) and 760 mm Hg. Therefore the reading obtained in calibrating a therapy unit must be corrected to standard conditions according to the following equation:

$$\underset{\substack{corrected\ for \\ temperature \\ and\ pressure}}{R/min} = \underset{reading}{`R'/min} \left(\frac{760}{P}\right)\left(\frac{273 + T}{295}\right)K \qquad (11)$$

where 'R' is the meter reading corrected for shutter time, P is the atmospheric pressure in mm Hg, T is the temperature in C, and K is the calibration factor for the meter. Finally, when a cone is used we must make an inverse square law correction according to equation (10).

ADDITIONAL PRECAUTIONS IN BEAM CALIBRATION

It is important to take certain precautions in the calibration of an X- or γ-ray beam, in addition to those already discussed.

1. At any particular treatment distance, the beam must be calibrated for each size cone or collimator opening.

2. Calibration must be done at each and every treatment distance.

3. The thimble must be in the center of the beam, oriented with its long axis perpendicular to the central ray.

4. We must avoid the presence of scattering material in the vicinity of the thimble chamber in obtaining the in-air exposure rate because scattered radiation would contribute additional ionization to the thimble and give a falsely high reading. Any

scattering medium, such as table, floor, or wall, must be at a distance from the thimble no less than four times the distance of the thimble from the source. The filter must also be at least 15 cm from the thimble at 200 kV in order that secondary radiation from the Al forefilter be absorbed in air before reaching the thimble.

5. The correct thimble chamber for the particular quality of radiation must be used, because the thimbles are **energy dependent.** They have been calibrated for a definite range of energies and if used at some other energy will give erroneous readings (see page 184). Where the discrepancy is not too great, correction tables may be used.

6. An X-ray therapy machine must be fully "warmed up" to the peak kV at which the calibration is to be done. Furthermore, the kV and mA must be watched closely during calibration. For example, an error of 5 kV at a 200-kV setting introduces an error of 5 or more percent in the exposure. An error of 1 mA in 10 causes an error of 10 percent in the exposure.

7. With beams of large size, say 10 cm × 10 cm or greater, additional exposure determinations should be made at the corners of the field. With circular beams, several readings should be made at the periphery in order to check the uniformity of the beam throughout its cross section.

8. Readings should also be made just outside the beam to determine the shielding efficiency of the cone or collimator.

9. The capacitor chambers and electrometer should be returned to the manufacturer periodically for recalibration.

UNITS OF RADIATION EXPOSURE AND DOSAGE

There are at the present time two units of physical and biological radiation dose that are of interest to the radiotherapist: the roentgen and the rad. A third unit, roentgen equivalent man or REM, is used in health physics and will be discussed in Chapter 17.

1. **Roentgen.** As defined above, 1 roentgen is a specific quantity of X rays or γ rays, which produces 2.08×10^9 ion pairs in 1 cc of air under strictly specified conditions. This may be derived as follows: 1 R produces 1 esu of charge of either sign in

1 cc of air (standard conditions, 0 C and 760 mm Hg). Since the charge on one ion is 4.8×10^{-10} esu,

$$\frac{1 \text{ esu}}{4.8 \times 10^{-10} \text{ esu}} = 2.08 \times 10^9 \text{ ion pairs/cm}^3$$

On the average, 33.7 electron volts are required to produce one ion pair in air. Therefore,

$$33.7 \text{ eV} \times 2.08 \times 10^9 = 7.01 \times 10^{10} \text{ eV}$$

representing the energy absorbed by 1 cc of standard air exposed to 1 R. This can be converted to the energy absorbed by 1 gram of air as follows:

1 cc air weighs 0.001293 g (under standard conditions)

$$\frac{1 \text{ cc}}{0.001293 \text{ g}} = 773.4 \text{ cc, the volume of 1 g air}$$

$$7.01 \times 10^{10} \times 773.4 = 5,421 \times 10^{10} = 5.42 \times 10^{13} \text{ eV,}$$
$$\text{energy absorbed by 1 g air}$$

Since $1 \text{ eV} = 1.6 \times 10^{-12}$ erg,

$$5.42 \times 10^{13} \times 1.6 \times 10^{-12} = 87 \text{ ergs absorbed by 1 g air}$$
$$\text{exposed to 1 R}$$

In summary, then, one roentgen is equivalent to the following physical units:

> *in 1 cc air* (O C and 760 mm Hg)
> 1 esu of ions liberated
> 2.08×10^9 ion pairs liberated
> 7.01×10^{10} eV of energy absorbed

> *in 1 g air* 1.61×10^{12} ion pairs liberated
> 5.42×10^{13} eV of energy absorbed
> 87 ergs of energy absorbed

> *in 1 kg air* 2.58×10^{-4} coulomb

2. *Rad.* In 1953, the Seventh International Congress of Radiology adopted a unit of absorbed dose, the *rad.* It is independent

of the type of radiation, and represents an absorbed dose of 100 ergs/g or 10^{-2} joules/kg (J/kg) of matter. More space will be devoted to the rad in Chapter 9.

FACTORS AFFECTING X-RAY EXPOSURE RATE

Several factors control the output of an X-ray machine. The output may be conveniently rated on the basis of the quantity of radiation per unit time, flowing through a unit cross section, as already described. This is designated as the intensity of radiation. However, in radiotherapy the exposure rate in R/min is generally used to denote intensity, rather than the more rigorous erg/cm^2-sec or joules/m^2-sec. Therefore, in the following discussion whenever the term intensity is used, reference is being made to the exposure rate in R/min, or R per unit time.

Tube Potential. As we increase the potential applied to the X-ray tube, the speed and kinetic energy of the electrons are increased. When 69.5 kV or more is applied to the conventional X-ray tube with a tungsten target, the kinetic energy of the electrons is sufficient to release K electrons and excite tungsten characteristic radiation. Furthermore, as the kV is increased the resulting brems radiation contains photons of higher energy and therefore has greater penetrating power.

Besides the increase in **photon energy** produced by larger tube potentials, there is also an increase in the intensity or **exposure rate.** This is due to the increase in the number of photons emitted per unit time as well as in their maximum energy as the tube potential is increased. The exposure rate is roughly proportional to the square of the applied kV in the orthovoltage region. For example, let us compare the output at 140 kV with that at 200 kV, keeping all other factors constant:

$$\frac{R/\text{min at 200 kV}}{R/\text{min at 140 kV}} = \frac{(200)^2}{(140)^2} = 2:1 \text{ (approximately)}$$

Thus, the exposure rate is approximately doubled as the tube potential is raised from 140 to 200 kV.

As a general rule, then, we may state that as tube potential is increased, there results (1) improved quality or penetrating power of the X-ray beam, and (2) increase in exposure rate.

It is interesting to observe that X-ray production is a relatively inefficient process. In the range 100 to 250 kV, less than 1 per cent of the electron energy in the X-ray tube is converted to useful X rays; the remainder degenerates to heat, creating the problem of dissipation of the unwanted heat in the anode. However, X-ray production becomes increasingly more efficient at higher potentials. Thus, at 20 MeV and above, the efficiency is so great that no special provision is made for heat dissipation in the traget.

Tube Current. As the tube current (milliamperage) is increased (by increasing the current and thermionic emission of the filament) the intensity of the X-ray beam changes almost in direct proportion. Any deviation from this rule is usually due to a change in the wave form of the tube potential associated with a change in tube current. The increased tube current means that more electrons strike the target per second, producing more X-ray photons per second, and therefore increasing the quantity of radiation per second, or the exposure rate (e.g. R/min). The penetrating power is not changed by altering the tube current alone, if the tube potential remains constant.

Time. The exposure in R is proportional to the time of exposure, with a given exposure rate. Thus,

$$Exposure = Exposure\ Rate \times Time$$

$$R = R/min \times min \tag{12}$$

Distance. The change in exposure rate at a given point in the beam, due to change in distance from the tube focus (or source of radiation), follows the inverse square law. It states that the exposure rate of radiation at a given point in the beam is inversely proportional to its distance squared, as measured from a point source. The law applies to a fair approximation with the usual focal spot in radiotherapy, but does not apply to brachytherapy with needles or plaques. A simple analogy is found by comparison with a shower head—the water droplets are farther apart at greater and greater distances from the shower head. Similarly,

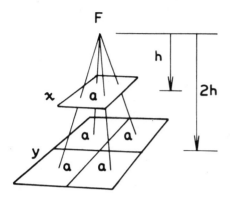

FIGURE 7.09. The inverse square law. At distance *h* the beam covers area *a*. At twice the distance (*2h*) the same beam covers area 4*a*. Therefore, the intensity of radiation, or the amount falling on a unit area, is 1/4 as great on plane *y* as on plane *x*.

the photons diverge as they move away from the focal spot. There are various ways of proving this law which, incidentally, applies to all forms of electromagnetic radiation.

Proof 1. Referring to Figure 7.09, note that four individual photons have been selected, originating at source or focal spot *F*. In plane *X*, the selected square surface *a* receives all four photons. Plane *Y* is at a distance from *F* twice that of plane *X* (*2h* and *h*, respectively). Due to divergence of the beam, only one photon strikes an area *a* in plane *Y*. In other words, the area *a* in plane *Y* receives ¼ the number of photons per second, and the intensity is accordingly ¼. Thus, if the distance is doubled, the intensity is $\frac{1}{2}^2 = \frac{1}{4}$, the initial value. Similarly, if the distance is tripled, the intensity is $\frac{1}{3}^2 = \frac{1}{9}$. On the other hand, if the distance is halved, the intensity becomes $1/(\frac{1}{2})^2 = 1/\frac{1}{4} = 4$ times the initial value.

Proof 2. The radiation leaves an X-ray tube in the form of a conical beam. In Figure 7.10 the upper plane is a circle of radius *r*, and the lower plane, at twice the distance, is a circle of radius *R*. All of the photons passing through plane *a* will also pass through plane *A*.

$$\pi r^2 = \text{area of plane } a$$

$$\pi R^2 = \text{area of plane } A$$

Since $R = 2r$,

$$\pi(2r)^2 = 4\pi r^2 = \text{area of plane } A$$

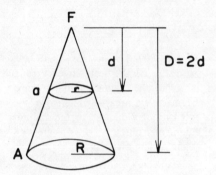

FIGURE 7.10. The inverse square law can be derived more rigorously by the use of a conical figure, since the beam has the form of a cone. (See text.)

Therefore, area of plane A is 4 times larger than that of plane a. Since the same amount of radiation falls on an area 4 times as large, each square centimeter of surface will now receive $\frac{1}{4}$ the radiation in unit time and the exposure rate will be $\frac{1}{4}$ as great.

Proof 3. Based on Figure 7.10, a more rigorous proof can be presented. Since a central vertical section through the cone of radiation is a triangle, and the intersections of the horizontal planes a and A with this triangle produce two similar triangles, we have the proportion

$$R/r = D/d$$

Squaring both sides,

$$R^2/r^2 = D^2/d^2$$

Multiplying the numerator and denominator of the left member by 4π,

$$4\pi R^2/4\pi r^2 = D^2/d^2$$

But $4\pi R^2$ is area A, and $4\pi r^2$ is area a. Therefore,

$$A/a = D^2/d^2 \tag{13}$$

Since the intensity of radiation is inversely proportional to the area which it covers,

$$I_A \text{ proportional to } \frac{1}{A}, \therefore A \text{ proportional to } \frac{1}{I_A}$$

$$I_a \text{ proportional to } \frac{1}{a}, \therefore a \text{ proportional to } \frac{1}{I_a}$$

where I_A is the intensity of radiation falling on plane A and I_a is the intensity of radiation falling on plane a.

Substituting these values in equation (13),

$$\frac{1/I_A}{1/I_a} = \frac{D^2}{d^2}$$

Therefore,

$$\frac{I_a}{I_A} = \frac{D^2}{d^2} \tag{14}$$

Stated in words, equation (14) means that the intensity of radiation on plane a is to the intensity of radiation on plane A as the distance squared of plane A is to the distance squared of plane a.

The reader is strongly urged to review the section in Chapter 1 dealing with the inverse square law. A *simplified method* of practical application is presented there, obviating the need of setting up the equation for the inverse square law, and thereby reducing the chance of error.

In practice, a therapy machine should be calibrated separately at various treatment distances because the radiation does not originate at a point source, but rather in a finite area on the target. However, the inverse square law serves to check the accuracy of such calibration.

Filtration. A filter is a sheet of metal placed in the X-ray beam to improve its quality. The function of a filter depends on the interaction of radiation with matter, as described in Chapter 4. As a result of this interaction, two processes occur in the filter:

a. *Absorption* of radiation (photons) by production of photo-electrons and recoil electrons which are absorbed in the filter material.

b. *Scattering* or deflection of photons out of the main beam. These processes affect both the quantity and the quality of the radiation. A filter decreases the exposure rate of a beam through the processes of absorption and scatter. With a given kV and mA, the thicker the filter and the higher its atomic number, the greater the reduction in exposure rate. However, just below the K absorption edge there is apparently abnormal transmission of low energy photons (see pages 205 to 206).

Since the X-ray beam is polyenergetic (wavelength hetero-geneous), and the lower energy photons are more readily removed from the beam by the filter than are the higher energy photons, there is a relative increase in the number of high energy photons in the emerging beam; in other words, its ***average penetrating power is increased.*** This influence of the filter on the quality of an X-ray beam will be treated in greater detail in the next chapter.

In summary, then, we may state that ***exposure rate***

1. Increases as the kV and mA are increased.
2. Decreases as the distance is increased, in inverse square proportion.
3. Decreases as the thickness and atomic number of the filter are increased.

FACTORS AFFECTING GAMMA RAY QUANTITY

The subject of the control of γ ray quantity and exposure rate is a complex one because of the variety of available sources: inter-stitial radium, telecurietherapy, radionuclides, etc. Therefore the factors affecting γ ray quantity will be discussed later in appro-priate sections.

Insofar as telecurietherapy beams such as ^{60}Co are concerned, the exposure rate is directly proportional to the activity of the source (curies), this being analogous to the potential and current of an X-ray tube. The γ-ray exposure rate is related to the distance between the source and the point of interest by the inverse square law as described for X-ray beams.

CHAPTER 8

X-ray Quality

FROM the strictly physical standpoint, the *quality* of an ordinary X-ray beam is completely specified by its *spectral distribution curve,* owing to the fact that such a beam is *polyenergetic,* being made up of photons of different energies (or wavelengths). The spectral distribution curve represents the relative intensities of photons of various energies.

Why is an X-ray beam polyenergetic? The answer may be found in the fundamental process of X-ray production, and includes the following factors:

1. *Fluctuation of Tube Potential.* The potential difference applied across the X-ray tube fluctuates widely from zero to a maximum, in step with the alternating current supply. (This range of variation is small in the constant potential circuit.) Therefore, the electrons in the tube are endowed with different velocities, and hence possess a range of kinetic energies. The resulting X-ray photons also have various energies, frequencies, and wavelengths.

2. *Brems Radiation.* The varying degrees of deceleration of electrons resulting from interaction with the strong nuclear electrostatic fields of the target atoms produce photons that vary in energy and wavelength.

3. *Characteristic Radiation.* If the applied kV is sufficiently high, characteristic radiation is excited in the target atoms, with the appearance of spectral lines (see Fig. 8.01).

4. *Multiple Interactions.* The electrons in the X-ray tube dissipate their kinetic energies either by single or multiple interactions with target atoms. Since different amounts of energy appear as photons, these too must have a range of energies.

ANALYSIS OF X-RAY BEAMS

When a polyenergetic beam is analyzed into its component photons by an X-ray spectrometer, and the relative intensities (e.g. exposure rates) are plotted as a function of their respective energies, a spectral distribution is obtained (see Fig. 8.01). Note that the curve has a high point or **maximum** which indicates the energy interval responsible for the maximum intensity or exposure rate. To the left and right of the maximum there is a progressive decrease in the radiation intensity corresponding to each energy interval. Such a continuous smooth curve describes the **general radiation** emitted by an X-ray tube. It is also known as "white radiation" by analogy with white light. The curve crosses the horizontal axis at the right corresponding to the maximum photon energy (minimum wavelength) in the beam in question. Maximum photon energy depends on the peak potential applied to the tube.

As described before, the kinetic energy (*K.E.*) of the electrons in an X-ray tube is changed, in part, to X-ray photons through

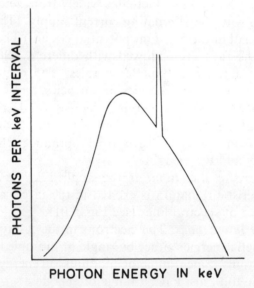

PHOTON ENERGY IN keV

FIGURE 8.01. Spectral distribution curve of a photon beam. The spike in the curve represents the *characteristic radiation* from a tungsten target superimposed on the *general radiation* (bremsstrahlung). A minimum energy of 69.5 keV is needed for the emission of tungsten *K*-characteristic radiation. Note that the characteristic radiation actually consists of a series of closely spaced lines and accounts for only a small fraction of the total radiation output (about 10 percent at 150 kV, decreasing rapidly above this kV).

the bremsstrahlung process. In the case of a small fraction of the electrons, their total K.E. is converted to photons of equal energy hv_{max} by head-on collision with nuclei of target atoms. Accordingly, any electron that happens to be accelerated by the peak tube potential (kVp) will have maximum *K.E.* and, during head-on collision with a nucleus, all of this *K.E.* will appear as a photon having maximum energy (or minimum wavelength) in this particular X-ray beam. Thus,

kVp = K.E. of fastest electron = hv_{max} (energy of most energetic photon)

In 1915 Duane and Hunt derived a simple equation expressing this relationship:

$$\lambda_{min} = \frac{12.4}{kVp} \qquad (1)$$

where λ_{min} is the minimum wavelength in Å and kVp is the peak kilovoltage applied to the tube. Equation (1) incidentally shows that as the kVp increases, the minimum wavelength of the generated X rays decreases. As a result, the frequency and hence the energy of the photons increases.

To find the energy of the most energetic photon in an X-ray beam, we substitute its energy hv_{max} for kVp in equation (1), and rearrange as follows:

$$hv_{max} = \frac{12.4}{\lambda_{min}}$$

where hv_{max} is in keV.

If the applied potential is high enough to dislodge K electrons of the tube target atoms, characteristic radiation is emitted, producing discontinuities in the curve of general radiation. At the energy intervals corresponding to the characteristic radiation, sharp peaks of intensity occur in the curve, as shown in Figure 8.01.

The dependence of the maximum photon energy on the energy of the electron producing it, can be demonstrated by a comparison of the two curves of general radiation obtained with the same tube operated at different potentials (see Fig. 8.02). It is obvious that at 200 kV, photons with higher maximum energy are produced than at 100 kV. Furthermore, the energy interval having the maximum intensity (peak of the curve) shifts to a higher energy. Finally, the relative exposure rate of the beam as a whole increases at higher kV, as shown by the greater area under curve B than under curve A.

It should be pointed out that the distribution of the photon energies, including the peak photon energy, in the *continuous spectrum* is governed solely by the *tube potential*. On the other hand, the *energy of the characteristic photons* increases with increasing *atomic number of the target element*. Interestingly enough, all other factors being equal, the radiation *intensity* is proportional to the atomic number of the target element. X-ray generating

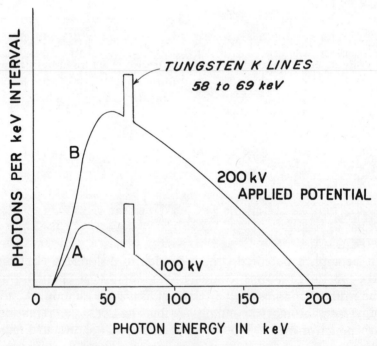

FIGURE 8.02. Comparison of spectral distribution curves for a tungsten target with applied potential of 100 and 200 kV, same filtration. Maximum photon energy increases with increasing applied potential. As indicated by the areas under the curves, total radiation output also increases with increasing operating potential.

equipment may be somewhat arbitrarily assigned the following kilovoltage ranges:

Grenz-ray therapy	10 to 20 kV
Superficial X-ray therapy	50 to 140 kV
Orthovoltage X-ray therapy	150 to 500 kV
Megavoltage X-ray therapy	1 MV and above

Some reserve the term megavoltage for photon energy of 1 to 2 MeV, and use the expression ultra-high voltage for higher energies than this.

MODIFICATION OF X-RAY BEAMS BY FILTERS

Let us now consider the effect of placing various thicknesses of absorbing material, called *filters,* in the X-ray beam. In general, a filter removes relatively more low than high energy photons, although all types of photons are removed to some extent. This change results from their interaction with atoms in the filter.

However, there is an apparent contradiction to the preceding statement in that filters display anomalous behavior in trans-mitting low energy photons under certain conditions. As we have already indicated, each electronic shell has a particular binding energy, and this is certainly true of the atoms of the filter. Upon passing through a filter, the continuous spectrum undergoes a change manifested by the appearance of sharp discontinuities or peaks at photon energies in the regions of the electronic binding energies of the filter atoms. These peaks occur just below *absorption edges* corresponding to the binding energies of inner shells. Furthermore, a filter may be "transparent" to photons of relatively low energy. How is this explained? Let us examine tin (used in the Thoraeus filter) whose *K absorption* edge is at 29.25 keV. The photons with energy just below 29.25 keV will not have enough energy to interact photoelectrically with K electrons and will have too much energy to interact significantly with L electrons. (Recall that photoelectric interaction has the greatest chance of occurring when the incident photons have energy just above the binding energy of the shell.) Therefore, such photons are transmitted through the filter. Furthermore, photons with energy just above the *K* shell will interact with *K* electrons, the resulting holes being filled by electron transitions (cascade) from higher energy levels with accompanying emission of tin characteristic radiation for the *K* shell, appearing as spikes in the spectral distribution curve of the radiation that has passed through the tin (see Fig. 8.03). Because of the "transparency" of tin below its *K* absorption edge a copper filter is used beyond the tin to absorb the transmitted, as well as characteristic, radiation.

With radiation in the orthovoltage region, except for the absorption edge effect, the *lower* the energy of the photons, the *larger* the total mass attenuation coefficient and, therefore, the *greater* the likelihood that the photons will be absorbed. Hence, the beam emerges from the filter with a larger percentage of high energy photons than it had upon entering the filter. Such a beam has a greater average penetrating power and is said to have been *hard-*

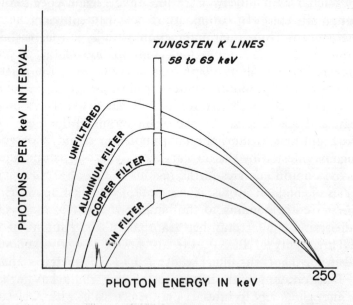

FIGURE 8.03. Spectral distribution curves with various filters, of a 250-kV beam, *tungsten* target. Filtration does not affect maximum photon energy—250 keV; it depends only on the applied kVp. An increase in the atomic number *Z* of a filter shifts the maximum of each curve (general radiation) to a higher photon energy, while the exposure rate decreases. Small spikes at the left end of the curve with the tin filter represent *tin K*-characteristic radiation.

ened by the filter. Figure 8.03 shows the approximate effect of filter atomic number on the hardening of an X-ray beam.

Note that as filtration is increased, the photon energy interval having the maximum intensity increases. Furthermore, heavier filtration does not change the maximum photon energy because, according to equation (1), this is a function of peak kV only. Finally, the exposure rate decreases as filtration increases because, in the passage of the beam through the filter, photons are absorbed or scattered, thereby reducing the total amount of radiation remaining in the beam.

What has just been stated in descriptive form can be considered also on the basis of *attenuation coefficients.* It will be recalled that the linear attenuation coefficient specifies the fractional decrease in the intensity of an X-ray beam per unit increase in thickness of absorber—the greater this attenuation coefficient the greater the fall in intensity of the beam per unit thickness of filter. Now, other factors remaining constant, the attenuation coefficient depends on the energy of the photons in the incident beam. Thus, if a polyenergetic beam of X rays enters a filter, except for the absorption edge effect (see above), *the attenuation coefficient is greater for the less energetic (longer wavelength) X rays than for the more energetic ones.* Therefore the former are absorbed to a relatively greater degree. However, just below the K absorption edge, and to a much smaller degree, the L absorption edge, there is an abrupt drop in the attenuation coefficient.

Summary. The foregoing discussion may be briefly summarized as follows:

1. The quality of an X-ray beam, from the standpoint of the *physicist,* is characterized by its spectral distribution curve of the energies of the constituent photons.

2. The quality of an X-ray beam, from the standpoint of the *therapeutic radiologist,* may be defined as its *penetrating power.*

3. The average penetrating power of an X-ray beam improves with increasing tube potential.

4. The quality of an X-ray beam improves with increasing thickness and atomic number of the filter. A filter removes relatively more low energy than high energy photons, with the exception of the edge phenomenon and the characteristic radiation emitted by the filter.

5. The continuous spectrum of an X-ray beam depends on the applied tube potential, whereas the characteristic radiation depends on the atomic number of the target element.

SPECIFICATION OF X-RAY QUALITY IN RADIOTHERAPY

Thus far, beam quality has been discussed entirely on the basis of its complete specification, but this is too cumbersome for radiation therapy. Because of the complexity of the various factors governing X-ray quality, some expression simpler than the complete spectral curve had to be devised to specify quality and to permit the radiologist to convey his treatment factors to his colleagues, either by direct communication or in published articles. Since the biologic effect of radiation is not greatly altered by small changes in beam quality, a less complex method than the distribution curve should suffice for radiation therapy.

The usual method of specifying beam quality in orthovoltage therapy include (1) the *half value layer* (*HVL*) and (2) the *accelerating potential* or applied voltage.

1. *Half Value Layer.* From the clinical standpoint, the quality of an X-ray beam may be defined as its *penetrating ability.* On this basis, let us see how a unit of quality may be derived. As we found in Chapter 4 (pages 105 to 109) and Figures 4.14 and 4.15, if a narrow *monoenergetic* beam passes through various thicknesses of the same filter, the exposure rate in R/min will decrease by equal fractions for each unit increase in thickness of filter—the linear (and mass) attenuation coefficient is *constant* (see Table 8.01).

TABLE 8.01
EFFECT OF FILTER THICKNESS ON THE TRANSMISSION OF A
MONOENERGETIC X-RAY BEAM, WHEN EACH MM OF ADDED FILTER
TRANSMITS 80 PER CENT OF THE RADIATION INCIDENT UPON IT.
FOR SIMPLICITY, IT IS ASSUMED THAT THE INITIAL EXPOSURE
RATE IS 100 R/MIN.

Filter Thickness	Transmitted Radiation
mm	*R/min*
1	100
1	80 ($= 0.8 \times 100$)
2	64 ($= 0.8 \times 80$)
3	51 ($= 0.8 \times 64$)
4	41 ($= 0.8 \times 51$)
5	33 ($= 0.8 \times 41$)

In actual practice, however, a beam of X rays. used in radiotherapy is always ***polyenergetic,*** for reasons already given. How
does such a beam behave toward various thicknesses of filter
material? Reference to Figures 4.17 and 8.04 shows that a semilog
plot of an attenuation curve of a polyenergetic beam filtered by
copper has a steeper initial slope, and then gradually flattens.
This is interpreted as follows: as more filter is added, the beam
becomes more nearly "monoenergetic." As a greater percentage
of the softer rays is absorbed, the relative number of harder rays
in the remaining beam increases while the attenuation coefficient
decreases.

As an extension of the concept of the linear attenuation coefficient, the half value layer can be more easily measured and is
a satisfactory way to specify the quality of an X-ray beam for
radiotherapy. The ***half value layer may be defined as that thickness***

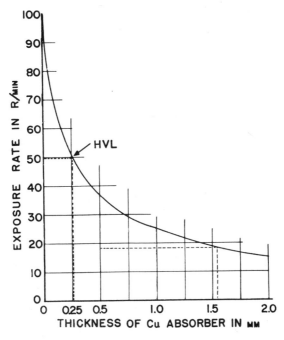

FIGURE 8.04. Transmission curve of a 200-kV beam showing that with increasing
filtration there is progressive increase in the HVL. Thus, with the unfiltered beam
the HVL is 0.25 mm Cu, whereas with an initial filter of 0.5 mm Cu the HVL is
approximately 1.5 mm − 0.5 mm = 1.0 mm Cu.

of a particular filter material which reduces the exposure rate of an X-ray beam to 50 percent of its initial value. The HVL serves as a practical measure of X-ray quality or penetrating ability. Obviously, a beam of harder quality requires a larger thickness of a given absorber for 50 percent attenuation than does one of softer quality. Thus, *the more penetrating beam has a higher HVL.*

Just as in the case of the linear attenuation coefficient, the HVL of a polyenergetic beam is not constant, but increases with increasing filtration. Table 8.02 and Figure 8.04 show that as

TABLE 8.02
EFFECT OF THICKNESS OF A COPPER FILTER ON THE TRANSMISSION OF A *POLYENERGETIC* (*HETEROGENEOUS*) X-RAY BEAM. FOR SIMPLICITY IT IS ASSUMED THAT THE INITIAL EXPOSURE RATE IS 100 R/MIN.

Filter Thickness	Transmitted Radiation
mm	*R/min*
0	100
0.25	50
0.50	37
1.0	25
1.5	19
2.0	15

filtration is increased from zero to 0.5 mm Cu, the HVL increases from 0.25 to 1 mm Cu. But a further increase in filtration by the same amount—from 0.5 to 1.0 mm Cu—would only raise the HVL from 1.0 to 1.2 mm Cu.

The *homogeneity coefficient* (*H.C.*) serves to denote how nearly homogeneous an X-ray beam is with respect to its photon energies. It is *defined as the ratio of the first HVL to the second HVL;* that is, the absorber thickness that decreases the initial exposure rate to one-half, divided by the absorber thickness that decreases the exposure rate from one-half to one-fourth:

$$H.C. = \frac{first\ HVL}{second\ HVL} \tag{2}$$

The *H.C.* of an inhomogeneous beam is a fraction, and it approaches unit the more homogeneous or the more nearly like a "monoenergetic" beam it becomes.

Note that as filtration is increased, the R/min output decreases. Therefore there is a practical limit of filter thickness in orthovoltage therapy with a given combination of kV, mA, and distance.

How is the half value layer of an X-ray beam measured? This can be done relatively simply, provided care is taken that the thimble chamber sees only primary photons that have passed through the filters, a condition called *narrow beam* or *good geometry* (see Fig. 8.05). A brief description of the method of measuring HVL will now be presented:

a. Select the technical factors of kV, mA, and filtration for the *initial beam* whose HVL is to be determined.

b. *Collimate* the beam to 5 cm (narrow beam geometry).

c. Place a *thimble ionization chamber* in the *center* of the beam at a *fixed distance* from the tube focus. To insure good geometry, this should be about 50 cm from the cone cap and filters, and at least several feet from other scattering objects such as table, floor, and walls.

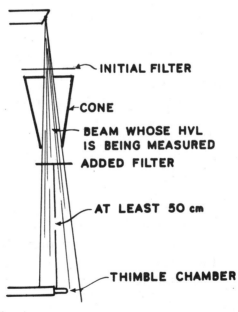

FIGURE 8.05. Arrangement exemplifying "good geometry" for measuring radiation output (exposure rate). Shown are the narrow beam, with the thimble ionization chamber at least 50 cm from the filter, and at least 1 meter from any scattering material.

d. **Measure the exposure rate** (e.g. R/min) with **inherent filtration** only (i.e. tube port, cooling oil, and bakelite cone cover). Tabulate this exposure rate under zero added filtration (i.e. initial beam) as in Table 8.02.

e. Repeat the procedure after adding a 0.25 mm copper filter with orthovoltage therapy, about 200 to 300 kV. All other technical factors remain constant.

f. Repeat the procedure for each of several further additions of copper filters. Assemble the results as in Table 8.02.

g. Plot the data graphically with exposure rate as a function of the total added filtration, as in Figure 8.04.

h. Locate the exposure rate corresponding to one-half the initial value on the vertical axis. Draw a horizontal line from this point to the curve, and then a vertical line from there to the horizontal axis to locate the thickness of copper that is responsible for halving the initial exposure rate. This halving thickness is, then, the HVL in copper.

Suppose now we wish to find the HVL of the beam when it has been filtered initially by 0.5 mm Cu. We first shift the vertical axis to coincide with the 0.5 mm Cu axis. The curve intersects this line at a value of 37 R/min. One half of this is 18.5. Reading across to the curve and then dropping a vertical line, we find the corresponding filter thickness to be about 1.5 mm Cu. But we must subtract from this the initial filter, so 1.5 mm − 0.5 mm = 1.0 mm Cu, the HVL when the initial filter is 0.5 mm Cu. Thus, we see again that an increase in the initial filtration produces a beam with a larger HVL—in other words, a harder beam.

Consideration must be given the kinds of material available for therapy filters. These are shown in Table 8.03. In addition, compound filters such as the Thoraeus filter (see page 244) have been designed for greater efficiency. In the 200 to 250 kV range, it has

TABLE 8.03
FILTER MATERIALS USED IN RADIATION THERAPY

kV Range	Basic Filter Material
below 20	Cellophane
20–150	Aluminum (Al)
150–500	Copper (Cu) or Tin (Sn)
1 MV–50 MV	Lead (Pb)

been found that tin (Sn) absorbs relatively more long wavelength X rays than does copper, with a smaller loss of R/min. A copper filter (called forefilter) is placed on the patient's side of the tin to absorb the characteristic radiation emitted by the tin as well as the radiation transmitted just below the *K*-absorption edge. An aluminum filter is then placed in front of the copper to absorb its characteristic radiation. At the usual treatment distances, the aluminum characteristic rays are absorbed by the intervening air. Even when copper is used without tin, aluminum is used as a forefilter to absorb its characteristic rays. Figure 8.06 is intended to clarify the relationship of the component parts of the compound filter.

2. *Tube Potential.* The HVL of an x-ray beam in a given material depends primarily on the applied potential—the higher the kV the larger the HVL. This is obvious, since a high kV X-ray beam with a relatively large percentage of high energy photons is harder, on the average, than a beam produced at lower kV. Similarly, X rays produced at a constant potential have a larger HVL than X rays produced at the same kV peak and a fluctuating potential. For example, the HVL of an X-ray beam produced at 160 kV by a constant potential generator is approximately the same as that produced at 200 kVp by a full wave generator, while a beam produced at 200 kVp by a Villard generator has a somewhat smaller HVL.

Although, for practical purposes, the HVL adequately specifies the quality of an orthovoltage X-ray beam, the therapist includes

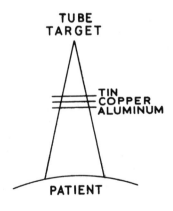

FIGURE 8.06. Thoraeus compound filter, showing the relationship of the component filters.

in his records the kVp and the total filtration (inherent filter + added filter). The reason is that it is possible to have a moderately filtered high kV beam with the same HVL as that of a more heavily filtered lower kV beam. This factor is ordinarily not significant in radiotherapy, and most tables in the literature state only the HVL, omitting reference to the kV. However, the International Commission on Radiation Units and Measurements (ICRU) recommended in 1963 that for radiotherapy up to 2 million volts, the kV or MV and the HVL be included in beam specification. Above 2 MV, the MV only need be stated.

X-ray beams may generally be regarded as "hard" or "soft" for clinical purposes:

a. *Hard beam*—high quality—good penetrating power produced by high tube potential, heavy filtration.

b. *Soft beam*—low quality—poor penetrating power produced by low tube potential, light filtration.

OTHER METHODS OF SPECIFYING X-RAY QUALITY

There are methods other than the HVL for specifying X-ray quality. Although rarely used at present in radiotherapy, they will be described briefly for the sake of completeness.

1. *Equivalent Constant Potential*—defined as the kV of a constant potential X-ray beam that best fits the attenuation curve of the beam in question. The equivalent constant potential method requires a set of standard absorption curves obtained experimentally for X-ray beams generated at various *constant* applied kV with various appropriate filters. Such curves for constant potentials ranging from 60 to 200 kV have been prepared by the U.S. Bureau of Standards. A complete attenuation curve is prepared with the unknown beam in increasing thicknesses of a suitable filter such as copper. The kV of the standard curve that most closely matches the one obtained with the unknown beam designates its equivalent constant potential, even though the unknown beam may have been produced with a fluctuating kV. For example, if the absorption curve of the unknown beam approximates most closely the standard curve (in the same filter

material) corresponding to a constant potential of 180 kV, then the equivalent constant potential of the unknown beam is 180 kV. This is evidently a more complicated method of specification than the HVL and offers no particular advantage in radiation therapy.

2. *Equivalent Energy*—defined as the energy of a monoenergetic beam that has the same HVL as the polyenergetic beam in question. It is derived from the total linear attenuation coefficient and the HVL. For example, the linear attenuation coefficient of copper for monoenergetic 200-keV X rays is 1.36/cm. The HVL is readily obtained from the linear attenuation coefficient μ_l as follows:

$$HVL = \frac{0.693}{\mu_l}$$

$$= \frac{0.693}{1.36} \tag{3}$$

$$HVL = 0.5 \text{ cm} = 5 \text{ mm Cu}$$

Thus, if an unknown polyenergetic beam of X rays has an HVL of 5 cm Cu, it can be said to have an equivalent energy of 200 keV. From this, we can derive the equivalent wavelength by modification of equation (1):

$$\lambda_e = \frac{12.4}{kV_e} \text{ Å}$$

where λ_e is the equivalent wavelength and kV_e is the equivalent energy. Therefore, in our example:

$$\lambda_e = \frac{12.4}{200} \text{ Å}$$

$$\lambda_e = 0.06 \text{ Å}$$

Table 8.04 shows the equivalent wavelength and equivalent photon energy of several typical heterogeneous (polyenergetic) X-ray beams used in radiation therapy. In general, the equivalent wavelength of a heterogeneous X-ray beam is approximately twice

TABLE 8.04
EQUIVALENT WAVELENGTH (λ_e) AND EQUIVALENT KILOVOLTAGE (kV$_e$)
FOR VARIOUS POLYENERGETIC BEAMS *

Half Value Layer Polyenergetic Beam	Equivalent Energy kV_e	Equivalent Wavelength λ_e
mm Cu	keV	$\overset{\circ}{A}$
0.5	50	0.24
1.0 (200 kVp)	80	0.15
2.0 (200 kVp)	110	0.11
3.0	140	0.088
4.0	165	0.075
5.0 (400 kVp)	200	0.062
6.0	250	0.050
8.0	370	0.033
10.0 (1000 kVp)	570	0.022

* After W. V. Mayneord, and L. F. Lamerton,[1] Courtesy of The British Institute of Radiology.

that of the minimum wavelength. Similarly, the equivalent photon energy or equivalent kV of a polyenergetic beam is about one-half the kVp. It should be pointed out that since the equivalent wavelength is derived from the HVL and the total linear attenuation coefficient of a particular absorber (filter), the HVL is an adequate expression of X-ray quality in clinical radiation therapy.

CHAPTER 9

Dosage in X-ray and Gamma-ray Therapy

ABSORBED DOSE

IN Chapter 7 we discussed in detail the important aspects of *exposure* as a measure of radiation quantity. We found that the unit of exposure—the roentgen (R)—is based on ionization in air under strictly specified conditions. Thus, 1 R represents an amount of radiation that liberates 1.6×10^{12} ion pairs per gram of air, expending energy of 33.7 ergs/ion pair. We shall now turn to another concept of radiation quantity—*absorbed dose.*

Absorbed Dose in Air. The therapeutic effect of radiation, depending as it does on physicochemical and biologic changes in tissues, is more nearly related to the *amount of energy absorbed* in the process of ionization and excitation, than on radiation exposure itself. In other words, only absorbed radiation is capable of inducing therapeutic or damaging effects on tissues. Since the roentgen is based simply on ionization, it does not specity directly the amount of energy absorption. Furthermore, various tissues exposed to 1 R of radiation of various energies absorb different amounts of energy. Finally, a unit of absorbed dose should be applicable over the entire range of radiation energies, whereas the roentgen is valid only for energies up to about 3 MeV.

How can exposure be converted to absorbed dose? It is well known from the interactions of penetrating radiation and matter that photons transfer energy to orbital electrons of irradiated atoms. When such electrons are released from the atom they are called *primary electrons* (sometimes secondary electrons), and they cause:

1. *Ionization,* with release of secondary electrons and formation of ion pairs. In general, the *ion density* along the ionization tracks of the electrons set in motion by photons determines the ultimate therapeutic effect. Thus, there is a unit, the *linear energy transfer (LET),* which is defined as the energy release per unit length of path of an ionizing particle (unit is 1 keV/μ).

2. *Atomic and molecular excitation* followed by emission of characteristic radiation, which may liberate Auger (*o'zhay*) electrons causing further ionization.

Only a small fraction of the energy released through ionization and excitation induces chemical and biologic changes. By far the largest part of the energy eventually appears as heat, the amount of heat production being a direct measure of the absorbed dose. In fact, this is one of the methods of direct determination of absorbed dose. However, the amount of heat produced is very small. For example, if the whole body were exposed to 500 R, usually a lethal amount, it would suffer a rise in temperature of only 0.001 C! Because of the difficulty inherent in the measurement of such minute amounts of heat, the calorimetric (heat) method of measuring absorbed dose, while useful in research, is not used directly in radiotherapy.

The problem of conversion of exposure to absorbed dose became especially important with the advent of high energy radiation, that is, above a few MeV where exposure in R *cannot* be measured. (Recall that the R is valid only for X- and γ-radiation up to 3 MeV and does not apply to particulate radiation.) Another unit of radiation quantity had to be devised that would be valid for all kinds of radiation, and would at the same time be related to energy absorption. Therefore the Seventh International Congress of Radiology (1953) adopted a unit of absorbed dosage, the *rad* (*R*adiation *A*bsorbed *D*ose), *defined as an absorbed dose of 100 ergs per gram of matter*. The general equation for absorbed dose is

$$D = E/m \qquad (1)$$

where E is the net energy deposited in a small mass m (the term net energy implies that the deposited energy must be corrected for any energy leaving the irradiated mass, such as bremsstrahlung).

Let us examine first the conversion of exposure in R to absorbed dose in rads (obviously, in the energy region where R is valid). This requires only simple arithmetic and certain well known experimental data :

1 R produces 1.61×10^{12} ion pairs/g air.

W (energy needed to produce in air 1 ion pair, including

energy expended on an average of 2.2 excitations per ionization, and the energy of released electrons) = 33.7 eV. 1 eV = 1.602×10^{-12} erg.

Therefore,

energy absorbed per g air exposed to 1 R = $\underset{\text{ion pairs/g}}{1.61 \times 10^{12}} \times \underset{\text{eV/ion pair}}{33.7} \times \underset{\text{erg/eV}}{1.602 \times 10^{-12}} = \underset{\text{erg/g}}{86.9}$

Since 1 rad is 100 ergs/g, it follows that 1 g of air exposed to 1 R absorbs a dose of 0.869 rad. The value 0.869 is the **conversion factor** of R to rads for air.

By simple computation we can show that R can also be converted to rads for matter in general (including tissues) as well as for air. The quantity of energy in ergs absorbed per gram of tissue equals the product of the energy E in the beam and the mass absorption coefficient μ_a/ρ:

$$energy\ absorption/g\ tissue = E(\mu_a/\rho)_{tissue} \qquad (2)$$

Similarly for air,

$$energy\ absorption/g\ air = E(\mu_a/\rho)_{air} \qquad (3)$$

Dividing equation (2) by equation (3),

$$\frac{energy\ absorption/g\ tissue}{energy\ absorption/g\ air} = \frac{E(\mu_a/\rho)_{tissue}}{E(\mu_a/\rho)_{air}} \qquad (4)$$

But we saw above that the energy absorption per gram of air = 0.869 rads per R. Substituting this in the denominator of the left side of equation (4), and canceling E in the right side because we are dealing with the same beam,

$$\frac{energy\ absorption/g\ tissue}{0.869\ rad/R} = \frac{(\mu_a/\rho)_{tissue}}{(\mu_a/\rho)_{air}}$$

Rearranging,

$$energy\ absorption/g\ tissue = \left[\frac{0.869(\mu_a/\rho)_{tissue}}{(\mu_a/\rho)_{air}}\right] rad/R$$

Substituting f for the ratio in brackets,

$$energy\ absorption/g\ tissue = f\ rad/R \qquad (5)$$

In general, the roentgen-to-rad conversion factors for various tissues exposed to radiation of different energies are designated by the symbol f. Typical values of f are shown in Table 9.01. The following equation gives this conversion:

$$D = f \cdot X\ rads \qquad (6)$$

where D is the absorbed dose in rads, f is the conversion factor, and X is the exposure in R. A practical consequence of the dependence of f on radiation energy and the nature of the absorber (i.e. its average atomic number) is that with X rays generated at 200 kV (HVL 1 mm Cu) an exposure of 100 R will produce an absorbed dose of 93 rads in muscle and 150 rads in compact bone; whereas, with ^{60}Co or ^{137}Cs γ rays 100 R will produce an absorbed dose of 96 rads in muscle and only 92 rads in compact bone.

Another radiation quantity is **_kerma_** (**K**inetic **E**nergy **R**eleased in **M**atter) which describes the first step in the interaction between photons and matter. Kerma is the **_total kinetic energy_** transferred to the ionizing particles (i.e. primary electrons) by the photons. The subsequent transfer of energy by the ionizing particles to

TABLE 9.01
ROENTGEN-TO-RAD CONVERSION FACTOR f FOR RADIATION OF
VARIOUS ENERGIES IN SOFT TISSUE, IN COMPACT BONE, AND IN
SOFT TISSUE WITHIN BONE (CAVITY SIZES 10 TO 50 μM)*

Radiation Quality in HVL	f		
	Soft Tissue	Compact Bone	Soft Tissue within Bone
1.0 mm Al	0.93	4.0	3.3
1.0 mm Cu	0.93	1.5	2.0
2.0 mm Cu	0.95	1.1	1.6
^{137}Cs γ rays (0.662 MeV)	0.957	0.925	1.15
^{226}Ra γ-ray Series (Av. 0.83 MeV)	0.957	0.92	1.05
^{60}Co γ rays (Av. 1.25 MeV)	0.957	0.92	1.05
4-MV X rays	0.956	0.921	1.05

*Based on data cited by Johns, H. E., and Cunningham, J. R.,[44] Massey, J. B.,[53] and Meredith, W. J., and Massey, J. B.[57]

the medium itself comprises the **absorbed dose.** Note that kerma and absorbed dose have the same meaning in the case of radiation with energy up to about 1 MeV, but with higher energy photons kerma may be larger than absorbed dose because of the escape of a fraction of the primary electrons' energy through bremsstrahlung.

Measurement of Absorbed Dose in Tissues—Bragg-Gray Cavity Theory. As we have seen, the measurement of exposure in R and conversion to absorbed dose in rads is reasonably straight-forward when the medium is air. However, in radiation therapy we treat a tissue volume and must be able to measure the absorbed dose there. Fortunately, the energy absorbed in a solid medium can be related to the ionization produced in a small air cavity within the medium by application of the **Bragg-Gray Cavity Theory.** According to this theory, the presence of a small air-filled cavity in a solid or liquid medium does not alter the distribution of primary electrons released within the medium when it is irradiated with X or γ rays. This holds true provided (1) the dimensions of the cavity are smaller than the average range of the electrons set in motion by the photons, (2) the thickness of the medium surrounding the cavity is greater than the range of the electrons, (3) the medium is homogeneous, and (4) the radiation field is uniform, without appreciable attenuation of the X or γ rays in traversing the air cavity. Under these conditions, the theory states that the energy E_m absorbed per unit mass of medium is to the energy E_g absorbed per unit mass of gas, as the mass stopping power S_m of the medium is to the mass stopping power S_g of the gas. We must include mass stopping power because different numbers of ions are produced in the gas and the medium by electrons of the same energy. (Mass stopping power is the loss of energy by an ionizing particle per unit length of path divided by the density of the medium and is therefore related to LET.) Thus, we have the simple proportion

$$\frac{E_m}{E_g} = \frac{S_m}{S_g}$$

$$E_m = \frac{S_m}{S_g} E_g \qquad (7)$$

Since E_g is the energy carried by the ions produced in the air cavity, it is simply the product of the number of ion pairs J_g per unit mass of gas, and the energy W carried per ion pair:

$$E_g = J_g W \tag{8}$$

Substituting this value of E_g from equation (8) in equation (7),

$$E_m = J_g W \frac{S_m}{S_g} \tag{9}$$

In equation (9) S_m/S_g is the average **stopping-power ratio** of the medium relative to air. Note that as the atomic number of the medium approaches that of air, this ratio approaches unity. Thus, the values of S_m/S_g with ^{60}Co γ rays is 1.002 for graphite, 1.133 for soft tissue, and 1.350 for water, relative to air. Assuming that $S_m/S_g = 1$, and substituting this value in equation (9),

$$E_m = J_g W$$

and since W is constant, the energy E_m released per unit mass of medium such as tissue (and therefore the absorbed dose) is proportional to the ionization in the gas-filled cavity.

Because of the validity of the Bragg-Gray Theory we can obtain the absorbed dose in radiation therapy from exposure measurements. We first immerse a properly designed thimble capacitor or similar chamber in a tissue-like phantom (water, masonite, rice, or equivalent) and measure the exposure at the point of interest. After applying appropriate correction factors (see pages 190 to 191) we convert the resulting exposure in R to absorbed dose in rads according to

$$D = f \cdot X \, rads \tag{10}$$

where again D is the absorbed dose in rads, f is the roentgen-to-rad conversion factor, and X is the corrected exposure in R. Values of f for radiation of different energies in soft tissues and bone are given in Table 9.01.

It should be pointed out that equation (10) applies only in the photon energy range up to about 3 MeV. Above this limit, only approximate conversion factors are available, relating the reading in R' of the dosimeter immersed in water phantom, to the ab-

TABLE 9.02
VALUES OF CONVERSION FACTOR C_λ IN RADS/R FOR DETERMINING
ABSORBED DOSE IN *WATER* USING ^{60}Co OR 2 MV X RAYS FOR EXPOSURE
CALIBRATION. C_λ VALUES AVERAGED FROM PUBLISHED DATA*

Radiation	C_λ
^{137}Cs	0.95
^{60}Co	0.95
2 MV	0.95
4 MV	0.94
20 MV	0.90

*ICRU *Report 14.*

sorbed dose D'. Values of this conversion factor, C_λ, are shown in Table 9.02. In using this conversion factor, we must also apply a calibration factor C of the ion chamber with reference to a standard such as cobalt 60:

$$D' = R'CC_\lambda \text{ rads} \tag{11}$$

Other Methods of Measuring Absorbed Dose. There are several methods of determining the absorbed dose of radiation besides ionization measurement. These will now be described briefly and their place in radiotherapy indicated.

Calorimetric dosimetry is based on the fact that virtually all the energy deposited in matter by X or γ rays appears as heat. Since the absorbed dose is proportional to the amount of heat produced per unit mass, measurement of heat production can be directly related to energy absorption by applying pertinent transformation factors. Unfortunately, the amount of heat liberated during radiation therapy is extremely small—about 10^{-3} to 10^{-5} calories per minute—so highly sensitive instruments are needed to achieve the required accuracy. The basic device is a semiconductor known as a ***thermistor*** whose resistance increases sharply with a small rise in temperature. A Wheatstone bridge is used to measure the change in resistance, from which the absorbed dose can be computed. Calorimetry is important at present in the calibration of ion chambers, especially for the measurement of absorbed dose from very high energy photons and electron beams. It is possible to achieve an accuracy of about 2 percent with calorimetric dosimetry.

Chemical dosimetry depends on the oxidation or reduction of certain chemicals by ionizing radiation. The *Fricke dosimeter* is based on this principle. It consists of a solution of ferrous sulfate, the ferrous (Fe^{++}) ion being oxidized to the ferric (Fe^{+++}) ion on exposure to radiation. After exposure, the amount of ferric ion in the solution is determined by the latter's optical density as measured by the absorption of light in the solution. From this the number of molecules of Fe^{+++} per unit mass can be determined. Using the G number, defined as the number of molecules changed per 100 eV absorbed, the absorbed dose in rads can be computed. Accuracy is of the order of about 3 percent. Since very large radiation doses are needed to produce significant oxidation of Fe^{++}; this type of dosimetry is used primarily for calibration of high energy electron beams.

Thermoluminescence dosimetry (*TLD*) depends on a property peculiar to certain crystals such as lithium fluoride (LiF). When LiF crystals containing impurities in their lattice structure are irradiated with X or γ photons, electrons are elevated to higher energy levels. While most of the electrons promptly return to their original shells (i.e. ground state), some are trapped at intermediate energy levels dictated by the impurities. The number of trapped electrons is proportional to the amount of energy initially absorbed from the radiation. After the first twenty-four hours, trapped electrons remain trapped indefinitely. When the crystals are subsequently heated, the trapped electrons absorb sufficient energy to raise them to the conduction band; they then return to ground state, accompanied by the emission of blue-green light. The emitted light is measured by an electronic system, the heart of which is a photomultiplier tube. By proper calibration against known absorbed doses of radiation the LiF dosimeter can be used to measure unknown doses. Since LiF has an effective atomic number very similar to that of soft tissue and air (8.2, 7.4, and 7.65, respectively) the absorbed dose per gram from equal exposures is virtually the same for LiF, soft tissue, and air. Therefore the LiF dosimeter is suitable for measuring absorbed dose in radiotherapy. LiF can be used as a powder in very small tubes, say, 1×6 mm; it may be prepared as solid rods or discs; or it may be fabricated in any desired shape and size. Although not yet so suitable as the thimble ionization chamber for general use in radiotherapy, TLD permits the measurement of absorbed dose in body cavities, or wherever there is a steep variation in dose rate such as we find near radium or cesium 137 needles or in the buildup region (see page 226) of teletherapy beams. Finally, this principle is used in modern personnel monitoring (see page 625). Accuracy of LiF dosimetry approaches 3 percent, the response being linear (proportional) with relation to the absorbed doses ranging from about 1 to a few hundred rads.

Photoluminescence dosimetry is another type of solid state dosimetry, using a special variety of glass that is silver activated. Stored light in this system is released by exposure to ultraviolet light (not heat, as with TLD). However, because of marked energy dependence, photoluminescent dosimeters are not widely used in radiation therapy, but are finding application in personnel monitoring.

Film dosimetry is not practicable in radiotherapy because of a number of factors, especially with very high energy beams. First of all, film is highly energy dependent, that is, its response depends not only on radiation exposure, but also on the energy of the photons. Second, it is very difficult to control not only the film thickness and composition of different batches of film, but also processing; while such control is perfectly adequate for radiography, it does not fulfill the strict requirements for dosimetry. However, film dosimetry is useful in procedures that do not require a high degree of accuracy, such as the determination of cross-sectional uniformity of teletherapy beams, coincidence of radiation beams and collimator lights, and alignment of beam directors. Finally, film dosimetry has been extremely useful in personnel monitoring.

DOSAGE DISTRIBUTION OF THE ENTERING BEAM

Given Dose. If a scattering medium such as a patient or a tissue-equivalent phantom is placed near a thimble ionization chamber as shown in Figure 9.01, the measured exposure rate in R/min will be greater than that obtained in air in the absence of the medium. This is especially important in orthovoltage therapy because a given exposure in air will give a larger skin ex-

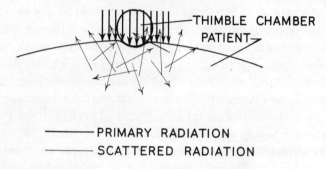

———— PRIMARY RADIATION

———— SCATTERED RADIATION

FIGURE 9.01. The thimble receives both primary radiation from the X-ray tube, and scattered radiation from the patient.

posure. With megavoltage radiation, maximum dosage is reached *below* the entrance surface.

1. *Backscatter Radiation.* Upon traversing the medium, X and γ rays scatter in various directions. Some are actually scattered back toward the entrance port of the beam as *backscatter radiation*, adding to the entrance dose. Backscatter is much more pronounced with orthovoltage than with megavoltage radiation.

2. *Electron Buildup.* As a *megavoltage* beam crosses the air-medium interface, primary electrons released by the photons build up to a maximum until *electronic equilibrium* is achieved. At this level, in a very small layer of medium whose thickness is at least equal to the range of the primary electrons, just as many electrons enter the layer (from interactions in the layer just behind) as leave the layer and enter the one beyond (see Fig. 9.02). The net effect is as though all the energy deposited in the small layer came from electrons set in motion by photons crossing the layer itself. However, if the primary photons undergo any significant attenuation as they cross the layer, more electrons will be freed as the photons enter than as they leave, and electronic equilibrium will not be achieved. The *equilibrium depth* is the depth below the surface at which electronic equilibrium is reached, and here lies the zone of *maximum ionization*. Between the surface and the equilibrium depth lies the *electron* or *dose buildup region*, as shown in Figure 9.02. It should be emphasized that electron equilibrium occurs virtually at the surface with kilovoltage radiation (about 200 to 300 kV), at a 5 mm depth with ^{60}Co γ ray (av energy 1.25

MeV), and at a 10 mm depth with 4-MV X rays. These depths correspond, incidentally, to the range of the electrons in the medium. A simplification of the buildup process is shown in Figure 9.03.

As the energy of the X- or γ-ray beam increases, the range of the primary electrons increases until there is significant attenuation of the photons over their range, and so true electronic equilibrium never occurs. However, up to about 3 MeV the error in assuming equilibrium conditions is insignificant in radiotherapy.

Thus, backscatter radiation contributes greatly to the surface dose with orthovoltage (200 to 300 kV) X rays, and there is virtually no electron buildup below the surface. On the other hand, with megavoltage X- or γ-ray beams, electron buildup significantly augments the absorbed dose below the surface at a depth related to the energy of the radiation; backscatter is very small, although not negligible.

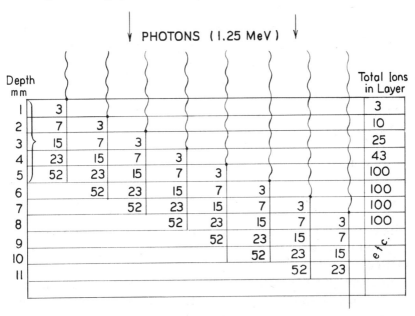

FIGURE 9.02. Cobalt 60 beam (av. energy 1.25 MeV). Electron buildup occurs between the surface and a plane about 5 mm below. Note the decreasing ion density, or dosage, beyond equilibrium depth. (*Adapted from Meredith, W. J., and Massey, J. B., Fundamental Physics of Radiology. Baltimore, Williams & Wilkins, 1972.*)

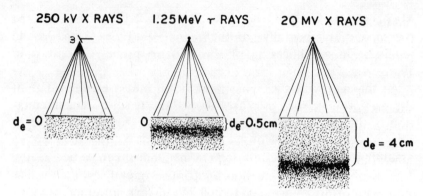

d_e Is Equilibrium Depth or Buildup Region

FIGURE 9.03. Simplified diagram showing the comparative electron buildup regions for radiation of various energies.

The term **given dose** refers to the absorbed dose at equilibrium depth, including backscatter.

Because the level of maximum ionization is reached at different equilibrium depths in the medium, depending on the energy of the radiation, we shall first discuss backscatter with orthovoltage beams, and then show how it differs from megavoltage beams.

With **orthovoltage radiation** (about 200 to 300 kV) maximum ionization occurs, for all practical purposes, at the skin or phantom surface, and so the "given" exposure rate is the **skin** or **surface exposure rate**, which may be defined as the in-air exposure rate at the treatment distance, plus the backscatter exposure rate,

$$X_0 = X + X_B \qquad (12)$$

where X_0 is the skin or surface exposure rate, X is the in-air exposure rate, and X_B is the backscatter exposure rate, all measured in R/min.

In actual practice we cannot measure backscatter itself. Instead, the in-air exposure rate is measured as already indicated (pages 188 to 192). The surface exposure rate under various conditions is measured directly by substituting a tissue-equivalent phantom for the patient. Phantom materials that have a scattering effect similar to human soft tissue (i.e. have a similar effective atomic number) include water, tempered Masonite, Mix D (a mixture of certain waxes), and a mixture of 60 percent rice flour and 40 percent sodium bicarbonate. In measuring the surface exposure rate we use the same procedure as in the determination of the in-air exposure rate, but the thimble ionization chamber is half submerged in the surface of the phantom for orthovoltage radiation, as shown in Figure 9.04. However, the procedure is fraught with errors and uncertainties. For example, if the stem of the ionization chamber is not tissue equivalent (as it is not in the Victoreen system), as much as 30 percent of the scattered radiation may be missed as a result of shielding by the stem. It is therefore preferable to obtain backscatter data from published tables.[8,44] However, we shall indicate how backscatter may be designated and computed, based on *exposure,* and assuming that the surface exposure data are correct.

Percentage backscatter can be obtained if the in-air exposure rate and surface exposure rate are known:

$$\% \ backscatter = \frac{X_o - X}{X} \tag{13}$$

where X_o is the measured surface exposure rate and X is the in-air exposure rate. For example, if $X_o = 60$ R/min, and $X = 50$ R/min,

$$\% \ backscatter = \frac{60 - 50}{50} \times 100 = 20\%$$

The *backscatter factor B* is simply the surface exposure rate divided by the in-air exposure rate,

$$B = \frac{X_o}{X} \tag{14}$$

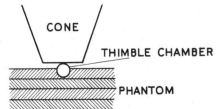

FIGURE 9.04. The thimble chamber should be half submerged in the phantom.

Thus, in the above example,

$$B = \frac{60}{50} = 1.2$$

The backscatter factor is the preferred way of expressing the degree of backscatter.

In a strict sense, the backscatter factor should be the ratio of the surface *absorbed dose rate* to the *in-air absorbed dose rate,* rather than the ratio of the corresponding exposure rates as just described. However, because direct measurement of absorbed doses is seldom feasible, we depend on careful exposure measurements with a small ion chamber under conditions in which absorbed dose is proportional to exposure.

In actual practice, an orthovoltage X-ray machine is simply calibrated for in-air exposure rates under various conditions of filtration, distance, and tube potential. The surface dose corresponding to 100 R in air under the stated conditions can readily be computed from data in published tables (see *Appendix*), as we shall proceed to show.

In the preceding discussion of orthovoltage radiation we obtained the backscatter factor from *exposure* measurements using a thimble ionization chamber with appropriate correction factors (see pages 190 to 191). Because it is preferable to express radiation dosage in terms of *absorbed dose,* and since the backscatter factors in published tables are ratios of dosage rather than exposures, we convert in-air exposure (or exposure rate) to absorbed dose (or absorbed dose rate) D in a small mass of tissue at the surface according to the following equation:

$$D = f \cdot X \text{ rads/min} \qquad (15)$$

where f is the R-to-rad conversion factor and X is the in-air exposure rate in R/min.

To find the *surface* absorbed dose rate D_0 we multiply the absorbed dose rate D by the backscatter factor B (obtained from tables,

$$D_0 = DB \qquad (16)$$

For example, suppose the corrected output of an X-ray machine at a particular distance in 82.2 R/min. From equation (15) the absorbed dose rate in a small mass of tissue at the surface is

$$D = 0.95 \times 82.2 = 78.1 \, \text{rads/min}$$

Now applying equation (16) to find the surface dose rate with full backscatter with a backscatter factor of 1.22,

$$D_0 = 78.1 \times 1.22 = 95.3 \, \text{rads/min}$$

Turning now to *megavoltage radiation,* we note that the *given exposure* is taken at *equilibrium depth,* that is, 5 mm for ^{60}Co γ rays, and 10 mm for 4-MV X rays. The measurement of exposure under these conditions is difficult and requires the use of a small, specially designed ionization chamber. In practice, a thimble capacitor chamber of appropriate thickness for the energy of the radiation is used to measure the exposure rate in R/min at a distance from the source equal to the source-skin distance (SSD) *plus the equilibrium depth.* Thus, for an 80 cm SSD, the in-air exposure rate is measured at a distance of 80.5 cm. This is then converted to the absorbed dose rate in a segregated small mass of tissue of equilibrium thickness, according to:

$$D = f \cdot X \cdot A \, \text{rads/min} \tag{17}$$

where f is the R-to-rad conversion factor for soft tissue, X is the in-air exposure rate in R/min, and A is the correction factor for the attenuation of the beam in tissue between the surface and the equilibrium depth (0.985 for ^{60}Co γ rays). To find the absorbed dose rate at equilibrium depth with full backscatter, we multiply the absorbed dose rate by the backscatter factor, available in published tables:

$$D_m = BD \tag{18}$$

where D_m is the absorbed dose rate at equilibrium depth with full backscatter, B is the backscatter factor, and D is again the absorbed dose rate in a segregated small mass of tissue at equilibrium depth. Note that *with megavoltage radiation the backscatter factor is the ratio of the absorbed dose rate (including backscatter) at equilibrium depth (D_m) to the absorbed dose rate (without backscatter) in a segregated small mass of tissue at the same location.*

In summary, then, to calibrate a ^{60}Co teletherapy unit in terms of "given" dose (that is, the absorbed dose at equilibrium depth, including backscatter) we first measure the output in "R"/min in air at the desired distance as described on pages 188 to 190, using a thimble chamber of suitable wall thickness (4 mm) for electronic equilibrium. This measured output must then be corrected for shutter time, temperature, atmospheric pressure, and instrument calibration factor (to correct for attenuation of the radiation in the wall). Finally, this corrected exposure rate R/min is converted to the given dose rate in rads/min.

An example of the required computations follows.

Suppose the measured output for a ^{60}Co teletherapy unit is 94.3 'R'/min when corrected only for shutter time, at a treatment distance of 80.5 cm (that is, source to equilibrium depth), with the center of the thimble chanber at this point in space. We have the following additional data:

Temperature   23 C (instrument calibrated initially at 22 C)
Pressure   758 mm Hg (instrument calibrated initially at
                           760 mm Hg)
f   0.957 rad/R
A   0.985 (attenuation factor of beam between surface and
            equilibrium depth)
Calibration Factor of R-meter   0.98 (correction by testing
                                       laboratory)

Then the finally corrected exposure rate is obtained as follows:

$$\text{In-air Exposure Rate} = 94.3 \text{ 'R'}/min \times \frac{273 + 23}{295} \times \frac{760}{758}$$
$$\text{(corrected)}$$

$$\times 0.98 = 92.97 \; R/min$$

$$\text{Given Dose Rate} = D_m = \text{In-air Exposure Rate} \times f \times A \times BSF$$

where *BSF* is the backscatter factor and the other terms are as above.

$$\text{Given Dose Rate} = 92.97 \text{ R/min} \times 0.957 \text{ rad/R} \times 0.985 \times BSF$$
$$= 87.4 \text{ rads/min} \times BSF$$

The given dose is obtained from the following relation:

$$\text{Given Dose} = \text{Given Dose Rate} \times \text{Time}$$

FACTORS AFFECTING BACKSCATTER

Let us now examine the various determinants of the back-scatter factor which, in turn, influences the given dose. These may be listed as follows: (1) area of treatment field, (2) depth of part irradiated, (3) quality of radiation, and (4) in the case of orthovoltage X rays, material constituting cone and its cap (not of practical importance when cone cover is ⅛ in. bakelite).

1. *Area of Treatment Field.* The backscatter factor increases as the area of the treatment port increases. Figure 9.05 is a graph showing this relationship with X rays (HVL 1 mm Cu) and ^{60}Co γ rays (HVL 12 mm Pb). The curves become progressively flatter as the area of the field increases, signifying that there is a greater increase in backscatter for a particular increase in field size when the field is small than when it is large. Also note the smaller effect of area on backscatter with a ^{60}Co beam. In general, the reason for the increase in backscatter with increasing field size is that the larger beam irradiates a larger volume of tissue, with a resulting larger component of scattered radiation. This, in turn, produces more backscatter, adding to the entrance dose (see Fig. 9.06).

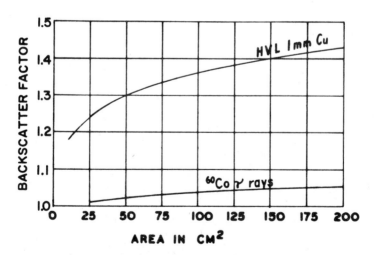

FIGURE 9.05. The backscatter factor increases with increasing field area. Note the smaller backscatter factors for ^{60}Co γ rays (HVL = 12 mm Pb) than for kilovoltage X rays (HVL = 1 mm Cu).

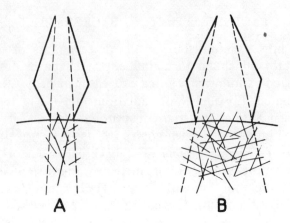

FIGURE 9.06. In *A*, the smaller port delimits a smaller irradiated volume and the amount of scattering is less than in *B* where a larger volume is irradiated.

2. ***Thickness of Irradiated Part.*** Only when the thickness of the irradiated part exceeds the range of the scattered radiation will full backscatter occur. This means that the backscatter factor will increase to a maximum as the thickness of the irradiated part increases to a critical value. After this thickness is reached, a further increase in thickness will contribute no additional backscatter. In general, if the irradiated part is thick enough for maximum backscatter, then the volume of tissue scattering radiation back to the skin is proportional to the area of the treatment field. On the other hand, as the thickness of irradiated tissue decreases below the critical value, the backscatter factor decreases, and a correction must be applied. For example, with radiation having a half value layer of 1.5 mm Cu, the depth for maximum backscatter is about 16 cm. If, with these factors, a structure 6 cm thick is irradiated, the backscatter will be 15 percent less than the maximum. Figure 9.07, based on data of Quimby and Laurence,[72] shows the variation in backscatter when the thickness of the irradiated part is less than that required for maximum backscatter. With megavoltage radiation there is so little backscatter that no serious error results if the part thickness is insufficient for full backscatter.

3. ***Quality of the Radiation.*** As the half value layer increases, backscatter increases until a maximum is reached at about HVL

= 1.0 mm Cu. Above this quality, Compton scattering occurs at progressively smaller angles (i.e. more and more in a "forward" direction). Consequently there is less backscatter, as shown in Figure 9.08 where the backscatter factor is plotted against HVL in copper, the treatment field being held constant at 100 cm². Since the HVL depends on the tube potential and filtration, these in turn determine the backscatter factor. With megavoltage radiation (^{60}Co γ rays and multimillion volt X rays) there is very little backscatter, even with large ports, because such high energy photons are scattered at small angles, as noted above. It should be emphasized that the percentage backscatter is not influenced by treatment distance. Reference to standard tables will readily show this to be true (see Depth Dose Tables in *Appendix*).

TISSUE OR TUMOR DOSE

In general, the exposure rate of radiation at a given point within the body (such as in treatment of a tumor) decreases

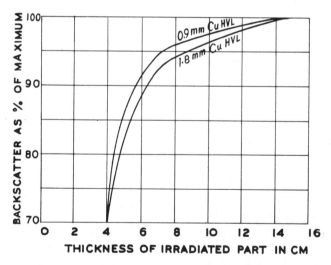

FIGURE 9.07. Relation of backscatter, as a percentage of maximum backscatter, to the thickness of the irradiated part. At HVL 1 mm Cu, backscatter is maximal when the depth of the underlying tissue is at least 16 cm. (Based on data of E. H. Quimby and G. C. Laurence.[72])

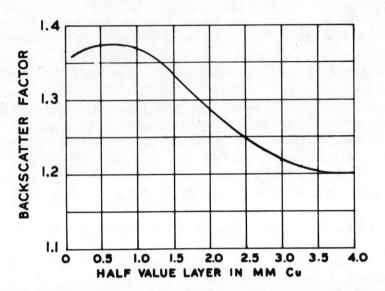

FIGURE 9.08. Backscatter factor reaches a maximum with a beam of about 0.5 mm Cu HVL, based on a field area of 100 cm[2]. Values averaged from published tables in H. E. Johns and J. R. Cunningham;[44] and P. N. Goodwin, E. H. Quimby, and R. H. Morgan.[35]

as its distance from the source or tube target increases. There are three causes for this *attenuation* or decrease in the intensity of the beam:

1. Absorption⎫
⎬ interaction of photons with matter
2. Scattering⎭

3. Distance—inverse square law

Consequently, the deeper a given beam penetrates into the body, the more it is attenuated and the smaller the dose rate in rads/min.

Absorbed Dose. It has already been pointed out that the therapeutic effect of radiation depends on the *quantity absorbed,* chiefly through the process of *ionization and excitation.* In other words, *only the absorbed radiation is capable of producing therapeutic or damaging effects on tissues.*

How can this absorbed energy be measured? It is well known, from the study of the interaction of X rays with matter, that the

X-ray photons transfer energy to orbital electrons of irradiated atoms. When set in motion in this manner, the primary electrons cause:

1. *Ionization,* with formation of ion pairs. In general, the ion density along the path of the primary electrons determines the therapeutic effect. The primary electrons may release secondary electrons by interaction with other atoms.

2. *Atomic and molecular excitation,* with emission of characteristic radiation and Auger electrons.

Most of the energy released through ionization eventually appears as heat, although a small fraction induces chemical changes. The amount of heat produced is a measure of the energy absorbed by the tissues, but it is actually so small that it cannot be measured practicably in radiotherapy (see page 223).

We have already seen that the roentgen, as a unit of exposure, is based on ionization produced in air. The roentgen does not indicate the amount of energy absorbed by the tissues and, besides, various types of tissues exposed to 1 R of various qualities of radiation absorb different amounts of energy. Therefore, radiation dosage is specified by *absorbed dose,* or simply *dose,* the unit of which is the *rad,* defined as an energy absorption of 100 ergs/g (see pages 218 to 220). The f factor applied in converting roentgens to rads varies slightly with the energy of the radiation and the effective atomic number of the absorber. For soft tissues it varies from 0.95 for kilovoltage (200 to 300 kV) X rays, to 0.957 for ^{60}Co γ rays. Another way of looking at the f factor is that it indicates the number of rads absorbed by a medium exposed to 1 R.

As explained earlier (see pages 220 to 221), the absorbed dose from 1 R in other tissues such as bone may vary significantly from that in soft tissues. For example, with *kilovoltage* radiation of HVL 2 mm Cu, the absorbed dose from 1 R in 1 g of compact bone is about 1.6 rads, or about 1½ times that in 1 g of soft tissue remote from bone. On the other hand, the *soft tissue elements* within small cavities in bone acquire about twice the absorbed dose in tissue in the absence of bone, a very important consideration in X-ray therapy. The reason for the preferential absorption of such kilovoltage radiation in bone is that in this energy region photoelectric absorption is still significant. Since the photoelectric absorption coefficient is nearly proportional to Z^3 (Z is atomic number) and the atomic number of the chief elements in bone is greater than that in soft tissues, greater absorption will occur in bone for equal exposures, gram for gram.

From tube potentials of 400 kV to 5 MeV, the Compton process predominates and since this is independent of Z, absorption per gram of bone is essentially the same as that per gram of soft tissues, from equal R exposures. Above this energy range, pair production becomes the main type of absorption. Since π_m is proportional to Z, absorption in bone again exceeds that in soft tissues for equal roentgen exposures.

At this point we should call attention to the absorbed dose in soft tissues at a *bone interface,* and *within bone.* Whereas this is not significantly different from absorbed dose in an equal mass of soft tissue (within a soft tissue medium) in the case of megavoltage radiation, the same cannot be said for kilovoltage radiation. With energy in the orthovoltage region the absorbed dose in soft tissue adjoining bone is *increased* by virtue of photoelectric interaction with elements of high atomic number (Ca and P) in bone.

Insofar as soft tissue elements *within bone* are concerned, the absorbed dose will depend on the size of the cavity in which they lie. Thus, individual osteocytes within lacunae (about 5 μ in diameter) will receive a dose nearly the same as that of bone of the same mass. However, the dose to cells in the center of larger cavities such as Haversian canals and cancellous bone will approach that for soft tissue elsewhere, although the cells lying near the wall of a cavity will receive a larger dose. There is no simple correction for these conditions, but in view of the almost universal replacement of orthovoltage by megavoltage therapy, this is no longer an important problem.

Central Axis Depth Dose. If the dose rate in rads per unit time is determined at various points along the central axis of a beam as it passes through a tissue equivalent phantom, it will be found to decrease progressively relative to the skin dose in the case of *orthovoltage* radiation. But with *megavoltage* radiation the dose rate will at first increase to a maximum value and then decrease. Depending on the quality of the radiation, the point of maximum absorbed dose rate will be located either in the skin or at some depth beneath. With radiation up to about 250 kV (HVL about 2 mm Cu), the primary electrons liberated in the interactions between the photons and tissue atoms have a short range, less than 1 mm. Therefore electronic equilibrium (see pages 226 to 228) is reached virtually at the skin surface. On the other hand, with megavoltage radiation such as ^{60}Co γ rays and 2-MV X rays the primary electrons have a longer range, approximately 5 mm in soft tissue, so that maximum ionization is reached at this depth, and that is where the maximum dose is delivered. These facts are reflected in depth dose tables which show the 100 per cent dose to lie virtually at the skin surface for kilovoltage X-ray beams (HVL 1 to 3 mm Cu), and at a point 5 mm below the surface for ^{60}Co γ rays. (Note that with X-ray beams of HVL 1 or 2 mm Cu and large ports, scattered radiation may cause the dose at 1 cm depth to exceed slightly the skin dose.) Table 9.03 shows the depth of maximum ionization and hence maximum dosage (D_{max} or D_m) for radiation of various qualities. The relation of beam quality to depth doses along the central axis is shown in Figure 9.09 which indicates also the site of maximum dosage in each instance.

The published depth dose tables are based on the measurement and computation of the absorbed dose at the indicated depth expressed as a percentage of the absorbed dose on the skin or at

TABLE 9.03
DEPTH OF MAXIMUM IONIZATION (ELECTRON EQUILIBRIUM OR
BUILDUP DEPTH) FOR RADIATION OF VARIOUS ENERGIES

	Energy	*Depth of Maximum Ionization*
		mm
X Rays	200 kV	<1
	2 MV	4
	4 MV	10
	6 MV	15
	15 MV	30
	22 MV	40
γ Rays	^{137}Cs (0.662 MeV)	4
	^{60}Co (av. 1.25 MeV)	5

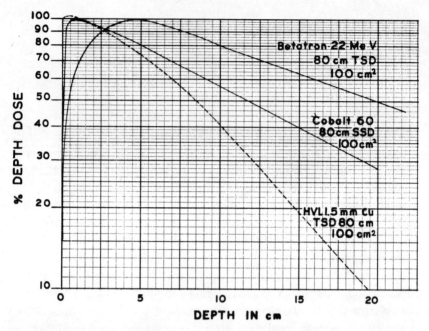

FIGURE 9.09. Depth doses curves for beams of various energies, based on data of H. E. Johns and J. R. Cunningham.[44] Note that the 100 percent depth dose occurs at progressively greater depths with increasing energy of the radiation. With kilovoltage radiation of HVL 1.5 mm Cu maximum dosage with large fields exceeds skin dose slightly because of large backscatter factor.

equilibrium depth for various combinations of field area, beam quality (energy or HVL), and source- or target-skin distance. The thickness of the irradiated part must be at least 16 cm and it must be several cm wider than the beam in all directions to simulate the conditions under which the depth dose tables were obtained. With kilovoltage therapy in the 200 to 250 kV range, the open end of the cone may be covered with organic material such as bakelite up to ⅛ in. thick without introducing an appreciable error. It must be borne in mind that such tables indicate the depth dose percentages along the **central axis** of the beam in **soft tissues.** The presence of fat, bone, or air containing organs may alter the depth dose from that indicated in the tables, but this is a complicated problem in the usual energy range of orthovoltage therapy

(200 to 300 kV) and will be taken up later. Furthermore, tables must be based on careful measurements, with attention to modifying factors. For example, there is progressive softening of the radiation at greater depths (mainly due to Compton scattering) and if an energy dependent measuring instrument is used, it will not reflect the true exposure rate at depths where there has been significant decrease in photon energy.

Published tables indicate the depth dose as a percentage of the **skin dose**, including backscatter for orthovoltage X-ray therapy, or as a percentage of the **dose at equilibrium depth** or D_{max} for megavoltage or telecurie therapy. In general, if no statement is made to the contrary, the **central axis depth dose is defined as the number of rads at a given depth in the tissues on the central axis per 100 rads on the skin including backscatter; or per 100 rads at equilibrium depth.** The distinction between orthovoltage therapy and megavoltage therapy must be made because, as already mentioned, ionization reaches a maximum nearly at the skin surface with orthovoltage therapy, and at some distance below the skin with megavoltage therapy. Most depth dose tables are set up in this manner, giving the number of rads at various depths on the central axis when the absorbed dose on the surface or at equilibrium depth is 100 rads. In other words, the depth dose appears in these tables as a percentage of the **given dose** (including backscatter). To find the **tumor dose** in rads at the center of a lesion, one has only to multiply the total given dose by the percentage depth dose:

$$tumor\ absorbed\ dose = given\ dose \times \%D.D. \qquad (19)$$

Unfortunately, published depth dose tables are not all in accord, and in any event they may not apply precisely to the equipment being used. The ICRU (*Handbook 87*) outlines a procedure for minimizing such discrepancies so that any standard set of depth dose tables may be used. The following is a summary of the recommended procedure:

1. **For each cone or collimator opening**, the exposure rate is measured with an appropriate thimble ionization chamber at a depth of 5 cm in a suitable tissue-equivalent phantom such as

Mix D or masonite, or in water. The R/min reading is corrected as described earlier (see pages 190 to 192).

2. Any recently published depth dose tables may be used, provided they apply to the radiation under study.

3. The surface exposure rate, including full backscatter, is then computed by dividing the exposure rate at 5 cm depth (step 1) by the percentage depth dose at 5 cm (from table).

4. From step 3 reasonably accurate exposure rates at other depths greater than about 4 cm can be determined by multiplying the calculated surface exposure rate by the appropriate percentage depth dose in the published table.

An example will now be given to demonstrate the procedure for obtaining the depth dose at any desired depth.

A. *Basic Data*

Technical factors: 10×10 cm^2 field; ^{60}Co beam; SSD 80 cm.

$$
\left.
\begin{array}{ll}
\text{Backscatter factor} & 1.035 \\
\%\text{Depth dose at 5 cm} & 78.5 \\
\%\text{Depth dose at 10 cm} & 55.6
\end{array}
\right\} \text{ from depth dose tables}
$$

B. *Depth Dose Determination*

Exposure rate at 5 cm depth = 82.2 R/min (measurement in phantom).

"Given" exposure rate including backscatter

$$\frac{82.2 \text{ R/min}}{0.785} = 104.7 \text{ R/min (calculation)}$$

Corrected exposure rate at 10 cm depth

$$104.7 \text{ R/min} \times 0.556 = 58.2 \text{ R/min (calculation)}$$

Dose rate at 10 cm depth

$$58.2 \text{ R/min} \times 0.96 \text{ rad/R} = 56 \text{ rads/min}$$

where 0.96 is the f value for a tissue-equivalent phantom.

It has been found with the above procedure that the difference in the depth dose rates among various published depth dose tables is reduced to the order of about 1 percent. With the older method of first measuring the in-air exposure rate and then calculating the depth exposure rate, the results may differ by about 8 to 10 per cent, depending on the tables used. However, the in-air exposure rate is still needed to calibrate and check the operation of the therapy equipment.

Factors in Percentage Depth Dose. There are four factors affecting the percentage depth dose: quality of beam, depth of lesion, area of treatment port, and source- or target-skin distance. These will be discussed individually.

1. *Beam Quality.* It has been stated a number of times that the quality of a beam of radiation refers to its penetrating power. Obviously, the more penetrating the beam, the greater the dose it will deliver at any particular point in the body relative to the given dose. But quality is determined by the photon energy or the HVL—the greater the photon energy or HVL, the greater the percentage depth dose (see Fig. 9.10). Since HVL depends on photon energy and, in the case of orthovoltage X rays, on filtration as well, an increase in either or both of these factors will increase the penetrating ability and percentage depth dose.

With X-ray beams, an increase in tube potential (e.g. kV) increases the relative number of higher energy photons with result-

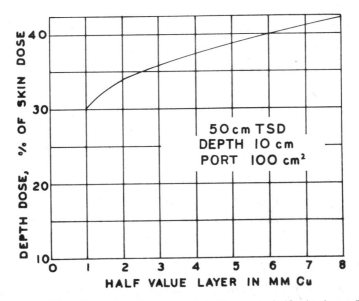

FIGURE 9.10. The relationship of percentage depth dose to half value layer. (Based on data from O. Glasser, *et al.*[33])

ing enhancement of the depth dose. Finally, filters of greater thickness and/or higher atomic number absorb relatively more low energy photons (except below the absorption edge), thereby improving the penetrating ability of the beam and increasing the depth dose.

In attempting to improve X-ray quality by increments of HVL, we must weigh the relatively slight gain in quality against the important economic factor of treatment time. Thus, the depth dose increases from 41 to 43 percent when the HVL is increased from 1 mm to 2 mm Cu, but this requires a three-fold increase in treatment time. Only by a drastic increase in HVL, as in megavoltage therapy, can treatment time be maintained at a reasonable level while the depth dose is significantly increased.

It is interesting to note that *compound filters* (*Thoraeus*) composed of tin, copper, and aluminum, are about 25 percent more efficient than simple copper and aluminum filters in removing the softer components of a 200 to 250 kV beam. This is explained by the fact that the lower energy photons (30 to 40 keV) are absorbed by photoelectric interaction with tin atoms because these photons have enough energy to dislodge K electrons. Radiation in this energy range is largely absorbed in the skin where it is of no value, and even causes harmful effects. That is why it is desirable to remove the softer components by adequate filtration. Just below about 29 keV (K absorption edge), photon energy is insufficient to dislodge tin K electrons and photoelectric absorption cannot occur; therefore, in this energy region tin is "transparent," permitting softer radiation to pass through. If copper is placed next to the tin as a secondary filter, it removes these softer components without absorbing a large fraction of the harder components. Furthermore, copper absorbs characteristic radiation emitted by the tin. Finally, aluminum is placed in front of the copper as a tertiary filter to remove the characteristic radiation of copper. Aluminum characteristic radiation is absorbed in a few cm of air. The arrangement of a Thoraeus filter in the X-ray beam was shown in Figure 8.06. A combination of thicknesses of the three metals may be selected such that a larger fraction of the beam is transmitted than with a copper and aluminum filter, the final beams having the same HVL in both cases. Thus, with a

Thoraeus filter, the same dose of radiation can be delivered in a shorter time than with an equivalent copper and aluminum filter.

It is important to know that the feasibility of improving the quality of an orthovoltage beam by increasing filtration is quite limited because the homogeneity coefficient (see page 210) very soon reaches unity; that is, large increases in filtration produce relatively little improvement in HVL. It is much more efficient to use megavoltage radiation.

2. *Depth of Lesion.* It is obvious that as the depth of the tumor increases, its absorbed dose decreases relative to the surface dose, or dose at equilibrium depth (i.e. given dose) provided the other factors remain constant. Figure 9.11 indicates this relationship in graphic form. Note that there is almost an inverse proportion between percentage depth dose and lesion depth.

It must be stressed that depth dose measurements may be subject to certain errors, depending on the method by which they were obtained. For example, depth dose tables based simply on thimble chamber measurements in a phantom do not necessarily

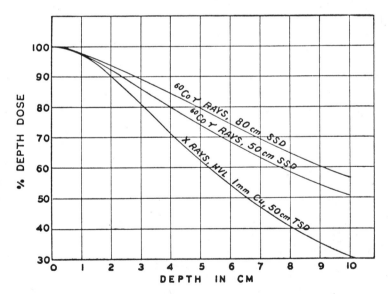

FIGURE 9.11. The percentage depth dose decreases progressively at increasing depths in the body, almost in inverse proportion. At any particular depth the percentage depth dose is larger with ^{60}Co γ rays than with kilovoltage X rays.

reflect the true exposure rates in the tissues below the surface because as the primary beam traverses the body there is progressive contamination of the beam by scattered and secondary radiation. Since this scattered radiation is of lower energy than the primary, and since the thimble chamber is energy dependent, sizable errors may result. Only when special precautions are taken to correct for the deterioration of the primary beam in the tissues, do the depth dose tables indicate the true values of percentage depth dose.

Mainly as the result of the work of Clarkson and Mayneord in England, information became available on the lengthening of wavelength of an X-ray beam as it traverses a thick absorber. They used a specially constructed double ionization chamber to study the relative amounts of primary and scattered radiation at various depths in a tissue equivalent phantom, with various combinations of HVL, field area, and depth. With very soft radiation, up to about 100 kV, the scattered radiation contributes less than $\frac{1}{3}$ of the total radiation in the beam beneath the surface. In orthovoltage X-ray therapy with an HVL of 2 to 4 mm Cu, the scattered radiation has sufficient energy to make a significant contribution to the beam. In fact, at a 3 cm depth the scattered radiation accounts for about $\frac{1}{3}$ the total for small fields, and $\frac{1}{2}$ the total for large fields. At a depth of 14 cm, the scattered radiation increases to $\frac{1}{2}$ the total for small fields and 4/5 the total for large

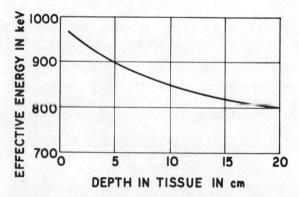

FIGURE 9.12. A ^{60}Co beam undergoes a small but gradual decrease in effective energy as the depth in the body increases. However, this is insufficient to cause a significant change in the f factor (R-to-rad conversion).

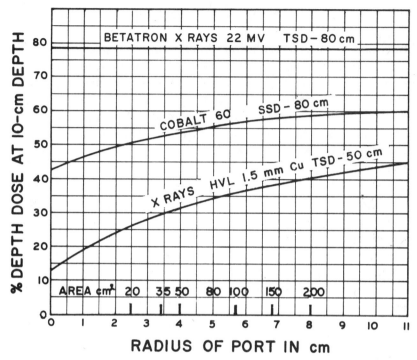

FIGURE 9.13. Relationship of the 10-cm percentage depth dose to field size, for beams of various qualities. Note that the higher the energy of the radiation, the less the field area affects the percentage depth dose. (From H. E. Johns, and Cunningham, J. R.[44])

fields. In the megavoltage region the scattered radiation is very penetrating, but its total amount is small relative to the primary beam, so that it contributes less to the total dose at a given depth. As indicated in Figure 9.12, even at a depth of 15 cm, a ^{60}Co beam has an effective energy of about 0.82 MeV, so that the *f* factor (R-to-rad conversion) is not changed significantly. The superiority of megavoltage over kilovoltage radiation with respect to depth dose is more pronounced for small ports than for large ones, as will be shown in the next section.

3. *Area of Treatment Field.* As the treatment port increases in area, there is a progressive increase in the central axis depth dose, more rapidly for the smaller areas, then more slowly with further increase in the area (see Fig. 9.13). We can explain this as follows: the volume of tissue irradiated is nearly proportional to the cross-

sectional area of the beam (i.e. to the area of the treatment field). Furthermore, the larger the irradiated volume, the larger the fraction of scattered radiation. Since tissue exposure is measured along the central axis of the beam, corresponding to the depth dose tables which are obtained in the same manner, the tissue dose is determined by the sum of the doses contributed by the primary radiation in the beam and the scattered radiation reaching the selected point on the central axis. Therefore, *the greater the area of the port the greater the amount of scattering and the larger the central axis tissue dose.* The effect of scattering, in boosting tissue dose, resembles the effect of backscatter in adding to the skin dose.

The influence of field area on depth dose varies with the quality of the beam (see Fig. 9.13). Scattered X rays associated with a low energy beam do not penetrate very far and so only a relatively small number can reach the central axis from points at an appreciable distance lateral to the axis; therefore, with soft X rays the depth dose does not increase materially with field area. In the 200 to 300 kV range, however, the scattered radiation is more energetic and therefore an increase in field area causes a pronounced increase in depth dose. Finally, in the megavoltage range, the highly energetic photons produce scatter almost entirely in a forward direction, in contrast to the orthovoltage beam which produces a large amount of lateral scatter. For this reason, field area does not have so great an effect on depth dose in megavoltage therapy as it does in kilovoltage (200 to 300 kV) therapy.

The relationship of depth dose to field area for various beam qualities may be appreciated by the study of depth dose tables (see *Appendix*). The first column in such tables includes depth dose values for "0" area. This refers to the primary beam only, without scatter. It should be noted that the surface dose and air dose for "0" area are the same, as would be anticipated. Comparison of the percentage depth dose at any depth for "0" area, with some particular area, immediately shows the contribution of scattered radiation under the stated conditions. For example, Table 9.04 shows that with radiation quality 1 mm Cu HVL and treatment distance of 50 cm, the 10 cm depth dose is 11 percent for "0" area (primary radiation), increasing to 33 per-

TABLE 9.04
PERCENTAGE DEPTH DOSES AT 10 CM WITH A TARGET-SKIN
OR SOURCE-SKIN DISTANCE OF 50 CM *

HVL	0	Field Area in cm² 100	200
1 mm Cu	11	33	43
12 mm Pb (^{60}Co)	38	50	55

* Based on data from Johns, H. E., and Cunningham, J. R.[44]

cent for a 100 cm² field. With radiation of 12 mm Pb HVL (^{60}Co γ rays) the corresponding figures are 38 and 50 percent, respectively. Thus, under these conditions, $\frac{2}{3}$ of the absorbed dose with the 1 mm Cu HVL beam is due to scattered radiation arising in the irradiated volume and joining the primary radiation in the central axis, whereas about $\frac{1}{4}$ of the tissue dose with the ^{60}Co beam is due to scattered radiation.

Furthermore, intercomparison of depth dose tables shows that larger treatment fields with megavoltage radiation do not improve the depth dose so much as with orthovoltage X-ray therapy. This is explained by the fact that there is less scattered radiation contributing to the beam in the megavoltage region.

The published depth dose tables apply to fields that are circular or nearly square. If one side of a rectangular field is more than twice the adjacent side, a correction factor must be introduced for the central axis dose, the reason being that with a highly elongated field, there is more contribution of scattered radiation to the central dose along the shorter dimension, and less along the longer dimension, than is found with a circular or nearly square field of the same area. To a reasonable approximation, a rectangular field can be converted to an equivalent square field for the purpose of dosage computation according to Sterling's method:

$$\frac{4 \times area\ of\ rectangle}{perimeter\ of\ rectangle} = side\ of\ equivalent\ square$$

For example, if the actual port measures 6 × 10 cm²,

$$4 \times area = 4 \times 6 \times 10 = 240\ cm^2$$

$$perimeter = 2(6 + 10) = 32\ cm$$

$$side\ of\ equivalent\ square = 240/32 = 7.5\ cm$$

The area to be used in finding the depth dose in this case is a square measuring 7.5×7.5 cm^2. Such a square does not appear in the usual depth dose table, but reasonably valid depth doses can be found by interpolation.

However, modern complete depth dose tables such as those published by the British Hospital Physicists' Association[8] give depth dose data for a variety of square and rectangular fields so that the desired depth doses can be obtained directly, with little or no interpolation. In any case, the appropriate rectangular field data should be used to minimize error in dosage computation.

4. *Treatment Distance.* In general, *depth dose increases with increasing source-skin distance.* With regard to the *primary beam alone,* this is strictly a geometric factor, being dependent on the inverse square law. In Figure 9.14 the dose at P with the shorter (50 cm) source-skin distance, as compared with the surface dose is:

$$\frac{D_n}{D} = \frac{(50)^2}{(60)^2} = \frac{25}{36} = 70 \text{ percent depth dose at } P$$

At the longer treatment distance, 80 cm:

$$\frac{D_n}{D} = \frac{(80)^2}{(90)^2} = \frac{64}{81} = 79 \text{ percent depth dose at } P$$

Thus, for the same skin dose and with the same field area, there is a greater depth dose obtained at the longer treatment distance. Incidentally, Figure 9.14 shows that at the shorter distance the rays are more divergent and therefore the radiation intensity falls off more rapidly relative to the dose at the surface.

Note that the foregoing discussion omits the factor of scattering. Obviously, the greater the amount of scattered radiation accompanying the primary beam, the less precisely the inverse square law will apply. In other words, the conversion of dose rates from one distance to another is complicated by the HVL of the radiation and the area of the treatment field. Deviation from the inverse square law is greater for larger fields and lower energy radiation, because under these conditions there is a larger contribution of scattered radiation. The greater the fraction of

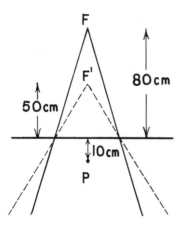

FIGURE 9.14. Percentage depth dose increases with increasing source-skin distance, as shown by less divergence of the rays at a longer distance. See text for mathematical proof.

scattered radiation in the beam, the less will be the improvement in depth dose with increasing treatment distance. Since there is no simple correction factor that can be applied to various combinations of HVL and area, it is essential that depth dose data be obtained directly from published tables, the inverse square law being applied only as an approximate check on the correctness of the treatment factors.

The improved depth dose with long treatment distance must be weighed against the increased treatment time. For example, when the source-skin distance is increased from 50 to 70 cm the depth dose increases by only 10 percent, but the treatment time must be doubled.

The depth dose factors may be summarized as follows:

1. The percentage depth dose *increases* with
    a. Increase in HVL or beam energy, provided the given dose (i.e. skin dose or dose at equilibrium depth) is maintained constant.
    b. Increase in area of treatment field.
    c. Increase in source-skin distance.
2. The percentage depth dose *decreases* with
    a. Increase in depth of the lesion.
    b. Decrease in HVL or beam energy.
    c. Decrease in area of treatment field.
    d. Decrease in source-skin distance.

TISSUE-AIR RATIO

Originally proposed by Johns for use in moving beam therapy, tissue-air ratio is now regarded as a general concept of which percentage depth dose is a special case. However, tissue-air ratios are based on depth dose data. Further details will be given on pages 295 to 304 with reference to moving beam therapy, but a brief summary of the relationship of tissue-air ratio to depth dose will be presented here. The tissue-air ratio R_t is expressed by

$$R_t = \frac{D_t}{D_a} \qquad (20)$$

where D_t is the absorbed dose at depth n within the scattering medium (in moving beam therapy, at axis of rotation), and D_a is the absorbed dose in a small segregated mass of the same medium at the same site (equilibrium thickness only, scattering medium removed) as shown in Figure 9.15. Then, according to the inverse square law,

$$\frac{D_m}{D_a} = \frac{F^2}{f^2} \cdot B \qquad (21)$$

where D_m is the absorbed dose at equilibrium depth, F is the distance from the source to depth n, f is the distance from the source to equilibrium depth (i.e. depth of maximum electron buildup), and B is the backscatter factor. Moreover,

$$\frac{D_t}{D_m} = P/100 \qquad (22)$$

where D_t is the dose at depth n in the medium, D_m is the dose at electron equilibrium depth as before, and P is the percentage depth dose, obtainable from published tables.

Multiplying equations (21) and (22),

$$\frac{D_t}{D_a} = R_t = \frac{F^2}{f^2} \cdot B \cdot P/100 \qquad (23)$$

Thus, according to equation (23) when $F = f$ (i.e. when n equals the equilibrium depth at maximum electron buildup) and P is 100 percent, the tissue-air ratio equals B, the backscatter factor.

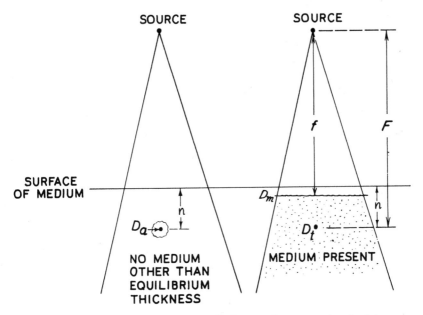

FIGURE 9.15. Diagram showing the terminology and concepts involved in computing *tissue-air ratio*. The left figure indicates the dose D_a to a segregated small mass of tissue or medium (just large enough for electronic equilibrium) at a point n cm below the surface; that is, there is *no* scattering medium and so D_a is the dose "in free space," (quoted from H. E. Johns[43]).

The right figure shows the dose D_t at the same point n cm below the surface, but with scattering medium present; that is, within the body or phantom. Thus, the tissue-air ratio = D_t/D_a.

f is the distance from the source to the level of maximum ionization D_m, and F is the distance from the source to the point n cm below the surface.

EXIT DOSE

It has already been pointed out that the depth dose tables available in the literature (Johns and Cunningham[44]; British Hospital Physicists' Association[8]), are based on a volume of phantom material sufficiently large to provide maximum scatter of the radiation beam. If the thickness of the irradiated structure is less than the critical value, the depth doses will be less than those indicated in the tables. The extreme case is the dose delivered on the skin surface directly opposite the portal of entry of the beam, that is, the zone through which the beam passes out

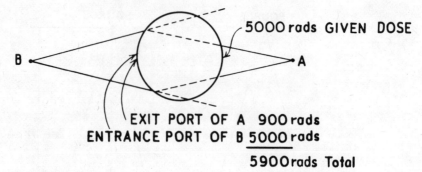

FIGURE 9.16. The exit dose must be added to the given dose to obtain the total entrance dose, an extremely important factor in planning radiotherapy.

of the body. This is called the **exit port**, and the dose delivered at its center is the **exit dose.** It is particularly important when opposing beams are used to crossfire a deeply situated tumor, because the exit dose must be added to the given dose (i.e. skin

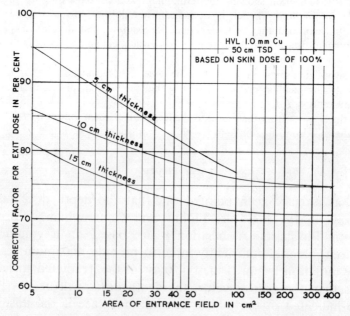

FIGURE 9.17. Correction factors by which depth dose must be multiplied to obtain the exit dose at the same level, for beam quality 1 to 2 mm Cu HVL. (Based on data from E. H. Quimby and G. C. Laurence.[72])

dose or dose at equilibrium depth) to obtain the total entrance dose:

$$total\ entrance\ dose = given\ dose + exit\ dose$$

Figure 9.16 illustrates the problem in diagrammatic form.

Although the exit dose is generally obtained by finding the depth dose at this level from standard depth dose tables, fairly large errors may result from this practice, but the error is on the side of safety. Actually, the exit dose is less than would be expected from the depth dose tables because there is no tissue equivalent scattering material beyond the exit port. Quimby and Laurence[72] have published the correction factors for X-ray therapy in the 200 to 250 kV range; these have been plotted graphically in Figure 9.17. With megavoltage radiation, backward scattering is of no great importance and the exit dose may be taken to be equal to the depth dose at that level, with only a small error, and this on the safe side.

ISODOSE CURVES

The data on absorbed dose computations from depth dose tables have thus far been concerned only with the dose to a lesion along the central axis of the beam. Assuming that a tumor lies in the center of the beam, we can obviously compute the absorbed dose only at the center of the tumor by this means. What about the doses in regions of the tumor located off center? The answer to this question is very important in planning effective radiotherapy because with most radiation beams there is significantly less dosage to points away from the center than at the center itself at a given depth due to less contribution from scattered radiation. To find the doses at points off the axis requires the use of *isodose curves* which are lines connecting points of identical percentage depth dose relative to the maximum or 100 percent dose. A typical isodose distribution is shown in Figure 9.18. This subject is discussed further on pages 274 to 284. However, we should note that it may be preferable to specify the tumor dose on the basis of the tumor volume enclosed by the 90 percent isodose line rather than the dose in the midline. If this is done, it should be clearly indicated in the patient's records. For example, with stationary opposed ports a dose of 6000 rads to the 90 percent isodose level is actually equivalent to 6600 rads in the midline. Similar considerations apply to rotation therapy.

There are several reasons for the smaller dose near the periphery of the beam as compared with that at the center. In the first place, the beam does not consist of parallel rays, but rather of a divergent cone of radiation so that at a given depth in the tissues, the peripheral rays have traveled a greater distance through the tissues and are more attenuated than the more central rays. Secondly, the more oblique peripheral rays have passed through the filter on a slant, thereby actually traversing a greater thickness of filter with resulting greater attenuation. Finally, there is less scatter near the edge of the beam than at the center because of the cut-off of the primary beam near its edge.

Thus, for complete specification of dosage throughout a tumor and the adjacent normal tissues, the dosage at various critical points, besides those at the center, must be determined. This is

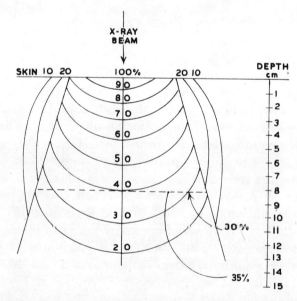

FIGURE 9.18. Isodose curves (distributions) for a kilovoltage X-ray beam (HVL 1 mm Cu). The curved lines connect all points receiving the same dose expressed as a percentage of the skin dose. Curved lines at the sides of the beam result from scattered radiation.

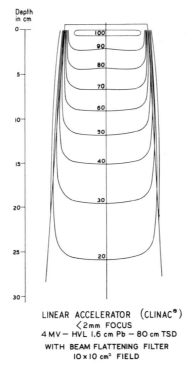

LINEAR ACCELERATOR (CLINAC®)
< 2mm FOCUS
4 MV – HVL 1.6 cm Pb – 80 cm TSD
WITH BEAM FLATTENING FILTER
10 x 10 cm² FIELD

FIGURE 9.19. Isodose curves (distributions) for a 4-MV linac, target-skin distance 80 cm. (Courtesy of Varian, data based on the Clinac 4®.)

no simple task and is one which cannot be carried out without very small, accurate ionization chambers and meticulous technic. The procedure is greatly facilitated by use of a computer. When the percentage depth dose has been charted for many points in the tissue equivalent phantom and the points of similar depth dose connected by lines, a series of *isodose curves* is obtained as shown in Figure 9.18. There is discontinuity at the edge of the beam because of the abrupt discontinuity of the primary beam and of the resulting scatter. A series of isodose curves must be obtained for every combination of beam quality, treatment distance, and field area. Fortunately, these are available for the majority of commonly used technical factors.[1,3].

If isodose curves are not available, a rough approximation may be made in the 200- to 250-kV therapy range. According to

Quimby,[33] the dose at any depth at a point 1.5 cm within the edge of the beam is about 10 to 15 percent less than the central axis depth dose for that level. Close to the edge of the beam, the depth dose falls to about one-half the midline dose for positions near the surface and to about two-thirds the central dose at greater depths. Beyond the edge of the beam the dose drops off abruptly, as stated above.

With megavoltage radiation the isodose curves are found to be flatter due to less variation in depth dose for off-center points (see Fig. 9.19). This is to be anticipated because of the smaller contribution of scattered radiation to the beam and the smaller effect of tissue absorption on the more oblique, though highly penetrating, peripheral rays. Further flattening can be achieved by the use of special filters (see pages 165; 318 to 319).

The application of isodose curves in radiotherapy will be discussed in detail in Chapter 10.

Therapy Planning

THE main purpose of any competent method of radiotherapy is the uniform and adequate irradiation of a tumor, including an adjacent "safe" zone of apparently normal tissue into which extension may have occurred. At the same time, the normal tissues must not suffer irreparable radiation injury. To accomplish this goal we must proceed with a definite plan of treatment which includes the following: (1) tumor localization and verification, (2) field selection and delineation, (3) accurate beam direction, and (4) delivery of the required radiation dosage to the tumor. Each of these factors will now be discussed.

TUMOR LOCALIZATION AND VERIFICATION

The first step in planning a course of external therapy directed to a deep-lying tumor is to ascertain the exact *position* of the tumor within the body. Once this has been determined, it can be related to surface landmarks, or to marks painted on the skin with stain such as Rorer's ® Castellani paint, or fluorescent ink that is visible only under a Wood's light.

Localization. Several methods are available for locating the position of a tumor. These include the following:

1. *Radiography.* Films are exposed in two mutually perpendicular planes with the patient in the same position as in therapy. If the organ of interest is radiotransparent as, for example, the esophagus or bladder, contrast medium will have to be used. The measured depth of the tumor on a film, from a selected treatment port, will then have to be corrected for magnification. Let us suppose that the esophagus is the site of the tumor and the patient has been radiographed in the anteroposterior and lateral views in the supine position. The tumor is first localized on the anteroposterior radiograph with relation to the anterior ends of the clavicles, and its length is measured. This can now be marked

259

on the patient's skin anteriorly. To determine the depth of the tumor, the lateral radiograph (made with a horizontal beam) is used. The anteroposterior diameter of the chest at the center of the tumor is measured on the radiograph, and is called D_R. It is also measured on the patient, and is called D_P. Next, the distance of the tumor from the anterior chest wall is measured on the radiograph, and is called T_R. The true distance of the tumor from the anterior chest wall, T_P, can now be computed by a simple proportion:

$$\frac{True\ tumor\ depth}{Tumor\ depth\ on\ radiograph} = \frac{AP\ diameter\ of\ patient}{AP\ diameter\ of\ radiograph} \quad (1)$$

$$\frac{T_P}{T_R} = \frac{D_P}{D_R}$$

$$T_P = \frac{D_P T_R}{D_R}$$

Let us apply this to an actual example. Suppose the anteroposterior diameter of the lateral radiograph is 20 cm, and of the patient, 15 cm. If the esophagus is 14 cm behind the anterior surface in the radiograph, what is its true depth beneath the anterior surface of the chest?

$$T_P = \frac{D_P T_R}{D_R}$$

$$T_P = \frac{15 \times 14}{20} = 10.5\ cm$$

Similarly, if the patient is to be treated in the prone position, the distance of the tumor in front of the posterior skin surface must be determined, because the relationship of the internal organs may change with a change in position of the body.

For beams that are to be directed at other angles than those corresponding to the above radiographs, a body contour is made with solid wire solder ⅛ in. thick and transferred to paper by means of a soft lead pencil or felt-tip pen. The depth of the lesion, after preliminary localization from the radiographs, can then be measured directly from this contour drawing (see Fig. 10.01).

In some instances, such as pelvic lesions, radiography may be used in conjunction with a pelvimeter to ascertain the actual depth of the tumor.

2. *Fluoroscopy.* With this method, each treatment port in succession is outlined with solid wire solder ⅛ in. thick and the wire adjusted until the lesion is adequately enclosed. The position of the wire is outlined on the skin with a felt-tip pen. It is important to have the patient in the actual treatment position for each port.

3. *Calipers.* In some instances, such as lesions of the cervix, special calipers can be used to measure the depth directly.

Verification. Whatever the method used to localize a tumor, it is essential that the accuracy of the localization be checked and adjusted radiographically. This can best be done by exposing films through each selected treatment port using the actual therapy beam or an X-ray simulator, each port being outlined with solid wire solder as above. A 200-kV therapy unit serves as an excellent simulator for a megavoltage unit when operated at the same distance; a simulator not only provides better radiographic contrast, but avoids the waste of megavoltage treatment time during localization procedures. Verification should be repeated periodically during a prolonged series of treatments to minimize the possibility of accidental shift in positioning.

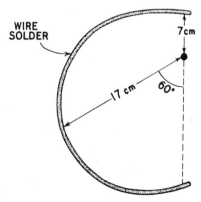

FIGURE 10.01. Wire solder used to obtain a body contour.

DELIMITATION OF FIELD SIZE AND PENUMBRA

An extremely important factor in planning radiation therapy is the selection of the *optimum field* or *port size*. This is based on two criteria:

1. Port size must be *large enough* to cover the lesion and include a suitable margin of apparently normal tissue.

2. Port size must not be so large as to irradiate an excessive volume of normal tissue.

The primary beam has a maximum diameter corresponding to any given source-skin or target-skin distance. As will be recalled, this is due to the divergence of the beam. To reduce the beam diameter for the treatment of lesions of various sizes, special field-limiting devices must be employed. With orthovoltage beams, these include principally cones, diaphragms, and lead shields. With megavoltage beams, specially designed *collimators* are used.

There is another important aspect of beam delimitation and that is *penumbra*. Since the source or focal spot has an appreciable area, a part of the radiation can undercut the edges of the collimator. Just as in radiography, this produces at the edge of the beam a poorly defined region of gradually decreasing intensity called *geometric penumbra* or *edge gradient:* the edge of the beam manifests a degree of *unsharpness.* Figure 10.02 shows the origin of geometric penumbra and includes pertinent terminology. For the sake of simplicity, we have replaced the collimator opening nearest the skin by a diaphragm. From the relationship of similar triangles, we see that

$$\frac{P}{s} = \frac{SD_eD - SCD}{SCD}$$

$$P = s\left(\frac{SD_eD - SCD}{SCD}\right) \tag{2}$$

where P is the geometric penumbra at depth d_e, s is the width of the source (or focal spot), SD_eD is the source-to-d_e distance, and SCD is the source-diaphragm (or distal collimator opening) distance. There are various practical measures of penumbra, one being the distance between the 90 percent and 10 percent isodose curves at the skin or at any particular depth. Note that geometric penumbra decreases with decreasing source width, decreasing distance of the collimator face from the skin or from any particular plane in the body, and increasing source-skin distance, provided, in the last instance, that the collimator-skin distance remains constant. Furthermore, geometric penumbra remains constant as port width is changed, but can be reduced by proper design and use of the collimator. However, it is very important to keep all material such as the collimator face, and beam trim-

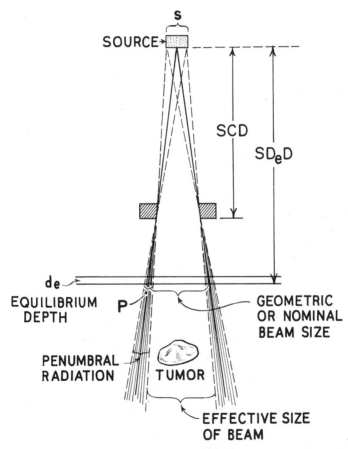

FIGURE 10.02. Terminology related to geometric penumbra and beam definition. Note how the penumbra grows as the depth increases.

mers and shapers, at no less than 15 cm from the skin to minimize the effects of electron contamination of the beam (see page 268).

Another important contributing influence on beam unsharpness is *scattered radiation,* consisting mainly of lateral or side scatter from within the irradiated volume. As we go from kilovoltage (e.g. 250 kV) to megavoltage radiation, lateral scatter decreases and beam sharpness improves. Beam unsharpness is evident in isodose curves (see Figs. 9.18 and 9.19) wherein the curves do not fuse at the beam edge but rather remain separated by finite distances. In general,

beam unsharpness = geometric penumbra + lateral scatter

By way of summary we can say that beam sharpness improves with an increase in the energy of the radiation, *SSD,* and efficiency of the collimator; and with a decrease in source diameter.

Because a radiation beam fades at its edges, usually over a distance of 1 or more cm, its width cannot be simply defined. One approach is to specify the *nominal width* of the beam as the distance between lines drawn from the center of the source through the edge of the diaphragm or distal collimator opening, measured at the depth of maximum buildup. Another convention is to describe beam width as the width of the 50 percent isodose curve at buildup depth. These two definitions of beam width give practically the same result.

Why is penumbra so important in radiation therapy? The answer may be seen in Figure 10.03A. A beam with a large penumbra will undertreat the edges of a tumor if the therapist ignores the decreased radiation exposure in the periphery of the beam. On the other hand, if the beam is enlarged sufficiently to encompass the entire tumor and a "safe" margin as in Figure 10.03B, an excessive amount of normal tissue will be needlessly irradiated, thereby impairing radiation tolerance. It is important to consider penumbra *at the depth of the tumor* because it increases with increasing depth. As a general rule, beams with the smallest available penumbra, preferably less than 1 cm at the skin, are essential for optimal irradiation therapy.

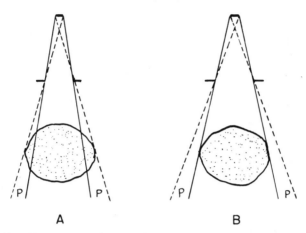

A B

FIGURE 10.03. Effect of penumbra on distribution of radiation. The stippled area indicates tumor plus margin of safety. *A*. Edge of tumor volume receives penumbral radiation *P* and is therefore undertreated. *B*. Collimator has been opened to include tumor volume in main beam (umbra), but now penumbra irradiates a significant volume of normal tissue. Obviously, the smaller the penumbra or edge gradient the smaller will be the volume of normal tissue irradiated.

The various types of megavoltage equipment have been discussed in Chapter 6. Aside from other differences we should realize that they differ significantly in source or focal spot size. With ^{60}Co the usual high intensity source has a diameter of 1.5 to 2 cm, although with very high specific activity this can be reduced to 1 cm. On the other hand, the focal spot in linacs is of the order of 0.2 to 0.3 cm, and in the Van de Graaff unit about 0.5 cm. The smallest focal spot of all is in the betatron, *0.2 mm!* Thus, geometric penumbra is significantly smaller with the high energy X-ray machines than with ^{60}Co, although proper collimation does improve the sharpness of the ^{60}Co beam.

Cones. The simplest type of cone, illustrated in Figure 10.04, is suitable for kilovoltage (200 to 300 kV) X-ray therapy. It consists of a lead aperture diaphragm with a thin metal cone attached, the entire unit being mounted directly below the tube aperture. If the cone wall is too light to absorb these particular X rays effectively, penumbral radiation arising from various points on

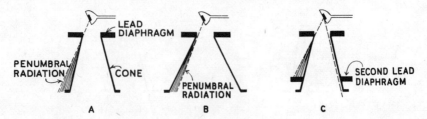

FIGURE 10.04. *A*. Penumbral radiation penetrates the side of the cone, striking the skin outside the treatment field. *B*. The lower opening is wider than the X-ray beam so that the periphery of the field is undertreated. *C*. An auxiliary lead diaphragm helps absorb penumbral radiation.

the focal spot pass through the cone wall, striking the patient's skin outside the selected field boundary, as shown in Figure 10.04A. On the other hand, if the cone is flared sufficiently to include the penumbral radiation, as in Figure 10.04B, the surface dose decreases near the edge of the field.

The problem cannot be solved by having the entire cone of sufficient lead thickness to absorb the penumbral radiation because of excessive weight. The most satisfactory solution is to place a second lead diaphragm around the cone just above the level of the skin as shown in Figure 10.04C.

Cone delimitation of a kilovoltage beam has many *advantages:*

1. *Fixed distance is assured;* there is no danger of approximating the tube any closer to the skin surface than the distance of the cone end.

2. *Penumbra can be reduced significantly.*

3. *Compression* by the bakelite-capped end of the cone reduces effective depth of the lesion in some cases, thereby increasing the depth dose. However, the thickness of the cone cover should not exceed ⅛ in. to avoid errors in depth dose determination.

4. *Immobilization* of the patient is facilitated by pressure contact with the end of the cone.

5. *Beam direction* is simplified. The central ray marked on the side of the cone may be alined with the center of the lesion.

Lead Shields. In the event that a field size is required for which no cone is available, the desired field may be delimited by the use of lead shields with the desired opening placed directly on the skin. The lead surrounding the field must be wide enough

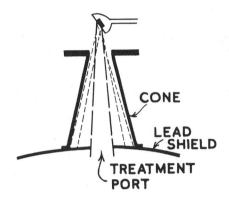

CONE

LEAD
SHIELD

TREATMENT
PORT

FIGURE 10.05. Delimitation of a kilovoltage beam by a lead shield of proper thickness.

to intercept all the unwanted radiation, as shown in Figure 10.05. An advantage of the lead shield is that one can use the central and more uniform portion of a larger X-ray beam to irradiate a relatively small field. One of the major disadvantages is that the lead is difficult to fit snugly against a curved body surface and its use is therefore restricted to flat areas.

One must be certain to use sheet lead of correct thickness for field demarcation—5/64 in. (2 mm) lead is required at 200 kV, HVL 1 mm Cu; about twice this thickness of lead is needed at 250 kV, HVL 3 mm Cu.

Collimators. The early ^{60}Co teletherapy units were provided with massive treatment cones to delimit the energetic γ-ray beams. However, not only were such cones unwieldy, but they were limited to only certain port sizes. A modern ^{60}Co teletherapy unit is equipped with a ***collimator*** consisting of a number of stacked lead or tungsten bars that are movable and interleaved. This type of collimator was originally designed by Johns, and is shown in Figure 10.06. One series of bars limits one dimension of the beam, while the opposite interleaving set limits the other dimension. Thus, a continuous range of rectangular ports from a minimum to a maximum is available. Because the inside edges of the bars are aligned with the source, penumbra is minimized. Further reduction of penumbra is accomplished by the addition of beam trimmers attached to the distal end of the collimator and moving

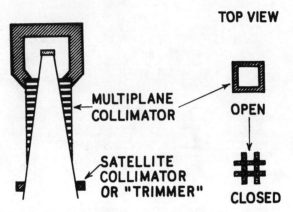

FIGURE 10.06. Function of a multiplane or multivane collimator for a megavoltage beam.

with the bars, as shown in Figure 10.06. A plastic tray may be used as a support for lead bars to permit additional beam shaping and penumbra control; however, neither the tray nor any of the bars should be closer than 15 cm to the patient's entrance port to reduce contamination of the therapy beam by secondary electrons (set free in the tray, etc.) which would be absorbed in the skin, causing an intensified reaction.

Within the collimator there is a *light localizer* consisting of a mirror and light system, designed to function as a rangefinder. Typically, rotation of a control knob causes a central light spot to coincide with a pair of intersecting crosshair images on the skin at the entrance port, when the preselected distance has been attained. Furthermore, when properly installed, the illumination of the port by light from within the collimator should coincide with the γ-ray beam so the treatment field can be visualized. Both the rangefinder, and coincidence of the illuminated port with the treatment field, should be checked periodically.

BEAM DIRECTION

To assure complete coverage of a deep-lying tumor we must have an accurate means of aiming the X- or γ-ray beam at the tumor, a process called *beam direction.* Inaccurate beam direction may result in serious underdosage of the tumor. In some instances, if the direction of the central ray is off by only a few degrees, the tumor may be missed entirely; or at best, be subjected to inadequate dosage at one edge due to off-centering. This type of error is known as a *geographic miss.* Auxiliary devices for beam direction are particularly important with small ports.

There are three main types of beam-directing devices: (1) protractor, (2) pin-and-arc, and (3) back pointer. The first two are known generally as *entrance directors.*

Protractor. Perfected by Demy,[17] this device indicates the angulation of the beam toward a tumor whose depth below the surface has been determined. It consists of a plastic or aluminum semicircle large enough to straddle the body, calibrated in degrees from zero at the center to 90 degrees at both ends as shown in Figure 10.07. The protractor is raised or lowered on the calibrated posts at its extremities until its *base* is at the level of the tumor. When the zero line of the protractor is placed directly over the tumor, every point on the *upper* edge of the protractor is located at a distance of 26 cm from the tumor, since this is the radius of the protractor. Furthermore, any beam directed along one of the graduations on the protractor will be aimed precisely

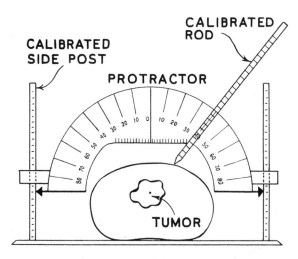

FIGURE 10.07. Schematic diagram of the Demy protractor method of beam direction. (For a more complete description of this method, please refer to N. G. Demy.[17]

at the tumor. Once the proper angles have been found and verified radiographically, they should be recorded for each treatment port for duplication in subsequent treatments. Naturally,
the angle indicator on the tube head itself must be accurate.

For any angular position of the beam, the depth of the tumor
below that particular treatment surface can be determined by
means of a calibrated rod, which is ruled in cm beginning with 26
at its lowest point and decreasing to zero above. Since the outer
margin of the protractor is a semicircle of 26 cm radius, every
point on its margin is 26 cm from the center of tumor. If the rod
is held in line with one of the graduations so that its tip contacts
the skin corresponding to that port of entry, the distance that the
rod projects above the arc is equal to the depth of the tumor below
the surface for that particular treatment port. This can be read
directly on the rod as illustrated in Figure 10.08. Thus the protractor method serves two purposes: it facilitates accurate direction of the beam, and it provides a simple method of determining
the depth of the tumor below every possible entrance port.

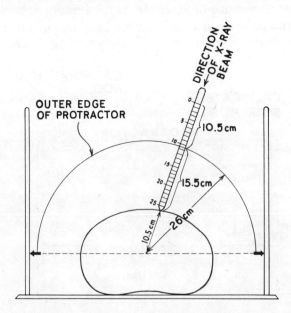

FIGURE 10.08. Determination of tumor depth for various points of entry, with the
Demy protractor.

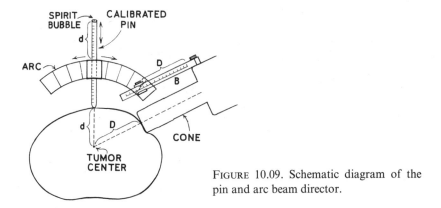

FIGURE 10.09. Schematic diagram of the pin and arc beam director.

Pin-and-Arc. A modification of the protractor method, the pin-and-arc is mounted on the tube housing, so the patient may be treated either recumbent or sitting. The arc consists of a segment of a circle calibrated in degrees. The pin is attached to the arc by means of a carrier that permits it to be slid along its axis, similar to the calibrated rod in the protractor method. First, the depth of the tumor below the center of the treatment port is determined. The pin is then slid out so that it projects above the arc by this same distance. Next, the desired angle between the pin and the beam axis is selected and the pin carrier moved so that the pin makes this angle with the beam axis. Finally, the tube head is angulated to bring the pin vertically over the center of the tumor, and at the same time, the position of the cone and the pin-and-arc is adjusted so the pin touches the skin (see Fig. 10.09). The vertical position of the pin is indicated by the central location of the spirit bubble. Now the beam is directed toward the tumor, the depth of which is indicated on the calibrated rack and pinion of the pin-and-arc.

Back Pointer. Also known as an exit director, the back pointer consists of a metal arc attached to the tube housing or collimator, partly encircling the anatomic part. A sliding metal rod, or pointer, is located at the opposite end in such a way that it points back directly through the central axis of the beam, as shown in Figure 10.10. In use, the cone or collimator is directed to the entrance port, and the patient so arranged that the pointer is aimed toward

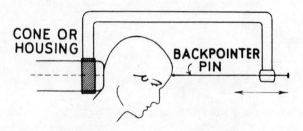

FIGURE 10.10. Diagram of a backpointer.

the center of the opposing exit port. If correctly localized in the first place, the tumor should lie on this axis. For precise utilization of this method, a plaster or plastic shell can be made to fit the anatomic area, such as the thorax in treatment of the esophagus. Once the position of the lesion has been verified radiographically with reference to fixed points on the shell, the treatment setup can be duplicated with satisfactory precision. A backpointer can be used only when the exit port is free; otherwise, the protractor or pin-and-arc is preferred.

DELIVERY OF PLANNED TUMOR DOSE

There are at least seven reasons why accurate dosage determination is necessary in executing a course of deep therapy:

1. To deliver a cancericidal dose of radiation to the tumor and its vicinity without irreparable injury to normal tissue.

2. To permit duplication or later modification in an effort to improve results.

3. To allow comparison with therapy methods at other institutions.

4. To transmit information to other radiologists.

5. To obtain information relative to the sensitivity and curability of various tumors.

6. To determine adequacy of therapy relative to recurrences and possible retreatment.

7. To provide complete records for scientific and medicolegal purposes.

Crossfire Radiation Technic. When a tumor lies at a considerable depth below the skin surface, it is impossible to deliver an adequate therapeutic dose through a single skin field without danger of excessive irradiation and irreparable damage to the skin and subcutaneous tissue, because the dose will be higher there than in the tumor. This may be avoided by dividing the total dose between two or more ports of entry and aiming each beam at the lesion, a procedure called *crossfiring.* This procedure, by distributing the calculated dose through two or more fields, spares the skin overlying each field and still concentrates an adequate dose of radiation on the deep seated tumor.

To apply the crossfire technic, we must have suitable *isodose curves.* However, we shall first consider the use of published depth dose tables as a first approximation. These data apply only if the size of the irradiated anatomic region resembles that of the phantom on which the tables are based, to assure full scatter in the tissues. In general, if the edge of the entire treatment field lies within a few cm of the edge of the anatomic part, the discrepancy is not significant.

To clarify the method of crossfire technic, an actual example will be used. Suppose we have a cylindrical structure 10 cm in diameter, the center point therefore lying 5 cm below the surface, as shown in Figure 10.11. Using a ^{60}Co beam at a source-skin distance of 80 cm and an 8×8 cm^2 port, we are to deliver a dose of 5000 rads at the center of the cylinder. However, we must not exceed a total entrance dose (given dose + exit dose) of 5500 rads in six weeks. From published data, the depth dose at 5 cm is 77 percent. Then

$$D_t = 0.77 \, D_m$$

$$tumor \ dose = 0.77 \times given \ dose$$

$$5,000 \ rads = 0.77 \, D_m$$

$$D_m = \frac{5,000}{0.77} = 6,500 \ rads$$

Thus, a tumor dose of 5,000 rads would require a total given dose of 6,500 rads. Obviously, this is far in excess of the permissible 5,500 rads.

Suppose, instead, we were to use two coaxial opposing beams as depicted in Figure 10.12. Each beam would now have to con-

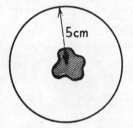

FIGURE 10.11. Diagram of a tumor located at the center of a cylindrical structure.

tribute half the tumor dose, or 2,500 rads. Obviously the given dose would also be reduced to one-half, or 3,250 rads. But we must add the exit dose contributed by the opposing beam. The uncorrected exit dose for a 64 cm² field is approximately equal to the depth dose at that level. In Figure 10.12 the dose at E contributed by beam 1 is taken at a depth of 10 cm, or 54 percent (see *Appendix*). Therefore,

$$3,250 \times 0.54 \approx 1,750 \text{ rads}$$

$$3,250 + 1,750 = 5,000 \text{ rads, } \textit{total entrance dose}$$

This is well within the specified entrance dose. Further reduction in the given dose could be attained by using three coplanar beams (i.e. axes in same plane), arranged about the axis at equal angles of 120°, as shown in Figure 10.13. Now the given dose would be one third of that required for a single port, or ⅓ × 6,500 rads = 2,170 rads. Each exit field would receive only part of the exit dose, as is evident in Figure 10.13.

Isodose Curves in Therapy Planning. In the preceding discussion, only the ***central axis*** depth doses have been considered and only the central tumor absorbed dose obtained. When the

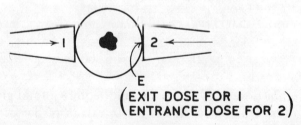

FIGURE 10.12. Directly opposed coaxial beams; the exit port of 1 coincides with the entrance port of 2.

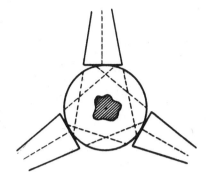

FIGURE 10.13. Three coplanar ports equidistant (120°) from each other. Note that the entrance and exit fields are only partly superimposed.

lesion is small, this method may be adequate. However, most lesions are of such a size that one must take into account the distribution of radiation at various critical points within the irradiated volume, to avoid points of over- or under-irradiation. Isodose curves are available to facilitate therapy planning on this basis (see pages 276 and 278). Such curves show, in detail, the distribution of percentage depth doses not only along the central axis, but at all points within the beam and outside the geometric edge of the beam. *Isodose curves* are composites of the actual measurements of percentage depth doses (relative to the maximum dose taken as 100 percent) of a particular beam at many points within a phantom. Lines are drawn connecting points of identical dosage, hence the term *iso* (same) plus *dose.* Figure 10.14 is an example of sets of isodose distributions, each curved line representing an isodose curve. Note that the percentage depth dose is higher along the central axis, at a given depth, than it is near the edge at the same depth. Thus, by constructing a horizontal line through the 40 percent depth dose curve intersection with the central axis, and extending it laterally, we find that it meets the 32 percent point near the edge of the field of the X-ray beam. This is due to the fact that scattered radiation adds to primary radiation along and near the central axis of the beam. However, scatter decreases near the edge of the beam, resulting in a lower percentage depth dose. Furthermore, the greater obliquity of the radiation near the edge makes for increased attenuation at a particular depth as compared with the straighter, more centrally disposed, radiation. *Lateral scatter* in

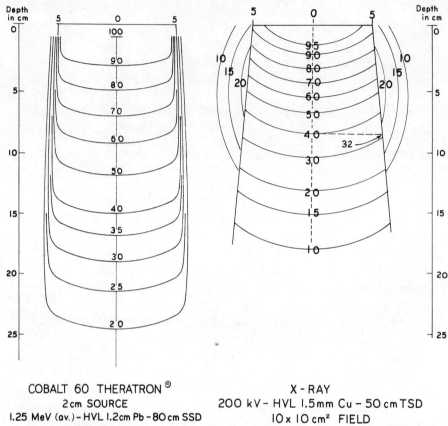

COBALT 60 THERATRON®
2 cm SOURCE
1.25 MeV (av.) – HVL 1.2 cm Pb – 80 cm SSD
10 x 10 cm² FIELD

X – RAY
200 kV – HVL 1.5 mm Cu – 50 cm TSD
10 x 10 cm² FIELD

FIGURE 10.14. Typical isodose curves. *A.* ^{60}Co beam (HVL 12 mm Pb). *B.* Kilovoltage X-ray beam (HVL 1.5 mm Cu). In each case, an infinite number of isodose distributions exist between any pair of curves.

the case of orthovoltage beams produces lateral bulging of the isodose curves, but with megavoltage beams lateral scatter is minimal and the lateral bulging is caused mainly by *penumbra* and, possibly, collimator leakage. The penumbra is significantly larger with ^{60}Co sources than with the small focal spots of megavoltage X-ray generators such as the 4-MV linac.

In practice, isodose curves, drawn to the same scale as the anatomic part being treated, are placed on a full scale drawing of that part at all entrance ports, and the points of intersection of the isodose curves are marked. Where any two or more curves intersect, the total depth dose is the sum of those represented by the intersecting curves. If each treatment port receives the *same* total given dose, such as D_m, then dose D_n at any point within the irradiated volume is:

$$D_n = D_m \times (isodose\ 1 + isodose\ 2 + isodose\ 3)$$

If *isodose* 1 is 40 percent, *isodose* 2 is 40 percent, and *isodose* 3 is 60 percent of the given dose, and if $D_m = 2,000$ rads, then the dose at the point of intersection would be:

$$D_n = 2,000\,(0.40 + 0.40 + 0.60) = 2,000 \times 1.40$$

$$D_n = 2,800\ \text{rads}$$

Let us see how we can plot isodose distributions for three coplanar beams when the lesion is centrally situated, equidistant from all the entrance ports. It may be stated, in general, that depth dose plotting with isodose curves takes two forms, either (1) determination of the doses at a great many points in the paths of the crossfiring beams by plotting composite isodose curves, or (2) determination of the dose only at certain critical points to insure adequate minimal dosage and, at the same time, avoid over-irradiation or "hot spots."

1. *Composite Isodose Curves.* The contour of the part to be irradiated is obtained first. A simple method is to wrap solid wire solder snugly around one-half the structure if it is symmetrical, as is usually the case. The contour so obtained is then traced on translucent paper placed over a large fluorescent illuminator (about 41 × 48 cm²). Next, the isodose chart corresponding to the required quality of radiation and beam size is placed under the outline in various positions to obtain the best arrangement. The central axis of the isodose curves must coincide, in each position, with the central axis of the entrance beam.

In the simple example we have selected we have decided to use three coplanar ports making angles of 120° with each other as shown in Figure 10.13. The isodose chart is applied and the curves traced on the contour outline sheet as in Figure 10.15, the percentage depth doses being marked for each curve. Next, the iso-

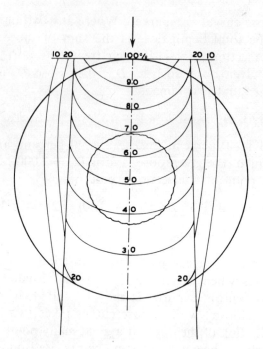

FIGURE 10.15. Isodose distribution under the first port.

dose chart is shifted around the contour 120° and the curves again traced in the new position. The points of intersection of the iso-dose curves are now marked as shown in Figure 10.16, preferably with ink of a different color, to show the total percentage depth dose at each point. The total is simply the addition of the two curves. For example, if a 50 percent curve intersects a 70 percent curve, that point is 50 + 70 = 120 percent of the dose contributed through **one port**, provided both ports receive the same total dose. The points of similar depth dose are then connected to obtain a composite depth dose curve for the two positions of the chart thus far plotted, as shown in Figure 10.17. To avoid confusion, one should prepare a new contour outline sheet showing these composite curves.

The new sheet is substituted for the old one on the illuminator and the isodose chart applied in the third position, the points of intersection between these curves and the composite curves being marked in ink of a third color. This step is depicted in

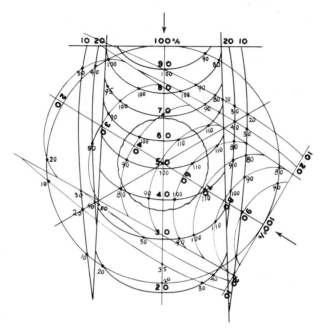

FIGURE 10.16. Superimposition of the isodose distribution under the second port, on those under the first port.

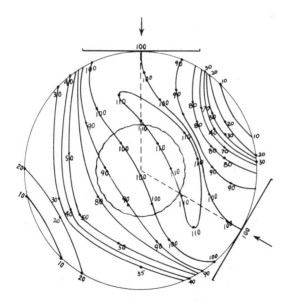

FIGURE 10.17. Summation of isodose curves at points of intersection.

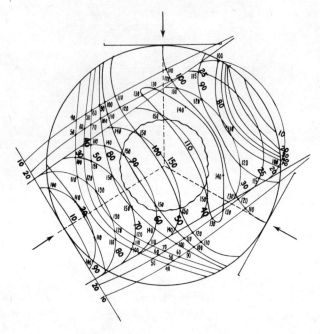

FIGURE 10.18. Superimposition of third set of isodose curves on the first two.

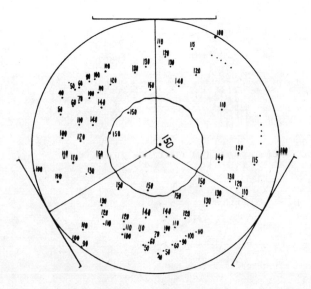

FIGURE 10.19. Summation of intersecting isodose curves under all three ports.

Figures 10.18 and 10.19. Again, all the intersecting points bearing the same total depth dose values are connected to obtain the final composite isodose curve shown in Figure 10.20. The procedure may be simplified by using a third contour outline sheet in preparing the final set of curves to avoid a multiplicity of intermediate lines.

The radiologist can readily determine, by studying the composite isodose curves, just how uniformly the lesion is being irradiated, how much normal tissue is being included at the periphery, and whether or not there are hot spots. Figure 10.20 shows that all portions of the tumor, including a safe margin, receive a 140 to 150 percent depth dose. For example, if each of the three fields receives 3,000 rads, the minimum tumor absorbed dose will be $3,000 \times 1.40 = 4,200$ rads.

Conversely, if we wish to deliver a 6,000 rad minimum dose to the tumor in six weeks, the total given dose to each field will be

$$D_m \times 1.40 = 6,000$$

$$D_m = \frac{6,000}{1.40} = 4,280 \text{ rads}$$

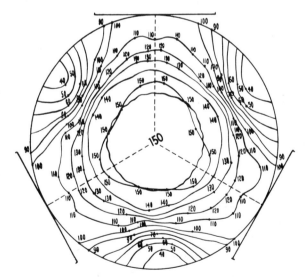

FIGURE 10.20. Completed isodose curves, composite of all three sets, made by connecting the points of same dosage in Figure 10.19. Note the uniformity of dosage in and near the tumor.

To determine the daily increment of dose to each field, assuming that there are five treatments per week, or a total of 30 cycles,

$$\frac{4,280}{30} = 143 \ rads/day, \ given \ dose$$

Plotting of the composite isodose curves, as well as the original one, is greatly facilitated by the use of special computerized devices.

2. **Determination of Dosage at Certain Critical Points Only.** By the application of isodose curves, we can obtain the percentage depth doses at selected important points only, in and about the tumor, as well as on the skin where entrance and exit ports may be superimposed. This method is especially suitable where the radiologist, through previous experience with complete isodose plotting of certain lesions, has become familiar with the critical points and therefore does not have to repeat a complete plot each time a similar lesion is to be treated.

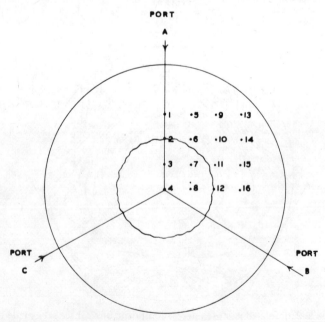

FIGURE 10.21. Basic plan for establishing summated depth doses at selected critical points, indicated by numbered points 1 cm apart.

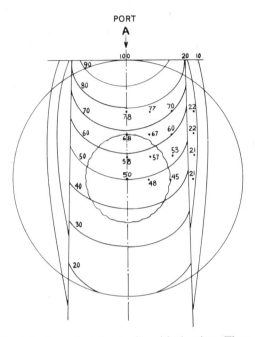

FIGURE 10.22. Contribution of port *A* to the critical points. These depth doses are entered in Table 10.01.

Using the same isodose curves as before, we first prepare a contour outline on translucent paper by means of wire solder. The central rays to the tumor from each port are marked and, from appropriate tables, the depth dose and given dose for each position of the beam are computed. If these are within the desired limits, the isodoses at critical points can now be determined. It is usually sufficient to plot the critical points 1 cm apart on one side of a symmetrically placed lesion, such as that used in our example. This is shown in Figure 10.21. Next, the isodose chart is placed successively in each selected position and the doses contributed to the critical points recorded in a table. The first step is shown in Figure 10.22. If a curve crosses a point exactly, the

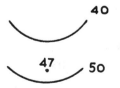

FIGURE 10.23. The depth dose between two isodose curves is estimated.

TABLE 10.01
PERCENTAGE DEPTH DOSES AT VARIOUS CRITICAL POINTS ONLY;
OBTAINED BY A PARTIAL ISODOSE PLOT, AS DESCRIBED IN THE TEXT

Port	Points															
	1	2	3	4	5	6	7	8	9	10	11	12	13	14	15	16
A	78	68	58	50	77	67	57	48	70	60	53	45	22	22	21	21
B	32	40	45	50	21	44	51	57	10	47	56	64	5	20	60	70
C	32	40	45	50	30	36	40	43	28	31	35	37	25	28	29	30
Total	142	148	148	150	128	147	148	148	108	138	144	146	52	70	110	121

depth dose is that represented by the curve. However, if the point lies between two curves, its corresponding dose is estimated, according to the example in Figure 10.23, where the dose is about 47 percent.

The isodose chart is now moved to the second position, 120° around the contour margin, and the depth doses at the same critical points again determined in the same manner (see Fig. 10.24). These data are entered in the table.

Finally, the isodose chart is shifted to the last position and the procedure repeated for each critical point as before (see Fig. 10.25). All of the data are now summated as in Table 10.01 and in Figure 10.26. It should be noted that the isodose distribution by this method is similar to that obtained by the complete plot (see Fig. 10.20). If the total depth doses contributed by the beam in the three positions are adequate and there are no zones of under- or over-irradiation, the plan is considered satisfactory.

With multiport therapy the central rays of all the ports should lie in the same plane. Such a *coplanar* arrangement facilitates isodose planning.

Arrangement of Crossfiring Beams. As a result of considerable experience with isodose distributions Paterson[66] has proposed certain criteria for the selection of crossfiring beams:

1. *Symmetrical arrangement* of treatment ports about at least one axis.

2. Each port added to an already existing arrangement moves the point of highest dosage *toward* itself.

3. Based on 1 and 2, if a lesion is irradiated by three coplanar beams arranged so that two are directly opposed and the third perpendicular to the common axis of the first two, the point of

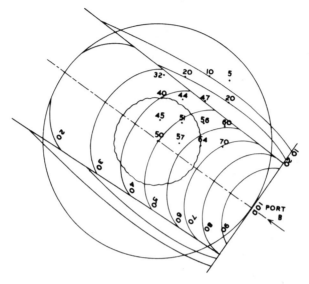

FIGURE 10.24. Contribution of port *B* to the critical points. These depth doses are entered in Table 10.01.

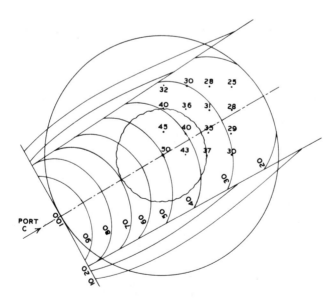

FIGURE 10.25. Contribution of port *C* to the critical points. These depth doses are entered in Table 10.01.

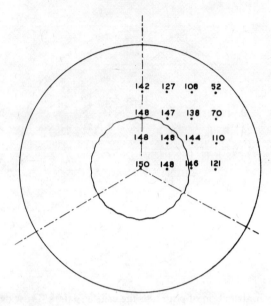

FIGURE 10.26. The summations of the contributed depth doses from all three fields are shown at the critical points. Note similarity to result obtained by the composite isodose curve method.

maximum dosage is **nearer** the latter port of entry, as shown in Figure 10.27. If this is not taken into account, the maximum radiation effect will not be located in the center of the tumor, and may even lie outside it.

4. Every effort should be made to **balance** the dosage contribution from all ports.

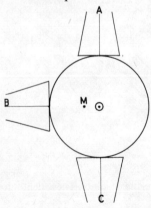

FIGURE 10.27. With this arrangement of ports the point of maximum dosage *M* is shifted toward the unopposed port.

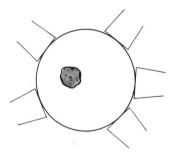

FIGURE 10.28. More ports are needed on the far side of an eccentric tumor to deliver the maximum dosage within the tumor.

5. If a tumor is off center, more fields should be added on the *far* side than on the near side to facilitate equalization (see Fig. 10.28).

6. Similarly, if two beams have their axes at an angle less than 180°, the maximum dose will be displaced toward the surface midway between them as in Figure 10.29. This combination has the same effect as a single field submerged in the tissues (see Fig. 10.29), with its axis on the bisector of the angle between the two beam axes. Paterson has named this the ***internal single field.***

Wedge filters are useful under certain conditions. When two beam axes intersect at an angle of less than 180° as in (6) of the preceding paragraph, a "hot spot" is produced at *M* in Figure 10.29. One method of compensating for this is to add a third port on the opposite side. However, this may not be possible. Another method is to overshoot the center of the tumor with the two beams to bring the hot spot nearer the center of the tumor. A more sophisticated approach is to use ***wedge filters***—wedge-shaped pieces of metal (usually aluminum, copper, brass, or lead, according to the energy of the radiation). Lead or brass is often used with ⁶⁰Co beams. The wedge filter distorts the isodose

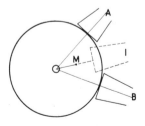

FIGURE 10.29. The effect of two ports whose central axes intersect at an angle of less than 180°, is that of an imaginary single field, 1, submerged in the tissues between the two ports. This is Paterson's *internal single field*, resulting in a "hot spot" at *M*.

curves, making them slope as in Figure 10.30. The **wedge angle is defined as the angle the 50 percent isodose curve makes with a line parallel to the surface.** In other words, the wedge is so designed that it produces the desired distortion of the isodose curves. Figure 10.31 shows the combination of two wedge filters to produce wedge fields for the irradiation of a larynx. Note the beautiful box-like pattern of uniform irradiation of the volume of interest. A similar pattern can be used for irradiation of a maxillary sinus. Also note, in this figure, the designation *hinge angle*— the angle between the central axes of the two wedge fields. As a general rule, *for an optimum pattern of homogeneous radiation, the wedge angle should be equal to 90° minus 1/2 the hinge angle.* Thus, in the example given for the larynx,

$$\text{wedge angle} = 90° - \text{hinge angle}°/2 \qquad (3)$$
$$= 90° - 45° = 45°$$

Several points of caution should be observed. First, the use of wedges depends on careful design, verification, and application, and should be done under the supervision of a well qualified person, preferably a physicist. Second, wedge filters should not be transferred between treatment units unless they have been verified beforehand. Third, the wedge should be at least 15 cm from the skin to minimize electron contamination of the beam at the skin surface.

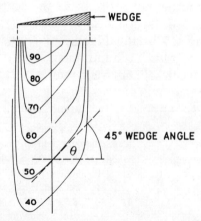

FIGURE 10.30. Distortion of isodose distribution by a wedge filter.

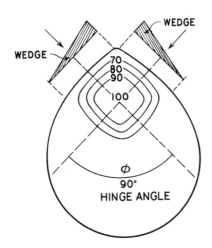

FIGURE 10.31. Combined isodose distribution obtained with a pair of beams with wedge filters. Note the box-like distribution without hot spots outside the volume of interest.

With directly opposing fields, the dose delivered by the beam leaving the skin opposite the entry portal is the *exit dose.* This has been regarded as roughly equal to the depth dose indicated in the usual tables for that particular depth, as though the exit port were completely surrounded by scattering material. Thus, the total skin dose for any treatment port equals the sum of the given dose (skin or equilibrium depth) and the exit dose.

Correction for Tissue Inhomogeneity (see also pages 304 to 307). Depth doses must be corrected for the various types of tissue being traversed by the beam. Recall that depth dose tables are based on phantoms with scattering properties equivalent to soft tissues of water density. The following approximate corrections usually suffice in radiation therapy:

1. In the lung, an anterior tumor would receive a reduced dose from an anterior port (less contributory scatter from surrounding air-filled lung), and an increased dose from a posterior port (greater transmission through air-filled lung). Thus, with ^{60}Co, the tumor dose increases on an average of 4 percent per cm of aerated lung. However, massive hilar tumors have so little air around them that no correction factor is needed.

2. If the beam traverses bone, about twice as much energy ab-

sorption occurs in bone as in soft tissues of equal masses when the quality if HVL 1 mm Cu. At 4 mm Cu HVL, absorption per gram of bone and soft tissue is about equal. This also holds true in the 1 to 2 MeV range. Above 10 MeV, bone absorption again exceeds that in soft tissue due to pair production, for which the mass attenuation coefficient is proportional to the atomic number. However, despite equal absorption of energy per unit mass of bone or soft tissue with ^{60}Co rays or 2 MV X rays, there is about twice as much absorption per unit *volume* of bone so that shadowing of high energy radiation does occur. Thus, when bone lies in the path of a beam in this energy range, the tumor dose beyond the bone computed from standard tables is decreased approximately 3.5 percent per cm of bone, up to a thickness of at least 3 cm.[43]

FIXED BEAM THERAPY THROUGH SLOPING SKIN SURFACES

In radiotherapy with fixed beams we often encounter skin surfaces which *slope* away from the normal cross-sectional plane of the beam. Several methods have been devised to compensate or correct for the resulting *air gap*, thereby permitting more accurate application of standard isodose curves. We shall limit our discussion to the more practical methods, including (1) bolus, (2) tissue-compensating filters, and (3) isodose shift.

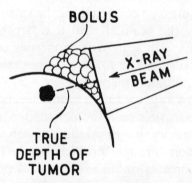

FIGURE 10.32. Bolus fills the air space between the flat surface of the cone and the curved surface of the body, to assure maximum scatter and permit application of isodose curves. (See page 291 for proper use of bolus.)

1. ***Bolus.*** Bags can be made up containing tissue equivalent material such as rice, small spherical sugar pellets, or a mixture of 60 percent rice flour and 40 percent sodium bicarbonate. Their absorbing and scattering properties simulate those of soft tissue, and they are therefore suitable as filling material between the end of the cone and the skin where the air gap occurs (see Fig. 10.32). Bolus is useful with ***kilovoltage radiation*** (200 to 300 kV) because we are not concerned with skin sparing and because depth dose tables are based on tissue equivalent phantoms whose surface is normal to the beam axis. Unless the air gap is filled with tissue equivalent material, the depth dose tables will yield erroneous results and the isodose curves will be distorted, as shown in Figure 10.33A. The true depth of the lesion is taken from the center of the free surface of the bolus. It must be emphasized that bolus should ***not*** be used with megavoltage radiation except to build up the dose in the skin, as in tangential therapy of the breast; otherwise, bolus defeats the skin-sparing property of high energy radiation.

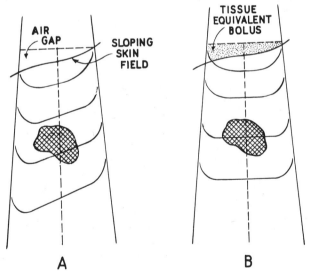

FIGURE 10.33. In *A* the isodose distribution is distorted when an air gap is present by virtue of a sloping field. In *B* the normal isodose distribution has been restored by the use of tissue equivalent bolus. This should be done only with kilovoltage radiation, since bolus negates skin sparing with megavoltage beams. (See Fig. 10.34 for the use of compensating filters.)

2. ***Tissue-compensating Filters.*** Various materials placed at some distance from the skin to preserve skin sparing by megavoltage radiation can be designed to compensate for the air gap in sloping fields. These include either tissue equivalent material such as Mix D, or high density material such as lead or brass so milled that absorption by the filter would equal that of the tissue missing from the air gap. Obviously such filters must be tapered to conform with the shape of the air gap (see Fig. 10.34). Any type of compensating filter used with megavoltage beams should be mounted at least 15 to 20 cm from the nearest point on the skin to minimize the effect of electron contamination of the beam. Compensation with appropriate filters allows the radiotherapist to apply standard isodose curves without further correction, provided the filters have been properly designed. However, it is extremely important to

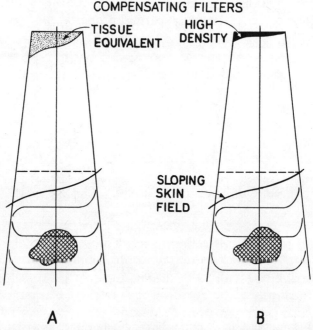

FIGURE 10.34. Compensating filters used to correct for the air gap in a sloping field. In *A* a tissue equivalent filter is placed at a sufficient distance from the skin to correct for the air gap and still maintain skin sparing with a megavoltage beam. In *B* a high density compensating filter of suitable dimensions is used for the same purpose.

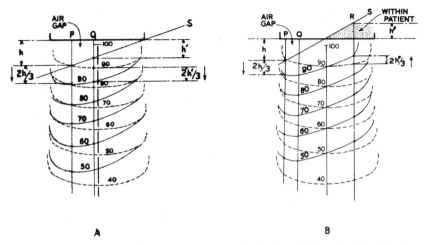

FIGURE 10.35. Correction of isodose curves by the isodose shift method for sloping fields. In *A* the source-skin distance (SSD) is taken at one *edge* of the field, and all corrections are in the same direction, the isodose curves being shifted distally point for point. In *B* the SSD is taken at the *center* of the sloping field and here the isodose curves are shifted distally under the air gap and proximally under the extra thickness of tissue. For ^{60}Co γ rays (1.25 MeV) the shift in each case is 2/3 of the thickness of the air gap or extra tissue thickness for each individual ray, such as P. Q. and R.

have a foolproof system of mounting and inserting the filter to avoid erroneous "compensation" of the wrong part of the treatment field.

3. *Isodose Shift Method.* There are several ways of modifying the application of isodose curves, some of which involve some form of computation such as the use of the inverse square law to correct for the air gap. Perhaps the easiest one is the *isodose shift method* wherein standard isodose curves are deliberately distorted by application of a correction factor. Figure 10.35A shows how this method operates when the source-skin distance (SSD) is chosen at the *highest edge* of the sloping field. As a general rule, with a ^{60}Co or a 4-MV beam we shift the isodose curves *distally* (deeper below the skin) over a distance equal to two-thirds the thickness of the air gap, along any individual γ-ray path. Several such points are plotted for each isodose distribution and a new curve drawn through them. If, as is more practical, we wish to choose the SSD at the *center* of the sloping field, one side will

have an air gap and the other an extra thickness of tissue, each being approximately wedged shaped, as shown in Figure 10.35B. Below the air gap we shift the isodose curves *distally* as in the preceding description, but below the added thickness of tissue we shift the isodose curves *proximally* (toward the skin) a distance equal to two-thirds the thickness of the extra tissue along each γ-ray path. Although the isodose shift method is approximate, it is entirely adequate for radiotherapy, provided the slope of the field does not exceed 45°. In any event, this method produces results comparable to those obtained by inverse square law computation.

Other methods of computing the dosage distribution through sloping fields include the *effective source-skin distance method* and the *effective coefficient attenuation method.* These are described in detail in *ICRU Handbook 87,* but since they are somewhat more difficult to apply than isodose shift and are not significantly more precise, they will not be discussed here.

SEPARATION OF ADJACENT PORTS

It goes without saying that whenever possible it is better to treat through a large single port than through separate adjacent ports; the latter arrangement makes it extremely difficult to avoid regions of over- or underdosage. However, there are occasions when the available beam is not large enough and two adjacent fields must be used.

For beams having significant penumbra such as we find in telecurie therapy, the preferred method is the *matching of isodose curves* at the desired depth when this is greater than 5 cm. Let us suppose we are using adjacent ports and the central axis depth dose with a single beam is 60 percent at 10 cm. The isodose curves are placed side-by-side with one-half the depth dose or 30 percent lines touching at a depth of 10 cm. The distance between the ports is then measured from the isodose distributions at the entrance surface. Table 10.02 shows the separation distances for ^{60}Co fields.

With beams having sharply defined edges, as with the linac, *geometric matching* at the desired depth may be used, separation

TABLE 10.02
SEPARATION DISTANCES OF ADJACENT PORTS FOR COBALT 60 BEAMS*

SSD (cm)	60		70		80	
Matching Depth (cm)	5	10	5	10	5	10
Average Field Width cm	cm	cm	cm	cm	cm	cm
10	1.5	2.5	1.0	2	0.5	1.0
15	1.8	3	1.3	2.5	0.7	1.5
20	2.0	3.5	1.7	3.3	1.0	2.2
25	2.2	4.0	2.0	3.5	1.2	3.0
30	—	—	—	—	1.5	3.5

* From *Physical Foundations of Radiology*,[35] by Goodwin, P. N., Quimby, E. H., and Morgan, R. H. Courtesy of the authors and Harper & Row, Publishers, New York, 1970. Separation should be checked for the particular collimator or trimmers at each treatment distance.

at the surface being adjusted to achieve fairly uniform isodose distribution in the zone of interest.

Of all the available methods, the least complicated one is the *shifting or double junction method.*[35] This provides a reasonably simple way of homogenizing the dosage distribution below the junction and is applicable to all depths, even those less than 5 cm. Here the separation of the ports is no greater than 0.5 cm. The junction is shifted 5 cm in one direction and then back 5 cm on alternate days. With this method reasonably uniform dosage distribution is achieved except for two small areas on the surface where the dose is about 10 percent higher than the midline maximum.

ROTATION THERAPY

The principle of rotation therapy is similar to that of crossfiring carried to the ultimate degree. Its objective is to maintain the beam centered on a deep seated tumor during rotation of the beam (or body). This is known as *isocentric radiotherapy.* The more superficial structures move past the beam, receiving significantly less radiation than the tumor itself. In practice this may be accomplished in two ways: (1) the patient is rotated in a standing or sitting position while the beam is aimed at the tumor, or (2) the recumbent patient is stationary as the beam is rotated about an axis and is continuously centered on the tumor. In effect, the tumor is crossfired from every conceivable direction on the body's circumference in the plane of rotation. Rotation may be complete or partial.

When properly carried out, rotation therapy delivers a considerably higher tumor dose than is possible with stationary beams. This is due to the relatively higher depth dose relative to given dose. In fact, the tumor dose with rotation therapy may be two or three times the given dose. However, the treatment fields must not be too wide relative to the thickness of the irradiated part because the depth dose advantage decreases as the width of the field increases. As the width of the beam approaches one-half the diameter of the anatomic part, the dose throughout the volume becomes almost uniform, thereby decreasing the percentage depth dose.

Tissue-air Ratio. In dosage determination for rotation therapy, the tissue-air ratio is the preferred approach. As indicated before on pages 252 to 253, the tissue-air ratio or tumor-air ratio R_t is defined by

$$R_t = D_t/D_a \tag{4}$$

where D_t is the absorbed dose at the site in question (e.g. axis, center of tumor), and D_a is the absorbed dose in a small mass of tissue (without scatter) at the same location. R_t was also shown to be described by the following equation:

$$R_t = \frac{F^2}{f^2} \cdot B \cdot P/100 \tag{5}$$

where, as before, (see Fig. 10.36) F is the distance from the source to the axis of rotation (n cm below the surface), f is the distance from the source to the level of maximum ionization (D_m), B is the backscatter factor, and P is the percent depth dose obtained from corrected tables.

Thus, the tissue-air ratio can readily be determined for a given therapy setup if the source-axis distance F, the tumor depth n, the backscatter factor B, and the percentage depth dose $\%D.D.$, are known. The last two values are obtainable from standard depth dose tables. Furthermore, with source-axis distances rang-

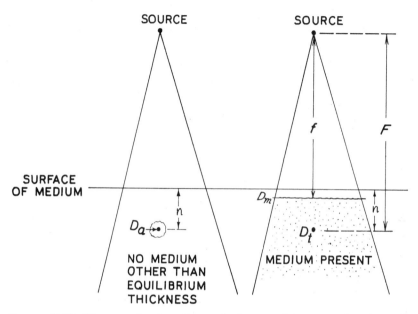

FIGURE 10.36. Diagram showing the terminology used in computing tissue-air ratio. D_m is the given dose (i.e. at equilibrium depth); D_t is the tumor dose within the body or tissue equivalent phantom; D_a is the dose to a small segregated mass of tissue at the level of the tumor (in absence of contributory scatter from surrounding tissue, i.e. dose in free space); F is the source-tumor distance; f is the source-skin or source-D_m distance; and n is the depth of the tumor. The point of reference here is the center of the tumor. Tumor-air ratio $R_t = D_t/D_a$.

ing from 40 to 100 cm the tissue-air ratio is independent of the distance with an accuracy of 1 to 2 percent, depending mainly on %D.D. and B. The reason for this is that the term F^2/f^2 in equation (5) increases in value as F decreases, at the same time that %D.D. decreases, so that the net value of the right member changes very little with a change in F. This applies only to hard radiation with HVL 2 mm Cu and above. Because of the dependence of tissue-air ratio on depth and on backscatter, as in equation (5), it is obvious that the tissue-air ratio increases with increasing field size, and with decreasing depth. Correction for elongated fields is made in the same manner as in stationary beam therapy.

Let us see now the application of tissue-air ratios in rotation therapy. First, a contour drawing is made of the part to be irradiated, in the same manner as in planning crossfire therapy. Solid wire solder is a satisfactory and readily available material for this purpose. With the tumor position marked on the drawing, radii are extended from the tumor center (axis of rotation) to the contour surface at intervals of 20°, as in Figure 10.37. Precision is improved with smaller intervals, but 20° is adequate. Each radius represents a particular tumor depth for a corresponding point of entry of the beam, the tissue-air ratio being readily found for each of these depths from the published tissue-air ratio tables of Johns and Cunningham,[44] (see Table 10.03). The tissue-air ratios for all the selected radii are averaged and called $\bar{R}_t$. For example, if, with a given combination of therapy factors, we find that $\bar{R}_t$ is 0.75, and the dose to a small mass of tissue (of equilibrium thickness) in free space at the position of the tumor is 40 rads,

$$\bar{R}_t = D_t/D_a$$

$$D_t = \bar{R}_t D_a$$

$$D_t = 0.75 \times 40 = 30 \text{ rads } tumor \ dose$$

If only partial rotation is carried out, the $\bar{R}_t$ is found only for the radii within the sector of rotation.

The determination of tissue-air ratios can be simplified by preparing a calibrated ruler for each combination of beam energy and field size, based on equation (5) or on data such as those in

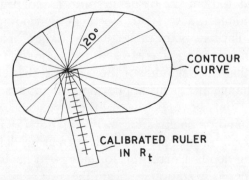

FIGURE 10.37. A transparent ruler calibrated in terms of tissue-air ratio at various depths for a given set of operating factors simplifies the derivation of the average tissue-air ratio.

TABLE 10.03
TISSUE-AIR RATIOS FOR RECTANGULAR FIELDS*

(Dose to a small mass of tissue at depth d, for a dose of 1 rad to the same mass of tissue at the same point in free space.)

Field size (cm × cm) at depth d, or axis of rotation

d (cm)	0×0	4×4	4×8	4×15	5×5	6×6	6×8	6×10	6×15	7×7	8×8	8×10	8×15	8×20	10×10	10×15	10×20	12×12	15×15	15×20	20×20	20×30	25×25	30×30	35×35
*0.5	1.00	1.01	1.02	1.03	1.02	1.02	1.03	1.03	1.03	1.03	1.03	1.03	1.04	1.04	1.03	1.04	1.05	1.04	1.05	1.06	1.06	1.07	1.07	1.08	1.08
1	.97	1.00	1.01	1.01	1.00	1.01	1.01	1.02	1.02	1.02	1.02	1.02	1.03	1.04	1.03	1.04	1.04	1.04	1.05	1.05	1.06	1.07	1.07	1.08	1.08
2	.91	.96	.97	.98	.97	.98	.98	.99	.99	.98	.99	1.00	.97	.98	.97	.98	.99	.98	1.00	1.01	1.02	1.03	1.03	1.04	1.04
3	.84	.91	.93	.94	.93	.94	.95	.95	.96	.95	.96	.97	.97	.98	.98	.98	.99	.99	1.00	1.01	1.02	1.03	1.03	1.04	1.04
4	.79	.87	.89	.90	.89	.90	.91	.92	.93	.91	.92	.93	.94	.95	.94	.95	.96	.95	.97	.98	.99	1.00	1.00	1.01	1.02
5	.74	.83	.85	.86	.85	.86	.87	.88	.89	.87	.89	.89	.91	.91	.90	.92	.92	.92	.94	.95	.96	.97	.97	.99	1.00
6	.69	.79	.81	.82	.80	.82	.83	.84	.85	.83	.85	.86	.87	.88	.87	.88	.89	.88	.90	.91	.92	.94	.94	.96	.97
7	.65	.74	.77	.78	.76	.78	.79	.80	.81	.79	.81	.82	.83	.84	.83	.84	.85	.84	.87	.88	.89	.91	.91	.93	.94
8	.61	.70	.72	.74	.72	.74	.75	.76	.77	.75	.77	.77	.79	.80	.79	.80	.82	.81	.83	.84	.86	.88	.88	.90	.91
9	.57	.66	.68	.70	.68	.69	.71	.72	.73	.71	.73	.73	.75	.76	.75	.77	.78	.77	.79	.81	.82	.84	.85	.87	.88
10	.53	.62	.64	.66	.64	.65	.67	.68	.69	.67	.68	.69	.71	.72	.71	.73	.74	.73	.76	.77	.79	.81	.82	.84	.85
11	.50	.58	.61	.62	.60	.62	.63	.64	.65	.63	.65	.66	.67	.68	.67	.69	.70	.69	.72	.74	.75	.78	.78	.80	.82
12	.47	.55	.57	.59	.56	.58	.59	.60	.62	.60	.61	.62	.64	.65	.64	.66	.67	.66	.68	.70	.72	.74	.75	.77	.79
13	.44	.51	.54	.55	.53	.55	.56	.57	.58	.56	.57	.59	.61	.62	.60	.62	.64	.63	.65	.67	.69	.71	.72	.74	.76
14	.41	.48	.50	.52	.50	.51	.53	.54	.55	.53	.54	.56	.57	.59	.57	.59	.61	.59	.62	.64	.66	.68	.69	.71	.73
15	.39	.45	.48	.49	.47	.48	.50	.51	.52	.50	.51	.53	.54	.56	.54	.56	.58	.56	.59	.61	.63	.66	.66	.69	.71
16	.36	.43	.45	.47	.44	.46	.47	.48	.49	.47	.48	.50	.52	.53	.51	.53	.55	.53	.56	.58	.60	.63	.63	.66	.68
17	.34	.40	.42	.44	.42	.43	.44	.45	.47	.44	.46	.47	.49	.50	.48	.51	.52	.51	.54	.55	.58	.60	.61	.63	.65
18	.32	.38	.40	.42	.39	.41	.42	.43	.44	.42	.44	.44	.46	.47	.46	.48	.49	.48	.51	.53	.57	.57	.58	.61	.63
19	.30	.35	.37	.39	.37	.38	.39	.40	.42	.40	.42	.42	.44	.45	.43	.45	.47	.45	.49	.50	.55	.55	.56	.58	.60
20	.28	.33	.35	.37	.36	.36	.37	.38	.39	.37	.40	.40	.41	.43	.41	.43	.44	.43	.46	.48	.53	.53	.53	.56	.58

*Adapted from data of Johns, H. E., and Cunningham, J. R.: The Physics of Radiology,[44] 1969. Courtesy of the authors and Charles C Thomas, Publisher, Springfield.

Table 10.03. Cleared X-ray film is suitable for this purpose. The appropriately calibrated ruler is then placed along each radius on the contour chart, as in Figure 10.37, and the R_t read directly on the ruler for each position. The average R_t is then computed in the usual manner. The preparation of these calibrated rulers is simplified by the fact, already pointed out, that a change in the tumor treatment distance F does not appreciably affect the value of R_t when F lies within the range of 40 to 100 cm, with ^{60}Co γ rays. Furthermore, we need only prepare calibrated rulers for the most frequently used treatment factors; tables for R_t may be consulted for the infrequently used factors. Note that R_t increases with beam area, and decreases nearly exponentially with depth.

To find the actual dose rate at a point on the axis, within the tumor, we first convert the in-air exposure rate at the axis to absorbed dose rate at the same point (in absence of body). Multiplying the product by the average corrected tissue-air ratio gives the dose rate at the axis point.

$$\textit{absorbed dose rate} = \textit{in-air exposure rate} \times f \times R_t$$
(at axis in tumor)   *(at axis)*

For example, if the in-air exposure rate is 84 R/min, f is 0.957 rad/R, and R_t is 0.51,

$$\textit{absorbed dose rate} = 84 \times 0.957 \times 0.51 = 41.0 \ \textit{rads}/\textit{min}$$
(at axis in tumor)

Computation of Doses for Points off the Axis. Despite the fact that the complete dosage distribution is not usually needed, we should be able to obtain the doses at certain selected points. These can be found by the use of isodose curves ***normalized*** to 100 percent at the axis of rotation (*ICRU Handbook 87*, method of Braestrup and Mooney). This means that the dose at any off-axis point can be compared with that at the axis taken as 100. Such a normalized curve is shown in Figure 10.38A. First the isodose pattern is laid over the body contour with its 100 percent point at the axis and the pattern is extended back through the body surface (see Fig. 10.38B). The procedure is then repeated for a number of angles of entry, say every 30°. In each position the percentage depth dose is recorded for the selected off-axis point. This "dose" is then multiplied by the tissue-air ratio for the particular angle of entry. The resulting corrected tissue-air ratios for all the angles of entry are computed to give the average for the point of interest. Similarly, tissue-air ratios can be found for other off-axis points. This method becomes less accurate as the skin level is approached and should therefore be used at depths no less than about 5 cm. We can now calculate the actual dose rate in the same manner as just described for points on the axis.

Rotation Isodose Distributions. Methods are available for determining isodose distributions in rotation therapy. They consist basically in summating a large number of single field isodose curves. However, this is an extremely tedious and time-

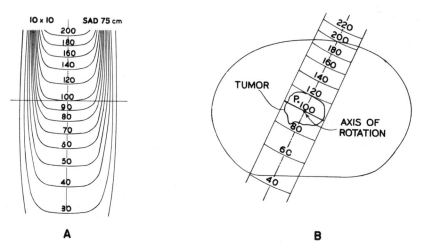

A   **B**

FIGURE 10.38. In *A* is shown an isodose pattern for ^{60}Co normalized to 100 percent at the axis of rotation (*isocenter*) when the source-axis distance (*SAD*) is 75 cm and the isocenter is 10 cm deep. While the dose rate depends on the depth of the isocenter, the percentage depth doses beyond the isocenter remain almost unchanged. Since the percentage depth doses near the surface do vary, another set of curves should be available for an isocenter depth of 5 cm, and probably 15 cm as well. (From P. N. Goodwin, E. H. Quimby, and R. H. Morgan,[35] by courtesy of the authors and Harper & Row, Publisher.) See also J. C. MacDonald: Simplified techniques in the employment of a rotational cobalt 60 beam therapy unit. *The American Journal of Roentgenology*, Vol. 86 [1961], p. 730.

In *B* is shown the application of such curves in rotation therapy. (Based on ICRU Handbook 87, and C. B. Braestrup and R. F. Mooney: Physical aspects of rotating telecobalt equipment. *Radiology*, Vol. 64 [1955], p. 17.)

consuming procedure and is not usually needed for routine therapy. Furthermore, a reasonable approximation may result from summating a limited number of single field isodose curves about the axis for selected critical points within and near the tumor volume.

In this section we shall discuss only the usual type of rotation in which the beam enters the body perpendicular to the skin surface. (In *conical rotation* the beam enters at some angle less than 90°.) The aim of rotation therapy is to provide **uniform dosage** throughout the tumor volume with **rapid fall-off** at its border, at the same time keeping skin dose at a minimum. A sharp fall-off in dosage at the edge of the tumor volume reduces dosage to normal tissues, thereby decreasing the integral dose. In fact, Johns[43] has stated that integral dose is a mathematical statement of the steepness of dosage fall-off or **edge gradient** at the border of the irradiated volume of interest.

There are several factors that influence the isodose pattern in rotation therapy, and these will now be pointed out as they pertain to the discussion in the last paragraph:

1. **Size of Port.** Maximum dosage prevails for some distance around the axis. In general, dosage to all points that remain continually within the beam is reasonably uniform, provided the penumbra is small. With small ports dosage gradient at the edge of the tumor volume is steeper than with large ports. At the same time, the region of uniform dose decreases with smaller ports. Furthermore, as port size increases, so does the skin dose, although this is not ordinarily significant. Thus, port size should be the smallest that will adequately include the tumor volume.

2. **Size of Penumbra.** As just mentioned, penumbral width affects the isodose pattern. With beams having a large penumbra, such as a wide ^{60}Co source, dosage distribution within the tumor volume is less uniform so that larger beams must be used to encompass the tumor adequately.

3. **Energy of Radiation.** As the energy of the radiation increases, the region of uniform dosage extends farther from the axis, this being especially significant in comparing kilovoltage and megavoltage beams. There is also a steeper dosage gradient at the edge

of the higher energy beam. Both of these characteristics are the result of the flatter isodose curves with higher energy radiation, which can be further improved by beam-flattening filters.

4. *Source-axis Distance (SAD).* An increase in *SAD* produces only a slight decrease in skin dose. However, the use of ^{60}Co beams at short distances should be avoided because of the large penumbra. In general, *SAD* does not significantly affect the isodose pattern within the tumor volume, provided the penumbra is small.

5. *Size of Patient.* A large patient affects isodose distribution in the tumor volume, and edge gradient, in much the same way as a large port. Therefore, we should use the longest practicable *SAD* with a beam of the highest available energy and the smallest penumbra.

6. *Shape of Patient.* When a cylindrical part is treated by full rotation (360°) and the tumor is on the axis, the isodose pattern is cylindrical. However, as the body cross section is usually elliptical the isodose pattern has the same configuration. Under these conditions the shape of the isodose pattern is also elliptical, but its major axis is perpendicular to the major axis of the body's cross section.

7. *Partial Rotation.* It is often desirable to use partial rotation in order to spare certain vital organs such as the spinal cord and the rectum. This can be nicely achieved by partial rotation. However this destroys symmetry, shifting the region of maximum dosage toward the irradiated sector (analogous to the situation with two stationary beams entering at a mutual angle of less than 90°). Correction can be made by past pointing and should be anticipated in the planning stage.

In summary, then, we can say that there are important differences between rotation and multiple port stationary therapy. Although some therapists are firm believers in rotation therapy, others are equally staunch advocates of the stationary method. Probably the wisest course is to select the one that best suits the problem at hand. In the long run, the choice of method depends on the training, experience, and judgment of those responsible for planning the therapy program.

CORRECTION FOR TISSUE INHOMOGENEITY
(VARIATION IN TISSUE DENSITY)

Tissue-air ratios, as we have just presented them, apply to tissues of **unit density,** that is, homogeneous soft tissues with a density similar to that of water. In practice, however, tissues are by no means uniform. For example, depth doses in the chest are greater than indicated in standard depth dose tables because of the greater transmission of radiation by the air-filled lungs (see pages 289 to 290).

It may be possible to obtain direct tumor doses which automatically correct for tissue inhomogeneity, as in the esophagus, by means of an appropriate detector. First the average tumor dose rate is measured with the detector inside the esophagus. Then this is related to the average given dose rate over the sector of rotation. The result may be called the (*tumor dose*)/(*given dose*) ratio which may be designated D_t/D_m. Once this is known, the tumor dose may be found by simply multiplying the given dose by the ratio in any given case in which the same combination of treatment factors prevails.

In 1952 Wachsmann[88] reported a method of dosage determination for rotation therapy, applicable also to fixed beam therapy, involving the measurement of exit doses opposite the entrance ports of the beam. These exit doses were designated as **transit doses.** We now use this method for the purpose of correcting for tissue inhomogeneity in the path of a radiation beam, that is, variations in tissue (bone, air, fat) from unit density (water, muscle). The setup is shown in Figure 10.39, where the radiation beam has passed through the patient and the transmitted or **transit dose** is measured with a closely collimated dosimeter at a point such as Q. Tight collimation minimizes the entrance of scattered radiation into the dosimeter. The collimator is of the focusing type, such as that used in radionuclide scanning, but must be 10 to 12 cm long for a ^{60}Co beam. With this procedure, the **percent transmission** is obtained for each beam axis:

$$\% \ transmission = \frac{transit \ dose \ with \ body \ in \ position}{transit \ dose \ in \ absence \ of \ body} \times 100 \quad (6)$$

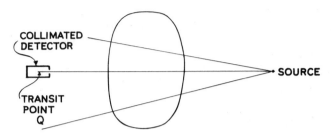

FIGURE 10.39. Measurement of the transit dose by a collimated detector. This can be extended to rotation therapy, the percentage transmission being obtained for each beam axis.

Obviously, the greater the density and thickness of the body along a particular axis, the smaller will be the transit dose and the percent transmission.

To correct for tissue inhomogeneity as in Figure 10.40, we first compute the total tumor dose contributed by both opposed beams, although the procedure to be described can be extended to rotation therapy. Standard depth dose tables are used for this computation. Next, we measure the transit dose along the beam axis and obtain the percent transmission according to equation (6). From Table 10.04 we find the equivalent thickness of unit density tissue and subtract this value from the actual thickness. The re-

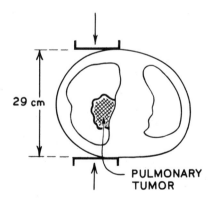

FIGURE 10.40. Cross-sectional diagram of a patient's chest to illustrate correction for increased transmission by air-filled lungs in computing tumor dose. Details in text.

TABLE 10.04
PERCENT TRANSMISSION OF A ^{60}Co BEAM THROUGH A UNIT
DENSITY PHANTOM UNDER CONDITIONS OF NO SCATTER *

Thickness cm	Transmission %	Thickness cm	Transmission %	Thickness cm	Transmission %
12	46.9	20	28.1	28	16.7
14	41.4	22	24.6	30	14.7
16	36.2	24	21.6	32	12.9
18	32.0	26	19.0	34	11.4

* Data of Fedoruk, S. O., and Johns, H. E.[26] Courtesy of *Brit. J. Radiol.*

sulting value is multiplied by one-half to obtain the average correction thickness to serve as a basis for correcting the tumor dose. Since attenuation of ^{60}Co γ rays is about 5 percent per cm of unit density tissue, we must multiply the average correction thickness by 5 percent and add the product *algebraically* to the initially calculated depth dose. (Algebraic addition is needed since a negative difference may result when the tumor is shadowed by bone.)

Let us now apply this method to an actual example, that in Figure 10.40. Suppose the computed tumor dose without correction is 80 rads. Bear in mind that different contributions were made by the two beams since one is traversing a larger thickness of air than the other. Suppose the transmission is found to be 19 percent. From Table 10.04 the equivalent thickness is 26 cm, whereas the patient's chest along the beam axis measures 29 cm. Then,

$$29 \text{ cm} - 26 \text{ cm} = 3 \text{ cm}$$

$$\frac{1}{2} \times 3 \text{ cm} = 1.5 \text{ cm}, \textit{ av. correction thickness}$$

$$1.5 \text{ cm} \times 5\%/\text{cm} = 7.5\%, \textit{ correction factor}$$

Since the tumor dose without inhomogeneity correction was 80 rads,

$$80 + \frac{(80 \times 7.5)}{100} = 86 \text{ rads}, \textit{ corrected dose}$$

A more accurate result is obtained by correcting for each of the two beams separately, but when the tumor is near the center of the irradiated volume, the above method in which the corrections are averaged is usually accurate to within about 1 to 2 percent.

An approximate correction that is reasonably accurate in radiotherapy, according to Meredith and Massey,[57] to be added for each cm of healthy lung is as follows:

$$300\text{-kV X rays} \quad +8\%$$

$$^{60}\text{Co } \gamma \text{ rays} \quad +4\%$$

$$4\text{-MV X rays} \quad +3\%$$

GRID THERAPY

Now infrequently used, grid therapy will be mentioned mainly for historical interest. It was first introduced by Köhler in 1909, and later revived for orthovoltage therapy by Marks in the United States, and by Jolles[45] in Great Britain. The principle may be briefly summarized as follows: a sheet of lead containing regularly spaced square holes and called a *sieve* or *grid* is placed on the skin at the entrance port of the X-ray beam. Radiation passes through the apertures only, to produce alternating irradiated and protected zones as shown in Figure 10.41. Even though radiation dosage in the unprotected areas is sufficient to produce a severe skin reaction, regeneration of skin proceeds outward from the adjacent protected areas. As a result, considerably higher doses of radiation can be delivered with relatively greater safety than with conventional therapy.

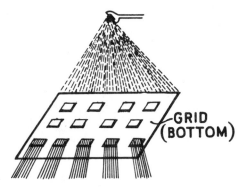

FIGURE 10.41. Diagram of the Jolles grid as seen from the underside. For simplicity, the rays passing through only one set of holes are shown.

The grid used by Marks is made of lead rubber and is perforated with squares ranging from 0.25 to 4 cm², with an average transmission of about 40 percent of the radiation striking the grid. The grid must be applied in the same position throughout the course of radiation, so the same areas are always exposed. The total exposure may be high; thus, Marks recommends a total exposure of no more than 10,000 R for large fields.

Jolles[11] has described in detail the theoretical basis of grid therapy, and has presented his views on its application. He uses a chessboard grid made of *sheet lead* which allows greater precision in duplicating position from day to day. The lead is backed by 1 mm Al to absorb the lead secondary radiation. Alternate squares are cut out, the optimum size varying from 0.5 to 1.0 cm in width. After about one half to two thirds of the total dose has been administered, the grid is replaced by one in which the open and closed areas are reversed; thus, the formerly protected areas are now irradiated, and conversely, the formerly irradiated areas are now protected. This second grid is called the *complementary grid.* In this manner, the usual exposure through one field totals 8,000 to 10,000 R in 3 to 5 weeks, depending on the size of the field, the half value layer of the radiation, and the location of the treatment field, much as with conventional therapy. Jolles admits that the beam of radiation leaving the grid is not strictly homogeneous, but states that with increasing depth it becomes more and more uniform. He even questions the necessity of insisting on homog-

TABLE 10.05
ERRORS IN DOSAGE DUE TO INACCURACIES IN
PHYSICAL FACTORS IN X-RAY THERAPY *

Factor	Best Possible Range	Error in Factor	Error in Dose	Range Probably Tolerated	Error in Factor	Error in Dose
kV	2 kV in 200 kV	1	2	5 kV in 200	2.5	5
mA	1 mA in 30 mA	3	3	1 mA in 10	10	10
Time	15 sec in 10 min	2.5	2.5	30 sec in 10 min	5	5
Distance	1 cm in 50 cm	2	4	2 cm in 50 cm	4	8
Total error in dose if all vary in same direction	±11.5%			±28%		

* From Glasser, O., *et al. Physical Foundations of Radiology,*[33] 1959. Courtesy of Paul B. Hoeber, Inc., Publisher, New York.

eneity, but this is contrary to the generally accepted view that the radiation delivered to a lesion be as uniformly distributed as possible.

Attempts have been made to determine the depth doses in grid therapy, but these have not been entirely successful. In most instances where this modality is used, dosage estimation is entirely or mainly empirical. In general, the grid is a useful adjunct in orthovoltage X-ray therapy where adequate dosage cannot be delivered by conventional methods, but this problem is much better handled with high energy radiation without grids.

SOURCES OF ERROR IN RADIATION THERAPY

H. Suit[81] has found mathematically that a 10 percent reduction in the dose that controls 90 percent of tumors of a given type, sharply decreases tumor control to only 5 percent! It is therefore imperative that utmost accuracy be attained in planning and executing a course of irradiation.

We shall now attempt to cover the more important errors that may arise in radiation therapy and the steps that can be taken to minimize them.

1. *Physical Factors.* Table 10.05, taken from Glasser and others,[33] shows errors in dosage resulting from variations in physical factors with kilovoltage X-ray equipment. While some of these may be compensating errors, it is just as likely that they may be in the same direction. Thus, a maximum error of ± 30 percent is possible. With ^{60}Co telecurie units we eliminate two sources of error—tube potential and current. On the other hand, with high-energy X-ray equipment the physical factors must be carefully adjusted, usually requiring the attention of a physicist or other qualified person.

2. *Treatment Timer.* As described on pages 190 to 191, therapy time must be corrected for "shutter" time. In addition, the operation of the timer itself should be checked regularly for accuracy by means of an appropriate interval timer.

3. *Source-skin or Source-tumor Distance.* Most modern therapy units are equipped with a light localizer and rangefinder system. However, these are subject to error. Distance should be checked

frequently with a stick or plumb line of appropriate length for each treatment distance. A small error in distance produces a disproportionate error in dosage because of the inverse square law.

4. *Beam Dimensions.* The light localizer should also ideally illuminate the treatment port, corresponding to the dimensions of the radiation beam. The coincidence of the two should be checked at regular intervals, since an unnoticed shift may occur. The beam dimensions must be large enough to encompass fully the tumor and a "safe" margin of normal tissue, within the selected isodose curves.

5. *Tumor Localization and Verification.* As already described on pages 259 to 261, a tumor must be carefully localized and its position verified radiologically, either by the treatment beam or a suitable simulator. This should be done during the planning stage and repeated as necessary. It goes without saying that improper localization may result in disaster for the patient.

6. *Beam Direction.* Unless accurate direction of the beam is achieved, a serious geographic miss can occur, with undertreatment of a portion or all of the lesion. In rotation therapy one must be certain that the axis of rotation is always at the desired point in the tumor.

7. *Calibration of Therapy Equipment.* Since all dosage computation depends on the accuracy of calibration of the radiation output, this should be done frequently by a radiation physicist. A plastic tray used as a support for beam-shaping blocks may attenuate the beam by as much as 10 percent, and it is therefore very important in giving the daily dose increment that the proper dosage chart (i.e. with or without the tray) be used. Furthermore, such trays, as well as other material, must be at a distance of at least 15 cm from the skin to minimize electron contamination of the beam at the skin level.

8. *Depth Dose and Other Tables.* Tumor doses computed in radiotherapy depend ultimately on published data. These have been obtained under experimental conditions and apply most precisely when conditions during therapy most nearly approach those under which the data were derived. Furthermore, the correct tables must be used for a particular dosage determination. In other words, published data should be used properly. Accu-

rate measurement of the patient is essential and should be consistent as to location—some therapists measure the body thickness at the center of the treatment port, whereas others prefer to measure the thickest part included in the beam.

From the preceding discussion it is obvious that radiation therapy requires minute attention to detail to avoid cumulative errors, with attendant risk of serious under- or overtreatment. All of the factors mentioned are subject to various probabilities of inherent or accidental error which must be kept to an absolute minimum. Even after a course of therapy has been started, it is good practice to review the patients' records weekly in an effort to uncover errors in planning and in everyday arithmetic.

COMPARISON OF KILOVOLTAGE (200 TO 300 kV) AND MEGAVOLTAGE RADIATION AS TO DEPTH DOSE

It goes without saying that a greater percentage depth dose is to be anticipated with *megavoltage* radiation than with *kilovoltage* (200 to 300 kV) X rays under similar conditions of source-skin distance and port area. This is true regardless of whether the megavoltage therapy is provided by ^{60}Co sources of adequate intensity, or multimillion volt X rays. Therefore, in the following discussion, any statement made concerning ^{60}Co applies to megavoltage X rays of comparable energy.

Table 10.06 compares ^{60}Co and kilovoltage X-ray depth doses. It is readily apparent that at a typical depth of 10 cm, there is a marked superiority of ^{60}Co over X rays with HVL as high as 4 mm Cu. Furthermore, there is an improvement in the depth dose with ^{60}Co as the source-skin distance (SSD) is increased from 50 cm to 80 cm; for example, for every 100 rads delivered at a 10 cm depth with a 50 cm SSD, 112 rads would be delivered with an 80-cm SSD, assuming the same given dose in each instance. This represents an improvement of 12 percent at the longer SSD.

Figure 10.42 has been included to show the isodose distribution obtained with ^{60}Co γ rays at an SSD of 80 cm; 4-MV X rays at 80 cm; ^{137}Cs γ rays at an SSD of 50 cm; and kilovoltage X rays of 1.5 mm Cu HVL at 50 cm. In each instance a treatment port of 10×10 cm^2 has been selected to facilitate comparison. Note how

TABLE 10.06
COMPARISON OF PERCENT DEPTH DOSE OF X RAYS, ^{60}Co γ RAYS,
AND BETATRON X RAYS. DATA ARE FOR A 100 CM^2 FIELD*

Depth	X Rays 2 mm Cu HVL 50 cm TSD	X Rays 2 mm Cu HVL 80 cm TSD	X Rays 4 mm Cu HVL 80 cm TSD	^{60}Co γ Rays 12 mm Pb HVL 80 cm SSD	Betatron 22 MV Compensating Filter 100 cm TSD
cm					
0	100.0	100.0	100.0	—	—
0.5	—	—	—	100.0	50.0
2	93.6	96.0	93.6	93.3	90.1
4	77.4	81.0	79.7	83.4	100.0
6	60.6	64.8	64.8	73.6	96.6
8	46.6	50.4	51.3	64.1	89.1
10	35.5	38.3	40.4	55.6	81.9
12	26.9	29.6	31.6	48.1	75.5
14	20.3	22.5	24.7	41.8	69.6
16	15.2	17.0	19.1	36.2	64.2
18	11.5	13.0	14.8	31.4	59.1
20	8.7	9.8	11.5	27.2	54.5

* From Johns, H. E., and Cunningham, J. R.: *The Physics of Radiation Therapy*,[44] 1969.
Courtesy of Charles C. Thomas, Publisher, Springfield, Illinois.

nearly alike are the percentage depth doses with ^{60}Co γ rays and 4-MV X rays, and how much greater they are than those with kilovoltage X rays. Also, observe the significantly better edge gradient of the linac 4-MV X-ray beam as compared with the ^{60}Co beam due to the small focal spot of the linac and the smaller associated penumbra. On the other hand, the ^{137}Cs beam has a relatively large penumbra, much like a kilovoltage X-ray beam, but with significantly higher percentage depth doses.

Let us now examine the advantages of megavoltage X-ray and ^{60}Co γ-ray therapy over kilovoltage X-ray therapy (1 to 4 mm Cu HVL). There are four such advantages:

1. *Skin-sparing Effect.* With kilovoltage X rays (HVL 1 to 4 mm Cu) the skin dose is contributed by primary radiation plus backscatter. Electronic equilibrium is reached so close to the skin surface that maximum ionization may be considered, for practical purposes, to be at the surface. In contrast, high energy ^{60}Co photons and megavoltage X rays possess greater energy than those produced in the 250 kV region, and therefore set free more energetic primary electrons with a correspondingly greater range. Electron equilibrium is not reached at the skin surface, but at a

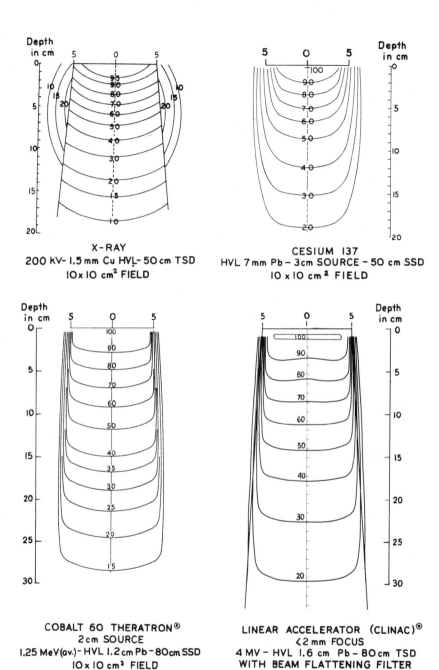

FIGURE 10.42. Comparison of isodose curves (distributions) for various teletherapy units under typical operating conditions. X-ray curves from H. E. Johns, and J. R. Cunningham,[44] by courtesy of the authors and Charles C Thomas, Publisher. Cesium 137 curves by courtesy of Picker Medical Products Division. Cobalt 60 curves by courtesy of Atomic Energy of Canada, Ltd. Clinac® curves by courtesy of Varian.

significant depth below, corresponding to the maximum range of the primary electrons (see pages 226 to 228). In the case of ^{60}Co this happens to be 5 mm. At greater depths, the dose is progressively attenuated because of absorption, scattering, and inverse square law. Table 10.07 shows the equilibrium depth for beams of different energies. This explains why depth dose tables for megavoltage and telecurie beams show the maximum or 100 percent dose to lie at some distance below the skin surface, depending on the photon energy of the primary beam. (This discussion should be compared with the equilibrium requirement for the free air and the thimble ionization chambers.) Since the maximum dose with megavoltage radiation is attained at a significant depth below the skin, severe *acute* skin reactions may be avoided even with intensive therapy.

2. *Higher Percentage Depth Dose.* Table 10.06 compares depth doses of kilovoltage X rays, with ^{60}Co γ rays and betatron X rays. At a 10 cm depth and 80 cm treatment distance, for example, the depth dose is 38 percent with 2 mm Cu HVL X rays and 56 percent with ^{60}Co, an improvement of 47 percent. Thus, for every 100 rads at a 10 cm depth with 2 mm Cu HVL X rays, the dose would be 147 rads with ^{60}Co γ rays.

3. *Equal Absorption in Bone and Soft Tissue.* The γ rays of ^{60}Co and the radium series with energies averaging 1.25 MeV and 0.8 MeV, respectively, are absorbed equally in equal *masses* of bone and soft tissue. With X-ray therapy at HVL 2 mm Cu, the absorption in bone may be almost $1\frac{1}{2}$ times as great as in soft tissues,

TABLE 10.07
DEPTH OF MAXIMUM IONIZATION (ELECTRON EQUILIBRIUM OR
BUILDUP DEPTH) FOR RADIATION OF VARIOUS ENERGIES

	Energy	Depth of Maximum Ionization
		mm
X Rays	200 kV	<1
	2 MV	4
	4 MV	10
	6 MV	15
	15 MV	30
	22 MV	40
γ Rays	^{137}Cs (0.662 MeV)	4
	^{60}Co (av. 1.25 MeV)	5

increasing the possibility of bone damage during intensive therapy. However, at 4 mm Cu HVL, X rays are of such quality that absorption in bone is approximately the same as in soft tissue, as shown in Figure 10.43. The photon energy in this figure is ex-

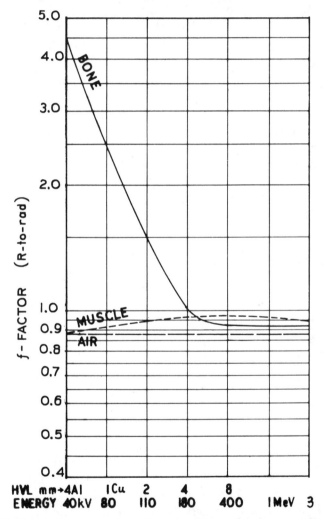

FIGURE 10.43. Relative energy absorption of radiation of various energies in bone and in muscle as indicated by the f factor (R-to-rad conversion). The peak potential of kV X rays is about twice that shown in the graph. Note that bone and soft tissue absorption in equal masses becomes approximately equal at HVL 4 mm Cu. The curves are not continued beyond 3 MeV because the roentgen and therefore the f-factor are no longer valid.

pressed in average values, the peak value for X rays being about double the average. Despite the equal absorption of energy in bone and soft tissue, gram for gram, with the higher energy photons, there is *greater absorption in bone than in soft tissue on a volume basis.* Therefore, bone lying in the path of the radiation beam causes "shadowing" of the tissues beyond. Johns[43] has computed the magnitude of this effect for ^{60}Co γ rays and found the reduction in depth dose to be about 3.5 percent per cm of bone. This correction must be taken into account in radiotherapy planning to avoid underdosage.

It is interesting to note that above 10 MeV, due to the predominance of absorption by pair production, the per gram absorption of energy in bone again exceeds that in soft tissues.

4. *More Forward and Less Lateral Scattering.* As we have learned in the discussion of the Compton Effect, the angle of scatter of photons decreases as the energy of the incident photons increases. Hence, there is a preponderance of forward scattering in the direction of the high energy primary beam as it passes through the body. With reduced side scatter, the edge of the beam is more sharply defined and the integral dose is reduced.

Let us now consider some of the *disadvantages* of high energy (megavoltage) radiation, although they are, by far, outweighed by the advantages.

1. *Skin-sparing Effect.* It is true that megavoltage therapy produces less skin effect than do kilovoltage X rays, and provides a genuine increase in depth dose. However, the maximum dose is no longer at the surface but about 5 or more mm below the surface where it produces an invisible reaction. This may result in late skin damage including fibrosis and ulceration. The clinician cannot use skin reaction as a guide to therapy, but must judge the maximum tolerance dose at the buildup depth, based on his training and experience. Moreover, therapy planning must be carried out with a high degree of accuracy.

2. *High Percentage Depth Dose.* One factor that has not been sufficiently taken into account, and about which complete data are lacking, is the relative biologic effectiveness of the γ photons of ^{60}Co and the photons of 2 mm Cu HVL X rays. According to Sinclair[78] the biological effectiveness is 10 to 20 percent higher

with kilovoltage X rays than with ^{60}Co γ rays, based on the 50 percent lethal dose in mice. Thus, if a tumor requires 5,000 rads of conventional X rays in five weeks, it will probably require 5,500 to 6,000 rads of ^{60}Co γ rays. Another problem concerns exit dose; this may be so high with megavoltage radiation, especially in small structures like the neck, that crossfire technics are limited. In any event, the exit dose must always be taken into account when opposed beams are used.

3. *Equal Absorption in Bone and Soft Tissue.* Friedman[31] has found essentially the same incidence of bone necrosis with megavoltage as with orthovoltage therapy despite equal absorption in bone and soft tissue, gram for gram. Corrigan explains this observation as follows: irradiation of bone to the same total dose as soft tissue causes swelling of the cellular elements which are confined by the bony walls. Consequently necrosis of cellular elements may still occur, even with megavoltage radiation.

4. *More-forward Scatter.* This is a real advantage of ^{60}Co and megavoltage X rays; but despite the reduction in lateral scatter, the large penumbra associated with the larger ^{60}Co sources increases the irradiated volume and also impairs to some degree the use of ^{60}Co in rotation therapy of small parts. However, 1.5 cm sources of high activity are now available. The focal spots of megavoltage X-ray therapy machines are much smaller than ^{60}Co sources, producing a much smaller penumbra, but the forward-peaked isodose distributions require the use of beam-flattening filters (see Fig. 10.44).

The *volume* or *integral dose* is less with megavoltage than with kilovoltage radiation on account of reduced lateral scatter and a larger exit dose at higher energies. However, in practice there may not be a large difference between the two kinds of radiation insofar as integral dose is concerned (see pages 322 to 324 for an actual example in which this comparison is made).

We may summarize the preceding discussion by stating that megavoltage therapy has distinct advantages over X-ray therapy of HVL 2 mm Cu. These include improved depth dose; conspicuous skin sparing; a somewhat smaller integral absorbed dose; and no preferential absorption in bone, probably decreasing the danger of bone necrosis, although this is not always so. The outstanding advantage of megavoltage therapy is the ease with which cancericidal doses may be delivered to deeply situated tumors, through fewer and smaller fields. On the other hand, these advantages are partly offset by a shift of the skin reaction to a point beneath the skin, the high exit dose, and the smaller biologic effectiveness. Furthermore, the therapist must take into account the fact that he is more often limited by the vulnerability of normal deep structures in the neighborhood of the tumor, than by skin tolerance. He must not blindly deliver a predetermined dose without regard to the sensitivity of adjacent structures. Finally, there is *no specificity* of action of megavoltage photon radiation on cancer cells, as compared with the kilovoltage photon.

BETATRON THERAPY

Almost in a class by itself (except for the 35-MeV linac) is the **betatron**, described on pages 162 to 165. It produces extremely high energy electron and X-ray beams.

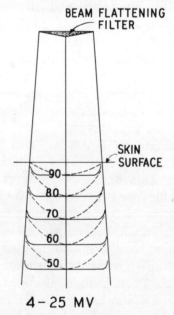

FIGURE 10.44. Flattening of isodose curves by use of filters. The broken lines show the forward-pointed curves in the absence of a filter. The solid lines represent the flattened isodose curves obtained with beam-flattening filters.

Being in the usual betatron therapy range of 22 to 25 MV, these X rays set in motion highly energetic primary electrons which reach maximum buildup at a much greater depth than that occurring with ordinary megavoltage radiation (e.g. 1 to 4 MV). Thus, the plane of maximum ionization and dosage is *4 cm* below the surface with 22-MV X rays. Figure 10.45 is based on the isodose curves of the M. D. Anderson Hospital and Tumor Institute betatron for a 100-cm target-skin distance. These curves were obtained with a copper beam-flattening filter to remove the sharp forward peak of the curves (see Fig. 10.44). Note again that the maximum depth dose—taken as 100 percent—is reached at a depth of *4 cm.* At 5 mm below the skin, the depth dose is 50 percent of the maximum dose. According to Johns and Cunningham,[44] the dose at the skin surface is 20 to 30 percent of the maximum. Thus, the depth dose percentage first increases progressively from the point of entry of the beam, to reach a maximum at a depth of

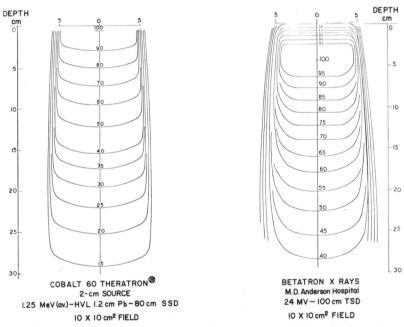

COBALT 60 THERATRON®
2-cm SOURCE
1.25 MeV (av.)–HVL 1.2 cm Pb–80 cm SSD
10 X 10 cm² FIELD

BETATRON X RAYS
M.D. Anderson Hospital
24 MV – 100 cm TSD
10 X 10 cm² FIELD

FIGURE 10.45. Comparison of isodose patterns with a ^{60}Co and a betatron beam. Note the greater depth of maximum dosage and the greater percentage depth dose with the betatron. (Isodose curves for betatron obtained through the courtesy of the M. D. Anderson Hospital and Tumor Institute, Houston, Texas.)

4 cm; it then decreases slowly at greater depths, the rate of decrease being less than that with lower energy radiation. The isodose curves for ^{60}Co are also included in Figure 10.45 for comparison. Table 10.06 presents comparative data for kilovoltage X rays, ^{60}Co γ rays, and betatron 22-MV X rays. From this table, we see that at comparable treatment distances and for a 100-cm^2 port, the percent depth doses are as follows:

$$
\begin{array}{ll}
\text{X rays (HVL 2 mm Cu)} & 38\% \\
^{60}\text{Co } \gamma \text{ rays} & 56\% \\
\text{betatron X rays (22 MV)} & 82\%
\end{array}
$$

It should be pointed out that with 22-MV betatron X rays, the field area does not influence significantly the depth dose because lateral scatter is negligible.

Since betatron X rays have an energy far above the 3 MV limit in the definition of the official roentgen, one cannot state exposure in terms of true roentgens. However, thimble chambers of appropriate wall thickness calibrated against ^{60}Co γ rays and used under rather complex conditions of measurement provide absorbed dose data for such high energy beams.

Finally, another factor that must be considered in betatron therapy is the absorption in bone. Since pair production becomes dominant above 10 MeV, there is greater absorption in bone than in soft tissue per gram (as the mass attenuation coefficient for pair production is nearly proportional to the atomic number of the medium). Thus, betatron X-ray therapy suffers from one of the same disadvantages as kilovoltage therapy, although to a lesser degree.

At the present time, the betatron is available in relatively few radiation centers. However, it has an important place in radiation therapy, especially since it produces high-energy electron beams as well as X rays.

ELECTRON BEAM THERAPY

The betatron and linac can provide high energy *electron beams.* Unfortunately, as we shall indicate, these have only limited application in radiotherapy because, as charged particles, they quickly dissipate their energy as they penetrate tissues. The length of path or range of the electrons depends on their initial energy. In fact, as a rule of thumb, the tissue penetration or range of an electron beam in cm is *numerically equal to about one-half the initial energy;* thus, a 10-MeV beam has a penetration of about 5 cm in tissue. Electron beams have a peculiar depth dose distribution because of their charge—the absorbed dose is nearly constant at first, over the electron range, beyond which there is a sharp decline. The higher the initial energy, the more gradual will be the fall in depth dose after the initial plateau. Figure 10.46 shows the depth dose curves for typical electron beams.

In the absence of a skin-sparing effect, the dose at the surface being virtually at the maximum, electron beam therapy is limited to lesions near the skin; for example, with a 20-MeV beam, the depth dose ranges from 100 percent at the surface to 90 percent at 5 cm, and drops to 50 percent at 8 cm. Typical isodose curves are shown in Figure 10.47. Note the rapid fall in depth dose below

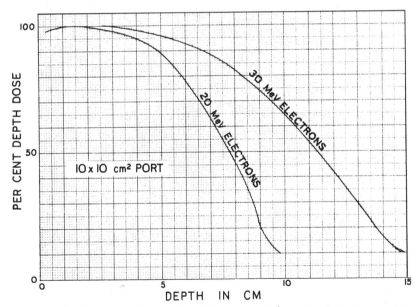

FIGURE 10.46. Depth dose curves for high energy electron beams. Based on data from H. E. Johns, and J. R. Cunningham, *The Physics of Radiology* (Springfield, Charles C Thomas, 1969).

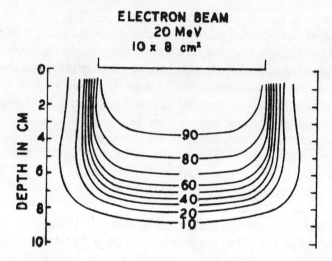

FIGURE 10.47. Isodose curves measured in a tissue equivalent phantom for a high-energy electron beam. A 0.010 lead foil filter has been used to broaden the beam. Note the large degree of scattering beyond the margins of the beam. (From P. Goodwin, E. H. Quimby, and R. H. Morgan,[35] by courtesy of the authors and Harper & Row, Publishers.

6 cm, and the lateral bulge of the isodose lines due to lateral scatter.

INTEGRAL DOSE

It has been known for many years that the irradiation of a patient through small ports is better tolerated than irradiation through large ports. In fact, a patient can tolerate only a certain maximum daily increment of radiation exposure, governed by the dose delivered to a given volume of tissue. This observation remained empirical until Mayneord, in 1940, placed it on a mathematical basis. His treatment of the problem is fairly complex, but a simple presentation will be given here.

He assumes, first of all, that irradiation of any portion of the body affects the body as a whole, the degree of this effect increasing with the mass of tissue irradiated and the dose delivered in a specified period of time. An arbitrary unit is selected—*1 gram-rad.* Since this unit is too small, Mayneord selected one a million times as large, the ***megagram-rad.***

The *integral dose*, measured in megagram-rads, is the summation of the absorbed doses in an extraordinarily large number (approaching infinity) of layers of tissue in the irradiated mass. For a single port, and assuming complete absorption of the beam (no exit dose), we have the following approximate equation for **kilovoltage** therapy:

$\frac{Integral}{dose}$ = 1.44 × *area* × *skin dose* × *depth at which dose is*
$\frac{1}{2}$ *the skin dose* × *correction for beam divergence*

$$I = 1.44\ AD_m\ d_{1/2}\left(1 + \frac{2.88\ d_{1/2}}{SSD}\right) gram\text{-}rads \qquad (7)$$

Division of gram-rads by 10^6 converts them to megagram-rads.

For example, if the skin dose is 3000 rads, the treatment port $10 \times 10\ cm^2$, $d_{1/2}$ 7.5 cm, and FSD 80 cm,

$$I = 1.44 \times 100 \times 3000 \times 7.5\left(1 + \frac{2.88 \times 7.5}{80}\right)$$

$$I = 4{,}100{,}000\ g\text{-}rads \text{ or } 4.1\ mega\text{-}g\text{-}rads$$

If four such fields are used, the total is

$$4 \times 4.1 = 16.4\ mega\text{-}g\text{-}rads$$

With **megavoltage** therapy there is usually a significant exit dose with a resulting smaller integral dose. Therefore the following correction factor must be applied to equation (10),

$$(1 - e^{-0.693 d/d_{1/2}})$$

where d is the thickness of the patient and e is the natural logarithmic base. The values for the various powers of e are given in Table 4.02. To deliver the same dose as in the above example, but using a ^{60}Co beam, say at a depth of 10 cm, we would have to use a given dose (D_m) of 2050 rads. The integral dose would then be

$$I = 1.44 \times 100 \times 2050 \times 11.5\left(1 + \frac{2.88 \times 11.5}{80}\right)$$

$$\times (1 - e^{-0.693 \times 20/11.5})$$

$$I = 3.35\ mega\text{-}g\text{-}rads$$

and for four fields, the total integral dose would be 13.4 mega-g-rads.

The integral dose is not widely used at present because it correlates poorly with clinical observation although it may serve as an approximate guide to probable systemic tolerance. However, as a result of typical calculations, it has been found that one reason for the superiority of megavoltage therapy over conventional therapy is the fact that smaller fields are employed and the skin dose is smaller, thereby reducing the integral dose. Johns[43] has stated that with identical HVL, treatment distance, and port size the integral dose is an index of the magnitude of the **penumbral radiation;** thus, the larger the focal spot or source size, all other factors being equal, the greater the penumbra and the resulting integral dose. A sharply defined beam with a very small penumbra has a steep dosage gradient at its edge, and Johns therefore suggests that another term such as **dosage gradient** be used instead of integral dose, since the former may be more important in radiotherapy.

DUTIES OF THE TECHNOLOGIST IN RADIOTHERAPY

It is essential that actual day to day treatment of the patient, including correct positioning, beam direction, and selection of therapy factors, should be under the direct supervision of the radiologist. What, then, should be the duties of the therapy technologist in external beam therapy? These may be conveniently divided into two categories: (1) establishment of proper rapport with the patient, and (2) participating as an assistant to the radiologist during therapy. Each will now be considered separately in some detail.

Establishment of Rapport with Patient. Whenever a new patient presents himself for external beam therapy, the technologist, by maintaining an air of confidence, and by explaining to the patient that the treatment is painless, can often mitigate the patient's fears and insure his cooperation. The technologist can emphasize that previous experience with others having similar disease has shown the treatment to be well tolerated. The patient may need to be told that his friends and neighbors, although they mean well, lack sufficient information about his condition and about the form of therapy being instituted, to advise the patient of possible consequences. By presenting a cheerful, sympathetic attitude, the technologist can make the daily treatment less of an ordeal to the patient, thereby securing his full cooperation.

Usually, the radiologist himself explains what is going to be done during therapy, including the pertinent details. However, the technologist should be sufficiently familiar with the procedure to be able to repeat the explanation, if necessary. The patient should be made as comfortable as possible on the treatment table, and should never be allowed to feel that he is being left alone, unsupervised during actual therapy. To this end, he should be watched through the observation window or television monitor, and made to realize that he is being so observed. Automatic timers and other safety devices should be shown to him so that he understands he is fully protected. The purpose of lead shields, treatment cones, and collimators should also be explained from the standpoint of the protection which they afford.

Under no circumstances should the technologist discuss with the patient any questions about his own or any other patient's disease, or with a third party. Any information available to the technologist should be kept in strict confidence. Questions of this sort, or any others pertaining to the patient's condition, should be referred to the radiologist.

Ulcerated areas on exposed parts should be covered with a dressing to conceal their unsightliness. If odor from such wounds cannot be controlled, the patient should be allowed to wait in a separate room away from others.

The technologist should constantly be on the alert for untoward reactions and report them immediately to the radiologist. Never, by word of mouth or by facial expression, should there be any indication that reaction to therapy is other than anticipated. However, any complaints should be called to the attention of the radiologist without delay. It should be pointed out that patients will often complain of such symptoms as diarrhea, urinary frequency, and nausea, to the technologist, or perhaps the secretary, bookkeeper, or maid, and yet fail to mention them to the radiologist.

Finally, the technologist should arrange appointments for follow-up examinations and blood counts, fill out appointment cards, and encourage the patients to return for followup examinations.

Assisting the Radiologist. The duties in this category include first, direct *assistance* in daily therapy—positioning, immobilization, and beam centering; second, checking the treatment factors; third, record keeping; and fourth, examination of patients.

The technologist is responsible for keeping clean linens or tissue paper on the therapy table. Where separate cones or special devices such as beam directors are used, the technologist arranges to have the proper devices selected and attached according to the radiologist's prescription. He helps to immobilize the patient in as comfortable a position as possible to prevent movement during therapy. The technologist usually manipulates the locks on the source housing and stand while the radiologist centers the beam.

The treatment factors in kilovoltage therapy prescribed by the radiologist should be checked before each treatment: kV, mA, filter, time, cone of proper size and length, and treatment field. After the radiologist has completed the positioning of the patient and has applied the treatment cone, and before the X-ray machine is turned on, all of the above factors should be checked again. Similar attention should be paid to preparation for treatment with megavoltage radiation. Only then should the actual treatment be started. During treatment, the technologist must pay close attention to both the control panel and the patient to see that the factors remain constant and the patient does not move out of position.

One of the most important responsibilities of the technologist is record keeping. According to the Seventh International Congress of Radiology (1953), such records should include:

1. *Nature of Beam.*

    a. Type: X-ray, ^{60}Co, ^{137}Cs, etc.
    b. kV, Mv or γ-ray energy in MeV.
    c. Inherent and added filter.

d. X-ray half value layer (HVL) in terms of:
Al 10–120 kV
Cu 120–400 kV
Pb above 1 MeV
(with megavoltage therapy and telecurie therapy some radiologists use half value thickness in terms of tissue, that is, the thickness of tissue that reduces the dose rate of the beam 50 percent.)

2. ***Technic or Dosage***

    a. Number, size, and location of ports.
    b. Source-skin distance.
    c. Time interval between fractionated treatments.
    d. Number of treatments in course.
    e. Total treatment time in days or weeks.
    f. Dose rate at suitable point in treatment beam.
    g. Any two of these:
      1) Air dose.
      2) Backscatter factor.
      3) Skin dose or dose at equilibrium depth, each treatment.
    h. Type and use of "bolus."
    i. Percentage depth dose along central axis.
    j. Tissue doses in rads as follows:
      1) Total given dose.
      2) Maximum dose in irradiated tissue.
      3) Maximum dose in tumor or tissue of interest.
      4) Minimum dose in tumor or tissue of interest.
    k. Outline of treatment ports on appropriate anatomic diagrams.

All of the above data are fundamentally the responsibility of the radiologist, being prescribed in the initial plan of treatment, but the daily record keeping is usually delegated to the technologist. The form of the therapy record varies from one department to another, although the standard form originally designed by the Radiological Society of North America is now widely used. The data which are recorded daily by the technologist, regardless of the precise form used, should include the following minimum factors for each area treated:

Date
Beam energy in kV, MV, or MeV
Milliamperage (mA)
Half value layer (HVL)
Target- or source-skin distance (TSD or SSD)
Area of treatment field in cm^2
Depth of tumor
Location of treatment field
Dose rate in air
Skin dose or dose at equilibrium depth (i.e. given dose) each day.
Given dose total to date
Tumor dose to date
Filter, when used, to be initialed daily by the technician after verification of correct filter.

It is advisable to check the records weekly in order to detect possible errors; if any are discovered, they should be reported to the radiologist immediately.

The records should include the dictated follow-up notes made by the radiologist at each visit of the patient following completion of therapy. Blood counts, other laboratory data, and all letters written by the radiologist to the referring physician and to others must also be incorporated in the chart. If a patient fails to keep an appointment, a note should be made on the progress sheet, and the patient sent another appointment. It is advisable to place a duplicate treatment record on the patient's hospital chart if an inpatient. All of the records, including port radiographs, should be placed in good order in a large envelope, with the patient's name plainly printed on the front, and filed.

Each time the equipment is calibrated, the technologist should see that the physicist's or radiologist's data are entered in a notebook under the correct date. The notebook should be available for reference at any time.

It is the therapy technologist's duty to aid the radiologist in the initial and follow-up examinations, particularly with female patients. The patient must be properly draped, instruments and materials set out, and chart available for review. During the examination of a female patient, a female technologist (or nurse) must *always* remain in the room. If a biopsy is to be taken, all required assistance is to be given. The biopsy specimen should be handled carefully; placed in the proper fixing solution; accurately labeled with the patient's name, date, and other pertinent data; and sent to the pathologist. The technologist should see that blood counts are done regularly on the patient as required by the radiologist, and that the patient is weighed periodically.

It is obvious, from the foregoing discussion, that the assistance provided by the technologist in radiotherapy is of inestimable value. A well-trained technologist not only aids the patient through the ordeal of a sometimes frightening form of therapy, but facilitates the radiologist's task in the day-to-day details of therapy.

CHAPTER 11

Radioactivity and Nuclear Physics

DEFINITION

RADIOACTIVITY may be defined as the spontaneous transformation of atomic nuclei with emission of particulate and/ or electromagnetic (photonic) radiations. These include mainly the following processes: α decay, β^- decay (negatron emission), β^+ decay (positron emission), γ radiation, electron capture, internal conversion, and isomeric transition. In fact, radioactivity involves the *de-excitation* (C. Craig Harris) of individual atomic nuclei. The term *decay* refers to the decline in the population of a radionuclide sample. Other types of nuclear de-excitation or decay have been discovered, but are as yet unimportant in nuclear medicine.

HISTORICAL BACKGROUND

In 1896 a French physicist, Henri Becquerel, discovered radioactivity during the accidental observation that *uranium* ore wrapped in black paper causes fogging of a photographic plate. Further study led him to the conclusion that uranium emits invisible rays which penetrate not only paper, but also thin sheets of metal. He later demonstrated that the same rays *ionize air* and discharge an electroscope. In 1898 G. C. Schmidt found that the element thorium, discovered sixty years earlier by Berzelius, also gives off rays. During the same year, two new radioactive elements, *polonium* and *radium,* were discovered by Marie and Pierre Curie in pitchblende ore. It is Marie Curie who is credited with having coined the term *radioactivity.* In 1899 a French physicist, A. Debierne, found another radioactive element, actinium, in pitchblende. Thus, by 1900 five radioactive elements were known: uranium, thorium, polonium, radium, and actinium.

In discovering these radioactive elements, scientists were bound to observe the various types of radiation emitted by them. Thus,

330

Becquerel, having previously discovered a penetrating form of radiation in uranium, found another kind of radiation, one that can be deflected by a magnetic or electric field in exactly the same manner as cathode rays. Therefore he decided that this type of radiation must consist of negatively charged particles. In summary, then, Becquerel recognized the emission of at least two different forms of radiation by naturally occurring radioactive elements: (1) a *highly penetrating ray* capable of passing through thin sheets of metal in the same manner as X rays, and (2) a less penetrating form of radiation consisting of *negatively charged particles*.

At about the same time E. Rutherford, a British physicist, observed two kinds of uranium radiation, one of which he found to be positively charged and capable of passing through only extremely thin sheets of aluminum (less than 0.002 cm thick); he named this α (alpha) radiation, later proving it to be particulate in nature (see pages 337 to 338), and therefore more correctly called α *particles*. The other type of uranium radiation could pass through greater thicknesses of aluminum and was identical with Becquerel's negative particles; Rutherford called this β (beta) radiation, more properly, β *particles*. In fact, the β particles are about 1,000 times more penetrating than the α. In 1900 Villard, in France, studied the third type of radiation already reported by Becquerel, and found it to be undeviated by a magnetic field. This was γ radiation which, along with X rays, belongs to the family of electromagnetic radiation. Thus, the naturally occurring radioactive elements emit one or more of the three types of radiation—α, β, and γ.

The preceding discussion has been based on the naturally occurring radioactive elements, over 40 of which are known. Their decay with emission of radiation is called *natural radioactivity*.

In 1934 Irene Curie and her husband Joliot accidentally discovered the phenomenon of *artificial radioactivity*. The nuclides which are capable of such behavior are *isotopes* created artificially from stable elements. Curie and Joliot found that aluminum foil irradiated with radium α particles emits two kinds of radiation—*neutrons* (previously discovered by Chadwick), and *positrons* (positively charged particles previously discovered by Anderson). They were surprised to find the positrons continuing to be emitted even after removal of the source of α particles. Further investigation revealed an exponential decrease in the intensity of these positron rays in the same manner as the radiation occurring in natural radioactive decay. In fact, the **half-life** of this decay process is three minutes. Curie and Joliot therefore concluded that they had induced **artificial radioactivity** in the aluminum foil. This reaction may be indicated as follows:

$$\underset{\substack{aluminum}}{{}^{27}_{13}\text{Al}} + \underset{\substack{\alpha\ particle}}{{}^{4}_{2}\text{He}} \longrightarrow \underset{\substack{radiophosphorus}}{{}^{30}_{15}\text{P}} + \underset{\substack{neutron}}{{}^{1}_{0}\text{n}}$$

$$\underset{\substack{radiophosphorus}}{{}^{30}_{15}\text{P}} \longrightarrow \underset{\substack{silicon}}{{}^{30}_{14}\text{Si}} + \underset{\substack{positron}}{{}^{0}_{+1}\text{e}} + \underset{\substack{neutrino}}{\nu}$$

Note that the phosphorus formed in this reaction is an artificially radioactive nuclide having a mass number of 30. It is an isotope of stable phosphorus which has a mass number of 31. This is an example of artificial **transmutation,** aluminum being changed to phosphorus. Curie and Joliot proposed the prefix **radio** for the radioactive isotopes, attaching it to the name of the stable element. Thus, any radioactive isotope of phosphorus is called **radiophosphorus.** Since 1934, more than 700 radionuclides have been produced; and, in addition, several entirely new elements beyond uranium have been created artificially—the transuranic elements.

The α particles from ordinary sources such as radium can induce radioactivity in lighter elements because they are able to penetrate their relatively weak nuclear potential barriers. On the other hand, in elements of high atomic number, that is, above potassium, the nuclear electric field (positive) is so powerful that it repels the relatively low energy, positively charged α particle. Therefore, a more energetic bombarding particle is required. Special devices, such as the cyclotron, synchrocyclotron, and proton-synchrotron, have been used to endow subatomic particles with sufficiently high kinetic energy to penetrate the strongly positive nuclear potential barriers of the heavier elements, with the result that one or more radioisotopes of all the known elements have been produced artificially. These particle accelerators have been discussed in Chapter 6. Of even greater practical importance is the use of reactor neutrons for inducing radioactivity (see pages 375 to 377).

Nuclides. The nouns "isotope" and "element" do not always imply a distinct species of atom. For example, nuclear isomers are isotopes, but their nuclei differ in energy content. The term *nuclide* has been introduced to specify completely a particular kind of atom on the basis of its *nuclear configuration. A nuclide may be defined as a species of atom whose nucleus has a characteristic number of protons, number of neutrons, and energy content.* To be a distinct nuclide, an atom must have more than transitory existence; thus, nuclear isomers are distinct nuclides, but ordinary excited nuclei which decay promptly to ground state, and intermediate products in nuclear reactions, are not considered distinct nuclides. If a nuclide happens to be radioactive, it is called a *radionuclide.*

FACTORS IN NUCLEAR STABILITY

Radioactivity is the physical manifestation of nuclear instability. What causes nuclei to be unstable and to break down (deexcite) spontaneously with the emission of radiation? Several factors are thought to be responsible for this sort of behavior of certain nuclides, but first it should be pointed out that the determination of instability depends on the sensitivity of the measuring technic. Thus, some nuclides which are now considered to be stable may eventually prove to be unstable when more sensitive measuring technics have been evolved; for example, lanthanum 128, once thought to be stable, was subsequently proved to be radioactive.

We may best approach the study of nuclear instability by considering those factors which govern *stability.* These factors are not completely understood, and some are still in the stage of hypothesis. However, a brief review of some of the more important concepts will now be presented.

1. *Neutron-proton Ratio.* If the ratios of neutrons to protons for various stable nuclides are plotted against atomic number, we find a ratio close to unity for the lightest nuclides (up to calcium 40), and a progressive increase in the n/p ratio with increasing

atomic number. In other words, as the atomic number increases, a progressively larger neutron excess (over protons) seems to be required for stability. For example, stable helium contains 2 protons and 2 neutrons in its nucleus, a ratio of 1. Stable lead 208 has 126 neutrons and 82 protons, a ratio of about 3/2.

2. *Odd-even Rules.* When the numbers of neutrons and protons of stable nuclides are studied, a curious relationship is found: the majority of stable nuclides contains *even* numbers of both neutrons and protons. The following list shows the number of stable nuclides with each of the 4 possible configurations, N representing the neutron number, and Z the proton (atomic) number.

even Z—even N	164 stable nuclides
odd Z—even N	50 stable nuclides
even Z—odd N	55 stable nuclides
odd Z—odd N	4 stable nuclides

It is apparent from this list that *even* numbers of protons and neutrons occur most frequently in stable nuclides, and that only a small percentage of stable nuclides contain odd numbers of both types of nucleons. An interesting point here is the fact that the α particle, consisting of a pair of protons and a pair of neutrons, is an exceedingly stable configuration probably because the nucleons form a closed system. However, the α particle is believed not to have an independent existence within a larger nucleus, but rather to be formed at the instant of ejection.

3. *Nuclear Binding Energy.* The energy holding the nucleons together in a nucleus is called the *nuclear binding energy.* This is defined as the energy required to separate a nucleus of atomic number Z into Z hydrogen atoms and $A - Z$ neutrons, where A is the mass number. (Since the definition specifies hydrogen atoms in the product particles, it also includes the electronic binding energy.) Thus,

$$BE = ZM_H + NM_n - M \tag{1}$$

where BE is the binding energy of the nucleus, Z is the atomic number of the nucleus, M_H is the atomic mass of hydrogen, N is the number of neutrons, M_n is the mass of a neutron, and M is the atomic mass of the isotope.

The derivation of the concept of nuclear binding energy has already been discussed on pages 48 to 49, being based on Einstein's equation for the mass-energy relationship, $E = mc^2$. If the individual masses of the particles—hydrogen atoms and neutrons—are added, the sum is greater than the mass of the nucleus as measured in a mass spectrograph. This is explained by the loss of mass during the formation of the nucleus. Since matter cannot be destroyed, the lost mass must have been converted to an equivalent amount of energy which was radiated from the nucleus. This energy constitutes the *nuclear binding energy.* To separate a nucleus into its component nucleons, the same amount of energy must now be added, and we may therefore regard the nuclear binding energy as a measure of nuclear stability. A convenient concept is the *binding energy per nucleon,* obtained by dividing the nuclear binding energy by the total number of nucleons (i.e. mass number). In general, the stable nuclides with a mass number exceeding 10 have a binding energy per nucleon averaging about 8 MeV (range about 7.5 to 9 MeV).

4. *Nuclear Forces.* The forces within the nucleus cannot be electrical because the protons would tend to repel each other. Nor can they be gravitational because this force is inadequate to account for the nuclear binding energy. Therefore, another type of force, simply called *nuclear force,* has been postulated. This operates over an extremely *short range,* becoming negligible at distances greater than 1 *fermi* $= 10^{-13}$ cm, or the diameter of the hydrogen nucleus. Nuclear force is probably about 100 times stronger than coulomb (electrical) force, or otherwise the protons would repel each other. Furthermore, nuclear force is about 10^{39} times stronger than gravitational force. The nuclear forces existing between two protons, a proton and a neutron, and two neutrons are approximately the same.

5. *Exchange Forces.* This is a highly theoretical concept, involving the rapid transfer of an appropriate π meson between a proton and a neutron, two protons, or two neutrons, as a result of which an attractive force is exerted between the nucleons.

The preceding discussion may be expanded as follows: nuclear stability requires a binding energy large enough to maintain the nucleus in that state. Conversely, if the binding energy is less than that required for stability, the nucleus de-excites in a manner typical of that particular nuclide. In every instance, the binding energy of the product nucleus exceeds that of the parent. *Neutron-deficient radionuclides* de-excite to stable nuclides, increasing the n/p ratio by one of the following processes: (1) emission of a positron and a neutrino as a proton changes to a neutron; (2) capture of a K (or L) electron, changing a proton to a neutron; or (3) emission of an α particle, probably by electrostatic repulsion by nuclear protons at the instant it is formed. Alpha decay occurs only in certain radionuclides whose atomic number exceeds 82.

On the other hand, *proton-deficient radionuclides* de-excite to stable nuclides by emitting a negative β particle and an antineutrino in the conversion of a neutron to a proton. A few nuclides such as ^{64}Cu have the unique property of emitting both positrons and negatrons; and ^{74}As de-excites by negatron emission, positron emission, and K-electron capture.

Artificial radioactive nuclides are usually created by the addition of a particle (proton, neutron, or deuteron) to the nucleus of a stable atom, resulting in nuclear instability. In the process of rearrangement of the nuclear constituents in a radionuclide as it arrives at a stable state, particles and/or photons are emitted exactly as in the case of naturally occurring radioactive elements.

At this point it will be of interest to define several terms that are often used to designate certain categories of nuclides. Recall that Z indicates atomic number, A is mass number, and N is neutron number. Based on nuclear composition:

Isotopes are atoms of the same element that differ in the number of nuclear neutrons. An example of an isotopic pair is $^{128}_{53}$I ($Z = 53$, $A = 128$, and $N = 75$) and $^{131}_{53}$I ($Z = 53$, $A = 131$, $N = 78$).

Isobars are atoms which have the same mass number, regardless of the nature of the nuclear constituents. An example of an isobaric pair is $^{24}_{11}$Na ($A = 24$) and $^{24}_{12}$Mg ($A = 24$).

Isotones are atoms that have the same number of nuclear neutrons, regardless of the other nuclear constituents. An example of an isotonic pair is $^{2}_{1}$H ($N = 1$) and $^{3}_{2}$He ($N = 1$).

TYPES OF NUCLEAR DE-EXCITATION (DECAY)

At this point, we shall review the types of radiation emitted by nuclei during radioactive decay. The more common types of nuclear de-excitation will be discussed briefly, since they have already been considered in detail in Chapter 3. During de-excitation, energy is released in the form of γ rays, or kinetic energy of particles. The total energy so released during nuclear de-excitation is called *transition energy.*

Alpha Decay. The nuclei of certain radioactive elements, for example, radium, decay with the emission of α *particles* by a process called α *decay.* These particles are identical with helium nuclei, consisting of 2 protons and 2 neutrons, and having two positive charges. Alpha particles are actually helium atoms stripped of orbital electrons, which means that they are the same as helium ions. With the emission of an α particle, the nucleus loses two units of atomic number (2 protons) and four units of atomic mass (2 protons and 2 neutrons), thereby changing to a nucleus of an entirely different element. This process represents one form of *nuclear transformation* or *transmutation.*

Because the massive α particle carries a double charge it can *readily ionize* atoms in its path. In this process, the electrical (coulomb) field of the α particle interacts with a loosely bound orbital electron, accelerating it sufficiently to drive it completely out of the atom. The freed electron and the residual positively charged atom together constitute an *ion pair.* The magnitude of the ionizing ability of α particles is evident from the fact that a 2-MeV radium α particle may produce about 60,000 ion pairs per cm of path in air (β particles with similar energy release only 50 ion pairs/cm). Instead of ionizing an atom, the α particle may simply raise an orbital electron to a higher energy level, producing *atomic excitation.* In both types of interaction—that is, ionization and excitation—the α particle gradually loses energy and slows down. Its ionizing ability (specific ionization) *increases* near the end of its path because it spends more time in the vicinity of an atom, a phenomenon known as the *Bragg peak.*

Two important characteristics of α particles are *velocity* and *range.* The initial velocities (and hence, energies) of α particles are essentially alike for all the atoms of a given radionuclide. Furthermore, the α particles from different radionuclides have different initial velocities. These vary from 1/20 to 1/10 the velocity of light. As indicated above, the velocity gradually decreases, and when the α particle comes almost to rest it annexes two electrons and becomes a neutral helium atom:

$$1 \text{ α particle} + 2 \text{ electrons} \longrightarrow 1 \text{ helium atom}$$
$$He^{++} \quad + \quad 2\,e^{-} \quad \longrightarrow He$$

The *range* of α particles is the distance they travel in a given medium. Since the initial velocities of α particles from a given source are nearly uniform, their kinetic energies and ranges are, too, except for "straggling." Thus, the range of α particles is characteristic of the emitting nuclide. As described in Chapter 3, the range of an α particle is proportional to the cube of its initial velocity. Furthermore, the shorter the half-life of an α emitter, the longer the range of the α particles because of their greater initial energy; this principle is embodied in the *Geiger-Nuttall Rule.*

Because of the strong ionization produced by α particles, their range in tissue is very short. Usually, they cannot even pass through the keratinized (outermost) layer of the skin.

Beta Decay. During nuclear de-excitation of certain radionuclides, electrons are emitted with energies ranging from zero to a maximum. These electrons are *β particles,* and their emission is usually referred to as *β decay.* There are two kinds of β decay, *negative* and *positive,* the former being far more common. Since β particles do not exist in a free state in the nucleus, how can we explain their origin?

Radionuclides such as ^{32}P, in which the n/p ratio is too high for nuclear stability, de-excite by $β^{-}$ decay:

$$^{32}_{15}P \longrightarrow \, ^{32}_{16}S + \, ^{\ \ 0}_{-1}β + \tilde{v}$$

Figure 11.04B shows the decay scheme of ^{32}P.

In $β^{-}$ decay a nuclear neutron changes to a proton, a $β^{-}$ particle (symbol $^{\ \ 0}_{-1}β$ or $^{\ \ 0}_{-1}e$) and an antineutrino ($^{0}_{0}\tilde{v}$). Whereas the proton remains in the nucleus, the β^- particle together with its antineutrino is ejected from the nucleus.

$$\underset{\text{neutron}}{^1_0 n} \longrightarrow \underset{\text{proton}}{^1_1 H} + \underset{\text{negatron}}{^{\ 0}_{-1} \beta} + \underset{\text{antineutrino}}{^0_0 \bar{\nu}}$$

Since the total energy carried by the β^- particle and its accompanying antineutrino must equal the maximum β-particle energy during the de-excitation, and since this total energy is constant for a particular path of decay of a given radionuclide, it is obvious that a high energy β^- particle is accompanied by a low energy antineutrino, and conversely:

$$E_{\text{max}} = energy_\beta + energy_{antineutrino} \qquad (2)$$

where E_{max} is the maximum β-particle energy.

The range and velocity of β^- particles depend on their individual energy. Some β^- particles can penetrate 1 cm or more of tissue. Most of the β^- particles emitted by radium are absorbed by 0.5 mm Pt.

Another variety of β decay, involving the emission of a positively charged electron—β^+ or positron (symbol $^0_{+1} \beta$ or $_{+1}^{\ 0} e$)— occurs with certain radionuclides such as ^{22}Na (see Fig. 11.01) in which the n/p ratio is too low for nuclear stability,

$$^{22}_{11} Na \longrightarrow {}^{22}_{10} Ne + {}^{\ 0}_{+1} \beta + \nu$$

In this process a nuclear proton gives rise to a neutron, a positron, and a neutrino:

$$\underset{\text{proton}}{^1_1 H} \longrightarrow \underset{\text{neutron}}{^1_0 n} + \underset{\text{positron}}{^{\ 0}_{+1} \beta} + \underset{\text{neutrino}}{\nu}$$

Positron emission requires an available energy of 1.02 MeV, this being the energy equivalent to the rest mass of the positron plus that of the electron lost from one of the atomic shells.

Internal Conversion. Some radionuclides de-excite to daughter nuclides that are still in an excited state. Usually these go to ground state by γ-ray emission. However, in the case of certain nuclides such as gold 198 (^{198}Au) this excess nuclear energy is

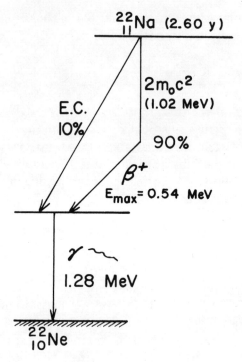

FIGURE 11.01. Decay scheme of sodium 22. This is an example of a radionuclide that de-excites by positron (β^+) emission (90%), although an alternate route is K capture (10%). Both modes arrive at the excited state of neon, which then de-excites by emission of a 1.28-MeV γ ray.

disposed of by the process of *internal conversion* in which an electron is ejected from one of the inner shells (most often the K shell) as the result of interaction between the excited nucleus and the electron. This process is summarized in the following equation:

$$KE_{ce} = h\nu - W_K \tag{3}$$

where KE_{ce} is the energy of the *conversion electron,* $h\nu$ is the excess nuclear energy, and W_K is the binding energy of the K shell harboring the conversion electron, in this instance the K shell. No γ ray is emitted; the unsophisticated interpretation is that the γ ray that might otherwise have been emitted ejects the conversion electron. The continuous β spectrum of the parent nucleus (e.g. ^{198}Au) has superimposed upon it discontinuous peaks representing the conversion electrons of the daughter nuclei. After emitting conversion electrons, the excited atoms return finally to ground state by the emission of characteristic X rays or Auger electrons. Thus,

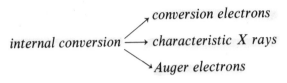

$$\textit{internal conversion} \longrightarrow \begin{cases} \textit{conversion electrons} \\ \textit{characteristic X rays} \\ \textit{Auger electrons} \end{cases}$$

Electron Capture. In 1938 another type of nuclear de-excitation was discovered, characterized by the transition of an orbital electron into the nucleus. It turns out that this process is more likely where, although the n/p ratio is too low for maximum nuclear stability, β^+ decay is impossible because the nuclear energy levels of the parent and daughter atoms do not differ by at least 1.02 MeV. Since capture usually involves an electron in the K shell, it is termed **K capture.** Much more rarely, **L capture** occurs, the electron dropping from the L shell into the nucleus. Upon entering the nucleus, the electron unites with a proton to form a neutron:

$$\underset{\textit{proton}}{{}^1_1\text{H}} \quad + \quad \underset{\substack{\textit{electron} \\ \textit{(usually K)}}}{{}^{\ 0}_{-1}\text{e}} \quad \longrightarrow \quad \underset{\textit{neutron}}{{}^1_0\text{n}} \quad + \quad \underset{\textit{neutrino}}{{}^0_0\nu}$$

The resulting atom has an atomic number one less than its parent (1 proton neutralized), and may be excited, emitting a γ ray in the process of reaching ground state. Electron capture leaves a hole in the respective shell, so the atom is excited. It returns to the ground state by emitting characteristic X rays and Auger electrons. Thus,

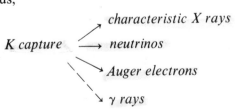

$$\textit{K capture} \longrightarrow \begin{cases} \textit{characteristic X rays} \\ \textit{neutrinos} \\ \textit{Auger electrons} \\ \gamma \textit{ rays} \end{cases}$$

Isomeric Transition. An excited nucleus usually decays to ground state by emitting a γ ray in 10^{-13} sec. However, in some instances γ emission takes appreciably longer, and such nuclei are called *isomers.* They usually occur in pairs, about 70 such isomeric pairs being known at present among artificial nuclides. As we have already indicated, there is ample evidence that *energy levels* are present inside the atomic nucleus just as there are outside. Transition of nuclear particles from one energy level to another is accompanied by the emission of energy (analogous to characteristic radiation during transition of orbital electrons). Thus, one nuclear isomer is in a higher energy state called the *metastable state* if its half-life exceeds 10^{-6} sec. It returns to the *ground level*, that is, it is converted to its other isomer, by radiating a γ ray. During this process, known as *isomeric transition,* there is no change in atomic number or mass number—there is simply a transition of particles in the nuclear isomer from a higher to a lower energy level, the difference in energy being emitted as a photon, in this case a γ ray and/or a conversion electron. Internal conversion may occur during isomeric transition as in the case of technetium 99m (^{99m}Tc), shown in Figure 11.02. Incidentally, this is an example of *branching transition* or *branching decay.* Note that in the minor branch α, the ratio of internal conversion electrons to γ photons, is high—

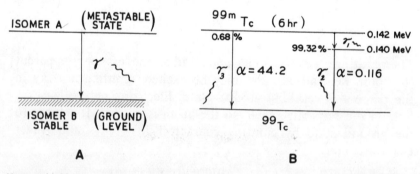

A   B

FIGURE 11.02. In *A* is shown the general decay scheme isomeric transition. Isomer A decays, with an appreciable half-life to ground state by emitting a γ ray. In *B* is an example of isomeric transition—the decay of technetium 99m (99ᵐTc), half-life 6 hr. A very small fraction de-excites directly by emission of a 142-keV photon (γ ray). The preponderant route or branch (99.32%) is de-excitation in two steps: first to the 140-keV level, thence to ground state of technetium 99. The symbol α is the ratio of the number of internal conversion electrons to the number of γ photons.

44.2; whereas in the major branch it is 0.116 which means that there are 11.6 conversion electrons for every 100 γ photons.

Gamma-ray Emission. We have already indicated that γ rays are a type of electromagnetic radiation similar to X rays. They travel with the speed of light and are highly penetrating. Because γ rays are neutral, they cannot be deflected by a magnetic or electrical field. Furthermore, like X rays they cannot be focused with a lens.

Gamma rays are emitted by certain radionuclides. Following the emission of particulate radiation, the nucleus may be left in an excited state; that is, it has not reached the ground or most stable form of that nucleus. To reach ground level, it radiates energy in the form of a γ ray whose energy is characteristic of the *daughter* nuclide. The emission of γ rays may occur in stages, producing a series.

Gamma radiation also accompanies certain nuclear reactions. For example, in radiative capture, a neutron is captured by a nucleus which becomes excited. In de-exciting to ground state, it emits a γ ray.

In summary, then, we can state that as the result of particle transitions between energy levels within the nucleus, or ejection of particles from the nucleus, excess bits of energy are emitted by the daughter nucleus in the form of characteristic γ rays.

The ionizing power of γ rays, because they are uncharged, is slight—about 1 to 2 ion pairs per cm in air. Ionization by γ rays is almost entirely indirect, occurring through the action of primary electrons which they release from atomic orbits.

ARTIFICIAL RADIOACTIVITY

Unstable isotopes can be produced artificially for all stable elements. The radioactivity of such unstable isotopes, having the same general characteristics as that found in the naturally occurring radioactive elements, is called *artificial radioactivity*. It is readily apparent that the distinction is not a fundamental one, but merely serves to classify radionuclides into two large groups: natural and artificial.

The reactions engendered in nuclei irradiated by certain types of particles have shed a tremendous amount of light on the internal structure and behavior of the heart of the atom. For example, such investigations led to the Nobel Prize-winning discovery of the neutron by Chadwick in 1932.

It will be instructive to examine the requirements for the production of an artificial radionuclides, that is, the **activation of nuclides.**

1. **Target Nucleus** of the element which is to be bombarded by subatomic particles.

2. **Projectile**, usually a particle having a fairly large mass and high speed, although these are not essential. A large charge on the bombarding particle may be more of a hindrance than a help, because of repulsion by the electrostatic (coulomb) field of the target nucleus. Various particles can be used as projectiles: neutrons, protons, deuterons, and α particles. Protons and deuterons can be accelerated to very high speeds by special devices such as the cyclotron, making them very efficient projectiles. Neutrons, since they have no charge, readily penetrate the target nuclei because nuclei do not present an electrostatic barrier to them. In Figure 11.03 a neutron is shown entering a nucleus. On the other hand, a proton would have to possess sufficient energy to exceed the energy of the barrier in order to enter the nucleus (although according to Gamow, such charged particles have a small probability of leaking through the barrier even if they have less than the required amount of energy). Alpha particles, with their two positive charges, require very high energy to overcome the repelling force of the electrostatic barrier.

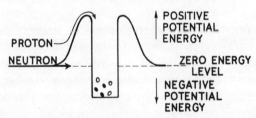

FIGURE 11.03. A proton usually requires energy in excess of the positive potential barrier of a nucleus in order to enter the nucleus. A neutron, on the other hand, being uncharged, does not confront such a barrier, so it easily enters the nucleus.

TABLE 11.01
ENERGY EXCHANGES IN NUCLEAR REACTIONS

Projectile Particle	Energy Carried by Particle	No. of Nucleons in Particle	Energy Needed to Separate Particle Into Nucleons	Net Energy Gained by Compound Nucleus
	MeV		*MeV*	*MeV*
α particle	32	4	28.2	3.8
proton	8	1	→	8
deuteron	16	2	2	14

Deuterons are much more efficient projectiles than α particles for various reasons. First, the target nucleus gains a net energy of about 14 MeV upon entrance of a deuteron. In contrast to this, the nucleus invaded by an α particle gains only 4 MeV. Therefore, the former type of reaction is more probable. Because only 8 MeV of energy is gained when a proton enters the nucleus, the probability of this reaction occupies an intermediate position. Table 11.01 summarizes the derivation of these energy relationships.

Second, deuterons may be regarded as made up of a proton and a neutron loosely associated, the binding energy of these two particles being about 2 MeV. If a deutron with kinetic energy greater than 2 MeV approaches a target nucleus, the positive electrical field of the latter may strongly repel the proton portion of the deuteron, leaving the neutron portion alone to enter the nucleus. This is known as the ***Oppenheimer-Phillips Mechanism*** or ***stripping reaction.***

3. ***Compound Nucleus*** is formed when a projectile enters a target nucleus. Such an overloaded nucleus is unstable, the degree of instability depending on the target nucleus and the entering projectile.

4. ***Disintegration of Compound Nucleus*** may occur by one of several routes. The energy brought into the nucleus by the projectile is shared by the nucleons present; one or a combination of nucleons may then acquire sufficient energy to escape through the nuclear electrostatic barrier (see below for exceptions). If the compound nucleus has a high atomic number, it will more probably eject a neutron, because this uncharged particle does not confront an electrostatic barrier. If the compound nucleus has a low atomic

number, it is more apt to emit a proton, since the electrostatic barrier is not too great and since a neutron is more firmly held by a nucleus of low atomic number. Alpha particles are emitted, with rare exceptions, only from nuclei with atomic number above 82 by "tunneling" through the electrostatic barrier; or when their energy is sufficiently greater than the electrostatic barrier. Deuterons are rarely emitted because very high energy is required. From this discussion we can see that the nuclear electrostatic barrier operates both ways—not only does it tend to protect the nucleus from entrance of positively charged projectiles, but it also tends to oppose the emission of positively charged particles from the nucleus.

The compound nucleus does not often emit β particles (positive or negative) because this is too slow a type of decay. It seems as though the compound nucleus is in a great hurry to get rid of its excess energy, this being accomplished much more rapidly by the expulsion of neutrons, deuterons, or protons. In some instances, the nucleus does not have sufficient energy to expel any kind of particle, and it therefore reaches stability by emitting a γ photon, a process called *radiative capture.* It occurs especially with entry of a slow neutron, this being *one of the most important types of nuclear reactions.*

The de-excitation of a compound nucleus, as already mentioned, takes place very rapidly—average life 10^{-14} to 10^{-12} sec —following the same laws as do any other radioactive nuclei. Usually, the product atom, after the decay of a compound nucleus, is also radioactive because nuclear stability has not yet been attained.

ACTIVATION OF ATOMS—NUCLEAR REACTIONS

Examples will now be given to illustrate not only the notation used, but also the varieties of reactions that can occur between projectiles and target nuclei. A given nuclide is completely specified by a *subscript* to indicate its atomic number and a *superscript* to specify its mass number. The sum of the superscripts of the reacting particles must equal the superscript of the product nucleus. The same applies to the subscripts.

1. *Alpha Particle Reactions.* Upon irradiating atmospheric nitrogen with α particles of radium, Rutherford (1919) discovered the production of an isotope of oxygen along with the liberation of protons, according to the following classical equation:

$$\underset{\text{nitrogen}}{{}^{14}_{7}\text{N}} \quad + \quad \underset{\alpha\ particle}{{}^{4}_{2}\text{He}} \quad \longrightarrow \quad \underset{\text{oxygen}}{{}^{17}_{8}\text{O}} \quad + \quad \underset{\text{proton}}{{}^{1}_{1}\text{H}}$$

This was the first instance of artificial *transmutation* of an element, but it must be noted that the product atoms are not radioactive. Incidentally, it may be designated as the ${}^{14}\text{N}(\alpha,\text{p}){}^{17}\text{O}$ reaction.

In 1930, Bothe and Becker made the historic observation that irradiation of a light metal such as beryllium with the α particles of polonium yields an extremely penetrating radiation, misinterpreted by Joliot and Curie as γ rays. However, in 1932 Chadwick proved these penetrating rays to be neutral particles—*neutrons.* The reaction is of the (α, n) type and occurs as follows:

$$\underset{\text{beryllium}}{{}^{9}_{4}\text{Be}} \quad + \quad \underset{\alpha\ particle}{{}^{4}_{2}\text{He}} \quad \longrightarrow \quad \underset{\text{carbon}}{{}^{12}_{6}\text{C}} \quad + \quad \underset{\text{neutron}}{{}^{1}_{0}\text{n}}$$

At present, α particles from natural sources are no longer used in the manufacture of artificial radionuclides because of their limited supply, the low probability of hits because of their large charge, and their low energies of 4 to 8 MeV.

2. *Neutron Reactions.* Since neutrons can be used to induce a great variety of nuclear reactions, they will be discussed in some detail. The principal source of neutrons for commercial purposes is the nuclear reactor. Additional sources for laboratory use include radium-beryllium mixtures; deuteron bombardment of heavy ice, heavy paraffin, or beryllium; and high energy γ irradiation of targets of low atomic number. Neutrons are arbitrarily classified on the basis of their kinetic energy: *fast neutrons* have an energy in excess of 100 keV, *intermediate neutrons* 100 eV to 100 keV, and *slow neutrons* 0.025 eV to 100 eV. The slowest neutrons with energy of about 0.025 eV are usually spoken of as *thermal neutrons* because their energy is approximately that of the average kinetic energy of gas molecules at ordinary tempera-

tures, although they move with great speed—about 2.2×10^5 cm/sec.

It is of interest that radionuclides produced by neutron irradiation, as in a nuclear reactor, have a neutron/proton (n/p) ratio that is too large for maximum nuclear stability; hence, such products decay by β^- emission.

a. *Radiative Capture—(n,γ) Reaction.* One of the most important of all induced nuclear reactions is radiative capture: a slow neutron, carrying no electric charge, readily enters the nucleus of a target atom. In fact, when it reaches a point within the range of nuclear force, it may even be attracted into the nucleus. The resulting compound nucleus may get rid of its excitation energy in various ways, the most common being the emission of a γ ray. Thus, nuclear reactions readily occur with thermal neutrons, constituting the most prolific source of artificial nuclides.

An example of the radiative capture reaction with slow neutrons is the following:

$$\underset{11}{23}\text{Na} + \underset{0}{1}\text{n} \longrightarrow \underset{11}{24}\text{Na} + \gamma \quad [^{23}\text{Na}\,(n,\gamma)\,^{24}\text{Na reaction}]$$
$$\underset{slow}{} \qquad \underset{unstable}{}$$

Note that in this case a *radioactive isotope of the target atom* is produced. In other instances, the product isotope may be stable. The ^{24}Na atom de-excites as follows:

$$\underset{11}{24}\text{Na} \longrightarrow \underset{12}{24}\text{Mg} + \underset{-1}{0}\text{e} + 2\gamma + \tilde{\nu}$$
$$\underset{\beta^- \; particle}{}$$

Although the radiative capture reaction may also occur with fast neutrons, this has a low order of probability. On the other hand, the probability of radiative capture of slow neutrons is high for almost every known nuclide, thus underlining the importance of this reaction.

b. *The (n,p) Reaction.* In this reaction a neutron enters the target nucleus and a charged particle, a proton, is emitted. Since the proton must have sufficient energy to escape the nuclear electrostatic barrier, this energy must be brought into the nucleus by the projectile neutron. Therefore, a fast or high-energy neutron is usually required for the (n,p) reaction. However, the product nucleus is usually a negative β emitter, and if the maximum β particle energy is low, the (n,p) reaction becomes possible even with slow neutrons. An example is the production of carbon 14, important in biologic research:

$$\underset{slow}{^{14}_{7}\text{N}} + {}^{1}_{0}\text{n} \longrightarrow \underset{unstable}{^{14}_{6}\text{C}} + {}^{1}_{1}\text{H} \quad [{}^{14}\text{N (n,p)} {}^{14}\text{C reaction}]$$

$$^{14}_{6}\text{C} \longrightarrow {}^{14}_{7}\text{N} + \underset{\beta^{-} \ particle}{_{-1}^{0}\text{e}} + \tilde{\nu}$$

(The energies of the emitted proton and the β particle have been omitted for the sake of simplicity, although they are important in nuclear physics.) In this reaction, known as a ***transmutation reaction,*** the product nucleus is an element different from the target.

c. ***The (n,α) Reaction.*** Just as in the (n,p) reaction, the energy of the projectile neutron in the (n,α) reaction must be high enough to permit the resulting α particle to escape the nuclear electrostatic barrier. However, the (n,α) reaction occurs more readily than the (n,p) because energy of about 8 MeV must be available to separate a proton from a nucleus, while only 4 MeV is needed to separate an α particle. When the target nucleus has a low atomic number, its electric potential is small and the (n,α) reaction becomes possible even with slow neutrons:

$$^{10}_{5}\text{B} + {}^{1}_{0}\text{n} \longrightarrow {}^{7}_{3}\text{Li} + {}^{4}_{2}\text{He} \qquad [{}^{10}\text{B(n,}\alpha\text{)}{}^{7}\text{Li reaction}]$$

3. ***Proton Reactions.*** Because the energy of the projectile proton must be high enough to allow it to penetrate the target's nuclear electrostatic barrier, proton reactions with nuclei become more probable with protons of high energy; or with nuclei of low atomic number when the protons are of low energy. High energy protons are usually obtained by acceleration in a cyclotron. It is of interest that since proton-induced reactions decrease the n/p ratio (i.e. increase p) below that needed for maximum nuclear stability, the product nuclei decay by positron emission or by electron capture.

a. ***Radiative Capture—(p,γ) Reaction.*** When protons are captured by nuclei of low atomic number, the compound nucleus may dissipate its excitation energy by emitting a γ ray in a manner analogous to the (n,γ) reaction:

$$^{27}_{13}Al + ^{1}_{1}H \longrightarrow ^{28}_{14}Si + \gamma \qquad [^{27}Al(p,\gamma)^{28}Si \text{ reaction}]$$

Note, however, that in this case the product is **not** an isotope of the target.

b. **The (p,n) Reaction.** This, too, becomes more probable with atoms of low atomic number:

$$^{23}_{11}Na + ^{1}_{1}H \longrightarrow ^{23}_{12}Mg + ^{1}_{0}n \qquad [^{23}Na(p,n)^{23}Mg \text{ reaction}]$$

4. **Deuteron Reactions.** Deuterons are very effective projectiles for nuclear transformations. The most common types of reactions include the (d,p) and the (d,n). The symbol for the deuteron is $^{2}_{1}H$. High energy deuterons are produced in a cyclotron.

a. **The (d,p) Reaction.** Because of the small binding energy of the deuteron, the target nucleus may repel the proton portion, allowing the neutron to slip in and form a compound nucleus— the so-called **stripping reaction** or **Oppenheimer-Phillips Mechanism.** This reaction has a high order of probability with low energy deuterons. An example is:

$$^{23}_{11}Na + ^{2}_{1}H \longrightarrow ^{24}_{11}Na + ^{1}_{1}H \quad [^{23}Na\,(d,p)\,^{24}Na \text{ reaction}]$$

^{24}Na is unstable and decays as described above. The (d,p) reaction yields the medically important radionuclide ^{32}P, but is no longer the principal source.

$$^{31}_{15}P + ^{2}_{1}H \longrightarrow \underset{unstable}{^{32}_{15}P} + ^{1}_{1}H \quad [^{31}P\,(d,p)\,^{32}P \text{ reaction}]$$

$$^{32}_{15}P \longrightarrow ^{32}_{16}S + \underset{\beta^- \; particle}{_{-1}^{0}e} + \tilde{v}$$

Note that with the (d,p) reaction, the product is an isotope of the target.

b. **The (d,n) Reaction.** When energetic deuterons approach a target the entire deuteron may enter the nucleus, followed by the ejection of an energetic neutron:

$$^{6}_{3}Li + ^{2}_{1}H \longrightarrow ^{7}_{4}Be + ^{1}_{0}n \qquad [^{6}Li(d,n)^{7}Be \text{ reaction}]$$

5. ***Photonuclear Reactions.*** We have already found that a high energy photon (threshold 1.02 MeV) may, in the vicinity of a nucleus, disappear and give rise to a negatron-positron pair. Another type of photonuclear interaction occurs with very high-energy photons, usually in excess of 10 MeV, in which nuclear particles such as neutrons and protons (less often α particles) are ejected from the nucleus. This threshold energy is equivalent to the binding energy of the proton and neutron in the nucleus. The daughter nucleus is often radioactive, although it typically has a short half-life of the order of a few minutes. This kind of nuclear reaction, called ***photodisintegration,*** may be especially important when the atmosphere is irradiated by high energy photons. For example, in the following (γ,n) reaction which requires a threshold energy of about 15.6 MeV:

$$^{16}_{8}O + \underset{15.6\ MeV}{\gamma} \longrightarrow {}^{15}_{8}O + {}^{1}_{0}n \quad [^{16}O\,(\gamma,n)\,^{15}O \text{ reaction}]$$

the daughter nucleus $^{15}_{8}O$ is radioactive, with a half-life of about 2 minutes.

In a few instances, exemplified by the following interaction, photodisintegration occurs with photons of somewhat lower energy:

$$\underset{deuterium}{^{2}_{1}H} + \underset{2.2\ MeV}{\gamma} \longrightarrow {}^{1}_{1}H + {}^{1}_{0}n \quad [^{2}H\,(\gamma,n)\,^{1}H \text{ reaction}]$$

Many other nuclear reactions may occur, but we have surveyed only a few of them to emphasize the more important ones. Worthy of special mention is the production of iodine 131, a very widely used radionuclide in medicine. ^{131}I can be made by two different nuclear reactions: bombardment of tellurium 130 with fast deuterons in the cyclotron, or slow neutrons in the nuclear reactor.

Cyclotron: $^{130}_{52}Te + {}^{2}_{1}H \longrightarrow {}^{131}_{53}I + {}^{1}_{0}n$ (d,n) reaction

Nuclear reactor: $^{130}_{52}Te + {}^{1}_{0}n \longrightarrow {}^{131}_{53}I + {}^{0}_{-1}e$ (n,β^{-}) reaction

Note that the identical radionuclide, $^{131}_{53}I$, results from both these reactions. The product disintegrates to stable xenon as follows:

$$\underset{\beta^{-}\ particle}{^{131}_{53}I \longrightarrow {}^{131}_{54}Xe + {}^{0}_{-1}e} + \gamma + \tilde{\nu}$$

However, the most abundant source commercially is from the separation of the *fission products* of the nuclear reactor. The medical use of ^{131}I will be considered later.

THE RADIOACTIVE DECAY PROCESS

We have seen that radionuclides, whether found in nature or produced artificially, undergo spontaneous nuclear transformation with the emission of radiation. This is designated as the *radioactive decay process.* Certain general characteristics of radioactive decay will now be considered.

Displacement Law. In 1902 E. Rutherford and F. Soddy discovered that during the transformation of naturally occurring radioactive elements, the daughter atoms differ from the parent not only in their nuclear structure, but also in their chemical nature. The change is predicated on the type of particle ejected by the nucleus.

1. *Alpha Emission.* When radium decays to radon by the emission of an α particle, the nucleus loses four atomic mass units and two atomic number units (contained in the α particle), being transformed into an entirely different element, *radon:*

$$^{226}_{88}Ra \longrightarrow {}^{222}_{86}Rn + \underset{\alpha \, particle}{{}^{4}_{2}He}$$

Since radon has two fewer positive charges on the nucleus than does radium, it loses two orbital electrons to become electrically neutral. At the same time, radon differs from radium in its chemical properties. As a matter of fact, *radium,* belonging to Group II elements in the Periodic Table, behaves very much like calcium and barium in chemical reactions. On the other hand, since *radon* is in Group O, it has no affinity for any element and therefore does not react chemically, resembling other inert elements such as helium, neon, argon, etc. (Heavier inert elements have been made to form compounds in minute amounts under exceptional conditions.)

2. *Beta Emission.* When a radionuclide decays by the emission of a β particle, as in the following reaction, it becomes a different element.

$$^{32}_{15}P - \underset{\beta^- \, particle}{{}^{32}_{16}S + {}^{0}_{-1}e} + {}^{0}_{0}\tilde{v}$$

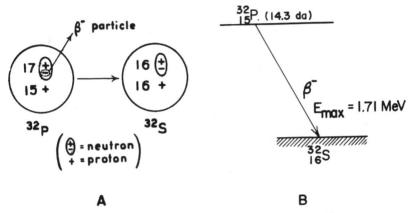

FIGURE 11.04. *A*. Radiophosphorus (^{32}P) decays to stable sulfur (^{32}S) by the emission of a β^- particle. *B*. Decay scheme of ^{32}P.

In this instance, radioactive phosphorus is changed to stable sulfur. How does this come about? Since the phosphorus nucleus contains 15 protons and 17 neutrons, and the β^- particle arises through the conversion of one neutron to a proton and an electron, this adds one nuclear positive charge increasing the atomic number from 15 to 16. The atomic number of sulfur is 16. Furthermore, the emission of one electron does not appreciably change the atomic mass, so the mass number of sulfur remains the same as that of radioactive phosphorus. Figure 11.04 illustrates this reaction.

3. *Gamma-ray Emission.* Following particle emission or nuclear bombardment, a γ ray may be emitted. There is no displacement of the atom in the Periodic Table as the result of the γ-ray emission itself, such displacement occurring only with the ejection of a charged particle.

In short, the Rutherford-Soddy Displacement Law predicts the shift in position of a daughter element relative to the parent in the Periodic Table of Elements when α particles or β particles are emitted. If an α particle is ejected, it carries away 2 atomic number units and the daughter element lies 2 places to the *left* in the Periodic Table. In β^- particle emission, a nuclear neutron is first converted to a proton, a negative electron, and an antineutrino; the electron is ejected as a β^- particle and the proton remains in the nucleus, increasing the nuclear charge by one. The daughter

354 The Basic Physics of Radiation Therapy

therefore has one more unit of atomic number, appearing one place to the *right* in the Periodic Table.

Applying the Displacement Law to the naturally occurring radioactive elements, Rutherford and Soddy grouped them, along with their descendants, into three families named after the longest lived member of each family: the uranium, thorium, and actinium series. A fourth such series, originating with the transuranic, artificially created element neptunium, is accordingly named the neptunium series; this series is not found in nature because it does not have a sufficiently long-lived member.

These *radioactive series*, as they are called, consist of a succession of *nuclides* ending with a stable element. The *parent* is the first member of the series (thus, uranium is a parent). The intermediate members arising by nuclear transformation are called daughters, and the final stable nucleus the end product. Whenever such a series of successive transformations characterizes the decay scheme of a radionuclide, the process is called *series decay*. Note that this differs from the transformation of a radionuclide in one or a few steps to a stable end product, for example, phosphorus 32 to stable sulfur 32.

Radioactive Decay Scheme. Physicists represent the transformation of a radioactive nuclide in schematic form to indicate (1) the parent nucleus with its half-life; (2) the radiation, particulate or photonic, that it emits; (3) the energy liberated; (4) the direction in which the atomic number (Z) changes, that is, larger or smaller; and (5) the end product. When Z increases as with β^- decay, the arrow points downward and to the right; but when Z decreases as with β^+ decay, the arrow points downward and to the left. When decay occurs by γ emission, there is no change in Z and the arrow points vertically downward. If decay occurs by alternate routes, that is, by *branching*, this is also indicated in the diagram (see Fig. 11.01).

Figure 6.01 shows the decay scheme of cobalt 60 (^{60}Co). When ^{60}Co is removed from the nuclear reactor it consists of two isomers, one with a half-life of 10.7 minutes and the other with a half-life of 5.3 years. Since the short-lived isomer changes to the 5.3-year isotope within a few hours, the commercial product is essentially 100 percent long-lived isomer. ^{60}Co emits a 0.31-MeV β^- particle and is transformed into an excited nickel atom (^{60}Ni) which reaches ground state by emitting two γ photons in succession. One has an energy of 1.17 MeV, and the other 1.33 MeV. Note that the γ rays are characteristic of ^{60}Ni, and not ^{60}Co.

It is of interest that the capture of slow neutrons by stable cobalt is a very efficient reaction, as mentioned earlier, because of its high capture cross section. The "half value layer" for slow neutrons is 2.3 mm Co, that is, this thickness of Co absorbs 50 percent of an incident beam of neutrons.

The nuclear decay scheme of radioactive cesium 137 (^{137}Cs) is shown in Figure 6.03 to illustrate decay by two alternate routes, that is, branching decay, either directly by emission of a 1.17-MeV β^- particle, or by emission of a 0.51-MeV β^- particle followed by a 0.66-MeV γ photon. In both cases the end product is the same, stable barium. Note that the expulsion of a β^- particle increases the positive charge on the Cs nucleus by one unit; thus, the daughter Ba lies one place to the right of Cs in the periodic table. In any particular sample of ^{137}Cs, 8 percent of the nuclei will de-excite by one route, and the remaining 92 percent by the other route, the ratio of the two being called the *branching ratio.*

The Radioactive Transformation or Decay Constant λ. Every radioactive sample decays *exponentially* at a *constant rate* which is typical of that particular nuclide. Since the decay rate of a given radionuclide is *constant,* it means that regardless of the number of such atoms originally present, *a certain fixed fraction decays in unit time.* For example, if the original number is 1 million atoms, and ½ decay per second, at the end of one second 500,000 atoms will have de-excited. In the next second, ½ of the remaining 500,000 atoms, or 250,000 will decay. This is illustrated in Table 11.02. Although the same fraction, ½, decays every second, the actual number of decaying atoms depends on the number initially present. This distinction must be firmly kept in mind if one is to understand thoroughly the decay process.

TABLE 11.02
THE DECAY OF A RADIONUCLIDE IN WHICH ONE-HALF
THE ATOMS DE-EXCITE EACH SECOND

Initial Number of Atoms	*Number Decaying in 1 Second*
1,000,000	500,000
500,000	250,000
250,000	125,000

Thus, the **transformation** or **decay constant** may be defined as the **fraction of the radioactive atoms present, decaying per unit interval of time.** In other words, it is the ratio of the number of atoms decaying in unit time, to the number present at the start:

$$\lambda = \frac{no.\ of\ atoms\ decaying\ per\ unit\ time}{no.\ of\ atoms\ initially\ present} \qquad (4)$$

The transformation or decay constant is expressed as a decimal fraction per second, or per hour, or some other convenient interval of time.

There is at present no practicable method of altering the decay constant which is always the same for a given radionuclide. It must be emphasized that it is impossible to predict which atoms of a radioactive sample will de-excite at a given moment, any more than one can state which kernel of corn will pop at any chosen instant. The decay rate is simply a **statistical** concept: of a given number of atoms, a certain definite fraction will undergo transformation per unit time. For example, radon (the first descendant of radium) decays at the rate of 16.6 percent per day. When calculated by the equation for radioactive decay, based in instantaneous values, the decay constant is 0.181 per day.

From the experimental observation that the number of nuclear transformations occurring in unit time ($\Delta N/\Delta t$) is proportional to the number of atoms present (N),

$$\frac{\Delta N}{\Delta t} \propto N \qquad (5)$$

Therefore,

$$\frac{\Delta N}{\Delta t} = -\lambda N \qquad (6)$$

where λ is the constant of proportionality, represented with a negative sign because there is a decrease in the number of atoms with the passing of time. Then, rearranging equation (6),

$$\frac{\Delta N/N}{\Delta t} = -\lambda \qquad (7)$$

we see that λ, the decay constant, is the fraction of atoms present decaying per given interval of time, Δt.

With the aid of calculus, equation (7) takes the familiar form of the law of radioactive decay,

$$N = N_0 e^{-\lambda t} \tag{8}$$

where N is the number of atoms remaining after a time t, N_0 is the initial number of atoms present, e is the base of natural logarithms (a constant), and λ is the decay constant. As indicated in Chapter 1, the values of $e^{-\lambda t}$ for desired values of λ and t can be found in appropriate tables (Table 4.02) and substituted in equation (8).

Instead of using the actual number of atoms in the equation, we can specify the quantity of radioactive material in terms of *activity,* the equation then being represented as

$$A = A_0 e^{-\lambda t} \tag{9}$$

where A is the activity of the radionuclide **remaining** after time t, and A_0 is the original activity of the nuclide.

From equation (9) we can derive the equation for A_d, the activity that has been **lost** in time t. Since

$$A_d = A_0 - A$$

substituting the value of A from equation (9),

$$A_d = A_0 - A_0 e^{-\lambda t}$$

and

$$A_d = A_0(1 - e^{-\lambda t})$$

Suppose we attempt to plot a curve of the decay of a radionuclide which decays at the rate of 50 percent per day. If the initial number of radioactive atoms is plotted on the vertical axis (ordinate), and time on the horizontal axis (abscissa), the resulting curve is that depicted in Figure 11.05. Note that the curve is not a straight line, but becomes less steep with the passing of equal intervals of time. If extremely short time intervals are selected for the measurement of the number of radioactive atoms

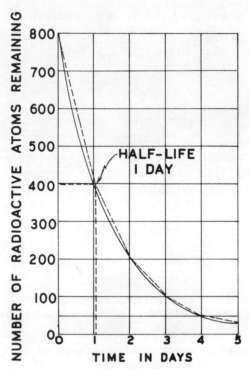

FIGURE 11.05. Decay curve of a hypothetical radionuclide. The dotted curve represents the daily fractional decay. The solid smooth curve follows the instantaneous rate of decay.

remaining, the curve becomes smooth, as shown in the same figure. Comparing the two graphs, we observe that even though the number of atoms remaining at the end of a relatively long interval of time, such as one day, is the same with both graphs, the number at some particular instant during this interval is less on the smooth curve. The reason for this lies in the very nature of the equation (8) which is known as an *exponential equation,* expressing the rate of decay per infinitesimal interval of time.

As we have already pointed out in Chapter 1, the plot of the decay process on ordinary graph paper is based on simple arithmetic intervals along both the vertical and horizontal axes. In other words, with equal intervals of time, although the *same fractional decrease* occurs in the number of radioactive atoms, the actual *number* of such atoms breaking down becomes less and less with the passing of time. Thus, in Figure 11.05 if we start with 800 atoms of a radionuclide having a half-life of 1 day, during the first day the number of atoms decreases 50 percent, from 800 to 400, a difference of $800 - 400 = 400$. During the second day, the number of atoms decreases from 400 to 200, a difference of 200. During the third day, the difference is $200 - 100 = 100$. In summary, then, there has been a numerical decrease from day to day as follows:

first day   400 radioactive atoms have decayed
second day   200 radioactive atoms have decayed
third day   100 radioactive atoms have decayed
etc.

If, instead of using ordinary graph paper, we select semilog graph paper in which the vertical axis is so scaled that each successive equal interval (beginning at the origin) represents the same *fraction* of the interval just above while the horizontal axis is laid off in numerically equal intervals, the resulting curve will be a straight line, as shown in Figure 11.06. There the lowest vertical division is 100 and the next above is 200; 100 is one half of 200. The next division is 200 and again, 200 is one-half of the one above, 400. Thus, the vertical divisions are numbered in geometric progression even though they are represented by equal distances on the axis, whereas the horizontal divisions are in ordinary simple arithmetic progression. Such a plot is called *semilogarithmic* or *log-linear*. A curve which appears as a straight line on a semilogarithmic plot is called an *exponential* or "dying away" curve. Note that the same general type of curve applies to the absorption of photons in matter, and to the fractional survival of cells in a culture subjected to irradiation.

Because decay is a random process, a tremendous number of radioactive atoms must be present for the decay equation to have statistical validity. This requirement is fulfilled under ordinary conditions.

Half-life. A very convenient concept, both in physics and in radiation therapy, is the *half-life* of a radionuclide. It may be defined as the *time required for one-half the atoms in a given quantity of a radionuclide to de-excite* (undergo transformation or "dis-

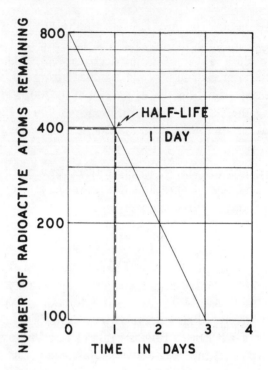

FIGURE 11.06. Decay curve of the same radionuclide as in Figure 11.07, plotted on semilogarithmic graph paper. Note that the curve now appears as a straight line.

integrate"). Thus, it is the time during which the *activity* (e.g. number of nuclear de-excitations/sec) of a radioactive sample decreases 50 percent. The half-life can be found by the use of the decay curve (see Figs. 11.05, 11.06 and 11.07). Select the point on the vertical axis representing one-half the initial activity. From this point, move horizontally to the curve, then down to the horizontal axis where the point of intersection corresponds to the half-life of the radionuclide. In Figure 11.07 the decay curve for radon shows its half-life to be about 3.8 days.

There is an interesting relationship between the half-life of a radionuclide and its decay constant λ. This is to be expected, for the greater the decay constant (i.e. the faster the decay rate) the shorter the half-life (i.e. the less time it takes for the activity to decrease 50 percent). In the equation for radioactive decay:

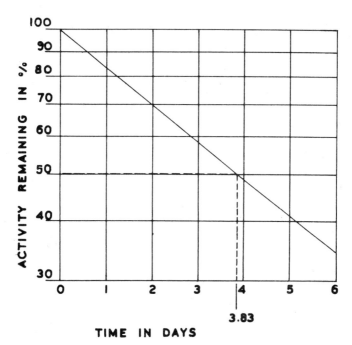

FIGURE 11.07. Decay curve of radon, semilogarithmic plot. The half-life is 3.83 days.

$$A = A_0 e^{-\lambda t}$$

let $A = A_0/2$ at time T where T is the half-life. Substituting,

$$\frac{A_0}{2} = A_0 e^{-\lambda T}$$

Dividing both terms of the equation by A_0:

$$\tfrac{1}{2} = e^{-\lambda T}$$

From the table for exponential functions (see Table 4.02), when $e^{-\lambda T} = \tfrac{1}{2}$,

$$\lambda T = 0.693$$

and

$$T = \frac{0.693}{\lambda} \tag{10}$$

Thus, if the half-life T is known, the decay constant λ can be found simply by dividing 0.693 by the half-life. (Note the similarity of this relation to that for HVL in terms of linear attenuation coefficient for a monoenergetic photon beam.)

We have mentioned that the decay constant is typical of a given radionuclide. From the preceding discussion, it is evident that the half-life, too, must be characteristic of any one nuclide because it is inversely proportional to the decay constant. If the half-life of an unknown radionuclide is determined, it can usually be used to identify the nuclide. Furthermore, the half-life of a particular radionuclide is constant, so a radioactive nuclide that is part of a chemical compound behaves exactly as the same quantity of the pure radionuclide (with rare exceptions).

By application of the principles of exponential decay, we can easily find the half-life and decay constant of any radionuclide. Since the semilogarithmic plot of the decay process is always a straight line, one need only determine two points (three for greater accuracy) to obtain the decay curve. Suppose we have a radioactive sample which measurement shows to have an activity of 100 units at a given instant (the unit of radioactivity will be taken up below). At the end of exactly twenty-four hours, the sample is again evaluated and found to have an activity of 83.4 units. At the end of another twenty-four hours, the activity has decreased to 69.6 units. Note that in each instance we are concerned with the amount of radioactivity **remaining**. These data are then plotted on semilog paper and a straight line drawn through the three points. The half-life may now be obtained by finding the time corresponding to 50 units, that is, half the original number of units (see Fig. 11.07). This is 3.83 days—radon. From this, the decay constant may be found by equation (10): $0.693/3.83 = 0.181$ per day.

Average Life. Since a given "population" of radioactive atoms behaves as a population of human beings in that there is a certain death rate (decay rate), we may conclude that there is also an average survival time of the atoms in a radioactive sample. In other words, what is the life expectancy of any particular atom in the sample? The rigorous mathematical derivation of average life requires the application of calculus. However, we can approximate this by the use of arithmetic to explain the meaning of average life. Suppose our radionuclide sample has a decay rate of 0.5 per day, and that we start with 1,000 atoms at time zero. Table 11.03 shows the arithmetic method of computing average

TABLE 11.03
ARITHMETIC METHOD OF DETERMINING THE AVERAGE LIFE OF
A RADIONUCLIDE. THE DECAY CONSTANT IS 0.5 PER DAY.

Time	No. of Atoms Remaining at Time t	Life of Atoms From 0 Time to Time t		
Days		Atom-Days		
0	1000	—		
1	500	500 ×	1 =	500
2	250	250 ×	2 =	500
3	125	125 ×	3 =	375
4	63	63 ×	4 =	252
5	31	31 ×	5 =	155
6	16	16 ×	6 =	96
7	8	8 ×	7 =	56
8	4	4 ×	8 =	32
9	2	2 ×	9 =	18
10	1	1 ×	10 =	10
		1000) 2000 atom-days		
		2 days, average life		

life. By dividing the ultimate number of atom-days by the number of atoms originally present, we obtain the average life, or life expectancy, in this case $2,000/1,000 = 2$ days. But the problem stated the decay constant to be 0.5. Therefore, it turns out that the average life is the reciprocal of the decay constant ($2 = 1/0.5$), a relationship which may be generalized algebraically as follows:

$$T_a = \frac{1}{\lambda} \tag{11}$$

where T_a is the average life, and λ is the decay constant.

Since we have already seen that $\lambda = 0.693/T$ (from equation 10), substituting this value of λ in equation (11),

$$T_a = \frac{1}{0.693/T}$$

$$T_a = \frac{T}{0.693} = 1.44T \tag{12}$$

Thus, if we know the half-life of a radionuclide, we can compute its average life by simply dividing by 0.693, or multiplying by 1.44.

For example, the half-life of radon is 3.83 days. Its average life is therefore $3.83/0.693 = 5.52$ days.

The Unit of Radioactivity. Thus far, we have been considering the various characteristics of the radioactive decay process. We must now turn to the *unit* in which *activity* is measured. This unit is the *curie* (Ci), defined as an activity of *3.7×10^{10} de-excitations per second.* In ordinary parlance, 1 Ci of a radionuclide is the amount decaying at the rate of 3.7×10^{10} atoms per second.

We shall now review the derivation of the Ci. To find the number of atoms of a particular radionuclide sample decaying in one second, usually abbreviated d/s, we must multiply the number of atoms present, N, by the fraction decaying per second,

$$d/s = N\lambda \tag{13}$$

According to the original definition of the Ci, it was the amount of radon in equilibrium with 1 gram of radium. Since this was formerly taken to represent 3.7×10^{10} d/s, the same unit was extended to include all radioactive nuclides. Although recent experiments have shown that 1 g of radium (Ra) undergoes fewer than 3.7×10^{10} d/s, the deviation is slight and will be neglected in this discussion. Let us first determine the number of atoms in 1 g Ra. We know that 1 gram-atomic weight of Ra is 226 g and that 1 gram-atom of any element contains 6.02×10^{23} atoms (Avogadro's number).

$$226 \text{ g Ra} = 1 \text{ gram-atom Ra}$$

Since 226 g Ra contains 6.02×10^{23} atoms Ra

$$1 \text{ g Ra contains } \frac{6.02 \times 10^{23}}{226} = 2.66 \times 10^{21} \text{ atoms}$$

or N in equation (13) $= 2.66 \times 10^{21}$ atoms

Since λ for Ra is about 1.38×10^{-11}/sec,

$$d/s \text{ for 1 g Ra} = N\lambda$$

$$= 2.66 \times 10^{21} \times 1.38 \times 10^{-11}$$

$$= 3.7 \times 10^{10} \text{ d/s}$$

Thus, 1 Ci, the activity of about 1 g Ra, always represents 3.7×10^{10} de-excitations/sec. The same unit may be employed for all radionuclides, both natural and artificial. In practice, it is often more convenient to use a smaller unit, the ***millicurie***, representing 3.7×10^7 d/s:

$$1 \text{ millicurie (mCi)} = 0.001 \text{ curie (Ci)}$$

It is obvious that 1 Ci of a rapidly decaying (high λ) radionuclide requires the presence of a smaller total number of atoms than of a slowly decaying one. As an example, let us compare Ra with radon (Rn). As just noted, 1 Ci specifies the activity of about 1 g Ra. How many grams of Rn have an activity of 1 Ci? First we must find the number of Rn atoms that must be present, of which 3.7×10^{10} will de-excite per sec. Let this number be N. Then

$$N\lambda = 3.7 \times 10^{10} \text{ d/s}$$

$$N = \frac{3.7 \times 10^{10}}{\lambda}$$

Since λ for Rn is 2.09×10^{-6} d/s,

$$N = \frac{3.7 \times 10^{10}}{2.09 \times 10^{-6}} = 1.77 \times 10^{16} \text{ atoms}$$

We must now find the mass of 1.77×10^{16} atoms of Rn. Since

$$1 \text{ gram-atom Rn} = 222 \text{ g}$$

and

$$1 \text{ gram-atom Rn contains } 6.02 \times 10^{23} \text{ atoms}$$

Therefore,

$$222 \text{ g Rn contains } 6.02 \times 10^{23} \text{ atoms}$$

$$1 \text{ atom of Rn weighs } 222/(6.02 \times 10^{23}) \text{ g}$$

The mass of 1.77×10^{16} Rn atoms is

$$1.77 \times 10^{16} \times \frac{222}{6.02 \times 10^{23}} = 6.5 \times 10^{-6} \text{ g}$$

Thus, 6.5 millionths of a gram (or 6.5 micrograms) of Rn has the same activity as about 1 gram of Ra—1 curie.

Because equal masses of different radioactive nuclides show different degrees of activity, there has been introduced the term *specific activity*, defined as the number of de-excitations per second per gram (d/s/g) of the radioactive nuclide. Specific activity is more often expressed in Ci/g. Accordingly,

$$\text{specific activity of radium} = 3.7 \times 10^{10} \text{ d/s/g} = 1 \text{ Ci/g}$$

$$\text{specific activity of radon} = \frac{N\lambda}{g}$$

where N/g is the number of radon atoms per gram.

$$\frac{N}{g} = \frac{6.02 \times 10^{23}}{222} = 2.71 \times 10^{21} \text{ atoms Rn/g}$$

Since λ for radon is 2.09×10^{-6} d/s,

$$\text{specific activity of Rn} = 2.71 \times 10^{21} \times 2.09 \times 10^{-6}$$

$$= 5.7 \times 10^{15} \text{ d/s/g}$$

or,

$$\text{specific activity of Rn} = \frac{5.7 \times 10^{15}}{3.7 \times 10^{10}} = 1.5 \times 10^5 \text{ Ci/g}$$

Table 11.04 compares some important constants of Ra and Rn. Note particularly the tremendous difference in the specific activities of these related radionuclides.

Specific Gamma-ray Constant Γ. A standard geometric setup is required for accurate measurement of the exposure rate of any particular γ-emitting radionuclide. Not only does this provide a sound basis for computing tissue doses in radiotherapy, but it

TABLE 11.04
COMPARISON OF CONSTANTS FOR RADIUM AND RADON

	Decay Constant (λ)	Half Life	Specific Activity	
	per sec	*days*	*d/s/g*	*Ci/g*
Radium	1.38×10^{-11}	5.84×10^5	3.7×10^{10}	1
Radon	2.09×10^{-6}	3.83	5.6×10^{15}	1.5×10^5

also allows precise intercomparison of various radionuclide substitutes for Ra (see pages 457 to 461). Unfortunately, there is some uncertainty as to how currently available exposure rate data have been obtained. In an effort to remedy this situation, the National Council on Radiation Protection and Measurements (NCRP) *Report No. 41* sets forth certain criteria for standardizing such measurements and for detailing specifications of radioactive sources. In particular, encapsulated γ-emitting sources for brachytherapy (i.e., radiotherapy with encapsulated radionuclides at a distance of a few cm by surface, interstitial, or intracavitary application) should be calibrated in terms of the exposure rate at a distance of 1 meter from, and perpendicular to, the long axis of the source at its center. Furthermore, at this distance the source should be essentially a point source, and the detector a point detector. After the exposure rate of any radionuclide has been made in this manner and the conversion ratio determined relative to that of Ra, it is a simple exercise to compute the exposure rate for any convenient distance.

There are two ways to specify the standard exposure rate from discrete radionuclide sources. One is the *specific gamma-ray constant* Γ, which refers to γ-ray emission only. This is usually stated for brachytherapy in terms of R per millicurie-hour at 1 cm. Mathematically, Γ is defined as follows:

$$\Gamma = \frac{R \cdot cm^2}{mCi\text{-}hr} \tag{14}$$

Note the term cm^2, required by the inverse square law. In the case of Ra, peculiarly, Γ pertains to encapsulation by 0.5 mm Pt. Published values of several well-known radionuclides appear in Table 11.05.

TABLE 11.05
SPECIFIC GAMMA-RAY CONSTANT Γ OF SOME IMPORTANT
MEDICAL RADIONUCLIDES*

Radionuclide	Γ
	R/mCi-hr at 1 cm
^{60}Co	13.07
Ra series (0.5 mm Pt filter)	8.25
^{137}Cs	3.2
^{131}I	2.18

* Except for ^{131}I, these data are from *NCRP Report No. 41, April 1974.*

The other method of specification is called the **exposure rate constant;** it includes not only γ radiation, but also characteristic radiation and internal bremsstrahlung with energy above a minimum value. This constant is usually expressed in R per curie-hour at 1 meter, and is less widely used than Γ in radiotherapy.

RADIOACTIVE EQUILIBRIUM

There are two types of radioactive equilibrium, **secular** and **transient.** These will be defined and explained in some detail.

1. **Secular Equilibrium.** If we take a sample of a **long-lived** radioactive element such as Ra and seal it in a leakproof container, we find a gradual accumulation of its descendants which comprise this radioactive series. Eventually (about one month in the case of Ra) the number of atoms of any given member undergoing decay will equal the number of new atoms of that member being formed from its parent, a condition known as **radioactive equilibrium.** For example, in the series

$$Ra \longrightarrow Rn \longrightarrow RaA \longrightarrow RaB \longrightarrow etc.$$

the number of RaA atoms being formed each second by the transformation of Rn, will be equal to the number of RaB atoms being formed per second by the transformation of RaA. This relationship holds for all members of the series. However, each member of the series has a different decay constant. For example, the Ra decay constant is 0.000428 per **year** and the Rn decay constant is 0.181 per **day.** At equilibrium, the number of Rn atoms decaying per second is equal to the number of Rn atoms appearing in the same time interval. Furthermore, the number of atoms of the next member, RaA, appearing in one second will be equal to the number of RaA atoms decaying per second.

Because the parent Ra has such an extremely long half-life, the activity of each of its descendants is nearly constant at equilibrium, at least relative to the human life span. Therefore, this is called **secular equilibrium.**

The concept of radioactive equilibrium may be clarified by a fictitious example presented in Table 11.06. Suppose we start with 1,000,000 radioactive atoms of a nuclide which decays at the con-

TABLE 11.06
HYPOTHETICAL EXAMPLE ILLUSTRATING THE PRINCIPLE OF
RADIOACTIVE EQUILIBRIUM WHEN THE PARENT IS A LONG-LIVED
NUCLIDE. THIS IS THEREFORE THE SECULAR TYPE OF EQUILIBRIUM.
IT IS ASSUMED THAT 10^6 ATOMS ARE PRESENT INITIALLY.
THE VALUES ARE ROUNDED TO THE NEAREST INTEGER.

	Parent A_1 ⟶		Daughter A_2 ⟶		Granddaughter A_3	
	Decay Rate 0.00001 Per Day		Decay Rate 0.5 Per Day		Decay Rate 0.3 Per Day	
	No. of Atoms Present	No. of Atoms Decaying	No. of Atoms Present	No. of Atoms Decaying	No. of Atoms Present	No. of Atoms Decaying
0–1	1,000,000	10	10	5	5	1
1–2	999,990	10	15	7	11	3
2–3	999,980	10	18	9	17	5
3–4	999,970	10	19	9	21	7
4–5	999,960	10	20	10	24	8
5–6	999,950	10	20	10	26	8
6–7	999,940	10	20	10	28	9
7–8	999,930	10	20	10	29	9
8–9	999,920	10	20	10	30	10
9–10	999,910	10	20	10	30	10

stant rate of 0.00001 per day, its daughter nuclide decays at the rate of 0.5 per day, and the next nuclide in the series decays at the rate of 0.3 per day. Table 11.06 shows that nuclides A_1 and A_2 reach equilibrium with each other on the sixth day and these attain equilibrium with A_3 on the tenth day. From the tenth day all three will remain in equilibrium, the same number of atoms, 10, of each member of the series decaying and forming every day until the parent element becomes depleted. The table also shows that the equilibrium amounts of each member of the series are different when radioactive equilibrium is established; thus, the equilibrium amount of A_2 is 20 atoms, while the corresponding equilibrium amount of A_3 is 30 atoms. Furthermore, it may be noted that element A_2, with the ***more rapid rate of decay***, is present in ***smaller quantity*** at equilibrium, than is element A_3 with slower decay rate.

The concept of secular radioactive equilibrium may also be shown by simple algebra. The number of atoms de-exciting per sec is equal to the number of atoms N present at the start, times the fraction λ de-exciting per sec,

$$d/s = N\lambda$$

In a radioactive series at equilibrium the number of atoms de-exciting per sec will be equal for all members of the series except for the final stable product. In other words, *$N\lambda$ will be the same for all members of the series:*

$$N_0\lambda_0 = N_1\lambda_1 = N_2\lambda_2 = N_3\lambda_3 = \ldots N_n\lambda_n$$

where each term represents the d/s of a member of the series. Taking any two intermediate members,

$$N_1\lambda_1 = N_2\lambda_2 \tag{15}$$

or,

$$\frac{N_1}{N_2} = \frac{\lambda_2}{\lambda_1} \tag{16}$$

Since λ_1 and λ_2 are both constants,

$$\frac{N_1}{N_2} = a\ constant \tag{17}$$

signifying that at equilibrium there is a constant ratio of the number of atoms of any two intermediate members of the series.

Equation (16) also states that the *equilibrium amounts of two radionuclides are inversely proportional to their decay constants;* that is, the more rapid the decay, the smaller the number of atoms of that nuclide at equilibrium.

Returning to equation (16), we can derive another useful relationship. We have already found that

$$\lambda = \frac{0.693}{T}$$

where T is the half-life. Therefore, λ is inversely proportional to T. Substituting $1/T$ for λ in equation (16):

$$\frac{N_1}{T_1} = \frac{N_2}{T_2}$$

$$\frac{N_1}{N_2} = \frac{T_1}{T_2} \tag{18}$$

Thus, the **equilibrium amounts of radionuclides are directly proportional to their half-lives,** or in other words, the longer the half-life the larger the equilibrium amount. Applying this to the Ra series, we note that Rn has a half-life of 3.83 days and RaC a half-life of 19.7 or roughly 20 minutes. Since 3.83 days are equivalent to about 5,500 minutes,

$$\frac{N_{Rn}}{N_{RaC}} = \frac{5,500}{20} = 275$$

which means that at equilibrium there are 275 times as many Rn atoms as there are RaC atoms.

We have thus far considered only the relative amounts of the various intermediate members of a radioactive series at equilibrium. What determines the actual **amount** of each? This obviously depends on the quantity of the parent radionuclide present, since the same fractional decay yields more product atoms when a larger number of parent atoms are present at the start. Therefore, when the parent atoms decay to half their initial quantity, the maximum amount of each daughter nuclide will decrease to one-half its initial equilibrium quantity. This leads to the important result that the **half-life of a radioactive series as a whole is the same as that of the parent element, provided the latter is sealed and has a longer half-life than any of its daughters.** For example, if we start with a sealed Rn tube, equilibrium is reached in a few hours; and even though we may be interested in the RaC for its γ rays, and even though the half life of RaC itself is 19.7 minutes, as long as it is in radioactive equilibrium in a sealed container, its effective half-life is the same as that of radon, 3.83 days.

In general, if the completely sealed parent radionuclide has a **long** half-life relative to its descendants as, for example, Ra, the activity of the radioactive source remains almost constant for practical purposes and we have a condition of **secular equilibrium,** that is, the equilibrium amounts of the daughter nuclides remain essentially constant during a human generation.

b. **Transient Equilibrium.** If a parent radionuclide such as radon, having a relatively **short** half-life, is sealed in a cell, maximum activity is reached in a few hours. Beyond this point the equilibrium amounts decrease at the same rate as the parent Rn because no additional Rn is being added. At equilibrium,

$$N_{Rn}\lambda_{Rn} = N_{RaA}\lambda_{RaA} \qquad (19)$$

In 3.83 days, N_{Rn} will have decreased by $\frac{1}{2}$. Therefore, $N_{Rn}\lambda_{Rn}$ or

TABLE 11.07

HYPOTHETICAL EXAMPLE OF TRANSIENT RADIOACTIVE EQUILIBRIUM ASSOCIATED WITH A SHORT-LIVED PARENT ELEMENT. IT IS ASSUMED THAT 10^6 ATOMS ARE PRESENT AT THE START. SIMILAR EQUILIBRIUM IS ESTABLISHED WITH FURTHER DESCENDANTS IN THE SERIES, BUT THESE ARE OMITTED FOR THE SAKE OF SIMPLICITY. THE VALUES SHOWN ARE ROUNDED TO THREE FIGURES.

| | Parent A_1 $\longrightarrow$ | | Daughter A_2 | |
| | Decay Rate 0.2 Per Day | | Decay Rate 0.99 Per Day | |
Day	No. of Atoms Present	No. of Atoms Decaying	No. of Atoms Present	No. of Atoms Decaying
0– 1	1,000,000	200,000	200,000	198,000
1– 2	800,000	160,000	162,000	160,000
2– 3	640,000	128,000	130,000	128,000
3– 4	512,000	102,000	103,000	102,000
4– 5	410,000	82,000	83,000	82,200
5– 6	328,000	65,600	66,400	65,800
6– 7	262,000	52,400	53,000	52,600
7– 8	210,000	42,000	42,500	42,100
8– 9	168,000	33,600	34,000	33,700
9–10	134,000	26,800	27,100	26,900
10–11	107,000	21,400	21,700	21,600
11–12	85,600	17,100	17,300	17,100
12–13	68,500	13,700	13,900	13,700
13–14	54,800	10,960	11,100	11,000
14–15	43,800	8,760	8,870	8,780
15–16	35,000	7,000	7,090	7,020
16–17	28,000	5,600	5,670	5,600
17–18	22,400	4,480	4,540	4,490
18–19	17,900	3,580	3,620	3,590
19–20	14,300	2,860	2,900	2,870
20–21	11,400	2,280	2,310	2,290
21–22	9,120	1,820	1,840	1,830
22–23	7,300	1,460	1,480	1,460
23–24	5,840	1,170	1,190	1,170
24–25	4,670	930	942	933
25–26	3,740	750	759	751
26–27	2,990	598	606	600
27–28	2,390	478	484	479
28–29	1,910	382	387	383
29–30	1,530	306	310	307
30–31	1,220	244	247	245
31–32	976	195	197	195
32–33	781	156	158	156
33–34	625	125	127	125
34–35	500	100	101	100
35–36	400	80	81	80
36–37	320	64	65	64

the **number** of de-excitations of radon per sec will have decreased $\frac{1}{2}$. According to equation (19), $N_{RaA}\lambda_{RaA}$ or the number of de-excitations of RaA per sec will also decrease by $\frac{1}{2}$. Thus, although equilibrium is maintained, it is **transitory** because the actual number of de-excitations per sec is decreasing according to the decay rate of Rn. Table 11.07 illustrates the principle of **transient equilibrium** based on a hypothetical example.

The practical result of the preceding discussion is as follows: the activity of a freshly separated sample of Rn increases to a maximum in about 5 hours. Beyond this time, it decreases at a constant rate of 16.5 percent per day; and at the end of about one month, decay has progressed to the point where residual activity approaches zero. This principle applies only if Rn is separated from Ra and sealed, as in a gold implant. It explains why Rn can be used in nonremovable implants; the dose is precalculated and practically all of its activity will have been lost in one month.

On the other hand, if we start with Ra sealed in a needle so that it remains accessible to its daughter elements, the γ-ray activity increases for 35 days, then becomes constant because secular equilibrium has been reached. Figure 11.08 shows the comparison between sealed Ra and Rn sources.

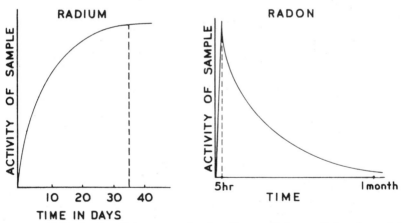

FIGURE 11.08. At the left is a curve showing the growth in γ activity of a sealed *radium* source as it reaches equilibrium with its decay products. The maximum activity is reached on the 35th day, and then declines slowly with the decay rate of Ra. At the right is a curve representing the γ activity of a sealed *radon* source, separated from its parent Ra. It reaches a maximum in about 5 hours, then decreases at the decay rate of Rn, becoming negligible in about 1 month.

Of great practical importance in nuclear medicine at the present time is the production of technetium 99m (^{99m}Tc) with a half-life of 6 hours, from the decay of molybdenum 99 (^{99}Mo) with a half-life of 66 hours, in the so-called "technetium cow." This is an excellent example of *transient equilibrium.* As the ^{99}Mo decays, ^{99m}Tc grows and reaches maximum activity in about 22 hours. Thereafter the parent and daughter (i.e. ^{99}Mo and ^{99m}Tc) in transient equilibrium decay along parallel curves as shown in Figure 11.09, with the same apparent half-life as the parent. Note that the activity of the ^{99m}Tc at any instant after transient equi-

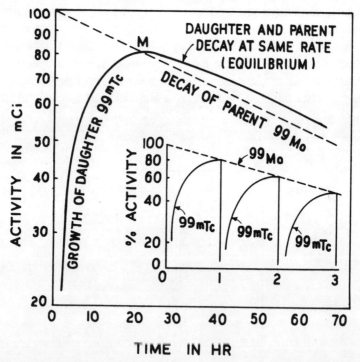

FIGURE 11.09. Transient equilibrium during the decay of molybdenum 99 (^{99}Mo) to ^{99m}Tc. Shown here are the growth curves of the daughter ^{99m}Tc and the decay of the initially pure ^{99}Mo. After the maximum activity of the parent ^{99}Mo becomes equal to that of the daughter ^{99m}Tc, both decay at the same rate—a condition of *transient equilibrium.* The inset shows how the curves are modified by daily milking of the ^{99}Mo "cow." (After H. E. Johns, and J. R. Cunningham, *The Physics of Radiology* [Springfield, Thomas, 1969].)

librium has been reached is slightly less than that of ^{99}Mo because about 14 percent of the latter decays directly to stable ^{99}Tc.

NUCLEAR REACTOR

If any single event may be credited with heralding the age of atomic energy, it is the discovery of the neutron by Chadwick in 1932. Although regarded at first as simply another nuclear particle, the neutron, as a powerful device for inducing nuclear reactions, has become the key to the tremendous energy locked in the atomic nucleus. This has brought about the atom bomb and the nuclear reactor.

Neutron Physics. Soon after its discovery, the neutron was found to be a particularly suitable projectile for bombarding atomic nuclei. Because of the absence of an electric charge on the neutron, it can readily enter a nucleus, inducing a reaction which depends on the atomic number of the nucleus and the kinetic energy of the neutron. In general, there is an arbitrary division of neutrons into four main categories, based on their kinetic energy:

fast neutrons—energy greater than 100 keV
intermediate —energy 100 eV to 100 keV
slow   energy 0.025 eV to 100 eV
thermal   energy about 0.025 eV

Thermal neutrons are often referred to as slow neutrons.

Slow-Neutron Reactions. The slowest neutrons are called *thermal neutrons* because their average kinetic energy is similar to that of gas molecules at ordinary temperatures. A slow neutron easily enters a nucleus; in fact, upon approaching a nucleus, a slow neutron is actually attracted by short range forces. Four different types of reactions may ensue. The first three have already been described on pages 347 to 349; they include radiative capture, proton emission, and α-particle emission. The fourth is *fission*, the splitting of certain heavy nuclei; it will be explained later on pages 377 to 381.

Fast-neutron Reactions. When *fast neutrons* with energy in excess of about 100 keV enter certain nuclei the resulting compound nucleus is endowed with a superabundance of energy. A sequence of events then takes place depending on the energy of the neutron and the atomic number of the target nucleus. Four principal types of reactions are initiated by fast neutrons.

1. *Elastic Scattering.* Moderately fast neutrons with energy appreciably less than 100 keV are unable to excite the nuclei of target atoms. Such neutrons bounce off the nuclei without loss of energy. This is analogous to the elastic collision between billiard balls. Elastic scattering is the most common type of interaction of moderately fast neutrons with matter.

2. *Inelastic Scattering.* The faster neutrons possess enough energy to excite the nuclei of many of the heavier atoms, about 100 keV or more being sufficient in most cases. Under these conditions, the scattered neutron has less kinetic energy after the collision, some of its energy having been expended in exciting the nucleus which then returns to zero energy state by emitting a γ ray.

3. *Transmutation Reaction.* When certain target nuclei are exposed to fast neutrons, the compound nucleus emits a proton in the first stage of its decay; in other instances, the compound nucleus emits an α particle. In either case, the neutron enters the nucleus, and a charged particle is expelled. Examples of the transmutation reaction follow:

$$\underset{16}{\overset{32}{}}S + \underset{0}{\overset{1}{}}n \ldots \rightarrow \quad [\underset{16}{\overset{33}{}}S] \quad \ldots \rightarrow \quad \underset{15}{\overset{32}{}}P \quad + \underset{1}{\overset{1}{}}H \; [(n,p) \text{ reaction}]$$

$$\begin{array}{cc} \textit{compound} & \textit{radio-} \\ \textit{nucleus} & \textit{phosphorus} \end{array}$$

$$\underset{20}{\overset{40}{}}Ca + \underset{0}{\overset{1}{}}n \ldots \rightarrow \quad [\underset{20}{\overset{41}{}}Ca] \quad \ldots \rightarrow \underset{18}{\overset{37}{}}Ar + \underset{2}{\overset{4}{}}He \; [(n,\alpha) \text{ reaction}]$$

$$\begin{array}{c} \textit{compound} \\ \textit{nucleus} \end{array}$$

4. *(n,2n) reaction.* When extremely high energy neutrons, 10 MeV or more, enter certain nuclei, the compound nucleus decays by the emission of two neutrons. There are many examples of this reaction, one being:

$$\underset{6}{\overset{12}{}}C + \underset{0}{\overset{1}{}}n \longrightarrow \underset{6}{\overset{11}{}}C + \underset{0}{\overset{1}{}}n + \underset{0}{\overset{1}{}}n$$

The product atom decays to stable boron by emitting a positron $_{+1}^{0}e$:

$$_{6}^{11}C \longrightarrow {} _{+1}^{0}e + {} _{5}^{11}B + v$$

The Fission Process. Up to this point we have been considering the type of reaction in which, after bombardment by neutrons, the target nuclei emit charged particles, neutrons, or γ rays. However, a remarkably different reaction was observed in 1934 by E. Fermi upon exposing uranium to slow neutrons. He thought he had produced elements of higher atomic number than uranium —the so-called *transuranic* elements. Yet, there were certain discrepancies in the results, unexplained by this assumption. Shortly thereafter, I. Noddack suggested an alternative explanation, namely, that the uranium, after exposure to neutrons, splits into several large fragments. For five years physicists sought the correct interpretation of Fermi's results, apparently having overlooked Noddack's publication. Finally, in 1939, O. Hahn and F. Strassman isolated atoms of intermediate atomic number among the products resulting from the slow bombardment of uranium. They found that when uranium, the last element in the periodic table, is subjected to *slow (thermal) neutrons,* a variety of γ-emitting radioactive nuclides is obtained. While these have a much smaller atomic number than uranium, the some 200 products of ^{235}U fission range in mass number from 72 to 160. These occur in two main groups: a "light" group (A = 85 to 104) and a "heavy" group (A = 130 to 149). Thus, the products of this type of reaction consist of atomic nuclei of intermediate mass, whereas the previously known nuclear reactions yield charged particles, neutrons, or γ rays and a product nucleus having an atomic number only slightly different from its parent atom.

L. Meitner and O. R. Frisch explained this new reaction in 1939 in the same manner as Noddack five years earlier: the uranium atom, after acquiring a low energy neutron, *splits* into two or more fragments. This process, called *fission, may be defined as the splitting of a heavy nucleus into two or more nuclei of intermediate atomic number.* On computing the total mass of the uranium atom plus the entering neutron, Meitner found it to exceed the sum of the masses of the product atoms and emitted neutrons; thus, there was a **mass deficit.** Using Einstein's equation for the equivalence of mass and energy, $E = mc^2$, she calculated that the "lost" mass was equivalent to a tremendous quantity of energy liberated per fission—about 200 MeV in the case of uranium 235 (^{235}U):

$$\frac{mass\ of}{uranium\ 235} + {}_0^1n = \frac{sum\ of\ masses}{of\ fission\ products} + 200\ MeV$$

The 200 MeV represents kinetic energy imparted to the **fission products** or **fragments,** heat, and emitted γ rays.

Note that **fissionable nuclei** invariably have a **high atomic number** and a **high mass number,** with the latter on the high side of the curve representing nuclear binding energy per nucleon.

The mechanism of nuclear splitting was explained by N. Bohr by analogy with a water droplet. The nucleus is maintained normally in a spherical form (similar to a drop of water) by the force of nuclear "surface tension." When a slow neutron enters the ^{235}U nucleus, a large amount of energy, approximately 6.5 MeV, is gained by the nucleus. This causes a deforming force, inducing oscillations of the nucleus which may at first become elongated and then assume a dumbbell shape, as shown in Figure 11.10. At this point the short range nuclear force becomes inoperative and the positive charges at both ends repel each other with sufficient force to cause the two portions to fly apart. The energy liberated in this disruptive reaction is about 200 MeV per event, as contrasted with a maximum of 10 MeV in ordinary nuclear reactions and 10 eV in a violent chemical reaction such as the explosion of one molecule of TNT.

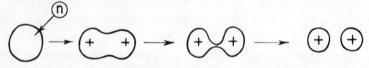

FIGURE 11.10. The water drop analogy in nuclear fission. The process is triggered by the capture of a neutron by a fissionable nucleus which rapidly assumes a dumbbell shape and subdivides into two almost equal fragments.

When this information reached Fermi, he suggested the possibility that since the fission fragments are unstable and carry an excess of neutrons, they may, in turn, liberate neutrons. In other words, for every neutron entering a uranium 235 atom, two or more neutrons plus about 200 MeV are produced. Such a tremendous liberation of energy presents unlimited potentialities for tapping atomic energy. This process, called a ***chain reaction***, is shown in Figure 11.11. Suppose one thermal neutron enters a ^{235}U nucleus and causes fission, during which one to three neutrons are liberated. These neutrons can enter other ^{235}U atoms, giving rise to three to nine more neutrons which, in turn, can produce fission in other ^{235}U atoms with liberation of still more neutrons until insufficient ^{235}U remains to continue the reaction. Thus, the original neutron which started the chain reaction behaved as a

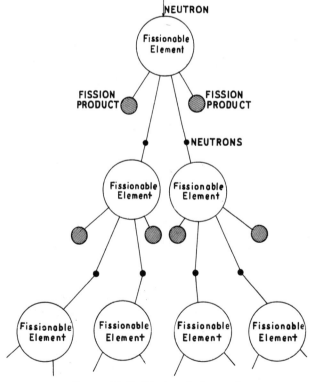

FIGURE 11.11. Nuclear chain reaction.

low energy trigger to set in motion the whole process of neutron and high energy release.

The following equation exemplifies the fission process with ^{235}U, although a great variety of daughter nuclides of intermediate mass number may be produced:

$$^{235}_{92}U + ^{1}_{0}n \rightarrow [^{236}_{92}U] \rightarrow ^{141}_{56}Ba + ^{92}_{36}Kr + 3^{1}_{0}n + 200 \text{ MeV}$$

Let us now review the energy exchange in the fission process. The thermal neutron entering the ^{235}U nucleus has a low kinetic energy of about 0.025 eV. This releases energy of about 200 MeV, a multiplication of energy by a factor of several billion in only one fission. Since the number of fissions in a chain reaction increases by geometric progression the multiplication of energy soon becomes astronomical. Furthermore, due to the extreme rapidity of the fission process, the tremendous release of energy occurs in about one millionth of a second. This, then, explains the devastating explosive power of the atom bomb.

Uranium Isotopes and Fission. Uranium consists of three natural isotopes—^{234}U, ^{235}U, and ^{238}U. To understand the operation of a nuclear reactor, we must first appreciate the reactions of two of these—^{235}U and ^{238}U—with neutrons. The probability of capture of a neutron by any nucleus is called its *cross section;* this is measured in units called *barns,* one barn being 10^{-24} cm^2 per nucleus. The barn is about the same size as the physical area of the average nucleus; however, it must be emphasized that the nuclear cross section in the above sense depends on the *energy of the incident neutron,* the *type of reaction,* and the *nature of the target element.* Thus, when the probability of a given nuclear reaction is high, it is said to have a large capture cross section; and when it is low, it has a small cross section. On this basis, ^{235}U *fission* has a large nuclear cross section for 0.025-eV slow neutrons, but a smaller cross section for fast neutrons. A *slow* neutron entering a ^{235}U nucleus releases 1 to 3 (average 2.3) neutrons per fission, therefore making possible a chain reaction. More than 99 percent of the neutrons are emitted instantaneously as *prompt neutrons,* while less than 1 percent appear later as *delayed neutrons.*

On the other hand, ^{238}U is fissionable only by *fast* neutrons having a relatively high energy of at least 1 MeV. However, the main neutron reaction of ^{238}U is the *nonfission* capture of intermediate neutrons, although even slow neutrons of the order of 0.025 eV may be captured; in both cases, the *transuranic element neptunium,* $^{239}_{93}Np$, is produced. This, in turn, decays by β^- emission to *plutonium,* $^{239}_{94}Pu$:

$$^{238}_{92}U + ^1_0n \underset{slow}{\longrightarrow} [^{239}_{92}U] \longrightarrow _{-1}^{0}\beta + ^{239}_{93}Np \longrightarrow _{-1}^{0}\beta + ^{239}_{94}Pu$$

The Graphite-Moderated Nuclear Reactor. As already noted, more than one neutron is liberated per fission of uranium, making possible a chain reaction with sustained release of nuclear energy. However, a certain minimum mass of uranium is required for a sustained reaction. Since ^{235}U is readily fissioned by thermal neutrons, it should be an excellent source of nuclear energy. Suppose we have a given minute mass of ^{235}U. A thermal (0.025 eV) neutron entering this mass causes fission of one atom. Since the selected mass of ^{235}U is so small, one or more of the neutrons produced during fission may escape before entering other ^{235}U atoms, so that no chain reaction occurs. If larger and larger pieces of ^{235}U are selected, the volume increases relative to the surface area and, at the same time, the rate of neutron production increases relative to the rate of neutron escape through the surface. *The minimum mass, such that the rate of neutron production just equals the rate of loss by escape is called the critical mass.* A mass smaller than this is *subcritical,* and a mass larger than the critical mass is *supercritical.* A supercritical mass of fissionable material goes out of control because the rate of formation of neutrons exceeds the rate of escape. Note that critical mass is not a fixed quantity, but depends on such factors as the nature and purity of the fissionable material, its geometric shape, and the energy of the neutrons.

The critical mass of ^{235}U is a sphere measuring nearly 10 cm in diameter. However, only about 0.07 percent (one part in 140) of naturally occurring uranium is ^{235}U, so it must be separated from the much larger amount of ^{238}U if a sufficient mass of pure

^{235}U is to be obtained. Since it is impossible to separate these isotopes chemically, various complicated processes such as electro-magnetic separation, thermal diffusion, gaseous diffusion, and other physical methods must be employed.

Sufficient ^{235}U was obtained to permit the manufacture of the first atom bomb. The principle of this device involves taking two masses of ^{235}U, each of which is below the critical mass, and suddenly combining them into a supercritical mass. This immediately initiates a chain reaction which releases a tremendous amount of energy in an extremely short interval of time. Actually, the explosion of an atom bomb occurs in about 10^{-6} sec, before all of the material has been fissioned, because it results from the sudden liberation of an immense amount of heat. The type of reaction in an atom bomb is called an **uncontrolled** reaction.

The possibility of devising a **controlled** chain reaction was suggested in 1942 by Fermi, using **natural uranium.** However, he had to contend with the strong affinity of the more abundant ^{238}U for the fast and intermediate neutrons produced in ^{235}U fission, removing them from further reaction with ^{235}U and thereby quenching the chain reaction. To solve this difficulty, Fermi introduced a material of low atomic number with little tendency to capture neutrons, but with the ability to slow them to thermal velocities after only a few collisions. These relatively slow neutrons can then react with ^{235}U nuclei in preference to ^{238}U which does not have a large cross section for slow neutrons. Thus, the trick is to prevent the fast and intermediate neutrons from being captured by ^{238}U by first slowing them sufficiently to cause fission of ^{235}U. Either heavy water or pure carbon (graphite) serves this purpose. Such materials, capable of slowing down neutrons without capturing them, are called **moderators.** Figure 11.12 summarizes the principles involved in the sustained fission process of ^{235}U.

A typical graphite-moderated uranium nuclear reactor is constructed of **graphite** building blocks stacked in layers like bricks (see Fig. 11.13). Each block is perforated to receive slugs of natural uranium or uranium artificially enriched with ^{235}U. The flow of neutrons—**neutron flux,** as it is called—must be controlled because the chain reaction, once initiated, would go on to completion, and the resulting heat would destroy the reactor. For

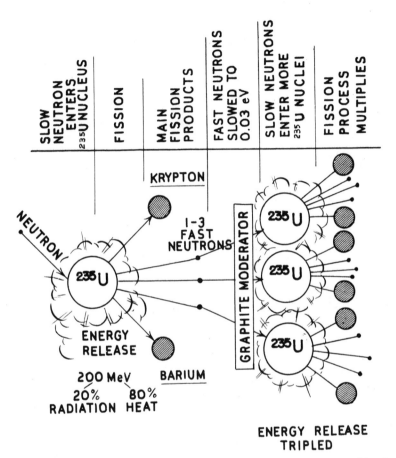

FIGURE 11.12. Fission of uranium 235 by slow (thermal) neutrons, resulting in a nuclear chain reaction.

proper function, the reactor should operate at a steady rate, each fission producing only one new fission. Since each fission normally would produce an average of 2.3 new ones, the process must be slowed down by the removal of excess neutrons through the use of a material which has a large capture cross section for slow neutrons. *Cadmium* and *boron-steel* both meet this requirement and are therefore suitable for controlling the reaction by absorbing excess neutrons. In actual use, the cadmium or boron-steel is fashioned into *control rods* which can be inserted into the reactor the proper depth to maintain a steady rate of fission; the greater

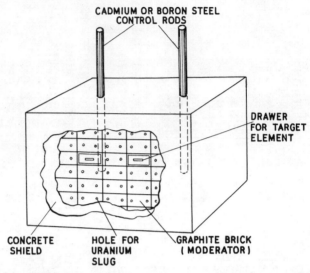

FIGURE 11.13. Simplified diagram of a graphite-moderated nuclear reactor utilizing uranium 235 (^{235}U) as the fuel.

the depth of insertion, the greater the absorption of neutrons and the slower the rate. One may define the ***fission rate*** as the number of fissions per second. This, in turn, depends on the ***multiplication*** or ***reproduction factor***, defined as the ratio of the number of neutrons in any one generation to the number in the generation just preceding it.

During the operation of a nuclear reactor, an atmospheric thermal neutron drifts into a uranium slug and selectively enters a ^{235}U atom, inducing fission. The emitted fast neutrons then pass into the graphite moderator and are slowed to thermal energy, whereupon they are capable of causing fission of other ^{235}U atoms. The chain reaction is regulated by adjusting the depth of the control rods. Thus, the amount of ^{235}U gradually decreases while the lighter fission products accumulate. Since these may capture neutrons, they impair the efficiency of operation of the reactor—they are said to poison the reactor. Furthermore, a great deal of heat is produced as ^{235}U and a small amount of ^{238}U are converted to fission products, and ^{238}U is gradually changed to [^{239}U]. As already indicated, [^{239}U] gives rise to neptunium and plutonium, the latter being fissionable by slow neutrons. Since it can readily be separated chemically from uranium, plutonium furnishes abundant fissionable material for use in special plutonium reactors for military purposes in the manufacture of bombs, and in fast power reactors.

An important factor in the control of the chain reaction is the presence of ***delayed neutrons*** arising during fission. These slow the buildup of neutron flux just enough to permit manual or automatic control of the reaction velocity by means of the control rods. Otherwise, the growth of neutron flux might destroy the reactor before the control rods could be inserted.

There is a certain minimum size required for a nuclear reactor, depending on the "fuel" (uranium, plutonium, etc.), energy of the neutrons, geometrical design, and other factors. If the reactor is too small, more neutrons will escape than are produced by fission, and the reaction will not be sustained. The ***critical size of a reactor*** is one in which neutron production equals neutron escape plus nonfission capture. A reactor larger than this is called supercritical. (Note similarity to critical mass of atom bomb.)

The ***graphite-moderated uranium nuclear reactor*** may be summarized as follows:

1. ***Essential Parts***
   a. Fuel—^{235}U and ^{238}U
   b. Moderator—pure graphite or heavy water
   c. Control rods—cadmium or boron-steel
   d. Protective barrier—concrete incorporating iron and barium ores

2. ***Operation***—fission of ^{235}U by thermal neutrons, slowing of resulting fast neutrons by moderator, fission of more ^{235}U (and to a slight extent ^{238}U by residual fast neutrons). Production of heat, fission products, and plutonium. Reaction buildup and decline not instantaneous, due to 0.75 percent of delayed neutrons, permitting time to regulate reaction by control rods.

Nuclear Fusion. In the preceding sections we discussed the release of energy when a nucleus undergoes fission into smaller fragments. The reverse process—the union or *fusion* of two or more light nuclei to form a heavier nucleus—is also accompanied by the release of energy because the product nucleus has less mass than the total mass of the fusing particles. Such atoms, when agitated by extremely high temperatures ranging from about 4×10^7 C to 1.5×10^8 C, are brought sufficiently close together for the short range nuclear forces to become effective, resulting in fusion. The following are but two examples of the fusion reaction:

$$\underset{deuteron}{{}^2_1\text{H}} + \underset{deuteron}{{}^2_1\text{H}} \rightarrow \underset{helium}{{}^3_2\text{He}} + \underset{neutron}{{}^1_0\text{n}} + \underset{energy}{3.3 \text{ MeV}}$$

$$\underset{deutron}{{}^2_1\text{H}} + \underset{triton}{{}^3_1\text{H}} \rightarrow \underset{helium}{{}^4_2\text{He}} + \underset{neutron}{{}^1_0\text{n}} + \underset{energy}{17.6 \text{ MeV}}$$

It must be emphasized that *fusionable nuclei* invariably are characterized by *low atomic number* and *low mass number*, the latter being on the low side of the curve representing nuclear binding energy per nucleon. The product nucleus has a higher binding energy per nucleon than either of the reacting nuclei. Recall that the reverse situation exists with regard to fissionable nuclei (see page 378).

At present the relatively new field of *plasma physics* is involved in experimental attempts to control the fusion process, especially with protons, deuterons, and tritons (tritium nuclei) to form helium. The high temperatures needed in fusion can be supplied by the fission of uranium, so this is often called the *fission-fusion process*.

Once fusion becomes economically feasible, it should provide an inexhaustible source of energy because of the almost unlimited supply of deuterium in the earth's water. An outstanding advantage of such an energy source is the absence of significant radioactive wastes with their attendant problem of safe disposal, aside from the at least equally important liberation of the United States from dependence on foreign countries for a large part of its energy requirements.

PRACTICAL APPLICATIONS OF NUCLEAR REACTOR

In recent years the principle of the nuclear reactor has been applied to the design of atomic submarines and industrial power generators. Essentially, this involves utilizing the heat produced in the reactor to operate a steam turbine. Other, more efficient means of converting nuclear energy to mechanical and electrical energy are being intensively studied and will not be considered further, except to point out that the disposal of radioactive waste in the conventional nuclear reactor promises to be an almost insurmountable problem.

The application of the nuclear reactor that is of interest to us is the wholesale manufacture of radionuclides for medical use. Because of the high neutron flux available in the reactor, radionuclides of almost every type and in nearly unlimited quantities can be readily produced. The element to be irradiated is placed in a metal can in a drawer which is slid into the reactor. After it has been exposed to the neutron flux for a suitable length of time, the target element is removed and the product nuclides processed and purified. All of this must be done behind shields that contain abundant hydrogen (water, paraffin), and by remote control to protect the operator from the high intensity radiation. The specific activity of the radionuclide depends on the density of neutron flux in the reactor and the time of irradiation of the element in the reactor.

We shall use the production of ^{32}P to exemplify two possible kinds of reactions in the nuclear reactor.

1. Radiative capture: (n,γ) reaction (Fig. 11.14)
2. Transmutation: (n,p) reaction (Fig. 11.15).

Note that in both types of reactions ^{32}P is the radionuclide product, but different target elements are used. In the (n,γ) reaction,

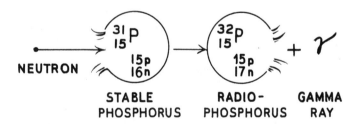

$$\text{NEATRON} \quad {}^{31}_{15}\text{P} \begin{array}{c} 15p \\ 16n \end{array} \longrightarrow {}^{32}_{15}\text{P} \begin{array}{c} 15p \\ 17n \end{array} + \gamma$$

STABLE   RADIO-   GAMMA
PHOSPHORUS   PHOSPHORUS   RAY

FIGURE 11.14. A neutron entering stable phosphorus renders it radioactive (^{32}P) by the (n, γ) reaction. The radiophosphorus is difficult to separate from the stable parent because of their chemical identity.

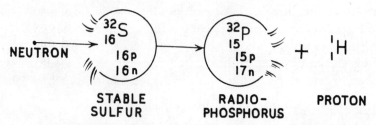

FIGURE 11.15. A neutron entering stable sulfur transmutes it to radiophosphorus (^{32}P) by the (n,p) reaction. The radiophosphorus can be separated chemically from the parent sulfur.

it is impossible to separate the stable and the radioactive phosphorus by chemical means. In the (n,p) reaction, where the target atom is sulfur, the product ^{32}P can easily be separated chemically from the sulfur. Therefore, the transmutation type of reaction is preferable, yielding ^{32}P of much greater specific activity since it is relatively uncontaminated by stable phosphorus. Such a radioactive isotope produced by transmutation is said to be *carrier free,* although a small amount of the stable element may be added as a carrier to facilitate its radiochemical handling.

Because of the high efficiency of the nuclear reactor, it is now the most productive source of radionuclides. The cyclotron is still useful in the manufacture of those nuclides which cannot be made in a nuclear reactor, or which have such short half-lives that they must be used close to their source of supply.

INTERNATIONAL SYSTEM OF UNITS (SI)

As we have already indicated in several places, the generally accepted units of exposure, absorbed dose, and activity were defined in the special units: roentgen (R), rad (rd), and curie (Ci), respectively, by the International Commission on Radiation Units and Measurements (ICRU) in 1962. During the same time that the ICRU was developing these units an international group of scientists was engaged in an effort to derive units that would fit into the metric system (the so-called Metre Convention). Finally, in 1960 the Eleventh General Conference of Weights and Measures adopted, as part of the Metre Convention, the **International System of Units (SI)** to which the USSR and the member nations of the European Economic Community have since become signatory.

Although it would seem at first sight that it would be desirable to bring all units into the metric system immediately, the conversion from the present units to the SI is fraught with great difficulties. First let us look at the exact equivalents of the units in the two systems:

1 roentgen (R) = 2.58×10^{-4} C·kg^{-1} (coulomb/kg) *exactly*
1 rad (rd)   = 0.01 J·kg^{-1} (joule/kg) *exactly*
1 curie (Ci)   = 3.7×10^{-10} s^{-1} *exactly*

The converse equivalents are:

exposure	1 coulomb/kg (C·kg^{-1}) $\approx$ 3876 R
exposure rate	1 ampere/kg (A·kg^{-1}) $\approx$ 3876 R/sec
absorbed dose	1 joule/kg (J·kg^{-1}) = 100 rad
absorbed dose rate	1 watt/kg (W·kg^{-1}) = 100 rad/sec
activity	1 per sec (s^{-1}) $\approx 2.703 \times 10^{-11}$ Ci

Although the SI recommendations have been to retain the R, rad, and curie for the present, the European Economic Community nations have already begun action to replace them with the new SI units.

As Lidén* has pointed out, the conversion is so complex that it may increase the possibility of error in radiotherapy. For example, the conversion from 6000 rad is readily made to 60 J·kg^{-1}. But in the case of absorbed dose rate, the fact that the watt is based on the second as the time unit may be concealed and lead to a large error. Lidén rightly thinks that the unit of absorbed dose rate should be J/(kg·s) or J/kg·min).

Insofar as activity is concerned, while the SI unit 1 s^{-1} is extremely small, and inconveniently so, multiple units are derived with difficulty when the strict rules are followed. Thus, an activity

*Lidén, K.: SI units in radiology and radiation measurement. *Radiol.*, *107:*463, 1973.

of 10^6s^{-1} (≈ 27 mCi) must be written as $1 \ \mu\text{s}^{-1}$ (1/microsec), and for 10^9s^{-1} (≈ 27 mCi) it is $1 \ \text{ns}^{-1}$ (1/nanosec).

Patient safety requires extreme care in the selection and application of units so as to minimize the possibility of error. As yet the SI has not been accepted here, although it is under consideration. It is quite possible that appropriate modifications will be effected in the SI to facilitate conversion from our present very convenient and practical system, and thereby render the SI acceptable on a worldwide basis.

CHAPTER 12

Implant Therapy with Radium, Radon, and Artificial Radionuclides

HISTORICAL SURVEY

IN 1901, five years after Becquerel discovered the emission of radiation by uranium, he accidentally incurred a skin burn while carrying a radium sample in his vest pocket. This is believed to be the first instance of a biologic effect resulting from such radiation. Soon afterward, Pierre Curie produced an experimental skin reaction on his arm by the application of radium, thereby confirming Becquerel's accidental observation.

The remarkable ability of uranium compounds to emit ionizing radiations capable of discharging an electroscope inspired Marie Curie to investigate this novel phenomenon. She soon found similar behavior in another element, thorium, an observation made independently by G. C. Schmidt a few weeks earlier.

On further study she found the intensity of the radiation emitted by pitchblende, a uranium ore, to be about four times greater than anticipated from its uranium content alone. Together with her husband Pierre, she embarked on a series of experiments to determine the source of the additional radiation.

The Curies used not only chemical methods of separation, but also a physical method of ionization measurement, employing Pierre's original highly sensitive and accurate piezo-electrometer. As each successive chemical fraction was obtained with the most tedious and painstaking technique, they measured its radiation intensity. Finally, in July, 1898, they announced the discovery of a radioactive element which they named *polonium,* in honor of Marie's native country Poland.

They soon found that another chemical fraction exhibited even greater activity and, after further chemical analysis, established another milestone in history by the discovery of *radium* in December, 1898. The specific γ-ray constant of radium is about 2 million times that of uranium.

The term ***radioactivity*** was coined by Marie Curie to specify the ability of certain elements to give off radiations spontaneously.

Soon after the discovery of radium, it was first employed in the therapy of superficial lesions by Danlos at the Paris St. Louis Hospital. In the United States, Robert Abbe (1905) first used radium enclosed in tubes for the interstitial treatment of malignant tumors; however, it is of interest that the American inventor, Alexander Graham Bell, had proposed this method of radiotherapy two years earlier in a letter to the editor of *American Medicine*.

Following the announcement of the Rutherford-Soddy theory of radioactive transformation in 1902, Duane suggested the use of ***radon*** in the therapy of malignant tumors. Not long afterward, Janeway prepared brass tubes containing radon gas, which he used successfully in therapy. This was modified by Joly and Stevenson who collected radon in tiny glass bulbs which could be inserted into hollow needles and replaced with fresh bulbs as needed. In 1924 Failla introduced the gold seed, a minute gold tube containing radon; such seeds could be implanted in a tumor in a planned pattern and left permanently because of the relatively rapid decay of radon. Gold implants proved to be a successful method of treating malignant tumors that were inaccessible to removable radium needles.

A number of years passed before the world supply of radium reached significant size, because tremendous amounts of ore had to be processed. In fact, the Curies obtained only 100 mg of radium after a prodigious amount of work, starting with one ton of pitchblende from which the uranium had previously been extracted. When sufficient amounts of radium became available commercially, several grams could be placed in a suitable "head" or "bomb" and used as an external source for therapy at a distance (telecurie therapy).

It is of historic interest that Janeway, who first used radon in therapy, introduced the "radium pack" in 1917; since then, considerable evolution in the design of teletherapy units has taken place. Thus, in effect, external "supervoltage" therapy dates back to 1917!

RADIUM

Contrary to popular opinion, radium is supplied commercially for therapy in the form of a salt—usually Ra sulfate or bromide —rather than as a pure metal. The reason for this is two-fold. First, the inherent radioactivity of Ra is not altered in any way by chemical combination, the intensity of the radiation being proportional to the Ra present in the compound. In the second place, the isolation of Ra as a pure metal is a very difficult, expensive, and unnecessary procedure for use in therapy. Although Marie Curie succeeded in obtaining the pure metal which tarnished rather rapidly, it is questionable whether this has ever been done again.

Pure metallic Ra is silvery white, resembling in its luster calcium or barium. It decomposes water, as does calcium, behaving chemically in other respects like the members of Group II in the Periodic Table. Its atomic number is 88, and its mass number 226.

DECAY AND RADIATIONS OF RADIUM

As we have already seen, Ra is an excellent example of an element exhibiting the peculiar property of radioactivity, that is, the spontaneous de-excitation or transformation of its nucleus with emission of ionizing radiation. The decay process is a **random** one, following the statistical laws of chance. As is true of other radioactive nuclides, decay is exponential with time, a certain fixed **fraction** of all the atoms present decaying per unit of time, regardless of the number initially present.

The types of radiation emitted by the Ra series have already been discussed in detail, but will be summarized here. Recall that these radiations are the prototypes of those given off by other radionuclides so that a thorough comprehension of their nature is essential in radiotherapy.

When a small specimen of Ra is placed in the bottom of a narrow well drilled in a block of lead, a narrow beam of radiation passes through the opening (see Fig. 12.01A). If the block is now placed in an electric field so the cathode is on the left and the anode on the right, the beam of rays is found to consist of three different

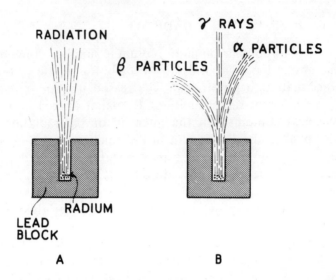

FIGURE 12.01. In *A* the radiation from a specimen of radium passes directly upward through the aperture in the lead block. In *B* the magnetic field (north pole below, south pole above the plane of this page) separates the α and β particles because of their different charges. The uncharged γ rays proceed straight upward.

groups. One group is deviated toward the cathode and hence must be positively charged; this constitutes the α particles. A second group is deflected toward the anode and must, therefore, be negatively charged; it consists of β particles. The third group is unaffected by the field, passing straight upward; therefore, it must be uncharged and, in fact, is known to consist of γ rays—electromagnetic radiation identical to X rays. Comparable results are obtained by the use of a magnetic field, verifying the nature of these radiations (see Fig. 12.01B).

A brief summary of the radiations emitted by the Ra series will now be presented (the appropriate sections in Chapter 3 should be reviewed).

1. *Alpha Particles.* The Ra series α particles, consisting of 2 protons and 2 neutrons, are identical to those present in other radionuclides. Furthermore, since its atomic number is 2 and its mass number is 4, the α particle is really a helium nucleus, that is, a helium ion bearing 2 positive charges.

$$\alpha \text{ particle} = He^{++}$$

The α particles of the various members of the Ra series are ejected with high velocities, approaching 1/20 ro 1/10 that of light (1.5 to 3 × 10^7 meters/sec). However, the initial velocities of all the α particles of a given radionuclide are the same, or occur in limited groups of velocities, carrying discrete amounts of energy away from the nucleus. The higher the initial velocity, obviously the greater will be the range or distance the α particles will travel in a given medium. In fact, the range is approximately proportional to the cube of the initial velocity. The α particles of the Ra series have an average range in *air* of about 3.3 cm, and a maximum of about 7 cm. They only penetrate about 0.05 mm (50 μ) of tissue, being almost completely absorbed by the outer layer of the skin or by an ordinary sheet of paper. Thus, because of their extremely short range in tissues, α particles are of little or no value in therapy (although they have been shown by Uhlmann to be useful, in the form of radon ointment, in the management of late radiation ulcers). Because of their large mass and high velocity, they carry about 90 percent of the energy emitted by Ra. Radium α particles have an energy of 4.66 MeV. One millicurie (mCi) of Ra emits 37 million (3.7 × 10^7) α particles per sec (by definition, and since one α particle is liberated per disintegration). Alpha particles, because of their double charge and large mass, are extremely powerful ionizing radiations; thus, one Ra α particle liberates about 140,000 ion pairs in its range of 3.3 cm in air.

2. *Beta Particles.* The β particles emitted by the Ra series are negatively charged electrons moving with velocities 1/3 to 9/10 that of light (1 × 10^8 to 2.7 × 10^8 meters/sec). They carry about 4 percent of the energy liberated by the Ra series, and do not occur in this series until Ra B appears (see Fig. 12.02). The range of β particles is not so uniform as that of α particles, but instead varies from zero to a maximum, corresponding to initial velocities which vary from zero to a maximum. The fastest β particles of the Ra series have a range of about 1.5 cm in tissue and are therefore about 300 times more penetrating than α particles. Almost all the β particles of the Ra series are stopped by 0.5 mm platinum or gold and, of course, this thickness also stops the α particles. The equivalent thicknesses of other materials are:

0.5 mm Pt or Au $\cong$ 1 mm Pb or Ag $\cong$ 2 mm brass

Therefore, these materials can be used interchangeably, in the thickness shown, as filters in Ra therapy. Beta particles, with only a single electric charge and a smaller mass than α particles, despite their higher velocity, are not so highly ionizing. Thus, the specific ionization (number of ion pairs liberated per unit length of path) of the radium β particles is about 1/500 that of the α particles.

Because of their poor penetrating ability, β particles cannot be employed in the treatment of deeply situated lesions. However, they are useful in the therapy of superficial skin lesions, especially to small areas.

3. *Gamma Rays.* Of the three types of radiation emitted by the Ra series, this is the only one that is electromagnetic in nature, belonging to the same category as light and X rays. The velocity of γ rays is constant in a given medium. 3×10^8 meters/sec (186,000 mi/sec) in air. Almost 7 percent of the radiant energy of the Ra series is emitted in the form of γ rays. They first appear in the series with daughter elements RaB and RaC (see Fig. 12.02) in a wide variety of spectral energies. Because of their electromagnetic nature, high average energy of about 0.83 MeV, and absence of charge, γ rays are the most penetrating of all the radiations emitted by Ra. In fact, their penetrating ability is more than 100 times that of β particles. Gamma rays are physically the same as X rays, differing only in their origin from atomic nuclei (it may be recalled that X rays are produced either during rapid deceleration of high speed electrons, or by transitions of orbital electrons). The application of Ra in therapy most often depends on the γ ray component of the emitted radiation, the α and β particles being absorbed by a suitable filter.

In Table 12.01 is presented a summary of the comparison of α, β, and γ radiations on the basis of penetrating power and ionizing ability in soft tissue.

The Radium Series. Radium is itself an intermediate member of one of the great families of naturally occurring radioelements —the *uranium series.* Since Ra is a long-lived radionuclide we customarily ignore its antecedents and assume that it is the parent of the so-called *radium series* (see Fig. 12.02).

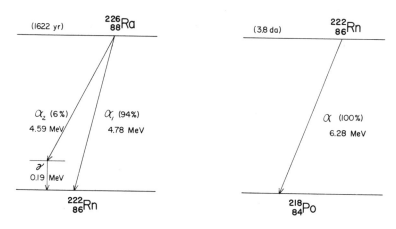

	URANIUM	RADIUM	RADON	RADIUM A	RADIUM B	RADIUM C	LEAD
				POLONIUM	LEAD	BISMUTH	
Atomic No.	92	88	86	84	82	83	82
Mass No.	238	226	222	218	214	214	206
Half Life	4.5×10^9 yr	1622 yr	3.8 da	3 min	26.8 min	19.7 min	stable

FIGURE 12.02. Relation of radium 226 to its decay products.

Top. The radium series, with successive product nuclides shown from left to right. These comprise the last part of the uranium series. Data on RaD, RaE, and RaF have been omitted.

Lower left. Decay scheme of radium 226. Note the low energy (0.19 MeV) γ ray which is of no importance in radiotherapy.

Lower right. Decay scheme of radon 222. No γ ray is emitted. The γ rays useful in therapy are emitted by RaB (^{214}Pb) and RaC (^{214}Bi).

TABLE 12.01
COMPARISON OF THE RADIATIONS EMITTED BY THE RADIUM SERIES

Radiation	Maximum Range in Soft Tissue	Specific Ionization in Soft Tissue
	cm	*ion pairs/μ*
α	0.005	3000
β	1.5	6
γ	indefinite (exponential absorption)	depends on energy of primary electrons

In Figure 12.02 we can see the operation of the Rutherford-Soddy Law, discussed earlier. When a Ra nucleus ejects an α particle, it loses mass units and atomic number units equal to those carried away by the α particle. Since the α particle has atomic number 2 and mass number 4, these must be subtracted from the corresponding values of the Ra nucleus:

$$^{226}_{88}\text{Ra} - {}^{4}_{2}\text{He} \rightarrow {}^{222}_{86}\text{Rn}$$

In this equation, the superscript 226 (mass number) of Ra minus the superscript 4 of the α particle equals the superscript 222 of the Rn atom. Similarly, the subscript 88 (atomic number) of radium minus the subscript 2 of the α particle equals the subscript 86 of Rn. So far the reasoning is obvious.

Now refer to RaB in Figure 12.02. For a nucleus of this radionuclide to emit a β particle (the γ ray may be neglected in this argument), one of the nuclear neutrons has to be converted to 1 proton and 1 negatron (and an antineutrino). Since the negatron is ejected as a β^- particle, the daughter nucleus, RaC, ends up with 1 more proton, or positive charge, than its parent. This added positive charge increases its atomic number by one unit. The mass number is unchanged because the β particle carries away only a minute fraction of a mass unit (about 1/1860).

$$^{214}_{82}\text{RaB} - {}^{0}_{-1}\beta \rightarrow {}^{214}_{83}\text{RaC}$$

In this equation, the mass number 214 of RaB minus the mass number 0 of the β particle gives a mass number of 214 for the daughter nuclide RaC. The atomic number 82 of RaB minus a minus 1 equals 83, the atomic number of RaC. Note that radium B is radioactive lead, $^{214}_{82}\text{Pb}$, and RaC is radioactive bismuth, $^{214}_{83}\text{Bi}$.

Thus, according to the Rutherford-Soddy law, if an α particle is ejected, the mass number decreases by 4, and the daughter nuclide shifts two places to the left (lower), in the Periodic Table. If a radionuclide decays by β^- emission, the daughter nuclide has the same mass number, but its atomic number is one place to the right (higher) in the Periodic Table.

Referring again to Figure 12.02, we note that Ra, Rn and RaA all emit α particles. The γ rays are emitted almost entirely by nuclides farther in the series: RaB and RaC (Ra itself gives off a very weak γ ray which may be neglected). Thus, it is incorrect, in a strict sense, to say that Ra gives off γ rays, if one has in mind the parent atom alone. Beta particles appear later in the series, arising from RaB and RaC. Thus, when we state that Ra emits all three types of radiation, we mean by implication the **radium series.** Since Rn gives rise eventually to the daughter nuclides RaB and RaC, it can be used in a sealed container as a **source** in γ-ray therapy.

Radioactive Constants of Radium. The general subject of specific γ-ray constants has already been discussed and the appropriate section in Chapter 11 should be reviewed. We shall now consider briefly the radium constants in particular.

1. **Decay Constant.** The decay or transformation constant λ of Ra is 0.0428 percent per year or, stated as a simple decimal, 0.000428 or 4.28×10^{-4} per year. Using the general equation for radioactive decay $A = A_0 e^{-\lambda t}$, we can determine A the activity of Ra **remaining** at time t, starting with activity A_0, by substituting the correct values in the equation. The values of $e^{-\lambda t}$ for various values of λt are shown in Table 4.02.

2. **Half-life.** As we have already indicated, the half-life of a radionuclide is the time in which one-half the atoms present at a given starting time will have decayed; or it is the time required for a given sample of a radionuclide to lose one-half its initial activity.

The half-life of radium can be obtained from the following equation derived on pages 360 to 361:

$$T = \frac{0.693}{\lambda} \tag{1}$$

where T = half-life.
Since, for radium, $\lambda = 0.000428$ (4.28×10^4) per year,

$$T = \frac{0.693}{0.000428} = 1,620 \text{ years}$$

It should be emphasized that equation (1) is important because it gives the decay constant when the half-life is known, and conversely.

Since Ra has such a long half-life, it can be used in radiation therapy without correction for decay. Once a sealed source has been prepared and secular equilibrium reached (in about one month), the activity remains almost constant during the professional lifetime of the user.

3. *Average Life.* A simple equation has already been presented (see Chapter 11) to show the relationship between the average life T_a and the decay constant,

$$T_a = \frac{1}{\lambda} \tag{2}$$

The average life of Ra is obtained by:

$$T_a = \frac{1}{0.000428}$$

$$T_a = 2.34 \text{ years}$$

The significance of average life is that it indicates the probable survival time of any individual atom of Ra in a sample. It is analogous to life insurance statistics on the probable survival of a given individual in a large population.

RADON

Source. When radium sulfate or radium bromide is kept in aqueous solution, radon gradually accumulates in and above the solution at a rate consistent with the decay rate of Ra. If the solution is then carefully heated, the resulting vapor contains Rn gas which can be collected and purified in a special type of apparatus known as a *radon plant.* It consists of an intricate system of glass tubing, as shown in Figure 12.03. The Rn is finally collected in a gold or glass capillary tube which is pinched off and sealed in short segments, usually a few mm in length. These Rn containing segments are called *seeds* or *implants;* they must be calibrated accurately before being used in therapy. It is an interesting fact that with Oddie's apparatus,[61] a solution of 2 grams Ra yields 1,000 mCi of Rn in slightly less than 48 hours. On account of the short half-life of Rn, the apparatus must be highly efficient to expedite the extraction process. In about 5 hours enough RaB and RaC will have accumulated to reach transient equilibrium, the γ-ray activity having reached a maximum by this time. Thus, freshly prepared Rn implants must be stored for 5 hours before use, to permit them to reach maximum strength. From this point on, decay occurs progressively as described below.

Properties. Radon is a heavy, colorless gas, with atomic number 86 and mass number 222, its symbol being $^{222}_{86}$Rn. It belongs to the family of inert elements which includes helium, neon, argon, etc. Rn is the first disintegration product of Ra,

$$^{226}_{88}\text{Ra} \longrightarrow \underset{\alpha \; particle}{^{222}_{86}\text{Rn} + {}^{4}_{2}\text{He}}$$

Referring to Figure 12.02, note that the gas Rn decays to RaA which is a solid, as are all the succeeding members of the series.

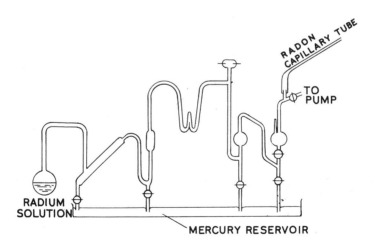

FIGURE 12.03. Simplified sketch of the Oddie radon plant.[61] (Courtesy of the British Institute of Radiology.)

Thus, if we start with a container of Rn gas, there soon results an accumulation of solid radioactive daughter nuclides known collectively as **active deposit**. The radiation emitted by Rn itself consists entirely of α particles:

$$^{222}_{86}\text{Rn} \longrightarrow \ ^{218}_{84}\text{RaA} + \ ^{4}_{2}\text{He}$$
$$\text{\tiny α particle}$$

However, the offspring, as already mentioned, emit collectively α and β^- particles, and γ rays. Therefore, sealed sources of **radon** may be used for γ-ray therapy provided (1) enough time has elapsed for radioactive equilibrium to occur, that is, about 5 hours; and (2) appropriate filters are used to absorb α and β particles.

Radioactive Constants. Just as in the case of other radionuclides, there are three important radioactive constants of radon:

1. **Decay Constant.** Radon decays at the rate of 16.5 percent per day. However, because of the exponential character of the decay process (same fraction of any initial quantity decaying per second), and because one day represents a relatively long period in the survival of a Rn atom, a much smaller time interval must be selected as the basis for the decay constant which, for Rn, is 2.1×10^{-6} per second or 0.181 per day.

2. **Half-life.** Using the equation for radioactive decay, we can find the half-life of Rn in the same way as we did for Ra:

$$T = \frac{0.693}{\lambda}$$

$$= \frac{0.693}{0.181}$$

$$= 3.83 \text{ days, } \textit{half-life of Rn}$$

3. **Average Life.** This may readily be found if the decay constant is known:

$$T_a = \frac{1}{\lambda}$$

$$= \frac{1}{0.181}$$

$$= 5.52 \text{ days or } 132.5 \text{ hr, } \textit{av. life of Rn}$$

RADIOACTIVE EQUILIBRIUM

This subject has been discussed in detail on pages 368 to 375 and should now be reviewed. However, we shall summarize it here with particular reference to radium and radon.

A radionuclide decay series is said to be in *radioactive equilibrium* when, in a sealed source, the rate of appearance of each daughter equals its rate of decay; that is, the amount being formed per second equals the amount decaying per second. However, a distinction is made between *secular* and *transient equilibrium.*

In *secular equilibrium* the parent nuclide has a much longer half-life than any of its daughters; Ra is an example. Because of the long half-life of Ra it furnishes a virtually inexhaustible supply of daughter nuclides. These accumulate until secular equilibrium has been established (about 35 days), provided the Ra was first sealed in a leakproof container such as a needle or tube. Now the daughters are present in constant amounts. Since the use of Ra in γ-ray therapy most often depends on RaB (radio-lead) and RaC (radiobismuth), and their amounts are constant at equilibrium, the specific γ-ray constant (Γ) of the sealed source is constant, thereby simplifying dosimetry. Furthermore, the half-life of the sealed source is the same as that of the parent Ra—1622 years.

Radon is an example of a radionuclide which reaches *transient equilibrium* with its descendants because it has a relatively *short half-life* of 3.83 days. Upon reaching transient equilibrium at about 5 hours after being sealed, Rn and its decay products continue to undergo rapid decay, with the same half-life as the parent Rn. Therefore, the γ-ray output decreases significantly during a course of Rn therapy. On the other hand, because of the extremely long half-life of Ra relative to treatment time, its γ-ray output remains virtually constant. As will be shown later, this difference between Ra and Rn must be taken into account in implant therapy.

GAMMA-RAY DOSAGE DETERMINATION

The following discussion will be limited to the surface, intra-cavitary, and interstitial application of γ-emitting radionuclides. Although the presentation is based on Ra and Rn, the same principles may be applied to other radioactive materials if appropriate correction factors are introduced.

With any system of γ-ray therapy, just as with X rays, we must ultimately find the radiation-absorbed dose in the lesion being treated (including a safe margin); more specifically, the **minimum absorbed dose.** The aim of therapy should be to deliver a minimum cancericidal dose (one which destroys practically an entire population of cancer cells). Any radiation above the minimum absorbed within the lesion itself is of no consequence because it is anticipated that the lesion will disappear. On the other hand, any portion of a tumor receiving less than the minimum cancericidal dose will not be entirely eradicated and is very likely to recur. Naturally, overirradiation of the normal tissues in the vicinity of the lesion must be avoided because they are needed in the repair process.

According to the Report of the ICRU,* the following data should be recorded whenever radioactive substances are used in surface, intracavitary, or interstitial therapy:

a. Description of treatment in detail, to permit duplication.

b. Physical characteristics of radioactive nuclide used—half-life, types of radiation emitted, energies of radiation emitted.

c. Filtration, including thickness and nature of all materials between the radionuclide and the lesion.

d. Initial activity, in mCi, of radionuclide, its spatial distribution, and time for each application.

e. Number and date of applications.

f. Total duration of treatments.

g. Dimensions and location of volume of interest.

h. Absorbed dose in rads, per treatment and for total treatment throughout the lesion itself and other significant exposed tissue.

On the basis of this outline, dosage systems have been constructed, modifiable for various therapy situations. Some of the factors mentioned in the ICRU recommendations, such as the detailed description of the treatment, are self-explanatory. We have already discussed, earlier in this chapter, the physical characteristics of radium and radon. We shall now consider those

---

*International Commission on Radiation Units and Measurements. *Handbook 62,* National Bureau of Standards (1956).

factors which are essential to the determination of the absorbed dose. Obviously, before we can arrive at a value for absorbed dose, the exposure in roentgens must be determined. Therefore, the following factors are essential:

1. Activity of the radioactive source in millicuries, and the time-intensity factor in mCi-hr.
2. Specific γ-ray constant Γ of the radioactive source.
3. Distribution of the sources in the volume of interest.
4. Absorbed dose in rads.

Modern dosage tables for radium indicate the absorbed dose directly, bypassing exposure in R.

ACTIVITY OF A RADIOACTIVE SOURCE

The Curie

Before an attempt is made to specify the absorbed dose in γ-ray therapy, we must first have a suitable unit of quantity of the particular radioactive nuclide. The first such unit to receive universal recognition was the *curie* (Ci), originally defined as that quantity of radon in equilibrium with 1 gram of radium element. As we have already implied, in short-term therapy lasting only a few hours, 1 gram of Ra delivers the same dose as 1 Ci of Rn. Obviously, if we have two containers, one of which holds 1 gram of Ra and the other 1 Ci of Rn, each will have the same amount of active deposit and therefore the same γ-ray intensity. Based on the modern definition of the Ci, 1 Ci of Ra or Rn is not exactly equivalent to 1 g of Ra, but the difference is not significant clinically.

Thus, the unit of activity of a Rn source is 1 Ci. In practical γ-ray therapy with interstitial sources, this is a rather large quantity and therefore 1/1,000 of a Ci or *1 millicurie* (mCi) is the conventional standard. Correspondingly, 1 milligram (mg) of Ra is the unit of quantity of Ra element for interstitial therapy. When Ra needles are purchased, it is advisable to have a National Bureau of Standards certificate which verifies their Ra content and purity, since certain short-lived radioactive contaminants such as mesothorium may give initially high γ-ray intensities.

However, since the mesothorium decays at the rate of 10 percent per year, the intensity of the γ radiation from such contaminated needles decreases significantly from year to year, in contrast to pure Ra needles which maintain their activity practically constant.

With the advent of artificial radionuclides in sufficient quantities for clinical application, it became necessary to find a unit of activity which could be used for all radionuclides. According to the accepted definition, I Ci is the activity of an amount of Rn in which exactly 3.7×10^{10} nuclei de-excite or decay in one second. The same unit is applied to all radionuclides:

$$1 \text{ curie (Ci)} = 3.70 \times 10^{10} \text{ d/s}$$
$$1 \text{ millicurie (mCi)} = 3.70 \times 10^{7} \text{ d/s}$$
$$1 \text{ microcurie } (\mu\text{Ci}) = 3.70 \times 10^{4} \text{ d/s}$$
$$(\text{d/s} = \text{de-excitations or disintegrations per sec})$$

Another unit has been suggested, though not widely accepted— the rutherford (Rd), defined as that quantity of a radionuclide such that it undergoes 10^6 (or 1 million) d/s.

COMPARATIVE RADIATION EXPOSURE WITH RADIUM AND RADON

Determination of Millicurie Hours

Before discussing the absorbed dose in rads during implant therapy we must first know something about the exposure rate of γ rays. This depends on the activity of the radionuclide (Ci or mCi) and the exposure time. However, there is an important difference between Ra and Rn in this regard, as explained above.

Since the half-life of radium is extremely long relative to treatment time, no correction need be made for its decay. Thus, the γ-ray activity of a Ra needle gradually increases during the first 35 days after being manufactured, as the daughter elements accumulate, following which the activity declines very slowly at the practically insignificant rate of only about 0.043 percent per year. Hence, insofar as radiation therapy is concerned, Ra activity is regarded as being constant.

The γ-ray output of a radium source is proportional to the number of milligrams or mCi, times the exposure time. Consequently, the total quantity of γ-radiation emitted by a low activity Ra needle placed in a tumor for a longer period of time is equivalent to that of a high activity needle for a shorter period of time, as, for example:

$$10 \text{ mg Ra} \times 4 \text{ hr} = 1 \text{ mg Ra} \times 40 \text{ hr} = 40 \text{ mg hr}$$

although it must be emphasized that the biologic effects may not be the same in both cases.

The situation is entirely different with a short-lived radionuclide such as **radon.** Its half-life is of the same order of magnitude as the usual treatment time, and therefore its decay must be taken into account. Because of the rapidly diminishing quantity of Rn in an implant over a period of days, we cannot simply multiply the mCi by the time to obtain the basis for computing γ-ray emission. Instead, in view of the fact that in any given sample of a radionuclide all of the atoms do not de-excite simultaneously, but do so in a random manner over a period of time, we can compute the **average life** of the atoms. It is over the average lifetime of a given quantity of Rn that it gives up practically all of its γ-radiation. Thus, if we start with 1 mCi of Rn and multiply this by its average life, we will obtain a value in mCi-hr whose γ-ray emission is equal to that from 1 mCi during "complete" or total decay.

Average life T_a is obtained from the following equation :

$$T_a = \frac{T}{0.693}$$

where T is the half-life. Thus, with Rn which has a T of 3.83 days,

$$T_a = \frac{3.98}{0.693} \times 24 = 133 \text{ hr}$$

This means that a 1 mCi permanent Rn implant would give the same total γ-ray emission to total decay as 1 mg Ra implanted for 133 hr. In common use is the expression

$$1 \text{ mCi destroyed} = 133 \text{ mCi-hr, or mg-hr}$$

In a treatment plan in which **permanent** Rn implants are inserted into the tissues and left to total decay, we simply multiply the mCi activity of the implants by 133 to obtain the mCi-hr. This would be the same mathematically, although not necessarily biologically, as the same number of mg-hr of Ra in removable needles. For example, if there are 8 seeds containing a total of 8 mCi of *radon,* the number of mCi-hr to total decay would be:

$$8 \times 133 = 1{,}060 \text{ mCi-hr}$$

But if 8 *radium* needles were used, containing a total of 8 mg, they would also have to be left in place 133 hr because

$$8 \times 133 = 1{,}060 \text{ mg-hr}$$

Since 1 mg Ra is equivalent to 1 mCi, the γ-ray exposure would be identical in both cases.

On the other hand, suppose 20 mCi Rn is applied, and then removed after exactly 48 hours. The total activity of Rn destroyed would then be the initial 20 mCi minus the mCi activity of the source at the time of removal. Referring to Table 12.02, we see that at the end of two days, 69.6 percent of the Rn is left. Then:

$$20 \times \frac{69.6}{100} = 13.9 \text{ mCi Rn remaining}$$

$$20 - 13.9 = 6.1 \text{ mCi destroyed}$$

$$6.1 \times 133 \approx 810 \text{ mCi-hr delivered during the}$$
$$\text{two days of treatment}$$

The 810 mCi-hr is equivalent to 810 mg-hr Ra. Thus, treatment with Rn in removable sources requires the use of a decay table to determine the exposure in mCi-hr.

Let us now consider a typical therapy problem. Suppose a treatment plan calls for 30 mg Ra in needles, to be left in place 168 hours. This would give $30 \times 168 = 5{,}040$ mg-hr. If we decided to use, instead, Rn in *permanent* seed implants, what total amount of Rn would be required? First, we know that the mCi-hr dose will be the same as with Ra because

$$5{,}040 \text{ mg-hr} = 5{,}040 \text{ mCi-hr}$$

Since 1 mCi destroyed = 133 mCi-hr, 5,040 mCi-hr would require a proportional number of mCi destroyed:

$$\frac{x}{1} = \frac{5,040}{133}$$

$$x = 38 \text{ mCi Rn required}$$

Thus, 38 mCi Rn left to total decay is equivalent physically to 30 mg Ra left in place for a total of 168 hr.

Finally, let us consider another type of problem in which we plan to use a *removable* Rn source. Suppose we use a Rn tube containing 25 mCi with which we need to deliver a total of 2,000 mCi-hr. How long must it be left in position in the lesion in order to fulfill this requirement? Dividing,

$$\frac{2,000 \text{ mCi-hr}}{25 \text{ mCi}} = 80 \text{ mCi-hr per initial mCi}$$

The table of Rn decay (see Table 12.02) shows that 80 mCi-hr per initial mCi is obtained at the end of 5 days and 3 hours. This, then, is the total treatment time required.

Since the advent of megavoltage therapy, and because of problems involved in obtaining accurately calibrated individual Rn implants, Rn therapy has suffered a marked decline. Furthermore, the hazards inherent in the use of Ra have spurred the search for artificial radionuclide substitutes.

Note that in the preceding discussion no attempt has been made to give the actual dose of radiation delivered; the discussion has been limited to the methods of arriving at the product of the strength of the radioactive source and the number of hours of application, that is, mCi-hr. This, by itself, is completely inadequate for the specification of γ-ray dosage and is, in fact, the final step in therapy planning with implants. We must first determine the required absorbed dose in rads for a given geometric pattern of radioactive sources. From this we compute the required number of mCi-hr or mg-hr from published tables.

TABLE 12.02
DECAY OF RADON (QUIMBY)*

Time Days	Hours	Percentage Remaining	mCi-hr Per Initial mCi	Time Days	Hours	Percentage Remaining	mCi-hr Per Initial mCi
0	0	100	0	2	20	59.82	53.42
	2	98.50	1.99	3	0	58.05	55.80
	4	97.02	3.96	3	6	55.47	59.26
	6	95.67	5.90	3	12	53.01	62.44
	8	94.14	7.82	3	18	50.71	65.60
0	10	92.72	9.62	4	0	48.42	68.60
	12	91.33	11.52	4	8	45.60	72.41
	14	89.98	13.33	4	16	43.57	75.07
	16	88.61	15.11	5	0	40.43	79.30
	18	87.28	16.96	5	8	38.02	82.52
0	20	85.98	18.64	5	16	35.78	85.40
	22	84.96	20.38	6	0	33.70	88.40
1	0	83.42	22.08	6	12	30.80	92.15
1	3	81.55	24.55	7	0	28.11	95.78
1	6	79.72	26.97	7	12	25.67	99.00
1	9	77.93	29.35	8	0	23.45	102.1
1	12	76.18	31.70	9	0	19.56	107.0
1	15	74.48	33.98	10	0	16.32	111.4
1	18	72.81	36.16	11	0	13.61	115.0
1	21	71.18	38.38	12	0	11.35	118.0
2	0	69.59	40.45	14	0	7.90	122.5
2	4	67.52	43.20	17	0	4.59	125.8
2	8	65.50	45.91	20	0	2.66	129.4
2	12	63.55	48.51	25	0	1.07	131.5
2	16	61.66	51.00	30	0	0.43	132.5

*From Glasser, O., et al.: Physical Foundations of Radiology,[33] 1959. Courtesy of Paul B. Hoeber, Inc., Publisher, New York.

DETERMINATION OF SPECIFIC GAMMA-RAY CONSTANT OF RADIUM

Having learned the meaning, importance, and limitations of the mCi-hr factor, we must now turn to the problem of determining the exposure in roentgens corresponding to a given number of mCi-hr of a particular radionuclide. This will then lay the groundwork for the use of dosage tables.

According to the international definition of the roentgen, no distinction is made between X rays and γ rays up to 3 MeV. But when it comes to the actual measurement of the γ-ray intensity of a given radionuclide by means of a free-air ionization chamber, certain practical difficulties arise. The electrons set in motion by the γ rays must dissipate their energy within the volume of interest. Furthermore, there must be a state of equilibrium between the number of electrons entering and leaving this volume. Therefore, the dimensions of the chamber must be of the same order as the range of the fastest primary electrons. (The chamber may actually be smaller than this because only a few of the primary electrons have the maximum range.) The long range of the electrons liberated by γ rays makes it impracticable to construct a suitable free-air ionization chamber. Furthermore, the problem of eliminating scattered γ rays is insurmountable, so that this source of error cannot be excluded.

A most ingenious method was suggested by Failla and Marinelli in 1937. This required a huge room in the center of which was placed a thin-walled ionization chamber. Because of the large dimensions of the irradiated volume, not only was the effect of scattered γ rays avoided, but the distance of the chamber from the radium source could be so chosen that electronic equilibrium was achieved (i.e. the same number of primary electrons left the measuring chamber as entered it from the outside). Friedrich and others finally applied this principle, using a room $100 \times 50 \times 22$ cubic meters. Their ionization chamber was a 40 cm cube of tissue paper, suspended in the center of the room. The result of their measurements agreed very well with the presently accepted value of the γ ray emission of Ra in roentgens per milligram-hour (R/mg-hr) at 1 cm.

Another method utilizes a pressure ionization chamber in which the principles of the open air ionization chamber apply, but in which compression of the air permits a decrease in chamber dimensions. This provides a greater number of molecules per cc than are available at atmospheric pressure. The pressure chamber allows measurement of radiation up to 1.5 MeV and is also adaptable to the measurement of radiation with energy as low as 350 keV.

In an earlier chapter we considered the measurement of X rays by means of air-wall chambers; the same method is applicable to γ rays if suitable modifications are introduced. It may be recalled that such chambers (also known as "thimble chambers") consist of a shell of material having the same effective atomic number as air, that is, 7.64. In effect, such a chamber simulates a compressed air ionization chamber. The air-wall chamber has the same effective atomic number as air, but is greater in density, just as is compressed air. The materials that can be used for thimble chambers in γ ray measurement may vary somewhat from the value 7.64 (6 to 13) because the primary electrons produced by γ rays are mainly recoil (Compton) electrons, and the Compton process is independent of the atomic number of the irradiated medium. Some of the materials that have been found suitable for air-wall chambers are graphite; perspex or celluloid coated with graphite to make it a conductor; composition of graphite and bakelite with a small amount of titanium or vanadium oxide; and "elektron" metal of Sievert. Wall thickness of such air-equivalent chambers must be great enough for electronic equilibrium, yet not so great as to absorb a significant amount of γ radiation. The γ rays of the Ra series require a chamber wall thickness of 4 mm. Air volume within the chamber must be small relative to the range of the primary electrons.

The measurement of γ rays by means of suitable thimble chambers is sufficiently accurate for clinical purposes and is a relatively simple method when compared with compressed air chambers and auditorium-size experimental procedures.

The most widely accepted value of γ-ray intensity at present is as follows: *a 1 mg point source of radium, filtered by 0.5 mm Pt, delivers 8.25 R per hour at a distance of 1 cm.* This definition underlies the general specification of emitted dose from other radionuclides. Thus, the *specific γ-ray constant* of a radionuclide is the exposure rate of the unfiltered γ rays from a point source of a defined activity of the nuclide at a defined distance. Accordingly, the specific γ-ray constant Γ is defined as the roentgens per millicurie-hour at 1 cm:

$$\Gamma = R/mCi\text{-}hr \text{ at } 1 \text{ cm}$$

With radium, a 0.5 mm Pt filter is included to eliminate α and β particles. Thus,

$$\Gamma_{Ra} = 8.25 \text{ R/mCi-hr at } 1 \text{ cm}$$

The Γ value for Ra decreases 2 percent for every 0.1 mm increase in Pt filtration, and conversely. Thus, with 1.0 mm Pt filtration, Γ for Ra is $8.25 - 10\%$ or 7.42 R/mCi-hr.

The Γ values for some of the more important radionuclide substitutes used in therapy will be given in Table 12.13. (See pages 366 to 367 regarding NCRP recommendations for measuring Γ.)

The preceding discussion may be summarized for a radioactive source of any size by a simple equation:

$$\text{exposure rate in } R/hr = \frac{m\Gamma}{d^2} \tag{3}$$

where m is the activity of the radioactive source in millicuries, d is the distance in cm, and Γ is the specific γ-ray constant of the radionuclide in question. The latter will be constant for a given radionuclide; as, for example, 8.25 R/mCi-hr for Ra. Suppose in equation (3), we double the value of m. Obviously, the value of the right member of the equation is doubled and the γ-ray intensity of the source is doubled. If the distance is doubled, the intensity is reduced to $\frac{1}{4}$ the initial value, in accord with the inverse square law.

Equation (3) can be converted to a form which gives, directly, the total exposure in R at a given point. To do this, intensity must be multiplied by the time during which the radium is applied:

$$\text{exposure in } R = \text{exposure rate in } R/hr \times \text{time in hr}$$

$$\text{exposure in } R = \frac{m\Gamma t}{d^2} \tag{4}$$

where t represents time in hours.

Let us apply equation (4) to a practical case. We have a 10 mg Ra applicator filtered by 0.5 mm Pt, at 3 cm from a skin lesion. The Ra is maintained in this position for 20 hours. What is the radiation exposure of the lesion (assume that we have a point source)? We see that

$$m = 10 \text{ mg}$$

$$t = 20 \text{ hr}$$

$$d = 3 \text{ cm}$$

$$\Gamma = 8.25 \text{ R/mg-hr at 1 cm}$$

Substituting in equation (4):

$$exposure = \frac{10 \times 8.25 \times 20}{3 \times 3} = 183 \text{ R}$$

It may be of interest to summarize equation (4) in words: the γ-ray exposure at a point source of any given radionuclide is:
1. Directly proportional to the activity (i.e. mCi).
2. Directly proportional to the time of exposure.
3. Inversely proportional to the square of the distance between the source and the point of interest.

A simple relation that has been found sufficiently accurate in protection problems is

$$exposure \text{ in } R = \frac{radium \text{ } in \text{ } grams \times time \text{ } in \text{ } hours}{(distance \text{ } in \text{ } yards)^2}$$

Although the Γ value for Ra may be subject to revision at some future data, it is unlikely that this would be large enough to be of clinical significance. However, the stated value of Γ is accurate for radium molds or other surface applicators only if there is at least 4 mm of tissue equivalent material between the Ra and the point of interest, this thickness being required for electronic equilibrium. Obviously, no added material is necessary for interstitial Ra therapy.

ABSORBED DOSE—THE RAD

It is essential that a clear distinction be made between the γ radiation to which anything is exposed, and the quantity of energy absorbed. The former is the *exposure* and is measured in *roentgens*. The latter is the absorbed dose and is measured in *rads*.

The reason for stressing this distinction is that the biologic or therapeutic effect of radiation is dependent on the *energy actually absorbed*, rather than the radiation to which the tissue has been exposed. For example, we may deliver identical exposure in R to bone and adjacent soft tissue, but the bone may absorb 1½ times as much energy per gram as the soft tissue, with X rays of HVL 2 mm Cu. This factor is unimportant in γ-ray therapy, however, because absorption per unit mass of bone and soft tissue is virtually the same in this energy region.

It should be recalled that the roentgen is a unit of **exposure** based on the ionization produced in air under certain well defined conditions. The ionization produced in tissue is not necessarily the same as in air, and the difference may be even greater with radiations of different energies. In general, the absorbed dose in a given material is proportional to the exposure; under conditions of electronic equilibrium:

$$D = f \cdot X$$

where D is the absorbed dose in rads, f is a constant for the given material, and X is the exposure in R. In air, f is equal to 0.87 rad/R for X or γ rays up to 3 MeV, so that

$$D_{air} = 0.87 X$$

Thus, for an exposure of 1 R there is an absorbed dose of 0.87 rad in air. Since, by definition, 1 rad is an absorbed dose of 100 ergs/g (ergs per gram), 1 R corresponds to an absorption of $100 \times 0.87 = 87$ ergs/g of air.

For other media, a different value of f must be used. Thus, for Ra γ rays in soft tissue, f equals 0.96 rad/R and

$$D_{tissue} = 0.96 X$$

Therefore, 1 gram of soft tissue exposed to 1 R of γ rays absorbs 0.96 rad. Since 1 rad is 100 ergs/g, 1 R gives rise to absorption equal to $0.96 \times 100 = 96$ ergs/g. Thus, with the γ rays of the **radium series,** as well as with $^{60}Co,$

1 R produces absorption of 0.87 rad or 87 ergs/g in air
1 R produces absorption of 0.96 rad or 96 ergs/g in soft tissue

Conversely, 1 rad corresponds to an exposure of 100/96 or 1.04 R (γ rays, soft tissue).

The precise calculation of absorbed dose is not difficult if the point of interest is surrounded by a homogeneous medium such as soft tissue. When kV radiation crosses boundaries between dissimilar tissues, such as bone and soft tissue, the problem is quite complicated. However, in the radium γ-ray energy region (av. 0.83 MeV) absorption is virtually the same in bone and soft tissue, gram for gram, so that the problem of absorbed dose at a boundary is negligible.

In summary, then, the absorbed dose in soft tissues can be derived with sufficient accuracy, for clinical purposes, from the ionization produced in air. Proper application of experimentally determined conversion factors, described above, permits derivation of the absorbed dose in rads or in ergs/g.

TYPES OF RADIUM APPLICATORS

For use in clinical therapy, Ra must be placed in a suitable container. Such a discrete, encapsulated quantity of a radioactive material is called a *source,* one or more sources being arranged in an appropriate pattern for the purpose of treating an accessible lesion. At the present time most Ra sources are enclosed in some type of metal: monel, brass, silver, gold, or platinum. These metals serve three purposes: (1) they act as filters; (2) they permit the application of radium in a particular form; and (3) they increase treatment distance.

Filtration. As we have noted previously, the three types of radiation emitted by Ra and its decay products have different penetrating abilities. Because the α particles have a very short range, any metal of appreciable thickness will completely absorb them. This is desirable in γ-ray therapy because the α particles are strongly ionizing and produce intense local reaction without delivering a significant depth dose. The β particles are more penetrating, and if they are to be used in superficial therapy, the container may be made of monel metal 0.05 mm thick. The monel acts as a filter, removing or screening out the α particles while allowing the β particles and γ rays to pass through. If only the γ rays are to be utilized, a 0.5 mm platinum or gold container enclosing the Ra will filter out all the α and almost all the β particles. Equivalent filtration is provided by 1 mm lead or silver, or 2 mm brass. Heavier filtration than this reduces the intensity, but causes only slight hardening of the γ radiation, (recall that exposure rate is reduced 2% per 0.1 mm Pt filter increase above 0.5 mm Pt).

Radium and Radon Containers. The various types of containers which are in general use will now be described.

1. *Implants* (*"seeds"*) are tiny, sealed capillary tubes about 0.75 mm by 3 mm, having a wall thickness of 0.3 mm gold. The activity of the contained **radon** should be measured accurately to insure correct dosage. Implants are usually left in the tissue as *permanent* implants. As already noted, the Rn loses almost all its activity in one month, the dosage being determined on this basis. The gold seeds remain in the tissues as non-irritating foreign bodies. Sometimes *removable* implants containing larger amounts of Rn are placed in or on a lesion and removed after a predetermined time to deliver the correct dose.

2. *Needles* are the most versatile type of Ra container, lending themselves to many different methods of application. They are hollow tubes provided with an eye at one end for threading and a point at the other. Radium is usually sealed inside the hollow shaft to form the *permanent* type needle (see Fig. 12.04). The needle wall consists of a platinum-iridium alloy, usually 0.5 mm thick. The *loading* of Ra needles, that is, the number of mg Ra/cm of active length has been more or less standardized. The most frequently used Ra loadings are 10 mg/cm for the so-called *high intensity* needles, and 0.66 mg/cm for the so-called *low intensity* needles. Other loadings are obtainable for special methods, such as the Manchester (Paterson-Parker) dosage system.

It must be emphasized that the external length of any Ra needle is always greater than its active length, that is, the length of the Ra within. The *active length,* being the true length of the Ra source, should be used in computing dosage.

3. *Tubes.* These are similar to needles, except for the absence of a point, but an eyelet is provided at one end for threading (see Fig. 12.04). Tubes are of two types, *permanent* and *sheath.* Ra is

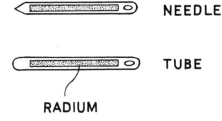

NEEDLE

TUBE

RADIUM

FIGURE 12.04. The construction of a permanent needle and tube.

sealed within the permanent tube, and is not removable. The sheath tube has a cap which can be unscrewed, and either Ra needles or Rn tubes inserted. Obviously, the sheath tube is a more versatile applicator than the permanent type and is, therefore, more widely used. The wall thickness is usually 0.5 or 1.0 mm platinum-iridium alloy.

4. *Plaques* are flat, hollow applicators with one face made of thin monel metal 0.05 mm in thickness, on the inner surface of which is permanently spread a layer of Ra (see Fig. 13.01). Plaques are available in various strengths and are used primarily for β therapy of superficial lesions.

DEFECTS IN RADIUM NEEDLES

Because of repeated use, Ra needles, as well as other containers, may be damaged to the extent that the air-tight seal is broken, permitting the escape of Rn gas. This may raise a serious problem of contamination. Therefore, any damaged Ra source should immediately be checked for *leakage* and, in any case, such tests should be made at least semiannually. A simple method is to place several needles or tubes in a glass container such as a test tube, insert a cotton ball in the top, and seal tightly with a rubber stopper. After 24 hours the absorbent material is tested with a survey meter by a method such as described by Rose (see page 629). Leaky sources should be sealed in unbreakable containers and returned to the manufacturer in accordance with his instructions. Obviously, when a damaged Ra source is found, the possibility of contamination of work areas, equipment, and personnel must be investigated.

Another type of defect in Ra sources is *faulty distribution* of the Ra salt, especially when it has been loaded as a powder. This may result from an error in fabrication, or from settling of the powdered salt near one end of a needle, especially when stored vertically. It can be detected by placing the needles on a sheet of film in the darkroom for one minute, then exposing briefly to a weak light directly above the film, the needles being left in position. This combines an autoradiograph of the Ra in the needles, with a photogram of the needles themselves to show the distribution of the Ra. Any needles showing serious non-uniformity of Ra distribution should be returned for repair. Incidentally, this same testing procedure may also detect radon leakage by showing a zone of fogging which spreads beyond the margin of the image produced by the γ radiation.

IMPLANT GAMMA-RAY THERAPY PLANNING

In introducing this important subject we must emphasize that implant therapy with discrete radioactive sources poses a serious radiation hazard for the therapist and the auxiliary personnel as well, especially in a busy practice. To minimize such exposure, various methods of **afterloading** have been designed in which the implant is made initially with empty devices such as metal or Teflon tubes. As soon as the therapist has achieved the desired distribution plan, he quickly introduces the radioactive sources into the hollow tubes.

We have already indicated that the Γ or specific γ-ray constant is based on a point source. However, in practical γ-ray therapy we are concerned with sources that have appreciable dimensions. The Γ of such finite sources will not be the same as that from a point source containing the same amount of Ra. In fact, the larger the source the smaller the R/mCi-hr at 1 cm, as will be proved later. The actual measurement of γ-ray exposure at various points on a Ra needle has only recently been accomplished by means of either a specially designed and calibrated scintillation probe or a thermoluminescent dosimeter, although it is usually possible to compute such doses on the basis of 8.25 R/mCi-hr at 1 cm. This may be done by considering a linear Ra source to be made up of an infinite number of discrete points, each of which is assumed to represent a point source (see Fig. 12.07). The exposure at any selected point P is then the summation of the exposures from all the points along the source. A complete summation can be made by the use of a computer. However, we can demonstrate this principle using simple arithmetic. In Figure 12.05 is shown a 1 cm Ra needle, and we are to determine the R/hr at point P at a distance of 1 cm on a line perpendicular to the needle at its center. The distances of P from various points along the needle

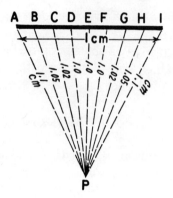

FIGURE 12.05. The distances of a given point P from various points in a linear radium source. The total exposure rate at P is the summation of the exposure rates from innumerable points in the source.

have been measured and are indicated in the diagram. We can now determine the R/mc-hr at P by means of the inverse square law, given that the Γ is 8.25 R/mCi-hr at 1 cm. For example, the contribution X from one end of needle A is obtained by setting up the following inverse square proportion:

$$\frac{X}{8.25} = \frac{1^2}{(1.1)^2}$$

$$X = \frac{1}{(1.1)^2} \times 8.25$$

$$X = \frac{8.25}{1.21} = 6.8 \text{ R/mCi-hr}$$

Similarly, we can find the R/mCi-hr contributions (neglecting oblique filtration) from various points along the needle to point P:

$$
\begin{array}{ll}
\text{A} & 6.8 \text{ R/mCi-hr} \\
\text{B} & 7.5 \\
\text{C} & 7.93 \\
\text{D} & 8.25 \\
\text{E} & 8.25 \\
\text{F} & 8.25 \\
\text{G} & 7.93 \\
\text{H} & 7.5 \\
\text{I} & \underline{6.8} \\
\end{array}
$$

9)69.21(7.7 av. R/mCi-hr

(Note the symmetry of the distributions on either side of the center of the needle.) Adding all these values and dividing by the number of points, 9 in this example, we obtain the average Γ for the 1 cm needle. This turns out to be 7.7 R/mCi-hr. The greater the number of points selected, the more accurate will be the average value of Γ.

In this computation we used the inverse square law. However, it should be emphasized that this law applies to a reasonable approximation only if the distance of P from the needle along the midline perpendicular is equal to or greater than twice the active length of the needle.

There is another correction that must be applied in the calculation of γ-ray dosage from a filtered linear applicator such as a tube or needle. Since the γ rays converge toward point P in the above example, those leaving near the ends of the source, as at A and I, travel more obliquely, passing through a greater thickness of filter and therefore undergoing more attenuation than would be expected on the basis of the inverse square law alone. An appropriate correction factor is therefore required for the average R/mCi derived above. Recently published tables of radium dosage include correction for oblique filtration. In addition, *radium isodose curves* may be plotted by computer.

The preceding discussion also explains why the exposure rate at point P is less than would be obtained if all the radium were concentrated at the needle's midpoint, in which case the Γ would be 8.25 R/mCi-hr.

Quimby System. Gamma-ray exposures at various points about linear sources, originally published by Quimby,[33] have been modified by Greenfield, Tichman, and Norman[36] and later converted to rads by Quimby and Goodwin[35] using a factor of 0.948 (see Table 12.03). To use these tables, we must understand the terminology employed. The letters across the top indicate various distances along the needle or tube, starting with A at the center. The left hand vertical column, headed "Distance from Tube (cm)" shows the shortest distance of the point of interest from the source. For example, in Figure 12.06 there is a 2 cm needle with the letters shown corresponding to the table. Point P is on a line perpendicular to the tube at point B. Referring to Table 12.03 we find that for a 2 cm tube, at a distance of 2 cm in the left column, the

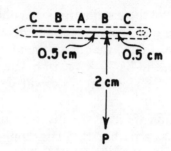

FIGURE 12.06. Explanation of terminology in Quimby's tables for linear sources.[33] This applies also to the modified tables in M. A. Greenfield, M. Tichman, and A. Norman.[36]

corresponding value under *B* is 1.75 rads/mg-hr, the γ-ray dose rate at point *P*. If the needle contains 10 mg Ra and is left in place for 8 hours, the absorbed dose will be $1.75 \times 10 \times 8 = 140$ rads. In other words, to obtain the dose, multiply the value shown in the table by the number of mg Ra in the tube and by the number of hours of exposure.

The same tables can be used for **radon** therapy if the treatment time is only a few hours. When therapy is longer than a few hours, we must find the mCi destroyed and convert to mCi-hr, by the familiar relationship:

$$\text{mCi destroyed} \times 133 \text{ hr} = \text{mCi-hr}$$

The mCi-hr may then be used in the same manner as mg-hr.

It must be emphasized that all γ-ray dosage systems are ultimately based on the dosage emitted by linear applicators. By mathematical consideration of various needle patterns, physicists have been able to arrive at fairly accurate systems of dosage. The two most widely used at the present time are:

1. Uniform placement of needles in rows, giving nonuniform radiation.

2. Placement of needles in a definite precalculated pattern, giving nearly uniform radiation.

These approaches to γ-ray dosimetry will be taken up separately for (1) surface applicators, (2) cavitary applicators, and (3) interstitial needles.

SURFACE RADIUM THERAPY

There are two general approaches in planning surface Ra therapy of superficial lesions. One is based on **uniform distribution** of sources according to the Quimby System, although this does **not** give uniform dosage. The other involves **nonuniform distribution** in specific patterns to achieve uniform dosage according to the Paterson-Parker (Manchester) System. These will now be described.

Quimby System. With this method we compute the doses at various critical points, using the data in the modified Quimby Table (12.03) for linear sources. Note that dose rates below the edges or corners of applicators with uniform distribution of radium may approach one-half those at the center. For example, in Figure 12.07, 4 radium tubes each with an active length of 3 cm and containing 3 mg Ra, are arranged in parallel rows covering an area of 9 cm². The problem is to find the doses at

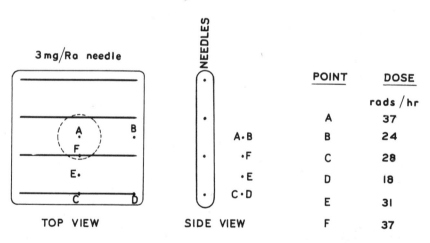

POINT	DOSE
	rads / hr
A	37
B	24
C	28
D	18
E	31
F	37

TOP VIEW   SIDE VIEW

POINTS A, B, C, D, E, F 1 cm BELOW PLANE OF NEEDLES.
MAXIMUM VARIATION IS BETWEEN A AND D, 100%.
CIRCLE ENCLOSES ZONE OF UNIFORM RADIATION DOSAGE.

FIGURE 12.07. Calculation of exposure rates at various points below a flat applicator, based on Quimby's modified tables for linear sources (see Table 12.03). Total dose at each point obtained by summation of doses from all the needles.

TABLE 12.03A
QUIMBY'S SYSTEM FOR LINEAR RADIUM SOURCES (MODIFIED)*
RADS PER MG-HR
0.5 mm Pt Filtration

Distance from tube (cm)	A	B	C	D	E	F	G	H	I	J	K
			Distance along tube axis (cm from center)								
	0	0.5	1.0	1.5	2.0	2.5	3.0	3.5	4.0	4.5	5.0
Active length 0.5 cm											
0.5	29.4	15.9	5.78	2.69	1.38	0.82	0.53	0.32	0.25	0.18	0.14
0.75	13.6	9.67	4.48	2.50	1.47	0.92	0.62	0.43	0.30	0.24	0.19
1.0	7.84	6.28	3.96	2.26	1.41	0.93	0.65	0.46	0.33	0.26	0.20
1.5	3.48	3.14	2.42	1.71	1.18	0.85	0.63	0.44	0.38	0.28	0.23
2.0	1.98	1.88	1.57	1.25	0.95	0.74	0.57	0.45	0.34	0.28	0.23
2.5	1.27	1.22	1.00	0.92	0.77	0.61	0.50	0.39	0.32	0.27	0.23
3.0	0.88	0.85	0.79	0.70	0.62	0.51	0.42	0.36	0.29	0.26	0.21
4.0	0.50	0.49	0.47	0.44	0.39	0.34	0.31	0.27	0.24	0.21	0.18
5.0	0.32	0.31	0.31	0.29	0.27	0.26	0.23	0.21	0.19	0.16	0.15
Active length 1.0 cm											
0.5	24.6	17.2	6.60	2.84	1.47	0.83	0.55	0.35	0.21	0.16	0.10
0.75	12.4	9.67	5.20	2.68	1.52	0.96	0.62	0.43	0.33	0.24	0.18
1.0	7.40	6.21	3.98	2.36	1.44	0.96	0.67	0.47	0.34	0.26	0.20
1.5	3.42	3.10	2.44	1.74	1.22	0.86	0.63	0.47	0.37	0.28	0.23
2.0	1.96	1.85	1.57	1.26	0.98	0.73	0.57	0.45	0.35	0.27	0.24
2.5	1.26	1.21	1.09	0.93	0.76	0.62	0.49	0.41	0.33	0.27	0.23
3.0	0.87	0.85	0.79	0.70	0.61	0.51	0.43	0.35	0.30	0.26	0.22
4.0	0.49	0.49	0.47	0.44	0.39	0.35	0.31	0.27	0.24	0.21	0.18
5.0	0.32	0.31	0.30	0.29	0.27	0.25	0.23	0.21	0.19	0.17	0.15
Active length 1.5 cm											
0.5	20.6	17.1	8.12	3.28	1.63	0.91	0.57	0.37	0.25	0.15	0.10
0.75	11.0	9.37	5.68	2.95	1.63	1.00	0.66	0.45	0.32	0.25	0.17
1.0	6.75	6.00	4.14	2.51	1.56	1.00	0.68	0.48	0.35	0.27	0.21
1.5	3.30	3.05	2.43	1.76	1.24	0.89	0.64	0.48	0.36	0.29	0.23
2.0	1.90	1.80	1.57	1.26	0.98	0.75	0.58	0.46	0.36	0.28	0.24
2.5	1.24	1.19	1.08	0.93	0.76	0.63	0.50	0.45	0.33	0.27	0.23
3.0	0.86	0.84	0.78	0.70	0.61	0.51	0.43	0.36	0.29	0.28	0.22
4.0	0.49	0.48	0.47	0.44	0.39	0.35	0.31	0.28	0.25	0.21	0.19
5.0	0.31	0.31	0.30	0.29	0.27	0.26	0.23	0.21	0.19	0.17	0.15
Active length 2.0 cm											
0.5	17.3	15.8	10.1	4.05	1.85	1.01	0.60	0.38	0.26	0.16	0.11
0.75	9.68	8.79	6.17	3.36	1.82	1.07	0.69	0.47	0.33	0.26	0.18
1.0	6.21	5.72	4.31	2.70	1.65	1.06	0.72	0.50	0.37	0.27	0.21
1.5	3.10	2.93	2.42	1.82	1.30	0.93	0.67	0.50	0.38	0.29	0.24
2.0	1.85	1.75	1.55	1.26	1.00	0.77	0.59	0.46	0.36	0.29	0.24
2.5	1.21	1.17	1.07	0.92	0.77	0.63	0.50	0.42	0.33	0.27	0.24
3.0	0.85	0.83	0.78	0.70	0.61	0.52	0.44	0.36	0.30	0.26	0.22
4.0	0.49	0.48	0.47	0.43	0.39	0.36	0.31	0.27	0.25	0.20	0.18
5.0	0.31	0.31	0.30	0.29	0.27	0.26	0.23	0.21	0.19	0.17	0.15

*From Goodwin, P. N., *et al.*: *Physical Foundations of Radiology,*[35] 1970. Courtesy of the authors and Harper & Row, Publishers, New York..

TABLE 12.03A (continued)
QUIMBY'S SYSTEM FOR LINEAR RADIUM SOURCES (MODIFIED)*
RADS PER MG-HR
0.5 mm Pt Filtration

Distance from tube (cm)	A	B	C	D	E	F	G	H	I	J	K
				Distance along tube axis (cm from center)							
	0	0.5	1.0	1.5	2.0	2.5	3.0	3.5	4.0	4.5	5.0
5.0	0.27	0.27	0.27	0.26	0.24	0.22	0.21	0.19	0.17	0.15	0.14
				Active length 2.5 cm							
0.5	14.6	13.9	11.0	5.33	2.24	1.16	0.65	0.42	0.27	0.18	0.12
0.75	8.53	8.05	6.40	3.89	2.08	1.19	0.75	0.50	0.35	0.25	0.19
1.0	5.65	5.33	4.35	2.96	1.82	1.15	0.76	0.53	0.38	0.28	0.22
1.5	2.96	2.80	2.40	1.87	1.36	0.96	0.70	0.51	0.40	0.30	0.25
2.0	1.77	1.72	1.53	1.27	1.01	0.80	0.61	0.47	0.37	0.29	0.25
2.5	1.19	1.15	1.05	0.91	0.78	0.64	0.51	0.41	0.34	0.27	0.23
3.0	0.84	0.82	0.77	0.69	0.61	0.52	0.44	0.37	0.31	0.26	0.22
4.0	0.48	0.47	0.46	0.43	0.39	0.36	0.31	0.28	0.25	0.21	0.19
5.0	0.31	0.31	0.30	0.28	0.27	0.25	0.23	0.21	0.19	0.17	0.16
				Active length 3.0 cm							
0.5	12.8	12.4	11.0	6.87	2.88	1.35	0.75	0.45	0.29	0.20	0.13
0.75	7.58	7.32	6.35	4.42	2.44	1.36	0.82	0.54	0.37	0.26	0.21
1.0	5.15	4.95	4.30	3.10	2.04	1.26	0.82	0.57	0.41	0.29	0.23
1.5	2.75	2.66	2.35	1.90	1.43	1.01	0.78	0.54	0.41	0.32	0.25
2.0	1.69	1.65	1.50	1.28	1.03	0.82	0.63	0.48	0.39	0.30	0.25
2.5	1.15	1.12	1.03	0.92	0.78	0.64	0.53	0.43	0.35	0.28	0.24
3.0	0.82	0.80	0.76	0.69	0.61	0.52	0.45	0.38	0.31	0.27	0.23
4.0	0.47	0.47	0.46	0.43	0.39	0.35	0.31	0.27	0.25	0.22	0.19
5.0	0.31	0.30	0.28	0.28	0.27	0.26	0.23	0.21	0.19	0.17	0.15
				Active length 4.0 cm							
0.5	10.1	10.0	9.47	8.32	5.27	2.21	1.04	0.59	0.35	0.24	0.16
0.75	6.17	6.05	5.72	5.92	3.42	1.92	1.07	0.66	0.44	0.30	0.22
1.0	4.31	4.22	3.94	3.39	2.49	1.60	1.01	0.66	0.47	0.34	0.25
1.5	2.42	2.38	2.24	1.93	1.54	1.16	0.83	0.61	0.46	0.34	0.27
2.0	1.55	1.51	1.42	1.26	1.08	0.86	0.67	0.53	0.41	0.33	0.27
2.5	1.07	1.04	0.99	0.90	0.79	0.66	0.55	0.46	0.37	0.30	0.25
3.0	0.78	0.78	0.77	0.73	0.67	0.61	0.46	0.39	0.32	0.27	0.23
4.0	0.47	0.46	0.44	0.42	0.39	0.35	0.31	0.28	0.25	0.22	0.19
5.0	0.30	0.30	0.29	0.28	0.27	0.25	0.23	0.21	0.19	0.17	0.16
				Active length 5.0 cm							
0.5	8.15	8.13	8.00	7.65	6.75	4.38	1.81	0.85	0.48	0.29	0.20
0.75	5.16	5.12	4.99	4.68	4.02	2.80	1.56	0.88	0.55	0.37	0.26
1.0	3.68	3.63	3.52	3.23	2.78	2.05	1.33	0.84	0.57	0.39	0.29
1.5	2.14	2.11	2.03	1.87	1.61	1.30	0.97	0.71	0.52	0.39	0.29
2.0	1.40	1.39	1.33	1.22	1.08	0.91	0.74	0.58	0.47	0.36	0.28
2.5	0.99	0.98	0.94	0.85	0.79	0.68	0.58	0.48	0.40	0.32	0.27
3.0	0.73	0.72	0.69	0.65	0.60	0.53	0.47	0.40	0.34	0.28	0.25
4.0	0.45	0.44	0.43	0.41	0.38	0.35	0.32	0.28	0.26	0.23	0.20
5.0	0.29	0.29	0.28	0.27	0.26	0.25	0.23	0.21	0.19	0.18	0.16

TABLE 12.03B
QUIMBY'S SYSTEM FOR LINEAR RADIUM SOURCES (MODIFIED)*
RADS PER MG-HR
1.0 mm Pt Filtration

Distance from tube (cm)	A	B	C	D	E	F	G	H	I	J	K
				Distance along tube axis (cm from center)							
	0	0.5	1.0	1.5	2.0	2.5	3.0	3.5	4.0	4.5	5.0
Active length 0.5 cm											
0.5	26.4	13.9	4.70	1.88	0.95	0.49	0.32	0.14	0.14	0.08	0.03
0.7	12.2	8.60	4.18	2.01	1.11	0.66	0.38	0.28	0.19	0.14	0.08
1.0	7.03	5.60	3.34	1.92	1.12	0.71	0.47	0.33	0.21	0.20	0.10
1.5	3.14	2.88	2.12	1.49	1.01	0.69	0.51	0.37	0.26	0.21	0.11
2.0	1.78	1.70	1.40	1.09	0.84	0.62	0.48	0.33	0.31	0.21	0.17
2.5	1.15	1.10	0.98	0.83	0.65	0.54	0.43	0.33	0.27	0.22	0.18
3.0	0.80	0.77	0.71	0.63	0.53	0.44	0.37	0.30	0.26	0.21	0.17
4.0	0.45	0.44	0.43	0.39	0.35	0.31	0.27	0.24	0.21	0.17	0.15
5.0	0.28	0.28	0.27	0.26	0.25	0.22	0.20	0.18	0.17	0.14	0.13
Active length 1.0 cm											
0.5	22.0	15.0	5.41	2.12	0.99	0.53	0.30	0.18	0.12	0.08	0.06
0.75	11.2	8.56	4.43	2.17	1.15	0.68	0.43	0.27	0.19	0.13	0.08
1.0	6.62	5.51	3.49	2.00	1.18	0.74	0.47	0.33	0.24	0.17	0.12
1.5	3.06	2.78	2.15	1.50	1.04	0.72	0.50	0.37	0.27	0.21	0.16
2.0	1.75	1.66	1.41	1.11	0.84	0.64	0.48	0.36	0.28	0.22	0.18
2.5	1.14	1.09	0.97	0.82	0.68	0.54	0.43	0.34	0.26	0.22	0.18
3.0	0.79	0.77	0.71	0.62	0.53	0.44	0.37	0.30	0.26	0.22	0.17
4.0	0.45	0.44	0.42	0.39	0.35	0.31	0.27	0.24	0.21	0.18	0.15
5.0	0.28	0.28	0.27	0.26	0.25	0.23	0.21	0.19	0.16	0.15	0.13
Active length 1.5 cm											
0.5	18.1	15.0	7.35	2.51	1.11	0.59	0.32	0.20	0.11	0.09	0.05
0.75	9.80	8.30	4.92	2.43	1.25	0.71	0.44	0.28	0.21	0.13	0.09
1.0	6.08	5.32	3.59	2.13	1.25	0.77	0.50	0.33	0.25	0.17	0.13
1.5	2.97	2.73	2.14	1.55	1.05	0.75	0.52	0.38	0.28	0.21	0.16
2.0	1.72	1.62	1.40	1.10	0.84	0.64	0.48	0.38	0.28	0.23	0.17
2.5	1.12	1.07	0.96	0.82	0.67	0.54	0.44	0.34	0.27	0.23	0.18
3.0	0.78	0.76	0.70	0.63	0.53	0.45	0.37	0.31	0.26	0.22	0.18
4.0	0.45	0.44	0.42	0.39	0.35	0.31	0.27	0.25	0.21	0.18	0.16
5.0	0.28	0.28	0.27	0.26	0.25	0.23	0.20	0.19	0.17	0.15	0.13
Active length 2.0 cm											
0.5	15.0	13.8	8.56	3.32	1.33	0.64	0.35	0.21	0.13	0.08	0.06
0.75	8.60	7.81	5.37	2.81	1.42	0.80	0.47	0.30	0.20	0.13	0.10
1.0	5.50	5.02	3.73	2.39	1.35	0.82	0.53	0.35	0.25	0.18	0.13
1.5	2.88	2.61	2.16	1.58	1.11	0.78	0.54	0.39	0.29	0.22	0.17
2.0	1.66	1.58	1.38	1.11	0.87	0.66	0.50	0.38	0.29	0.23	0.19
2.5	1.09	1.05	0.96	0.82	0.67	0.56	0.44	0.35	0.28	0.23	0.18
3.0	0.77	0.75	0.69	0.62	0.54	0.46	0.37	0.31	0.27	0.22	0.18
4.0	0.44	0.44	0.42	0.39	0.35	0.31	0.27	0.25	0.21	0.18	0.16
5.0	0.28	0.28	0.27	0.26	0.25	0.22	0.21	0.19	0.17	0.15	0.13

*From Goodwin, P. N., *et al.*: *Physical Foundations of Radiology*,[35] 1970. Courtesy of the authors and Harper & Row, Publishers, New York.

TABLE 12.03B (continued)
QUIMBY'S SYSTEM FOR LINEAR RADIUM SOURCES (MODIFIED)*
RADS PER MG-HR
1.0 mm Pt Filtration

Distance from tube (cm)	A	B	C	D	E	F	G	H	I	J	K
				Distance along tube axis (cm from center)							
	0	0.5	1.0	1.5	2.0	2.5	3.0	3.5	4.0	4.5	5.0
				Active length 2.5 cm							
0.5	12.6	12.1	9.58	4.41	1.67	0.76	0.48	0.24	0.14	0.08	0.06
0.75	7.54	7.11	5.63	3.31	1.66	0.88	0.52	0.33	0.21	0.15	0.10
1.0	4.99	4.67	3.79	2.53	1.51	0.91	0.57	0.38	0.27	0.19	0.14
1.5	2.63	2.48	2.11	1.62	1.16	0.82	0.57	0.41	0.30	0.22	0.17
2.0	1.59	1.53	1.35	1.13	0.88	0.68	0.52	0.39	0.30	0.23	0.19
2.5	1.06	1.02	0.94	0.82	0.68	0.56	0.45	0.36	0.28	0.23	0.19
3.0	0.75	0.74	0.69	0.62	0.53	0.46	0.38	0.32	0.27	0.22	0.18
4.0	0.44	0.43	0.41	0.38	0.35	0.31	0.27	0.25	0.21	0.18	0.16
5.0	0.28	0.27	0.27	0.26	0.24	0.23	0.21	0.19	0.17	0.15	0.13
				Active length 3.0 cm							
0.5	10.9	10.5	9.48	5.90	2.26	0.95	0.47	0.27	0.16	0.09	0.07
0.75	6.69	7.37	5.56	3.80	2.01	0.96	0.59	0.36	0.23	0.16	0.11
1.0	4.49	4.33	3.73	2.73	1.84	1.09	0.63	0.45	0.27	0.20	0.15
1.5	2.46	2.36	2.08	1.66	1.22	0.86	0.62	0.44	0.29	0.24	0.18
2.0	1.53	1.47	1.33	1.12	0.90	0.70	0.53	0.41	0.31	0.25	0.19
2.5	1.02	1.00	0.92	0.82	0.68	0.56	0.47	0.37	0.29	0.24	0.19
3.0	0.74	0.72	0.67	0.61	0.53	0.46	0.38	0.32	0.27	0.22	0.19
4.0	0.43	0.43	0.41	0.38	0.35	0.31	0.27	0.25	0.21	0.19	0.16
5.0	0.28	0.27	0.27	0.26	0.24	0.23	0.21	0.19	0.17	0.15	0.13
				Active length 4.0 cm							
0.5	8.57	8.50	8.19	7.20	4.44	1.73	0.73	0.37	0.30	0.12	0.08
0.75	5.40	5.29	4.99	4.28	2.93	1.55	0.82	0.47	0.28	0.19	0.13
1.0	3.73	3.66	3.42	2.92	2.13	1.33	0.83	0.50	0.33	0.23	0.16
1.5	2.14	2.09	1.95	1.69	1.34	0.99	0.70	0.50	0.36	0.26	0.20
2.0	1.37	1.35	1.25	1.12	0.94	0.74	0.57	0.45	0.33	0.27	0.21
2.5	0.96	0.94	0.88	0.80	0.69	0.58	0.47	0.39	0.31	0.25	0.20
3.0	0.69	0.68	0.65	0.60	0.53	0.47	0.40	0.33	0.27	0.23	0.19
4.0	0.38	0.41	0.40	0.37	0.34	0.31	0.27	0.25	0.22	0.19	0.16
				Active length 5.0 cm							
0.5	7.00	6.96	6.86	6.48	5.78	3.58	1.38	0.59	0.29	0.17	0.09
0.75	4.48	4.44	4.32	3.83	3.47	2.37	1.26	0.66	0.38	0.24	0.16
1.0	3.16	3.13	3.03	2.81	2.39	1.73	1.10	0.66	0.42	0.27	0.19
1.5	1.88	1.85	1.78	1.63	1.40	1.11	0.82	0.58	0.42	0.30	0.22
2.0	1.24	1.22	1.18	1.07	0.95	0.79	0.63	0.48	0.38	0.29	0.23
2.5	0.88	0.87	0.83	0.77	0.69	0.60	0.51	0.41	0.34	0.27	0.22
3.0	0.65	0.64	0.62	0.58	0.53	0.47	0.41	0.34	0.28	0.24	0.21
4.0	0.40	0.40	0.38	0.36	0.34	0.31	0.28	0.25	0.22	0.20	0.17
5.0	0.27	0.27	0.26	0.29	0.24	0.22	0.21	0.19	0.17	0.15	0.14

various points in a plane 1 cm from the tubes. This would correspond to a clinical problem in which a 3×3 cm^2 Ra plaque is applied at 1 cm from the skin, parallel to its surface. We would need to know the doses delivered at various points on the skin beneath the plaque. Using Quimby's tables for linear sources (see Table 12.03), we calculate the contribution of each tube separately to given points such as A, B, C, D, E, and F. The dose rates from each tube to point A are first added and divided by 4 to obtain the average rads/mg-hr. This is then multiplied by the total mg-hr to obtain the actual dose in rads at point A. Similarly, the doses at the other points can be computed. It is evident that the lowest dose rate is under the corners of the active area of the plaque, corresponding to D, where it is 20 rads/mg-hr. Under the center of plaque, A, the dose rate is 37 rads/mg-hr. Thus, the dose beneath the corners of the plaque is about one-half that beneath the center.

Note that the area of the plaque is 9 cm^2. This irradiates uniformly an 0.8 cm^2 area directly beneath the center, but at a distance of only 0.5 cm beyond this area, the dose has already dropped off about 15 percent. Obviously, this method of surface irradiation can be utilized properly only if the therapist is fully aware of its limitations. In the example just quoted, the treatment time would have to be increased 12 percent over that required for adequate irradiation of the center, to irradiate adequately point C. In order to irradiate point D with a sufficient dose, the dose under A would have to be doubled. Crossing the inactive ends of the sources improves significantly the uniformity of dosage distribution below the applicator.

Paterson-Parker (Manchester) System. To improve the homogeneity of irradiation by discrete sources, Paterson and Parker[64] published, in 1934, a new dosage system in which the Ra sources are distributed in nonuniform patterns. With this method, the maximum variation in dosage over the treated *surface* does not exceed ± 10 percent, provided their rules are carefully observed. If a particular distribution pattern falls within 25 percent of the ideal according to this system, homogeneity of irradiation is not significantly impaired.

The applicator's active surface must be parallel to the treated surface at any selected treatment distance. Furthermore, the treatment distance must be accurately measured and maintained because even slight errors in distance introduce large errors in dosage. The specific rules for external flat applicators follow.

1. **Circles.** Whenever possible, the applicator should be circular. The Ra tubes are arranged uniformly about the circumference, with the ends of the tubes no farther apart than the treatment distance. A minimum of 6 tubes is required. The distribution of additional Ra within the circle depends on the ratio of the diameter of the circular applicator to the treatment distance *h*. The following rules hold:

    a. *Diameter/h* = less than 3—all Ra at periphery
    b. *Diameter/h* = 3 to 6—5% of Ra at center
                      95% of Ra at periphery
    c. *Diameter/h* = more than 6—Ra in 2 concentric circles
                                and center, as follows:

        1) 3% of Ra at center
        2) Percent of Ra in outer circle according to the following scheme:
            if outer diameter = 6*h*, outer circles 80% of Ra
            if outer diameter = 7.5*h*, outer circle 75% of Ra
            if outer diameter = 10*h*, outer circle 70% of Ra
        3) Inner circle gets remainder of Ra, its diameter being ½ the outer circle

These relationships are shown schematically in Figure 12.08. In general, for circular surface applicators, distribution is optimal when **distance/h = 2.83.**

The Paterson-Parker System is impractical at very short distances when the diameter is more than 6*h*. However, a simple modification by Paterson, shown in Figure 12.09, is applicable although it is not accurate within the ± 10 percent variation specified for the system.

Oddie[62] has shown that small circular lesions no larger than 2.5 cm in diameter can be uniformly irradiated at a distance of 0.5 or 1.0 cm by 3 needles arranged in an equilateral triangle. The needles must have an active length equal to the diameter of the circle, while the sides of the triangle are 1⅓ times the length

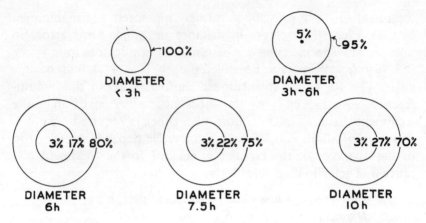

FIGURE 12.08. Distribution of radium in circular surface applicators, depending on the ratio of the applicator diameter to height (*h*) above the lesion. Paterson-Parker system.[64]

of the needles, the ends being open (see Fig. 12.10). Special tables are required.

2. *Squares.* Radium distributed uniformly about perimeter. Disregard space between ends if not greater than the treatment distance *h*.

    a. Side no greater than 2*h*, place all Ra at perimeter.
    b. Side greater than 2*h*, add parallel lines of Ra, dividing area into strips = 2*h*.
        1) If one added line, its linear density in mg/cm should be 1/2 that of periphery.
        2) If two added lines, their linear density in mg/cm should be 2/3 that of the periphery.

These relationships are illustrated in Figure 12.11.

3. *Rectangles.* Same rules as for squares, but add lines parallel to long side and correct for elongation according to the following rule:

        Ratio of Sides 2:1   add 5% mg-hr
        Ratio of Sides 3:1   add 9% mg-hr
        Ratio of Sides 4:1   add 12% mg-hr

4. *Irregular Areas.* If the shape approaches a rectangle, use

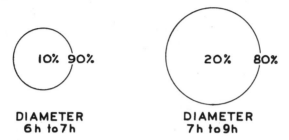

FIGURE 12.09. Modification of Paterson-Parker System for surface applicators at very short distances.[66]

the rules for rectangles. If the shape is elliptical, treat as a circle, averaging the major and minor diameters of the ellipse.

For *curved applicators,* the rules are as follows:

1. *Convex Areas.* For curves up to a hemisphere or semi-cylinder, the rules for flat surfaces apply, with this modification: the amount of Ra should be determined from the tables for the treated area, but it should be distributed over the larger but corresponding surface of the applicator, as shown in Figure 12.12.

2. *Concave areas.* In this case, the area of the applicator itself is used to arrive at the dosage, regardless of the size of the lesion. If the area treated is much larger than the area of the applicator (i.e. a highly curved surface) it may be preferable to use a tube or a point source at a longer distance *h*.

Having determined the size and shape of the applicator, treatment distance, and distribution of the Ra, we can now find the actual dosage from Paterson-Parker Tables for surface therapy (see Table 12.04). If the plan has been carried out according to the above rules, we have only to find the *area* in the left vertical

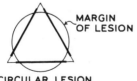

CIRCULAR LESION
DIAMETER < 2.5 cm
h = 0.5 or 1.0 cm
TUBES OR NEEDLES IN TRIANGLE
ACTIVE LENGTH = DIAMETER
LENGTH OF SIDE OF TRIANGLE = 1⅓ DIAMETER

FIGURE 12.10. Oddie's modification of the Paterson-Parker system for uniform irradiation at very short distances (0.5 to 1.0 cm) with applicators smaller than 2.5 cm in diameter.[62]

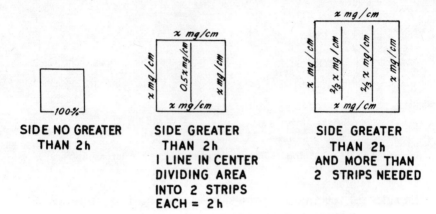

FIGURE 12.11. Distribution of radium in square applicators, depending on the ratio of the length of the side of the applicator to the height (*h*) above the lesion. Paterson-Parker system.[64]

column and read the number below ***treatment distance*** corresponding to this area. The number shown in the table is the number of mg-hr for 1,000 rads at the treatment distance, the variation over the treated surface falling within ± 10 percent. An example may help to clarify this. Suppose we have a 2 cm lesion on the skin, to be treated by a flat radium mold 4 cm in diameter. The surface dose is to be 5,500 rads in 8 days, with the mold at a distance of 1 cm for about 8 hours daily. Then:

Treatment area is $\pi r^2 = 3.14 \times 2 \times 2 = 12.6 \text{ cm}^2$
From Table 12.04, at 1 cm distance,
    1,000 rads requires 525 mg-hr (by interpolation)
    5,500 rads requires $5.5 \times 525 \approx 2890$ mg-hr

Since the mold is to be applied approximately 8 hours per day for 8 days, the total exposure time is 64 hrs and the applicator will contain about 2,890/64 = 45 mg Ra.

The ratio of the diameter to the distance is 4/1; therefore, a single circle with 95 percent and a central spot with 5 percent are required.

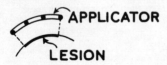

APPLICATOR

LESION

FIGURE 12.12. For a convex area, radium calculated for lesion area is distributed over larger applicator area.

The circumference of the applicator is $2\pi r = 12.6$ cm. Eight 5-mg tubes (active length 0.85 cm) may be placed on circle = 40 mg, with active ends less than 1 cm apart (see Fig. 12.13). The central Ra, c, may be found as follows:

$$c = 0.05 \times total\ Ra$$
$$c = 0.05(c + 40)\ \text{mg}$$
$$c = 0.05c + 2.20\ \text{mg}$$
$$0.95c = 2.20\ \text{mg}$$
$$c \approx 2\ \text{mg, to a sufficient degree of accuracy.}$$

Hence, two 1-mg tubes may be placed at the center. The total Ra actually used is 42 mg, slightly less than that approximated above,

TABLE 12.04
AREA SOURCES
MANCHESTER SYSTEM OF RADIUM DOSAGE*
PATERSON AND PARKER TABLES SHOWING MG-HR PER 1000 RADS FOR
SURFACE APPLICATORS OF DIFFERENT SIZES, AND VARIOUS
TREATMENT DISTANCES MEASURED ALONG A LINE
PERPENDICULAR TO THE CENTER OF THE SOURCE.
Filtration = 0.5 mm Pt

			Treatment Distance in cm					
Area	0.5	1.0	1.5	2.0	2.5	3.0		
cm^2							*Filtration Corrections*	
0	32	127	285	506	792	1140		
1	72	182					*(Multiply mg-hr for 0.5 mm*	
2	103	227	399	636	920	1274	*Pt by Factor Shown, to*	
3	128	263					*Obtain Correct mg-hr*	
4	150	296	492	743	1032	1389	*for Any Given Filter)*	
5	171	326						
6	188	354	570	832	1134	1495	*Filter*	
7	204	382					*Used*	*Correction*
8	219	409	637	910	1229	1596	*mm Pt*	*Factor*
9	235	434						
10	250	461	697	982	1314	1692	0.3	0.96
11	264	485					0.5	1.00
12	278	511	755	1053	1396	1780	0.8	1.06
13	292	534					1.0	1.10
14	306	558	813	1120	1475	1865	1.5	1.20
15	321	581					2.0	1.30
16	335	602	866	1184	1553	1947		
17	349	622						
18	364	644	918	1245	1623	2027		
19	378	663						
20	392	682	968	1303	1690	2106		

*From Meredith, W. J.: *Radium Dosage. The Manchester System*,[56] 1958. By permission of E. & S. Livingstone, Ltd., Publisher, Edinburgh and London. The original data have been multiplied by the factor 1.064, to correct for the latest value of Ra Γ (8.25 R/mg-hr at 1 cm) and to convert to rads ($f_{Ra} = 0.957$). Larger areas and distances have been omitted because teletherapy is more likely to be used.

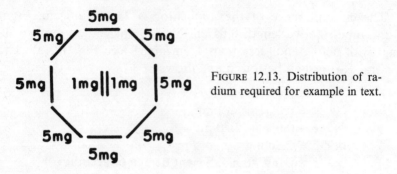

FIGURE 12.13. Distribution of radium required for example in text.

and filtration is 1 mm Pt. Therefore the exposure time must be increased 10 percent for the smaller Ra loading, and another 10 percent for increased filtration, for a total of $64 \times (1.10)^2 \doteq 77$ hr. As the mold is to be applied daily for 8 days, each application will be $77/8 = 9.6$ hr daily. The final distribution of the Ra appears in Figure 12.13.

Several important points need to be emphasized in the application of the Paterson-Parker System in surface therapy:

1. The *radium sources* available in the Radiology Department may not be suitable because there is not a sufficient variety to fulfill the distribution laws in all cases. As a matter of fact, this is one of the weaknesses inherent in the Paterson-Parker System, namely, that it requires a large variety of tubes or needles, both as to the Ra content and linear density. This may be handled in part by preparing a few standard applicators to serve for the usual type of lesion to be treated.

2. *Filtration* is a very important consideration, as with other systems. The tables are based on 0.5 mm Pt or its equivalent. Correction factors for various filters are shown in Table 12.05 for surface therapy only.

3. The *area* of the applicator should be such that it extends 1 to 2 cm beyond the edge of the lesion to insure irradiation of an adequate margin. Whenever possible, arrange to have the diameter of the applicator 2.8 to 3 times the treatment distance to permit all the Ra to be placed at the periphery in the form of a ring. A hole cut in the center of the applicator permits observation of the lesion.

4. The Paterson-Parker System specifies nonuniform distribu-

TABLE 12.05
SURFACE THERAPY
CORRECTION FACTORS TO BE APPLIED WHEN MATERIALS OR
THICKNESSES OTHER THAN 0.5 MM PT ARE USED AS FILTERS
WITH RADIUM SOURCES. TO FIND THE CORRECT MG-HR,
MULTIPLY THE MG-HR INDICATED FOR 0.5 MM PT
FILTRATION BY THE CORRECTION FACTOR

Metal	Thickness	Correction Factor
	mm	
	0.3	0.96
	0.5	1.00
Platinum or Gold	0.8	1.06
	1.0	1.10
	1.5	1.20
	2.0	1.30
	0.5	0.90
Lead or Silver	1.0	1.00
	2.0	1.10
	3.0	1.20
	0.5	0.65
Brass, Copper,	1.0	0.96
Monel, Steel	2.0	1.04
	3.0	1.10

tion of Ra to give reasonably uniform irradiation of even larger lesions. On the other hand, the Quimby System tends to over-irradiate the center of large lesions, and its use should therefore be limited to lesions only a few centimeters in diameter. However, a higher central dose may be advantageous because of the greater probability of hypoxia and impaired radiosensitivity of the tumor core. Also, the Quimby System is more practicable in the United States because of the limited loadings of Ra needles ordinarily available.

5. The Paterson-Parker System gives the actual dose, when modified for the latest value of Γ—8.25 R/mg-hr at 1 cm—and converted to rads by the f factor 0.957. As shown in Table 12.04, these corrections are made by multiplying the original Paterson-Parker values by 1.064. Note that this gives a dose 6.4 percent larger numerically than the exposure in R obtained from the original tables, a factor which should not be neglected in planning.

6. To find the dose at some depth below the surface, add this depth d to the distance of the applicator from the surface, the total being $d + h$. This new distance may be used to compute the

depth dose from the tables in the same way as the surface dose, since the small degree of absorption over the short distances involved is virtually compensated for by multiple scatter. However, the radiation delivered at a depth below the skin may not be so homogeneous as that on the surface.

INTRACAVITARY RADIUM THERAPY

Radium or radon γ-ray therapy may be applied through natural or artificial body cavities. The applicators are often in the form of tubes or needles, either single or multiple. In the latter, tubes may be strung in a row of sufficient length to cover the lesion. The arrangement of radioactive centers should be carefully planned to irradiate the lesion as uniformly as possible. Furthermore, since the percentage depth dose increases with increasing distance of the source from the surface, one should surround the radium applicator with the maximum convenient thickness of spacing material. Platinum filtration varies from 0.5 to 2 mm, but the added thickness beyond 0.5 mm probably contributes more to distance than to hardening of the γ rays. A material of low or medium atomic number, such as rubber or brass, may be used as a *secondary filter* to absorb the platinum secondary radiation.

With the usual linear intracavitary applicators, dosage calculations may be obtained from Paterson-Parker Tables for linear sources (see Table 12.06). It should be noted that these tables specify 0.5 mm and 1.0 mm Pt filtration. The data are in mg-hr for 1,000 rads, for tubes of various lengths, at various distances along a line perpendicular to the tube at its center. For example, let us find the dose delivered at a point 1.5 cm from the center of a tube with a 5 cm active length and 1.0 mm Pt filtration. According to the table, 536 mg-hr will be required for 1,000 rads (see Fig. 12.14). Note that this table does not specify the dosage anywhere other than that shown in Figure 12.14. It does not indicate the dose delivered opposite some other point along the tube axis, such as the end of the tube. *Filtration correction factors are not available for this table.*

As we have shown earlier in this chapter, Quimby's Table for linear sources provides much more information since it gives the

TABLE 12.06
LINEAR SOURCES
MANCHESTER SYSTEM OF RADIUM DOSAGE*
PATERSON AND PARKER TABLES SHOWING MG-HR PER 1000 RADS FOR DIFFERENT ACTIVE LENGTHS, AND
VARIOUS TREATMENT DISTANCES ALONG A LINE PERPENDICULAR TO THE CENTER OF THE SOURCE

Filtration 0.5 mm Pt

Active Length	Treatment Distance in cm						
	0.5	0.75	1.0	1.5	2.0	2.7	3.0
0.0	32	70	127	285	506	792	1140
0.5	35	74	129	289	509	795	1142
1.0	40	82	135	295	515	801	1151
1.5	50	92	147	305	529	813	1165
2.0	59	104	163	320	535	830	1185
2.5	68	119	179	340	569	851	1210
3.0	79	133	196	365	593	877	1237
3.5	89	149	216	392	620	908	1268
4.0	100	163	234	417	650	943	1300
4.5	112	180	254	444	683	980	1337
5.0	123	195	276	471	718	1018	1377
5.5	135	213	296	500	753	1068	1420
6.0	147	228	316	530	789	1101	1466
6.5	157	245	337	560	827	1145	1515
7.0	169	260	359	588	864	1190	1564
7.5	181	276	381	620	904	1234	1615
8.0	192	292	404	651	944	1281	1668
8.5	202	309	426	683	983	1328	1722
9.0	213	327	448	714	1025	1375	1776
9.5	224	343	470	747	1066	1424	1830
10.0	235	359	493	778	1109	1473	1888

Filtration 1.0 mm Pt

Active Length	Treatment Distance in cm						
	0.5	0.75	1.0	1.5	2.0	2.5	3.0
0.0	35	79	140	317	562	878	1264
0.5	42	83	144	321	567	882	1267
1.0	50	90	152	330	576	890	1277
1.5	59	103	166	340	589	903	1293
2.0	69	119	183	362	609	922	1313
2.5	80	136	202	384	633	950	1341
3.0	92	152	224	411	662	983	1372
3.5	106	171	247	442	696	1019	1409
4.0	119	188	270	471	732	1059	1450
4.5	132	206	295	504	769	1100	1495
5.0	146	227	319	536	812	1146	1545
5.5	160	246	344	571	853	1192	1596
6.0	172	265	369	606	898	1242	1651
6.5	185	284	394	643	943	1294	1709
7.0	199	304	420	679	990	1347	1768
7.5	213	324	446	715	1035	1403	1829
8.0	227	346	472	754	1084	1459	1890
8.5	240	366	499	792	1131	1514	1952
9.0	253	387	527	830	1181	1574	2015
9.5	268	408	553	869	1229	1631	2080
10.0	282	428	581	908	1277	1691	2149

* From Meredith, W. J.: *Radium Dosage. The Manchester System*, 1958.[56] By permission of E & S. Livingstone, Ltd., Publisher, Edinburgh and London. The original data have been multiplied by the factor 1.064, to correct for the latest value of Ra Γ (8.25 R/mg-hr at 1 cm) and to convert to rads ($f_{Ra} = 0.957$). The original tables include lengths greater than 10 cm.

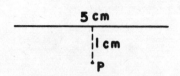

FIGURE 12.14. Paterson-Parker tables for linear sources give the number of mg-hr required to deliver 1,000 *R* at various distances, such as *P*, from the *center* of the source only.

dose rates at various distances on perpendiculars to a source of given length at 0.5 cm intervals along the axis of the source, and *even beyond its active length.* Furthermore, the data are inherently corrected for oblique passage of radiation through the filter. That section should be reviewed carefully and compared with Paterson-Parker Table for tube sources.

Data for linear sources are valuable in γ-ray therapy of such structures as cervix, uterine fundus, vagina, rectum, and maxillary sinuses. The diameter of the applicator should be as large as the patient can tolerate in order to improve the depth dose and to reduce the large error in dose that may result from small errors in distance. The Ra applicator may be placed at the center, surrounded by an adequate thickness of rubber or plastic. Noncompressible material should always be used so that the measured distance can be accurately maintained.

The dosage at various points in the volume of interest can be determined by the use of these charts even with various combinations of linear applicators. For example, most systems of Ra therapy for *carcinoma of the cervix* require (1) a linear source in the cervicouterine canal, and (2) a group of tube applicators deployed about the vaginal portion of the cervix. The majority

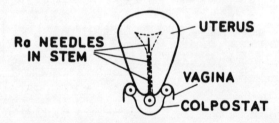

FIGURE 12.15. French method of irradiating the uterine cervix. Three needles are arranged in tandem in the cervicouterine canal, and three in the crossarm and colpostat against the cervix. All sources are alike in activity and active length.

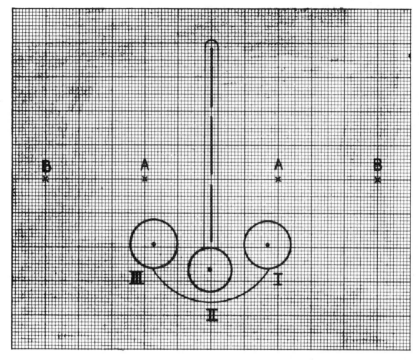

FIGURE 12.16. French type applicator for irradiation of the cervix. The doses at Tod's points A and B can be obtained by computation of the total doses contributed from the tandem and from the vaginal sources I, II, and III. A better concept of the dosage distribution is obtained by isodose plotting with a computer.

of present-day systems of cervical irradiation such as the Manchester Method[56] and the Ernst Applicator, specifying continuous irradiation or short term fractionation, are modifications of the original Paris Method of Regaud reported in 1929. The latter is the simplest, as shown in Figure 12.15. Dosage at various critical points may be computed from data for linear sources (see Table 12.06) or from published radium isodose curves. However, it is preferable to obtain dosage data by actual measurement in a tissue equivalent phantom for the type of applicator in use, by means of special dosimeters such as the thermoluminescent type, especially with the aid of a computer.

In 1938 Tod and Meredith[83] in England showed that the dosage to two particular points, known as Tod's points *A* and *B*, is

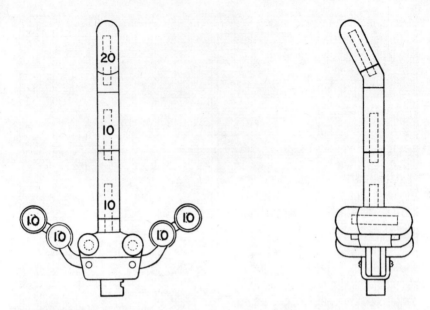

FIGURE 12.17. Diagram of Ernst expanding type cervicouterine applicator, with a useful loading for irradiation of carcinoma of the cervix. *A*. Front view. *B*. Side view.

critical for control of cervicouterine cancer (see Fig. 12.16). These points are defined as follows:

> ***Point A***—2 cm lateral to and above the external os.
> ***Point B***—3 cm directly lateral to point *A* (i.e. 5 cm lateral to the cervical axis)

It should be emphasized that these points are only a useful guide to therapy and do not, by any means, have absolute significance. In fact, they may fail when normal anatomic relationships are distorted by the bulk or position of the tumor.

The Ernst applicator is a very useful modification of the original Paris applicator, It has a segmented stem portion and an expanding vaginal portion that can be brought into close proximity to the lateral fornices. While it is extremely adaptable to the great majority of cervix cancers with only little or no adjustment, it is sometimes unsatisfactory for bulky or highly asymmetrical tumors. Figure 12.17 shows the applicator diagrammatically and includes a useful loading for carcinoma of the cervix in the earlier stages. Ernst originally published the exposure rates in R/hr at various points in the vicinity of the applicator with many different radium loadings. These data were obtained by actual measurement with a calibrated scintillation probe in a water phantom. However, there was an error of at least ± 7 percent. Included in the *Appendix* are a number of useful loadings with isodose distributions in rads per hour, obtained with the aid of a computer.

INTERSTITIAL RADIUM THERAPY

Although largely superseded by teletherapy with ^{60}Co and megavoltage X rays, interstitial therapy with discrete sources is still very useful in certain lesions such as those of the lip, skin, and oral cavity. Less often it may be used in the urethra and anus. Radium sources in the form of needles (or radon seeds) can be implanted directly into the tumor if it is reasonably small. As with surface Ra therapy, we should aim to distribute the sources so as to provide as homogeneous radiation as possible throughout the mass. Obviously we cannot entirely avoid zones of high dosage, called "hot spots," close to the sources; nor can we avoid zones of underdosage elsewhere. The objective of an acceptable system of interstitial therapy should be to attain an effective minimum dose, one which is cancericidal (destroys virtually all the cancer cells), without at the same time exceeding tissue tolerance in the vicinity of the hot spots. Ordinarily, when the hot spots are within the neoplasm, they may be disregarded. It is only when the points of maximum dosage fall within normal tissues that one must decide whether it is "safe" for those particular tissues.

A satisfactory system of interstitial therapy should provide reasonably homogeneous irradiation with a relatively simple plan of distribution of sources. Because of the inherent difficulty in implanting a tumor with mathematical exactness, the plan should not be so critical that a slight shift in the position of a source results in a large error in dosage. The distribution rules of the system should be so designed that the minimum dose can be readily computed without resorting to actual dosage measurement. In other words, the system should furnish the dosage data.

The problem is somewhat simplified in interstitial therapy by the fact that Ra γ-ray absorption by soft tissues almost equals the radiation scattered to them in the first few centimeters from the source. Therefore, the presence of tissues may be neglected in computing dosage, the Γ values in all being applicable without significant error. Thus, while the systems to be described were originally based on the old values of Γ for radium γ rays, these have been brought up-to-date by applying the latest value of Ra $\Gamma = 8.25$ R/mg-hr at 1 cm, and converting R to rads by the factor $f_{Ra} = 0.957$, for the Paterson-Parker System. Secondary X rays arising from the metal walls of the radium needles or seeds are difficult to measure and are disregarded.

It is impractical, in day-to-day clinical radiotherapy, to measure the dosage delivered by interstitial sources. Similarly, if we were to place Ra needles at random within the neoplasm and then try to calculate minimum dosage by summation of doses delivered by the needles according to the linear source tables, the task would be formidable, unless a computer were available. If an attempt is made to reconstruct needle distribution by means of models, this too becomes a time-consuming procedure which is of questionable value in routine therapy, although it may have educational merit for the student or resident.

Modern systems of interstitial Ra therapy obviate the problems mentioned above. There are at present three such systems. They all specify the distribution of the sources, area, or volume to be implanted, filtration, and number of milligram-hours required to deliver a certain minimum number of R or rads in the volume of interest. We shall devote the remainder of this section to a discussion of the three systems: (1) Paterson-Parker, (2) Martin, and (3) Quimby.

1. **Paterson-Parker System.** Using a method analogous to that proposed for surface therapy, Paterson and Parker[67] (1938) evolved a system based on the distribution of Ra according to very specific rules. If these are followed, the minimum dose is obtainable from appropriate tables (see Table 12.07) which Paterson and Parker derived mathematically. According to this system, two main types of implants are employed, one for needles distributed in one or more planes, and the other for sources imbedded in a volume of tissue in a definite pattern.

a. **Planar Implant.** The needles are arranged in either a single plane or in two parallel planes, to treat a flat, spreading lesion such as one might encounter in or near a surface. When the im-

TABLE 12.07
PLANAR IMPLANTS
MANCHESTER SYSTEM OF RADIUM DOSAGE *
PATERSON AND PARKER TABLES FOR INTERSTITIAL NEEDLE IMPLANTS
FILTRATION CORRECTION FACTORS HAVE BEEN MODIFIED
Filtration = 0.5 mm Pt

Area in cm²	mg-hr per 1000 rads	
0	32	**FILTRATION CORRECTIONS**
2	103	
4	150	*(Multiply mg-hr for 0.5 mm Pt by*
6	188	*Factor Shown, to Obtain Correct*
8	219	*mg-hr for Any Given Filter)*
10	250	
12	278	*Filter Used* · · *Correction*
14	306	*mm Pt* · · *Factor*
16	335	
18	364	0.3 · · 0.96
20	392	0.5 · · 1.00
22	418	0.8 · · 1.06
24	444	1.0 · · 1.10
26	470	
28	496	
30	521	
32	546	
34	571	
36	594	**TWO PLANE**
38	618	**SEPARATION FACTORS**
40	642	
42	664	*Separation* · · *Facto*
44	685	
46	708	1.5 cm · · 1.25
48	729	2.0 cm · · 1.4
50	750	2.5 cm · · 1.5

* From Meredith, W. J.: *Radium Dosage. The Manchester System,*[56] 1958. By permission of E. & S. Livingstone, Ltd., Publisher, Edinburgh and London. The original data have been multiplied by the factor 1.064, to correct for the latest value of Ra Γ (8.25 R/mg-hr at 1 cm) and to convert to rads (f_{Ra} = 0.957).

planted slab measures less than 1 cm in thickness, a single plane implant is adequate; if the slab measures 1 to 2.5 cm in thickness, a two-plane implant is required. For greater thicknesses, a volume implant should be done.

In a single plane implant, the minimum dose read from Table 12.07 applies to a slab of tissue 1 cm thick, with the needle plane in its center (see Fig. 12.18). The table indicates the number of mg-hr needed to deliver 1,000 rads ± 10 percent when the filtration is 0.5 mm Pt, correction being required for other filtrations. The same table also gives the minimum dose for two-plane implants, referable to the slab of tissue between needle planes, provided the separation between the planes is 1 cm. Correction must be made for other separations.

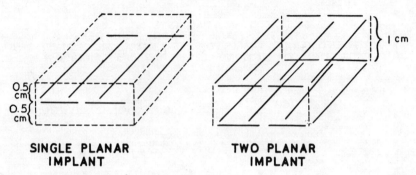

SINGLE PLANAR
IMPLANT

TWO PLANAR
IMPLANT

FIGURE 12.18. Single and two-plane interstitial radium implants according to the Paterson-Parker system.[67]

Distribution for planar implants depends on the area to be treated. If it is less than 25 cm², ⅔ of the Ra is placed around the margin and ⅓ is spread evenly over the area itself. For areas between 25 and 100 cm², ½ the Ra is placed around the margin and the other ½ evenly spread over the area itself. If the area exceeds 100 cm², ⅓ the Ra is placed around the margin and ⅔ is spread evenly through the area itself. The rules are shown diagrammatically in Figure 12.19.

The needles are to be arranged parallel to each other within the plane and, whenever possible, the ends should be crossed by needles at right angles. The parallel needles should be no more than 1 cm from one another or from the crossing ends (these distances refer to the active deposits within the needles). If the

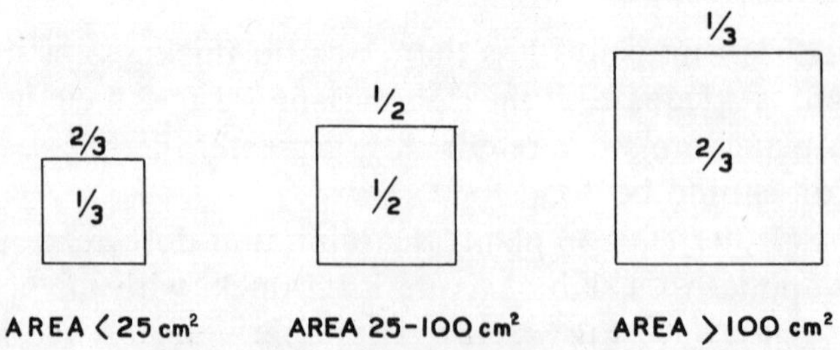

AREA < 25 cm²   AREA 25-100 cm²   AREA > 100 cm²

RADIUM DISTRIBUTION

	AREA < 25 cm²	AREA 25-100 cm²	AREA > 100 cm²
PERIMETER	⅔	½	⅓
CENTER	⅓	½	⅔

FIGURE 12.19. Distribution rules for interstitial radium according to the Paterson-Parker system.[67]

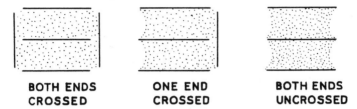

**BOTH ENDS
CROSSED**

**ONE END
CROSSED**

**BOTH ENDS
UNCROSSED**

FIGURE 12.20. Approximate radiation distribution depending on the crossing of the ends of the needles.

ends cannot be crossed, 10 percent must be deducted from the adequately irradiated area for each uncrossed end (see Fig. 12.20). When Rn seeds are used, they should be spaced about 1 cm apart in parallel rows.

In a two plane implant, the above rules hold for each plane. The space between the parallel planes should preferably be 1 cm, Table 12.07 indicating the minimum dose for this arrangement. For other separations, a correction factor is shown; the number of mg-hr for 1,000 rads must be multiplied by the appropriate correction factor. However, beyond 1.5 cm separation of the planes, homogeneity is impaired and therefore the tables show the percentage by which the midplane dosage (between the needle planes) is low. If both planes differ in area, the area for dosage purposes is the average of the two, and the Ra is distributed in proportion to each area.

Example 1. Single plane implant. Suppose we have a skin lesion and safe margin measuring 4×5 cm^2 and about 7 mm thick to be implanted with a single layer of radium needles. We wish to deliver 6,000 rads in about 7 days. Referring to Table 12.07 we find that a 20 cm^2 area requires 392 mg-hr per 1,000 rads for a single plane implant. Then

$$6{,}000 \text{ rads require } 392 \times 6 = 2{,}352 \text{ mg-hr}$$

$$\frac{2{,}352}{7 \times 24} = 14 \text{ mg Ra needed}$$

Since the area is less than 25 cm^2, $\frac{2}{3}$ must be placed at periphery.

$$\frac{2}{3} \times 14 \text{ is about 9 mg around margin}$$
$$\frac{1}{3} \times 14 \text{ is about 5 mg in lesion}$$

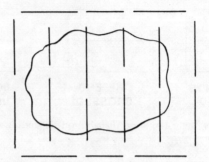

SINGLE PLANAR IMPLANT 4 x 5 cm²
0.5 mg/cm on periphery
0.33 mg/cm in center

FIGURE 12.21. Interstitial distribution of radium in example given in text.

These quantities of Ra may be arranged as shown in Figure 12.21, computed as follows:

> Perimeter of treated area = $(2 \times 4) + (2 \times 5) = 18$ cm
> Linear density of perimeter needles = 9 mg/18 cm = 0.5 mg/cm
> Center distribution 4 rows × 3 cm each = 12 cm total
> Linear density of central needles = 4 mg/12 cm = 0.33 mg/cm

Since we found above, on the basis of the Paterson-Parker Tables, that 2,352 mg-hr is needed to deliver a minimum dose of 6,000 rads in this problem, the total treatment time using 13 mg Ra (instead of 14 mg) is 2,352/13 or 180 hours.

If needles with the linear densities recommended in the preceding problem are not available, it may be possible to use other needles with appropriate distribution. Suppose, in the same example, only 0.66 mg/cm needles are available. Then, with 9 mg total needed for the periphery, and with the ends of the active deposits no more than 0.5 cm apart, the arrangement shown in Figure 12.22 may be used. The periphery will contain 14 cm of active length and $14 \times 0.66 = 9.24$ mg Ra.

The center can be covered by 8 needles of 1 cm active length, and will contain $8 \times 0.66 = 5.28$ mg Ra. The total amount of radium used is now $9.24 + 5.28 = 14.52$ mg. Since 2,352 mg-hr was required initially, the total treatment time is 2,352/14.52 = 162 hr with 14.52 mg Ra in the available needles.

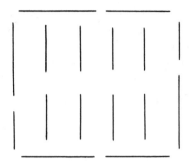

SINGLE PLANAR IMPLANT 4 x 5 cm²
ALL NEEDLES 0.66 mg/cm

FIGURE 12.22. Interstitial distribution of radium in same example as in Figure 12.21, modified for available needles.

It should be emphasized that it is not always possible to satisfy the requirements of the Paterson-Parker System unless a variety of needles with different linear densities are available. However, if a sufficient number of needles are stocked, having linear densities of 0.66 and 0.33 mg per cm, most planar lesions can be satisfactorily implanted.

Example 2. Two-plane implant. The calculations are similar to that for a single plant implant. If the distance between the planes is 1 cm, Table 12.07 gives the minimum dose midway between the planes. Suppose, in the preceding example, we had two planes separated by 1.5 cm. Then the dose would have to be multiplied by the factor 1.25. This would call for 2,352 mg-hr × 1.25 = 2,940 mg-hr. Since two planes are used instead of one, the linear density of the radium needles would have to be one-half that in a single plane implant, for a total treatment time of 2,940 mg-hr/14.5 mg = 203 hr, using 0.33 mg/cm needles throughout.

b. *Volume implant.* Since the two-planar implant does not provide homogeneous irradiation of lesions more than 2.5 cm thick, Paterson and Parker extended their system to include volume implants.[65] This applies to tumors in which the three dimensions are almost the same, and the tumor can be completely enclosed by Ra sources. Such lesions include, for example, tumors of the tongue or accessible lesions elsewhere. The most convenient shapes are the sphere, cube, and cylinder, the latter being most often employed. Homogeneity is represented by a 20 percent variation in dosage, except for localized hot spots near the radioactive sources. It must be emphasized that significant errors may arise during actual distribution of the needles because of the difficulty of conforming to the required geometric shape in every case.

Information in the Paterson-Parker Table for volume implants (see Table 12.08) is expressed, as before, in mg-hr per 1,000 rads, filtration being 0.5 mm Pt. The volume means the volume actually implanted and not the tumor itself.

TABLE 12.08
VOLUME IMPLANTS
MANCHESTER SYSTEM OF RADIUM DOSAGE*
PATERSON AND PARKER TABLES SHOWING MG-HR PER 1000 RADS WITH
CYLINDERS OF DIFFERENT VOLUMES. FILTRATION CORRECTION
FACTORS HAVE BEEN MODIFIED
Filtration = 0.5 mm Pt

Volume in cm³	mg-hr per 1000 rads	Elongation Factor	Elongation Correction
1	36		
2	58	1½	+3%
3	75	2	6%
4	91	2½	10%
5	106	3	15%
10	168		
15	220		
20	267		
25	311		
30	350		
40	425		**FILTRATION CORRECTIONS**
50	493		
60	556		*(Multiply mg-hr for 0.5 mm Pt by*
70	616		*Factor Shown, to Obtain Correct*
80	673		*mg-hr for Any Given Filter)*
90	729		
100	782		*Filter Used mm Pt* — *Correction Factor*
110	833		
120	883		
140	979		0.3 — 0.96
160	1069		0.5 — 1.00
180	1157		0.8 — 1.06
200	1240		1.0 — 1.10

*From Meredith, W. J.: *Radium Dosage. The Manchester System,*[56] 1958. By permission of E. & S. Livingstone, Ltd., Publisher, Edinburgh and London. The original data have been multiplied by the factor 1.064 to correct for the latest value of Ra Γ (8.25 R/mg-hr at 1 cm) and to convert to rads ($f_{Ra} = 0.957$). The original tables include volumes larger than 200 cm³.

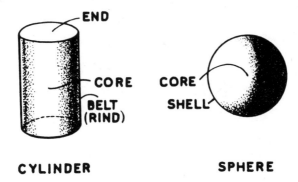

CYLINDER   SPHERE

FIGURE 12.23. Terminology used in the Paterson-Parker system for volume im-
implants.[65]

For distribution purposes, the cylinder comprises two zones,
an outer surface or **rind,** and an inner volume or **core.** The rind
includes the curved surface or **belt** and the two flat ends, as shown
in Figure 12.23. Needles, because of their length, are best distributed in a cylindrical pattern. If accurately calibrated radon
seeds are available, they may be distributed in a spherical volume.
The sphere is considered as having two parts, an outer surface or
shell and an inner volume or **core** (see Fig. 12.23).

In a cylinder, the total Ra is apportioned as in Table 12.09.

TABLE 12.09
DISTRIBUTION RULES FOR CYLINDERS, WITH VARIOUS
ARRANGEMENTS OF NEEDLES *

	Relative Distribution of Radium				*Computation of Volume*
Cylinder Type	*Belt*	*Core*	*End 1*	*End 2*	
Conventional cylinder (ends cross at *active* end of belt)	4	2	1	1	As outlined by belt and ends
Open end cylinder	4	2	1	0	Apparent volume minus 7½%
Cylinder, 2 open ends	4	2	0	0	Apparent volume minus 15%
Cylinder ends crossed at *inactive* tips of belt needles	4	2	2	2	Apparent volume
Cylinder tips crossed at 1 open end	4	2	2	0	Apparent volume minus 7½%

* From Morgan, R. H., and Corrigan, K. E.: *Handbook of Radiology,* 1955. Courtesy
of The Year Book Publishers, Inc., Chicago.

For example, if both ends of the implant can be crossed, distribution of Ra is as follows:

> Belt   4 parts (50%)
> Core   2 parts (25%)
> End I   1 part   (12.5%)
> End II   1 part   (12.5%)

The original system specifies that the needles in the end zones cross the **active ends** of the belt needles.

It is more practical to cross the **inactive tips** of the belt needles. Meredith and Stephenson[58] have accordingly modified the distribution of the radium sources as follows:

> Belt   4 parts (40%)
> Core   2 parts (20%)
> End I   2 parts (20%)
> End II   2 parts (20%)

The two types of arrangements are shown in Figure 12.24.

All sources must be spaced as evenly as possible around the belt, inside the implanted volume itself, and at the ends. At least 8 needles are required in the belt and at least 4 in the core. None of the sources should be closer than 1 to 1.5 cm. If the cylinder cannot be closed at one end, the adequately irradiated volume is decreased by 7.5 percent. If both ends must be left uncrossed,

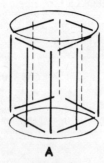
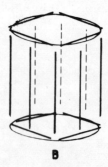

A   **B**

FIGURE 12.24. Distribution of radium needles in a cylindrical volume implant. The core needles have been omitted for simplicity. In *A* the active ends of the sources are crossed by the end needles, according to the original Paterson-Parker system.[65] In *B* the more practical method of crossing the inactive ends of the needles is shown, according to the modification of W. J. Meredith, and S. K. Stephenson.[58]

the adequately irradiated volume is reduced by 15 percent. Table 12.09 summarizes the distribution rules. The belt needles should extend well beyond the lesion at the open end to insure adequate irradiation of that portion of the tumor.

For cylinders in which the height is less than 1.5 times the diameter, no correction is needed, but with long narrow cylinders in which the height exceeds 1.5 times the diameter, the number of mg-hr must be increased by the corresponding elongation correction factor in Table 12.08. For example, a cylinder with a volume of 100 cm^3 requires 782 mg-hr per 1,000 rads. It has a height twice its diameter, or an elongation factor of 2. According to Table 12.08 this requires a correction of +6 percent:

$$782 \times 1.06 = 829 \text{ mg-hr, } corrected$$

If one has access to accurately calibrated radon seeds, a spherical volume containing the tumor may be implanted. The shell or outer surface of the sphere receives 75 percent of the total quantity of radon, the remaining 25 percent being distributed throughout the volume itself. The seeds should be spaced as evenly as possible, about 1 to 1.5 cm apart, on the surface and in the core.

Example. Volume implant—cylinder. A cancer of the tongue is to be treated in about 7 days, with a dose of 6,000 rads. The implanted volume will be a cylinder with a diameter of 3 cm and a height of 4 cm. Only the top can be closed, the needles crossing the inactive tips of the belt. Therefore, 7.5 percent is to be deducted from the volume of the cylinder to obtain the effective volume. The volume of the cylinder is found from the relation

$$V = \pi r^2 h$$

where V is volume, r is radius, and h is height of the cylinder.

$$V = 3.14(1.5 \text{ cm} \times 1.5 \text{ cm} \times 4 \text{ cm})$$

$$V = 28 \text{ cm}^3$$

The corrected volume after deducting 7.5 percent is 26 cm^3. According to Table 12.08, this volume by interpolation requires 319 mg-hr per 1,000 rads. Then 6,000 rads will require 6 × 319 or 1914 mg-hr. For a treatment time of about 7 days or 168 hours,

$1914 \div 168 \approx 12$ mg Ra is needed, distributed in the cylinder as follows:

Belt	$\frac{1}{2} \times 12 = 6$	mg
Core	$\frac{1}{4} \times 12 = 3$	mg
1 End	$\frac{1}{8} \times 12 = 1.5$	mg

The actual implant is derived as follows:

Belt—8 needles, each 4 cm long, active length 3 cm. If each needle contains 1 mg Ra, the total Ra content will be 8 mg, sufficiently close to the required 6 mg. Linear density is 1 mg/3 cm = 0.33 mg/cm.

Core—4 needles each 4 cm long, active length 3 cm. If each contains 1 mg Ra, the total in the core will be 4 mg, sufficiently close to the required 3 mg. Linear density 1 mg/3 cm = 0.33 mg/cm, same as in belt.

End—2 needles, 2 cm active length, each containing 1 mg Ra, for a total of 2 mg Ra. This approximates sufficiently the specified 1.5 mg. Linear density 1 mg/2 cm = 0.5 mg/cm.

Note that only two types of needles 0.33 mg/cm, and 0.5 mg/cm are required. The distribution is indicated diagrammatically in Figure 12.25. Since the total practical implant contains 10.5 mg Ra instead of a theoretical implant of 12 mg, the final treatment time will be 1914 mg-hr/10.5 mg = 182 hr.

A carcinoma surrounding a cavity such as the rectum or vagina can be treated by a combination of a cylindrical needle implant (belt) and a tube source in the center (core). The belt needles are inserted in the most peripheral part of the growth according to the rules for cylinder implants, and contain four parts of Ra.

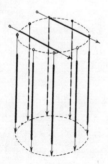

FIGURE 12.25. Distribution of radium needles in cylindrical volume implant, example in text. Belt—8 needles, each 1 mg in active length 3 cm. Core—4 needles, same as belt. End—2 needles, each 2 mg in active length 3 cm.

The tube source in the center should be surrounded by rubber or plastic so that its overall diameter is at least one-half the diameter of the whole cylinder, and should contain two parts of Ra. However, it is impossible in practice to leave the tube applicator in position in the rectum for longer than 48 hours, and it must therefore contain additional Ra to provide the correct mg-hr. This type of implant is rarely used at present except for small lesions or in palliative therapy of larger lesions.

2. *Quimby System.* Because of the already mentioned complexities of the Paterson-Parker System, and because it cannot be used for small lesions, requiring at least 8 needles in the belt and 4 in the core, Quimby[33] devised a method of interstitial volume therapy in which needles are distributed uniformly throughout the volume of interest. This sort of distribution produces a relatively greater central dose, but with small volumes the dosage difference between the center and the periphery of the implant may not be clinically significant. Furthermore, a larger dose at the center may be advantageous because, as will be shown later (see pages 569 to 571), the central zone of a tumor is likely to be anoxic and require a larger curative dose than the peripheral better oxygenated zone. In any case, if more uniform dosage is desired, the Paterson-Parker system should be used. Table 12.10 summarizes the data for the Quimby system. (See also Table 12.03.)

TABLE 12.10
MG-HR OF INTERSTITIAL RADIUM REQUIRED TO DELIVER 1000 RADS
IN VARIOUS VOLUMES, WITH FILTRATION OF 0.5 mm Pt (QUIMBY)*

Volume	Mg-hr 1000 rads	Diameter of Sphere	Mg-hr 1000 rads
cc		cm	
5	210	1.0	43
10	340	1.5	106
15	410	2.0	190
20	470	2.5	300
30	570	3.0	410
40	660	3.5	500
60	800	4.0	610
80	920	4.5	720
100	1060	5.0	840
125	1190	6.0	1140
150	1330	7.0	1490

* Originally published in *Physical Foundations of Radiology*[33] (Glasser, O., and others), 1959. Courtesy of Hoeber, Publisher, New York. The original data have been multiplied by 1.064 to correct for the latest value of Γ for Ra, and to convert to rads.

TABLE 12.11
STANDARD AMERICAN DIRECT-LOADED NEEDLES, LOW ACTIVITY
(COMPARE WITH TABLE 12.12)

Type	Radium	Active Length	Linear Density	Total Length
	mg	cm	mg/cm	cm
Short	1	1.6	0.66	2.77
Medium	2	3.2	0.66	4.4
Long	3	4.8	0.66	6.0

An advantage of the Quimby system is that any type of uniformly loaded needle can be used. It is particularly suited to the standard American needles in which linear density is 0.66 mg/cm for all sizes. Table 12.11 gives the specifications for low intensity needles.

For planar implants Quimby recommends uniform parallel arrangement of needles about 1 to 1.5 cm apart, or accurately calibrated Rn seeds 1 to 1.5 cm apart, The doses at certain critical points are determined from the table for linear sources (see Table 12.03). A minimum dose of 6,000 rads in one week is preferred, as with the other systems. The tolerance of the maximum dose or hot spots in a given implant must be determined by clinical judgment. When the low activity needles specified in Table 12.11 are used in a Quimby implant, it will be found that a minimum dose of 6,000 rads will be delivered in 7 days.

In volume implants based on Quimby's data, the needles should be uniformly distributed 1 to 1.5 cm apart either in plane layers, or in a cylinder. The space between planes should be no greater than 2 cm, and preferably 1.5 cm. The outermost needles should be at the tumor surface or just outside it. They should be long enough to extend beyond the lesion, and the ends should be crossed when possible. It must be emphasized that the dose read from the table is the minimum, and refers to the actual volume implanted. In a cylindrical implant, the height is the active length of the needles, and the diameter is outlined by the outermost needles in the implant. The same correction factors for uncrossed ends and for elongation of cylinders should be applied as in the Paterson-Parker System.

3. *Martin System.*[52] Just as with Quimby's System, the purpose of this system is to obviate the complexities inherent in the Pater-

TABLE 12.12
SPECIFICATION OF LOW ACTIVITY RADIUM NEEDLES
(CHARLES L MARTIN[52])

Type	Radium	Active Length	Linear Density	Total Length
	mg	cm	mg/cm	cm
Short	0.66	0.5	1.32	1.1
Medium	1.33	1.5	0.9	2.7
Long	2.4	4.0	0.6	5.1
Extra Long	3.0	4.5	0.67	6.0

son-Parker distribution requiring intricate planning and a stock of needles with various loadings. Martin's needles are specified in Table 12.12. Although it is not readily apparent, these needles represent uniform loading when actually implanted in the tissues. Figure 12.26 shows this in diagrammatic form. If a series of four short needles are lined up in a row with *inactive* ends touching, and a series of two medium needles arranged in similar fashion, almost the same number of mg Ra lies between the farthest separated active ends in each case. The overall linear density

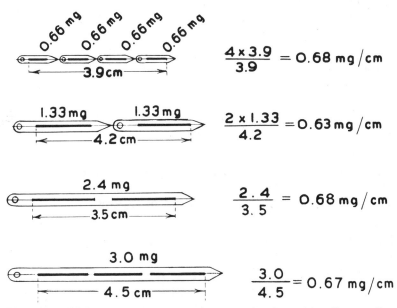

FIGURE 12.26. Average linear intensities of Martin's low intensity radium needles, when arranged end to end.

will therefore be nearly the same, provided the needles are applied end to end. They must not be inserted so that the active end of one needle meets the active end of the next needle because this would obviously result in a greater linear density. In fact, if the short needles were lined up without a space between the active ends, the linear density would be about twice as great.

The reason for uniform effective loading in Martin's technique is that the treatment time is constant, 168 hours. He has calculated that with these low intensity needles, arranged in parallel rows 1 cm apart, the minimum exposure of a slab of tissue 0.5 cm thick with the needle plane in its center, is 6,000 R. The maximum may be 12,000 R which he has found to be within tissue tolerance, especially since the hot spots occur within the tumor or close to its edge. For thicker lesions the needles can be inserted in two parallel planes, separated by a distance of 1.5 cm.

Thus, the Martin System furnishes a method of interstitial therapy that is relatively simple to execute, provides safe and adequate dosage in a conventional constant time, 168 hours, and does not require charts or complicated mathematical exercises once the operator has gained practical experience with it. However, unless the ends are crossed, the dosage falls significantly toward the open ends of the implant. If the ends cannot be crossed, *the implant length must be increased so the ends of the lesion receive adequate dosage* (see Fig. 12.07).

Martin also combines this type of interstitial radium implant (6,000 R) with about 2,000 R of 200-kV therapy delivered in 2 weeks.

Before leaving the subject under discussion, we may consider briefly the choice of 6,000 R in 168 hours as a standard exposure. Martin has shown that this exposure and time combination produces the same tissue effect as about 3.2 threshold erythema doses (T.E.D.) given within a few hours. Almost the same exposure in terms of T.E.D. is required with 200-kV X rays, which he showed clinically to be cancericidal for epidermoid carcinoma. Paterson and Parker also accept 6,000 R in 7 days as curative for most epidermoid cancers. Therefore, Martin adopted the standard 6,000 R in 168 hours, or 3.2 T.E.D., as the minimum cancericidal exposure for this type of tumor. Of course, if one wishes to deliver

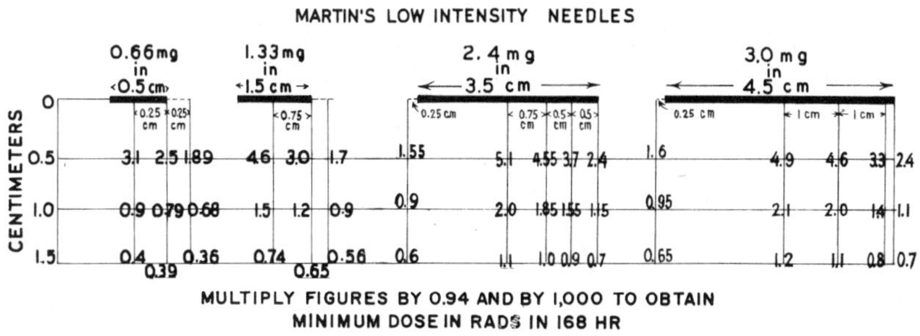

FIGURE 12.27. Depth doses obtained with Martin's low intensity radium needles, based on earlier value of Γ. To convert to modern R and to rads, multiply the indicated exposures by 0.94. (From Martin, C. L. and Martin, J. A.[52] (Courtesy of Charles C Thomas, Publisher, Springfield, Illinois.)

a larger minimum exposure, the total treatment time may be extended, but due care must be taken that the hot spots in normal tissue do not receive more than 12,000 R. This maximum holds good in the oral cavity and vagina. Rectal mucosa should not be subjected to more than 10,000 R in 168 hours. The doses at various points in the tissue can be readily calculated by summation from each needle, on the basis of Martin's[58] data (see Fig. 12.27), and conversion to the best value of R and to rads by multiplying by the factor 0.94.

IMPLANT THERAPY WITH ARTIFICIAL RADIONUCLIDES

In recent years, various radionuclides with sufficiently long half-lives have been used as substitutes for Ra in interstitial therapy. These include cobalt 60, cesium 137, gold 198, tantalum 182, and iridium 192. The same distribution systems that have been designed for Ra and Rn may be used with these radionuclides, provided dosage is modified for differences in filtration and Γ factors (see Table 12.13). However, the validity of at least some of the published Γ factors has been questioned (see pages 367 to 368).

The *advantages* of the radionuclide substitutes over Ra include:

1. *Availability* in a greater variety of forms, such as rods, wires, or beads. Ra is usually prepared as a powder which tends to pack toward one end of a needle or tube.

TABLE 12.13
SPECIFIC GAMMA-RAY CONSTANTS (Γ) FOR SOME RADIUM SUBSTITUTES

Radionuclide	Γ
	R/mCi-hr at 1 cm
Cobalt 60 (^{60}Co)	13.07
Cesium 137 (^{137}Cs)	3.24
Gold 198 (^{198}Au)	2.34
Tantalum 182 (^{182}Ta)	6.8
Iridium 192 (^{192}Ir)	5.1
Radium 226 (^{226}Ra)	8.25

2. **Safer** than **Ra.** Recall that Ra gives off a gas, Rn, which introduces the hazard of leakage through a damaged needle or tube. Similarly, breakage of a needle would permit the spill of the powdered Ra salt.

3. **Dimensions** comparable to Ra for encapsulation. By specifying the loading of the sources in terms of mCi Ra equivalent, dosage computation is greatly simplified. To find the number of mCi of any radionuclide equivalent to 1 mg Ra, we simply divide the Γ factor for radium by the Γ factor for the radionuclide. Thus,

$$\frac{\Gamma_{Ra}}{\Gamma_X} = \text{conversion factor}$$

where X is a particular radionuclide. Then,

$$1 \text{ mg Ra} \cong \text{mCi}_X \times \text{conversion factor}$$

Cobalt 60 should be used only when permanently sealed in a durable material such as 0.2 mm hyperchrome steel to prevent flaking of cobalt oxide with resulting contamination of instruments and environs. Because of the relatively light filtration and higher average γ-ray energy (av. 1.25 MeV), the oblique rays are less attenuated than the γ rays of the Ra series through platinum walls. Since the Γ factor for ^{60}Co is 13.07 R/mCi-hr at 1 cm, the Ra-to-^{60}Co conversion factor is 8.25/13.07 = 0.63. Hence,

$$1 \text{ mg Ra} \cong 0.63 \text{ mCi } ^{60}\text{Co}$$

so that when using the Paterson-Parker System with ^{60}Co needles or tubes, we must multiply the indicated mg-hr by 0.63. On the other hand, with the Quimby System, the rads/mg-hr must be divided by 0.63. However, if the ^{60}Co sources are expressed in terms of mg Ra equivalent, the tables for these systems may be used directly with an error of only a few percent. Since ^{60}Co has a half-life of only 5.3 years the output of the sources must be corrected at least every three months, decay being about 3.2 percent per quarter. This requires a complex inventory system, especially when new needles are added from time to time. Therefore this radionuclide is no longer highly regarded as a substitute for Ra.

Cesium 137 is becoming one of the more widely used substitutes for radium in implant therapy. It is usually prepared in the form of microspheres imbedded in ceramic and encased in stainless steel needles with 1.0 mm wall thickness. Its relatively long half-life of 30 years, with a decay factor of 2 percent per year, gives it a distinct advantage over ^{60}Co and other short-lived radionuclides which require frequent adjustment of exposure times and complicated inventory. Since the Γ factor for ^{137}Cs filtered by 1.0 mm stainless steel is 3.24 R/mCi-hr at 1 cm, the Ra-to-^{137}Cs conversion factor is 8.25/3.24 = 2.55. Thus,

$$1 \text{ mg Ra} \cong 2.55 \text{ mCi } ^{137}\text{Cs}$$

The data just given are from Krishnaswamy[49] who has published tables of dose distributions from ^{137}Cs sources in tissue. These are for needles of various lengths and are in the same format as the Quimby Tables for linear sources.

Cesium 137 emits γ rays with an energy of 0.662 MeV. While their transmission in soft tissues is nearly the same as that of Ra γ rays (av. energy 0.83 MeV), shielding is less difficult because of the absence of high-energy components.

Gold 198 is available in the form of "seeds" for implant therapy in much the same way as radon. The Γ factor for ^{198}Au is 2.34 R/mCi-hr at 1 cm, so that Ra-to-^{198}Au conversion factor is 8.25/2.34 = 3.53. Thus,

$$1 \text{ mg Ra} \cong 3.53 \text{ mCi } ^{198}\text{Au}$$

However, the seeds have a very short half-life of 2.7 days, and we must therefore compute the dosage on the basis of mCi destroyed.

The average life T_a of ^{198}Au may be obtained from the half-life T (64.8 hr) as follows:

$$T_a = \frac{64.8}{0.693} = 93.5 \text{ hr}$$

so if 1 mCi were implanted permanently, as is usually the case, it would give off the same total amount of radiation as if it had maintained constant activity over its average life. Hence,

1 mCi ^{198}Au destroyed = 93.5 mCi-hr

Since the Ra conversion factor was found above to be 3.53,

$$1 \text{ mCi } ^{198}\text{Au destroyed} = \frac{93.5}{3.53} = 26.5 \text{ mg-hr Ra}$$

or,

1 mg-hr Ra = 1/26.5 = 0.04 mCi ^{198}Au destroyed

Tantalum 182 has been used as a Ra substitute, but because of its short half-life of 115 days, it cannot be stored except for short periods of time. It emits β^- particles which must be removed by filtration, and a spectrum of γ rays from 0.05 to 1.24 MeV. Its Γ factor is 6.8 R/mCi-hr at 1 cm. Therefore the conversion factor from Ra to ^{182}Ta is 8.25/6.8 = 1.2 and

1 mg Ra $\cong$ 1.2 mCi ^{182}Ta

Tantalum 182 is prepared in the form of wires about 0.2 mm thick, usually in the shape of hairpins, ensheathed in 0.1 mm platinum. This is the form in which it has been used in the treatment of localized bladder tumors, although not so widely as teletherapy with megavoltage radiation.

Iridium 192 is suitable as a Ra substitute in interstitial therapy. It has a half-life of 74 days and decays by the emission of β^- particles (maximum energy 0.66 MeV) and a spectrum of γ rays with an average energy of about 0.34 MeV. Supplied in the form of stainless steel, ensheathed seeds measuring about 0.5 mm in diameter by 3 mm in length, the ^{192}Ir can readily be loaded into removable nylon ribbons at 1 cm intervals for threading into and through an accessible lesion. Dosimetry requires slight modification of the Paterson-Parker System because the lower energy of the γ radiation demands the implantation of a somewhat larger volume for a given lesion size. The β particles are absorbed by the stainless steel sheath. Since the Γ of ^{192}Ir is 5.1 R/mCi-hr at 1 cm, the Ra-to-^{192}Ir conversion factor is 8.25/5.1 = 1.6. Thus,

$$1 \text{ mg Ra} = 1.6 \text{ mCi } ^{192}\text{Ir}$$

Protection is faciliated by the small half value layer, 3 mm Pb. However, it is too early to estimate to what extent ^{192}Ir will replace Ra or be replaced by ^{137}Cs, in interstitial therapy.

Californium 252 ($^{252}_{98}$Cf), a transuranic element, is a completely different kind of source for implant therapy. Decaying by **spontaneous fission,** with a half-life of 2.6 years, ^{252}Cf yields **fast neutrons** and γ rays. About 2.4×10^{12} neutrons are emitted per sec per gram. A typical source[91] is in the form of a needle containing 1 μg of ^{252}Cf electroplated on a Pt-Ir rod which is enclosed in a cell and a Pt-Ir needle. The neutron spectrum shows a peak at 1 MeV, but about 7 percent have an energy of 6 MeV. The γ-ray peak occurs at about 0.2 MeV. Measurement of dosage in a phantom indicates a contribution of about 20 percent from γ rays and 80 percent from neutrons. Comparison with radium shows the dose rate with a 1 μg ^{252}Cf needle to be similar to that with a 1 mg Ra needle (0.5 mm Pt filter), both needles having an active length of 2 cm. However, recent studies[39] have revealed that the relative biologic effectiveness with this combined neutron-γ-ray source varies inversely with the dose rate, RBE values as high as 12 having been found. Besides, distance is less effective in protection than in the case of Ra. Therefore the use of ^{252}Cf should be approached with extreme caution.

METHODS OF CHECKING ACCURACY OF IMPLANT

Due to various factors, it is often impossible to obtain ideal distribution of radium or other radioactive sources in actual clinical practice. In order to visualize the true position of the needles or seeds in an implant, it is advisable to make two radiographs perpendicular to each other, one of which is made, if possible, in a direction perpendicular to the major axis of a cylinder implant or the main surface of a plane implant. Since the length of the needles is known, the degree of magnification can be determined. However, this may not be accurate because of foreshortening of the needle images on the radiographs. A better method of assessing magnification is to place a metal ring with a known diameter on the skin surface nearest the implant. Since it is impossible to foreshorten all the diameters of a ring by projection, the ratio of the largest diameter of the ring as measured on the radiograph, to the actual diameter of the ring, gives the magnification factor for needles in the plane of the ring; further correction is needed for other planes. From this, one can arrive at the actual spatial separation of the needles. Adjustment of the implant can be made if it is considered unsatisfactory, or the treatment time may have to be modified (see Meredith[56]).

A better idea of the general orientation of the sources can be obtained by making stereoscopic radiographs of the implant. However, this cannot be used to determine the true distances between sources unless a precision stereoscope is available.

Reconstruction methods, such as those of Nuttall and Spiers,[60] using the tube shift method, provide a relatively accurate method of obtaining an actual model of an implant. This may be a very valuable exercise for the resident in radiology, and to obtain ideal experience in radium therapy, but it is extremely time-consuming and probably of no significant advantage over the simpler methods described above for routine therapy, once sufficient experience has been acquired.

CHAPTER 13

Surface Therapy with Beta Particles

S INCE the β particles emitted by radionuclides have a mean range of only a few millimeters in soft tissues, they cannot be used in the treatment of deep-seated neoplasms by surface application. However, the short range of β particles is advantageous in the therapy of a limited number of very superficial lesions including certain disorders of the anterior surface of the eye such as pterygium, corneal vascularization, or epithelioma; and occational skin keratoses and hemangiomas.

Beta applicators are calibrated in rads per minute at the surface. Such data are furnished at the time of purchase of the applicator, although it is desirable to verify this, preferably by the National Bureau of Standards. It is also advisable to check the uniformity of distribution of the radionuclide by film dosimetry.

In summary, we may state the advantages and disadvantages of β applicators as follows:

Advantages
1. High intensity, permitting short treatment time.
2. Extremely small depth dose, limiting significant dosage to a few mm of tissue and preserving the deeper structures.

Disadvantages
1. Exposure time critical because of high output.
2. Depth dose falls sharply with depth; hence, estimation of thickness of lesion is critical for cure.
3. Hazard of cataract induction is not completely eliminated in treatment of eye lesions.

The various types of radioactive materials used in surface or contact β therapy will now be described. In general, they may be divided into two categories, depending on whether they are natural or artificial radionuclides. The β-particle energies of these nuclides are given in Table 13.01.

TABLE 13.01
THE ENERGIES OF β PARTICLES EMITTED BY VARIOUS RADIONUCLIDES

Radionuclide	Maximum Energy	Half-life
Natural	*MeV*	
Ra D series	0.025	22 years
Ra E	1.17	5 days
Ra B series	0.65	26.8 minutes
Ra C	3.15	19.7 minutes
Artificial		
^{90}Sr series	0.61	28 years
^{90}Y	2.2	61 hours
^{32}P	1.7	14.3 days

NATURAL BETA-PARTICLE EMITTERS

Radium Series. The earliest source of β particles for surface therapy was the *radium plaque.* Such β plaques are available in two *standard* sizes—the full strength plaque containing 5 mg Ra per cm^2, and the half strength plaque containing 2.5 mg Ra per cm^2 of surface. Resembling a flat box, the plaque consists of 2 mm brass at the top and four sides to absorb the β particles. The bottom or front of the plaque, through which the β particles are to pass, is 0.05 mm monel metal backed by a thin sheet of mica 0.01 mm in thickness, coated with a mixture of radium sulfate and magnesium oxide. A typical plaque, shown diagramatically in Figure 13.01, is hermetically sealed to prevent the escape of radon. Uniformity of distribution of the Ra can be determined by film dosimetry. One of the dangers with this type of applicator is the possible leakage of Rn. Therefore, plaques must be checked every six months for leakage (see Chapter 12).

An advantage of the Ra plaque is its long, useful life because of its very long half-life. Actually, all of the β particles are emitted

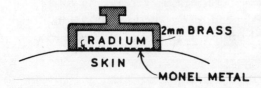

FIGURE 13.01. Sectional diagram of a radium surface plaque.

by RaB, C, and E in the active deposit, rather than by Ra itself. Such plaques also emit γ rays (α particles are absorbed by the monel filter), but the β-particle intensity is so great that in the usual short treatment time, the biologic effect is due almost entirely to the β particles. However, the γ-ray effect on the underlying tissues should not be overlooked. A full strength β plaque filtered by 0.1 mm monel delivers about 5,000 rads/hr at the surface.

Radium β plaques have been used in the treatment of certain types of hemangiomas, keratoses, and very superficial basal cell cancers. However, most superficial malignant lesions amenable to radiation therapy are better and more safely treated with γ rays, contact X-ray therapy, or low voltage X-ray therapy. The β applicator formerly used in treatment of nasopharyngeal lymphoid hyperplasia has deservedly fallen into disrepute.

Radon. When Rn is filtered by a sufficient thickness of material to absorb the α particles, it becomes a practical source of β particles. Such Rn applicators, in the form of glass bulbs, have been used in the therapy of superficial lesions of the eye. One of these, introduced by Burnam in 1940, was superior to the previously used sources of β particles for eye lesions. However, despite the excellence of Rn, there are certain disadvantages. Because of the short half-life (3.83 days) a Rn plant must be located within a reasonable distance to supply the Rn when needed. Gamma radiation accompanies the β particles, just as with the Ra plaque. Since the bulbs enclosing the Rn vary in thickness, inaccuracy of dosage is almost unavoidable. For these reasons, the use of Rn bulb therapy has been limited in extent, although most of the early experience in radiotherapy of the eye was based on Rn.

Radium (D + E). For extremely superficial lesions such as those on the anterior surface of the eye, applicators containing RaD have proved useful. The half-life of RaD, a pure β emitter, is 22 years. Its descendant, RaE, with a half-life of 4.9 days, emits β particles and soft γ rays. When the radiation from such an applicator filtered by 0.05 mm Al is measured, it is found to be effective at a depth in the tissues of only a fraction of a millimeter, since the 1 mm depth dose is only 10 percent (see Fig. 13.02). An Ra(D + E) applicator containing 10 mCi of the element filtered by 0.05 mm

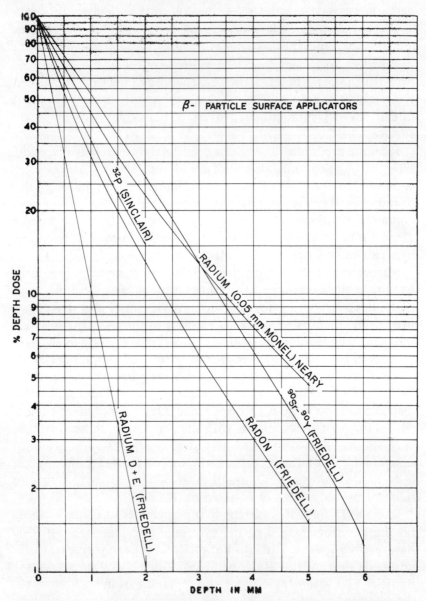

FIGURE 13.02. Depth dose curves for various types of surface β applicators. (Data from H. L. Friedell, C. I. Thomas, and J. S. Krohmer;[30] W. K. Sinclair and L. H. Blondal;[79] and G. J. Neary.[59]) Radon data based on Burnham applicator.

Al delivers approximately 600 rads in 70 sec. Because of the relatively low energy of the Ra(D + E) β particles, 0.025 MeV and 1.17 MeV, respectively, only the most superficial lesions are amenable to therapy. Furthermore, these radionuclides are difficult to obtain and are expensive. Finally, a relatively bulky applicator is required for sufficient Ra(D + E) to provide a conveniently short treatment time.

ARTIFICIAL BETA-PARTICLE EMITTING RADIONUCLIDES

Strontium 90-Yttrium 90 (^{90}Sr-^{90}Y). Among the host of artificial radioactive nuclides there should be one which has the characteristics required for β therapy. Friedell and co-workers[30] found strontium 90 (^{90}Sr) to be the nuclide of choice for the following reasons:

a. It has a long half-life—28 years—obviating frequent replenishment of the applicator.

b. It decays to yttrium 90 which emits energetic β particles—2.2 MeV.

c. There is no accompanying γ radiation, thereby simplifying protection.

d. It has suitable physical and chemical properties, such as ease of manipulation, purity, and high specific activity. The decay scheme of ^{90}Sr is shown in Figure 13.03. It may be summarized as follows:

$$^{90}_{38}\text{Strontium} \xrightarrow[\substack{28\text{-yr} \\ \text{half life}}]{} {}^{90}_{39}\text{Yttrium} + {}^{0}_{-1}\beta \ (0.61 \text{ MeV}) + \tilde{v}$$
$$(maximum)$$

$$^{90}_{39}\text{Yttrium} \xrightarrow[\substack{2.7\text{ days} \\ \text{half life}}]{} {}^{90}_{40}\text{Zirconium} + {}^{0}_{-1}\beta \ (2.2 \text{ MeV}) + \tilde{v}$$
$$(stable) \qquad (maximum)$$

According to the decay scheme, the more effective source of β particles at equilibrium is the yttrium 90 because of the greater maximum energy 2.2 MeV, as contrasted with the ^{90}Sr β-particle energy of 0.61 MeV, this being absorbed by the source casing. The end product zirconium is stable.

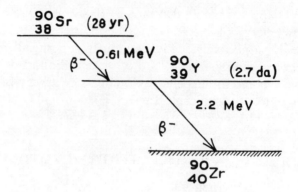

FIGURE 13.03. Decay scheme of radiostrontium (^{90}Sr).

Because of the desirable features of the ^{90}Sr-^{90}Y source, it has become the most prevalent form of β therapy of lesions on the surface of the eye, although it can also be applied to other very superficial lesions on body surfaces. The standard form of this applicator is shown in Figure 13.04.

In practice we are concerned mainly with the *surface* dose rate at the center of the applicator, and this must be determined experimentally by means of an extrapolation ionization chamber. However, this information is supplied at the time of purchase. Furthermore, the decay rate dictates that β output should be corrected annually on the basis of the decay schedule for this nuclide.

In the Tracerlab ® applicator, the radioactive material, ^{90}Sr-^{90}Y, is covered by a protective layer 100 mg per cm^2, consisting of a filter of stainless steel 2 mils (0.05 mm) thick and aluminum 10 mils

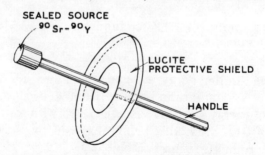

FIGURE 13.04. Diagram of Tracerlab® ^{90}Sr applicator.

(0.25 mm) thick, sealed by a double hermetic seal. The source has an active diameter of 5 mm and an outside diameter of 12.7 mm. Two loadings are available, 40 mCi and 100 mCi. Each instrument is individually calibrated by the manufacturer, the dosage at the *surface* of the applicator being stated in rads per second. For example, the 40 mCi applicator is rated at approximately 45 rads per second at full contact.

It must be emphasized that because of the poor penetrating ability of β particles, their energy is not uniformly distributed in the underlying tissues, being maximal near the surface of the applicator and falling almost to zero at a depth of 9 mm. However, absorbed dose at the surface is a convenient statement of dosage, allowing the duplication of treatment, evaluation and correlation of results with dosage, and intercomparison of data. Reference to Figure 13.02 shows the comparative depth dose curves of various types of β emitters. It is evident that ^{90}Sr-^{90}Y shows favorable depth dose characteristics for superficial therapy of the eye; the HVL in tissue is seen to be 1 mm, the dose at 5 mm being only 3 percent of the surface dose. The lens receives approximately 5 percent of the corneal surface dose; thus, with a corneal dose of 6,000 rads, the lens should receive about 300 rads a dose that carries a definite risk of cataractogenesis.

Recent studies by Jones and Dermentzoglu[46] have been conducted with both a convential ^{90}Sr applicator and one specially designed with a thin silver filter. The authors point out that an applicator with too wide a diameter may make full contact only at the center of the treated area, a tear-filled gap occurring at the periphery. This may reduce the peripheral dose by as much as 32 percent. Better contact is achieved with a small applicator, especially because the depth dose falls off more rapidly. A slightly concave applicator gives even more uniform contact. Since the applicator must be placed at the limbus in most cases, and the most sensitive cells lie about 3 mm from the limbus, an effective lens dose as high as 25 percent of the surface dose may be reached.

Some interesting data have been presented by Friedell.[30] He found that the β particles from various sources compared very favorably with each other and with 44-kV (Philips) contact therapy, as to the degree of skin reaction produced by equivalent doses of radiation. On the other hand, 6,000 rads with a β applicator is equivalent to about 3,000 rads of 100-kV X rays.

The problem of protection in the use of ^{90}Sr-^{90}Y is minimized by the absence of γ radiation. However, brems radiation is produced when the high energy β particles of ^{90}Y interact with atoms in their paths. At a distance of one foot from the storage box (Tracerlab), a significant intensity of X radiation (brems) can be detected. Exposure to the unshielded source should be avoided, since the β-particle range is about 8 meters in air. Because of the extremely short treatment time, less than 1 minute in the vast majority of instances, the radiation reaching the therapist is negligible when the plexiglass shield is in place, and the applicator is held by the upper end of the handle.

One must be extremely careful not to damage the plaque. In any case, a wipe test must be done every six months to test for leakage. The instructions, material, and processing of wipe tests should comply with the requirements of health authorities (see method of Rose, page 629).

Radiophosphorus (^{32}P). Since ^{32}P is a pure β-particle emitter, it has been employed to a small extent, mainly experimentally, in the treatment of superficial lesions. A method was first proposed by Low-Beer in 1947, using a solution of a definite quantity of ^{32}P absorbed in blotting paper and applied directly to the lesion. He developed an empirical system of treatment for skin lesions, based on a certain number of microcuries of ^{32}P per cm^2 of a given type of lesion. In England, Sinclair[79] employed ^{32}P incorporated in polystyrene plastic sheets. However, this radionuclide has not been widely used for surface therapy because of its short half-life and the problems of preparation and handling. The depth dose curve follows rather closely that of Rn β particles, the HVL in tissue being approximately 0.5 mm. Only about 15 percent of the surface dose reaches a depth of 2 mm (see Fig. 13.02).

Superficial Electron Beam Therapy. Another method of electron beam therapy, of artificial origin, should be mentioned here. As early as 1953, Trump[85] used the *electrons* accelerated in a Van de Graaff generator to about 2.5 MeV, in the treatment of selected skin lesions. The interesting facts about this beam include:

(1) the maximum dose is delivered at a point 2 to 4 mm below the surface; (2) the surface dose is about 75 percent of this maximum; and (3) the maximum range of these electrons in the tissues is about 7 mm. Consequently, a layer of tissue about 4 mm thick just beneath the skin receives reasonably uniform irradiation. A thicker layer of tissue can be given uniform dosage by increasing the energy of the electrons, so that the thickness of tissue treated can be controlled by the electron beam energy. More recently, **high energy** electron beam therapy ranging up to about 20 MeV is being used for certain superficial neoplasms. The characteristics of such beams are described briefly on pages 320 to 322.

CHAPTER 14

Medical Use of Radionuclides

WHEN ordinary stable nuclides are exposed to subatomic particles in devices such as the cyclotron or nuclear reactor, stable or radioactive nuclides of slightly different mass numbers are produced. These may have the same atomic number as the bombarded target atoms, and therefore exhibit identical chemical, physiological, and biological properties; or they may acquire the atomic number of an entirely different element. Consequently, we have a powerful means of producing *radioactive isotopes* of stable atoms. A number of radionuclides have also been obtained as by-products of uranium fission in the nuclear reactor. The availability of a variety of radionuclides in profusion has spawned the rapidly expanding field of *nuclear medicine.*

As indicated in Chapter 11 the *purity* of a radionuclide sample depends on how it was produced. If a pure element such as cobalt is irradiated with slow neutrons in a nuclear reactor, the resulting radiocobalt cannot be separated from its nonradioactive isotope by *chemical* means, the resulting product being a mixture of the two isotopes. The stable cobalt is called a *carrier.* The specific activity, up to a maximum, depends on the total exposure of the parent cobalt to the neutron flux.

On the other hand, if we start with tellurium and irradiate it with slow neutrons, the product is radioiodine, which is an entirely different element from tellurium and can be separated from it chemically. The product ^{131}I can therefore be obtained almost free of stable iodine and is said to be *carrier free.* However, the *fission products* of the nuclear reactor still serve as the major source of ^{131}I from which it is separated by distillation.

Radionuclides such as radiocesium (^{137}Cs)—products of uranium fission—may be contaminated with a large amount of stable

472

carrier. Furthermore, the situation is one of "taking what you can get" because fission products are incidental to uranium fission, in contrast to the controlled irradiation of elements such as cobalt in the nuclear reactor.

As we have already seen, radionuclides decay in a characteristic pattern—each decays at its own constant rate and has a characteristic half-life, average life, decay constant, etc. Artificial radioactive isotopes most often emit β particles and neutrinos, or γ rays, or all three.

Our discussion of the medical use of radionuclides will concentrate on therapy, although their application in diagnosis will be considered briefly. Wherever possible, fundamental principles will be stressed. Available instruments will be described in some detail.

The following outline summarizes the medical uses of radionuclides according to various indications:

1. *Diagnosis*—general procedure

  a. Compound tagged with radionuclide (radioactive isotope of a normal element substituted for it in the compound).

  b. Injected or ingested in tracer amount—small enough to be diagnostic, but not large enough to deliver intolerable radiation exposure.

  c. Body cannot distinguish between radioactively tagged compound and its stable counterpart.

  d. Fate of tagged element determined by counting with special instruments (GM counter; scintillation counter; scintiscanner; gamma camera)

   (1) Externally as with ^{131}I, thyroid gland; ^{99m}Tc or ^{197}Hg, brain; ^{197}Hg, kidney; ^{99m}Tc or ^{198}Au, liver; ^{99m}Tc, lungs, bone.

   (2) Internally as in probing internal organs such as brain.

   (3) Excretions as in counting urine in Schilling test (^{57}CoB$_{12}$) for pernicious anemia.

   (4) Secretions as in measuring ^{131}I output in saliva.

   (5) Hematology, ^{59}Fe and ^{51}Cr in tagging of erythrocytes.

2. ***Therapy***—methods

   a. *Chemical*

   (1) Selective absorption as ^{131}I in thyroid gland: ^{131}I given orally in therapeutic amount; selectively absorbed in target organ—thyroid—which is irradiated by deposited radionuclide, in this instance, 90 percent of therapeutic dose from β particles, 10 percent from γ rays.
   (2) Differential absorption as ^{32}P in malignant tumors.
   (3) Colloidal dispersion as ^{198}Au in the reticuloendothelial system.

   b. *Physical*

   (1) External as ^{60}Co and ^{137}Cs in teletherapy, shown in Figure 6.04; and ^{90}Sr in contact therapy, shown in Figure 13.04.
   (2) Interstitial as ^{60}Co needles or wires; ^{137}Cs needles; ^{192}Ir wires; ^{198}Au seeds.
   (3) Intracavitary as ^{60}Co needles or wires; ^{137}Cs needles; ^{32}P-chromic phosphate or ^{198}Au in pleural or peritoneal malignant effusions.

RADIONUCLIDES IN MEDICAL DIAGNOSIS

To study the absorption, distribution, and fate of a given chemical compound in the human body, we first prepare a sample of the compound in which one or more atoms has been replaced by one of its radioactive isotopes. This is called a ***tagged*** compound. Because the stable element and its radioactive isotope have identical chemical and physiological properties, the living organism cannot distinguish between them, and so it utilizes either of them indiscriminately. (Exceptions are ordinary hydrogen and its isotopes —deuterium and tritium—because of the large relative difference in their atomic masses and consequent difference in mobility.) Due to its emission of penetrating radiation, the tagged compound may be detected in the organs or body fluids by appropriate methods. If the behavior of such a tagged compound is first determined in *normal* individuals, it can then be used to ascertain the functional status of various organs in patients. This is the fundamental principle of the medical use of radionuclides not only in diagnosis but in treatment as well.

There are two main procedures for detecting the *localization* of a radionuclide within the body. The first requires a *special detector* connected to a counting device. This serves both to localize the radionuclide and to determine its quantity by comparison with a known standard. A similar procedure can be used to find the amount of radionuclide present in body fluids.

Autoradiography. Another method, used mainly in clinical research, is a photographic process called *autoradiography* or *radioautography*. The patient is first given a suitable dose of radionuclide. After an appropriate interval, the organ under investigation (e.g. the thyroid gland following the administration of radioiodine) is removed surgically. A slice of the organ is placed in contact with X-ray or special film in the dark for a suitable length of time. After being processed, the film will show areas of darkening where it has been in contact with zones of tissue containing a sufficient concentration of radioisotope (see Fig. 14.01).

A modification of radioautography, utilizing histologic sections, is termed *microradioautography*. After the patient has been given a measured dose of radionuclide, the removed organ or tissue is fixed in methanol, or in Bouin's or Carnoy's solution. To prevent diffusion of radionuclide, especially ^{131}I and ^{32}P, the tissue may be fixed in cold propylene glycol and imbedded in Carbowax.® After the fixed tissue is sectioned, slides are prepared in the usual

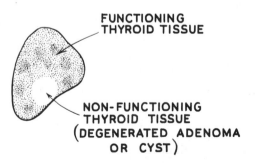

FUNCTIONING
THYROID TISSUE

NON-FUNCTIONING
THYROID TISSUE
(DEGENERATED ADENOMA
OR CYST)

FIGURE 14.01. Radioautograph of a thyroid slice containing a functionless nodule.

manner. Then, in the darkroom, several slides are placed in firm pressure contact with a photographic plate (such as lantern slide type) or with Kodak® autoradiographic permeable base stripping film and stored in darkness for a time depending on the total counts per cm² of slide surface. Usually, a total of 5×10^6 counts per cm² is adequate, requiring several weeks, but it is advisable to expose for various lengths of time to be assured of at least one satisfactory radioautograph. The slides are then processed, the best one being selected by observation under a microscope. Areas of darkening are compared with a slide bearing a section of the same specimen stained in the usual manner, so that the site of concentration of the radionuclide in the cells can be determined. Control slides of tissues without radionuclides and with emulsion alone, should be processed together with the test slides to detect excess background radiation or artifacts. An alternate method is to immerse the cleared histologic section (on the slide) in liquid emulsion such as Kodak NTB-2 or NTB-3, leaving a thin layer. After sufficient exposure, which may have to be determined by trial and error as before, the slide is immersed in developer and is then rinsed, fixed, and washed.

Radioautographic methods are not quantitative, but do show exactly where certain radionuclides may be concentrated on a cellular or histologic level. For additional details, several references are cited in the Bibliography (Rogers,[75] Fields and Seed.[28]

We shall now return to the *physical methods* of determining the amount of a radionuclides in organs or body fluids. These require instruments known as *pulse counters*. of which there are three types: *proportional counters, Geiger-Müller tubes*, and *scintillation detectors*. Essential to the operation of such detectors are the auxiliary recording devices which include *rate meters* and *scalers*. The following sections will take up the essential principles and construction of G-M tubes and scintillation counters.

GEIGER-MÜLLER TUBES

Under certain well-defined conditions, the activity of a radionuclide can be determined by counting the number of emitted ionizing particles or γ photons detected by a pulse counter in unit time. We found in an earlier chapter that the unit of activity of a radionuclide is based on the number of **nuclear transformations** or **de-excitations per second.** Since each such event ejects one or more particles and/or photons, the activity of the radionuclide may be found by comparison with a known standard of the same radionuclide. Thus, if the radionuclide in an organ or fluid, and the same nuclide in a standard sample, are counted under **identical geometric conditions,** then the amount of nuclide in the sample may be determined by the following simple proportion after the counting rates have been corrected for background:

$$\frac{millicuries\ in\ unknown}{millicuries\ in\ standard} = \frac{net\ counts/min\ of\ unknown}{net\ counts/min\ of\ standard}$$

or

$$mCi\ unknown = \frac{mCi\ standard \times net\ c/min\ of\ unknown}{net\ c/min\ of\ standard}$$

The net sample count rate R_N is the difference between the total count rate R_T and the background count rate R_B.

$$R_N = R_T - R_B \qquad (1)$$

The background count rate is obtained with the sample and all other known radioactive sources removed from the counting range of the detector. A count rate is the quotient of the total count by the elapsed time. Background should always be taken into account unless it is so small as to be negligible.

One of the devices that actually counts the number of particles or photons reaching it from a radioactive source is the **Geiger-Müller** or **G-M tube.**

Principle. Before describing the construction of a G-M tube, let us first look into its underlying principle. During the passage of penetrating radiation a gas becomes conductive due to ionization of its atoms. Thus α, β, γ, and X rays have the ability to strip orbital electrons from the gas atoms, the latter remaining as positively charged ions. The electrons exist free for only a short period of time, ionizing other atoms along their paths. Thus, in essence, the passage of ionizing radiation such as that emitted by radionuclides causes the formation of positive and negative ions, or **ion pairs,** in the gas.

The density of the ion pairs per cm of path is called *specific ionization,* the number of ion pairs depending on the energy of the ionizing agent. Alpha particles, because of their relatively slow speed and double charge, produce high specific ionization. Beta particles, with a higher speed and smaller charge than alphas, yield about 1/1000 the specific ionization of α particles, but the path of β particles is correspondingly longer so that nearly the same *total* number of ion pairs is produced by both types of particles with similar energies. An average energy of 33.7 electron volts is required to liberate one ion pair. Gamma and X rays cause ionization indirectly by freeing and setting in motion electrons from atomic orbits. These primary electrons in turn ionize atoms in the same manner as β particles. Neutrons also cause ionization, *indirectly,* through recoil of atomic nuclei with which they collide.

We may regard detectors used in nuclear medicine as (1) locating radioactive nuclides and (2) determining their quantity by actually counting a certain fraction of the particles or photons received from the radionuclide in unit time, under carefully controlled conditions. Usually, the amount is stated in *counts per minute* (c/min). How are these particles detected? We have just seen that the particles have the ability to ionize gases through which they pass. The detector is a *modified ionization chamber* which, as will be recalled, consists of two electrodes with an applied voltage that is too small to cause a current to flow between the electrodes until ionizing particles enter the chamber and produce pairs of ions. The potential difference between the electrodes then causes positive ions to move to the negative electrode (cathode) and negative ions to move to the positive electrode (anode), this movement of ions constituting a flow of current in the tube. An auxiliary system measures the current carried by the ions.

A Geiger-Müller (G-M) tube is really a type of ionization chamber or diode operating under special conditions for the purpose of detecting and counting ionizing particles or photons. It consists of a *negatively charged cylindrical electrode* (cathode) and a *positively charged coaxial wire electrode* (anode), as shown in Figure 14.02.

G-M TUBE

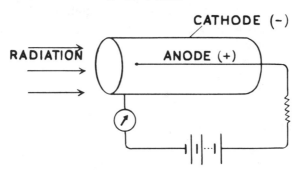

FIGURE 14.02. Schematic diagram of a Geiger-Mueller tube.

We shall now investigate the response of a G-M tube to received ionizing particles or photons at various applied voltages, as embodied in a G-M characteristic curve (see Fig. 14.03). When the applied voltage is *zero,* all the ions liberated during passage of the radiation into the tube recombine to form neutral atoms, as in Zone I. No current flows through the tube. As the voltage is increased to about 500, more and more of the ions are separated before they can recombine, the electrons moving to the positive central wire, and the positive ions to the negative cylinder (Zone II). At saturation voltage, all the ions are separated immediately after being formed and none are able to recombine. However, the negative electrical pulses generated by the electrons arriving at the anode are too weak to be detected by the counter. Thus, in Zone II the instrument behaves as an *ionization chamber.*

A further increase above the ***starting potential*** of about 800 volts causes a sharp increase in the size of the pulses so that they can be detected by deflection of a meter needle, or by an audible "pop" if an audio circuit is included. This turn of events is explained as follows: above the starting potential each primary ion is speeded up sufficiently to cause ionization of other gas atoms by collision, a process called ***avalanche*** or ***Townsend Cascade.*** The resulting extremely large number of secondary ions are responsible for the detectibly large electric pulse. Furthermore, in this region— Zone III—the avalanche of secondary ions spreads farther along the anode wire as the applied voltage is increased, generating a larger pulse for a particular ionizing event. In fact, the ratio of the total number of ions produced to the number of primary ions is called the **gas amplification factor**, representing the magnification of the pulse due to ionization by collision.

$$\text{gas amplification factor} = \frac{total\ ions\ produced}{number\ of\ primary\ ions}$$

Because of amplification in this manner, more and more weak pulses become detectable as the applied voltage is increased. Hence the count rate increases in proportion to the voltage, and Zone III is therefore known as the **proportional region.** A counter operating in Zone III is a **proportional counter.**

A further increase in voltage carries the curve into Zone IV, wherein the gas amplification factor may be 10^5 or 10^6. This is known as the regional of **limited proportionality.** It has no practical application at present.

At the **Geiger-Müller threshold,** usually about 1,000 volts, depending on the particular tube and counting system, we find the

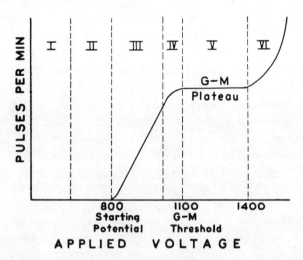

FIGURE 14.03. Variation in pulses per minute with applied voltage in an ionization chamber. In Zone II, below the starting potential, the chamber operates as a simple ionization chamber. Zone V is important for pulse counting of radionuclide activity (G-M region).

beginning of the *G-M plateau* in which the counts per minute remain nearly constant for a given radiation field as the voltage is increased. This corresponds to Zone V in Figure 14.03. In the G-M plateau almost any ionizing particle which enters the tube initiates an avalanche with an amplification factor of about 10^8 or *one hundred million times.* The avalanche spreads along the entire length of the wire almost instantaneously. Thus, regardless of the specific ionization of the entering particle or photon, the same high, negative electrical pulse is generated at the wire anode. The size of the pulse is large and is independent of the number of primary ions produced by the radiation entering the tube. Therefore, in the G-M region no distinction can be made between various types of ionizing radiation, unless some form of external shielding is employed. Similarly, the number of pulses is independent of the energy of the ionizing radiation. The G-M tube operating on its plateau simply counts the ionizing particles or photons indiscriminately.

The *slope* of the plateau is defined as the change in the count rate, under identical conditions, per 100 volt increase. This may be 1 or 2 percent in satisfactorily operating counters. It is caused by imperfect quenching (see page 482); and by surface irregularities in the central wire and in the chamber wall, giving rise to spurious discharges that increase slightly with increasing voltage. The length of the plateau is usually about 300 volts. In order to avoid the possibility of operating the G-M tube near the threshold or near the upper end of the plateau where a slight fluctuation in voltage may cause a large change in counting rate, one should select the midpoint voltage of the plateau as the operating voltage. However, the plateau should be reviewed periodically because it may become shorter as the tube ages.

At the upper end of the plateau, a further increase in voltage produces a sharp rise in the counting rate, eventually leading to a *continuous discharge* which may ruin the tube. Therefore in testing a G-M tube to determine its plateau, one should discontinue the procedure as soon as a small rise in voltage, near the end of the plateau, causes a large increase in the counting rate.

Dead Time. Let us look a little more closely into the operation of a G-M tube in the plateau region. When an ionizing particle

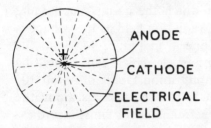

ANODE

CATHODE

ELECTRICAL
FIELD

FIGURE 14.04. Cross section of a G-M tube. The electric field is stronger near the central wire anode due to the field's convergence from the cylindrical cathode.

or photon enters the tube, it liberates from the wall and contained gas primary ion pairs consisting of negative electrons and an equal number of positive ions. An avalanche results from ionization by collision close to the central positively charged wire, because here the electric field is stronger than it is near the broader surface of the cathode, as shown in Figure 14.04. The avalanche, it may be recalled, travels the full length of the wire. There are now many electrons and positive ions in the vicinity of the wire. Because of their smaller mass, the electrons are rapidly drawn to the central wire anode in less than one millionth of a second. But the positive ions are heavier and move more slowly as an ion cloud or space charge in the opposite direction (toward the cathode) in about 1/10,000 sec. The positive space charge, lingering near the central wire anode after the electrons have reached it, temporarily decreases the strength of the electric field near the wire, preventing further ionization by collision and thereby rendering the counter insensitive to radiation. During this short, insensitive interval, known as the ***dead time,*** entering particles and photons are not detected. The dead time of most G-M tubes is about 200 microseconds (2×10^{-4} sec).

Quenching. Two events occur when the positive ions finally reach the cathode: (1) each ion is neutralized by taking up an electron which enters one of its higher energy levels, causing the atom to be in an excited state; (2) immediately, this electron drops to zero energy level, radiating a series of photons, some of which are in the ultraviolet region and are sufficiently energetic to liberate photoelectrons from the cathode metal. These photoelectrons can then set off a second avalanche, with repetition of the entire process to produce a continuous discharge. Obviously a G-M tube, under these conditions, would be unsuitable for counting the particles emitted by a radionuclide because each entering particle would initiate an endless series of discharges.

To overcome this difficulty, G-M tubes are **gas filled,** a suitable gas being selected to prevent the initiation of secondary avalanches. Such tubes are **self-quenched.** One type of G-M self-quenched tube is filled with 10 percent ethyl alcohol vapor and 90 percent argon at a pressure of about 10 cm of mercury (about $\frac{1}{8}$ atmosphere). Argon ions formed during the avalanche ionize alcohol molecules which then drift toward the cathode where they pick up electrons and dissociate into smaller molecules. This avoids the liberation of characteristic ultraviolet radiation by alcohol, preventing the occurrence of a secondary avalanche. Furthermore, alcohol is a good absorber of ultraviolet light. If argon ions happen to reach the cathode, spurious discharges may occur, increasing in number with the applied voltage; this accounts, in part, for the slow rise in the slope of the G-M plateau.

The finite quantity of alcohol in the G-M tube limits its useful life. Since there are about 10^{20} alcohol molecules in a new tube and about 10^{10} break down with each pulse, the alcohol disappears after $10^{20} \div 10^{10} = 10^{10}$ pulses. For practical purposes, however, the life of the average self-quenched tube is about 10^8 pulses or counts. This is really an extremely high number. For example, in a typical 24 hr radioiodine uptake study, there may be about 120 counts per minute at 20 cm. If the count is taken for 5 minutes, this represents a total of 600 counts.

$$\frac{10^8 \; counts \; per \; tube \; life}{600 \; counts \; per \; test} = 1.7 \times 10^5 \; tests$$

Thus, about 170,000 such tests could be made within the lifetime of the tube, if there were no other factors operating to shorten its life.

In summary, then, we may state that to prevent secondary avalanche in a G-M tube, a gas must be introduced to quench the discharge. A G-M counter of this type is said to be **self-quenching.** A quenching gas should have three properties: (1) it should **dissociate** rather than emit radiation when excited; (2) it should have a **low ionizing energy** relative to the main gas in the tube;

and (3) it should have a ***strong absorption affinity for ultraviolet light.*** Alcohol vapor fulfills these specifications. Incidentally, the last requirement also reduces the likelihood that ultraviolet light entering the tube from the outside will produce spurious counts.

Another type of quenching, known as ***external*** or ***nonself-quenching***, requires an auxiliary electronic circuit. Immediately following the avalanche, a resistor in the circuit drops the voltage and resulting gas amplification factor to such a low value that a second avalanche cannot occur. The counter remains insensitive for the brief interval while the voltage is at this low level, but the voltage quickly returns to its original value, again rendering the counter sensitive.

Construction of G-M Counters. An ordinary G-M tube consists of a cylindrical cathode, usually in the form of a thin layer of silver or copper flashed on the internal surface of a glass tube. These metals have a low photoelectric efficiency, which means that they have a very small tendency to emit photoelectrons when struck by ultraviolet light, and so are relatively non-light sensitive. Obviously, it is undesirable for G-M tubes to respond to ordinary light, since special shielding would be required to avoid erros in counting. The cylindrical cathode is usually 1 to 10 cm in diameter by 2 to 20 cm in length. The central tungsten wire anode measuring 0.025 cm or less in diameter must have an exceedingly smooth and flawless surface to avoid irregular electrical fields which might nullify the characteristic plateau in the G-M curve.

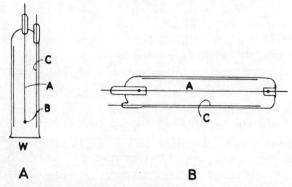

FIGURE 14.05. A. End window type of G-M counter. B. Side window type. *A* is anode, *B* is bead, *C* is cathode, *W* is window.

Two principal forms of G-M counter are available. The ***end window*** or ***bell counter*** (see Fig. 14.05A) is used principally for counting β particles. The cathode may be either a metallic cylinder or a suitable metal coating flashed on the inside of the glass tube. Since the glass and metal would absorb the softer β particles, a very thin window of mica about 1 to 2 mg/cm^2 is placed at one end of the tube. This transmits a large percentage of β particles and also renders the counter directional. The wire anode is supported at one end only, its free end being directed toward the window and terminating in a glass bead to avoid a strong electric field at its sharp end. In the conventional type G-M counter, the window is 2 cm in diameter, but a diameter up to 6 cm is available for special purposes. The operating voltage (midpoint of plateau) may be in the vicinity of 1,100 to 1,500 volts for an end-window G-M counter.

The other form of G-M tube is the thin walled ***cylindrical type,*** shown in Figure 14.05B. It is not directional, in contrast to the open-end type, and is made of extremely thin glass coated on the inside with a very thin layer of metal. It is used to measure energetic β particles of about 1 to 2 MeV, like those emitted by ^{32}P. Even though some of the β particles may be absorbed by the glass, they may initiate brems radiation and, besides, a sufficient number reach the interior of the tube and are counted. The wire anode at the center is attached at both ends in the cylindrical G-M tube.

As already mentioned, the G-M tube is usually filled with quenching gases, the most inexpensive and most widely used being argon and alcohol vapor. The argon must contain a trace of impurities to make it more suitable for the quenching process.

A conventional G-M counter exhibits only slight efficiency in counting X and γ rays (about 1%) due to their low specific ionization. But a special bismuth cathode increases efficiency to nearly 10 percent because the X or γ rays, on striking the bismuth, eject orbital electrons which then initiate an avalanche. This type of G-M counter is called a bismuth or ***high efficiency*** γ-ray counter. On the other hand, an ordinary G-M tube has a high efficiency, approaching 100 percent, for β particles with sufficient energy to pass through the window of the tube.

Another special type of G-M device is the ***gas flow counter*** used

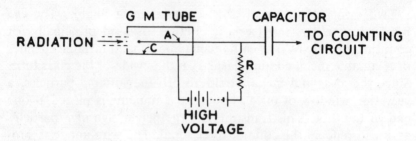

FIGURE 14.06. Simplified counting circuit for a G-M tube.

in counting very low energy β particles. The radionuclide sample is placed inside this counter and measurements are made while a slow stream of special gas flows through.

G-M Counter Circuits. Counters are connected to suitable electronic circuits to amplify each electrical pulse. Since the electrons move swiftly to the central wire anode, a negative pulse is generated there by each avalanche. The negative pulse, lasting about 10^{-4} sec, is actually similar to a high frequency alternating current which can be transmitted by a capacitor of low capacitance, as shown in Figure 14.06. The pulse can also be fed into the counting circuit of a rate meter or scaler, as will be described below.

SCINTILLATION COUNTERS

Early in his investigation of radioactivity, Rutherford used a zinc sulfide screen to detect α particles. When struck by α particles zinc sulfide gives off visible flashes of light known as *scintillations.* This method was abandoned after the G-M counter was invented, but the scintillation method has been revived and perfected to such high efficiency that it has almost completely replaced the G-M counter in quantitative studies in nuclear medicine. The combination of a scintillator in the form of a *crystal phosphor* and a *photomultiplier tube* to detect the light flashes constitutes the *scintillation counter* (see Fig. 14.07). The crystal phosphor may be zinc sulfide for counting α particles. Anthracene is most often used for β particles, and thallium-activated sodium iodide for γ rays.

When ionizing radiations enter a scintillation crystal, two processes ensue. One is the simple passage of radiation through the crystal without interaction. Such transmitted radiation escapes detection by the crystal. The other, more important, process is the interaction between the incident radiation and the atoms within the crystal causing excitation (displacement of orbital electrons). As the excited atoms return to the ground state, low-energy photons in the visible and ultraviolet region of the spectrum are emitted in flashes of extremely short duration. These light photons are conducted through a lucite block to the photosensitive **cathode** of the **photomultiplier tube** where **photoelectrons** are ejected. Now the first anode or **dynode** attracts the photoelectrons which eject additional electrons. This process is repeated, with progressive acceleration and multiplication of electrons from dynode to dynode through about 10 stages, with an amplification factor of 3 or 4 at each stage. The resulting total **amplification factor** may reach 3^{10} or 4^{10} (60,000 to 1 million times). **Dead time** is extremely short, so that several hundred thousand counts/min can be detected without loss of counts. For example, scintillation counters have a dead time of about 10 microsec, as contrasted with G-M counters which have a dead time of about 200 microsec.

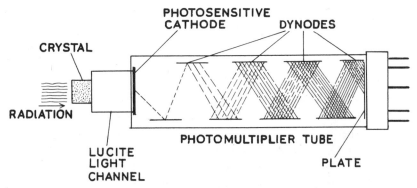

CRYSTAL

RADIATION

PHOTOSENSITIVE
CATHODE   DYNODES

LUCITE
LIGHT
CHANNEL

PHOTOMULTIPLIER TUBE

PLATE

FIGURE 14.07. Diagram of a scintillation detector used in radioactivity studies. Incoming radiation causes scintillations in the crystal. The light is conducted by the lucite to the light-sensitive cathode where photoelectrons are emitted. These are accelerated by a series of anodes and are detected as pulses by the counting circuit after they strike the plate.

Miniature scintillation detectors are available, equipped with organic phosphors such as anthracene, having an effective atomic number similar to air. Such detectors can be used to determine radiation dosage in the 150 keV to 3 MeV energy range.

As mentioned before, the photomultiplier tube converts the light flashes in the scintillator to electrical pulses. However, these *output signals* or pulses leaving the photomultiplier are too small to be counted, and therefore need further amplification. But first they must be passed through a *preamplifier* to shape them properly and avoid excessive weakening on transmission through the co-axial cable on the way to the amplifier. This is accomplished by matching the impedance of the photomultiplier tube to that of the *amplifier*. Upon arrival, the pulse energy or signal size is increased, the resulting *amplifier gain* being the quotient of the voltage of the output signal by that of the input signal of the amplifier.

But the amplifier output signals are still not ready to be counted. They vary in size because this is proportional to the energy released in the scintillator by the incoming photons or particles. Furthermore, spurious signals arise from background radiation and circuitry noise. Therefore, a *pulse height analyzer* or *spectrometer* is introduced into the circuit to limit the counting or display to signals in a certain desired range, corresponding to the particular range of the energy spectrum of the radiation being measured in the first place. The spectrometer consists of a lower level and a higher level *discriminator*, so arranged electronically that signals of a size smaller or larger than the selected range are rejected. The range of photon energies detected is called the *window* for that particular radionuclide. Window width must be selected carefully. If it is too narrow, precision improves, but the counting rate may become too small; besides, error may be introduced by analyzer instability. On the other hand, if the window is too wide, too much background and circuitry noise is included, with loss of precision. Optimally, the width of the window should be adjusted to include about 85 percent of the counts in the total-absorption peak (i.e. the region in which the photon energy is completely absorbed in the detector crystal).

When the count rate of a scintillation detector is plotted against the applied voltage, a plateau is obtained. This resembles the plateau of a G-M tube, but has a different cause. Unlike the pulses in a G-M tube, the light flashes in a crystal detector vary in intensity with the energy of the ionizing particle or photon. Thus, there will be a variation in the energy of the electrical pulses transmitted by the photomultiplier tube. Now two factors come into play. First, if a lower level discriminator is included it passes only those electrical impulses whose energy exceeds a certain minimum value. This eliminates circuitry and background "noise" as described above. Thus, only ionizing particles or photons above a minimum energy are counted. In the second place, the sensitivity of the photomultiplier tube increases with an increase in the applied voltage: as the voltage is increased, more and more of the low intensity light flashes are counted because the electric impulses they initiate are amplified to the point where they can pass the discriminator. Thus, as the voltage applied to the scintillation detector is increased, the ***threshold of the plateau*** is reached where all light flashes produce pulses large enough to pass the discriminator. A further increase in voltage in the plateau region does not produce any significant increase in the count rate. If no upper level discriminator is included in the circuit, a further increase in applied voltage causes the appearance of circuitry noise of sufficient energy to pass the lower level discriminator and the curve rises abruptly; obviously, this region is unsuited to counting. The scintillation detector is properly used at about the middle of the plateau so that small fluctuations in voltage will produce no significant change in the count rate.

The ***sensitivity***, *S*, of a counter may be defined as the quotient of the counting rate, *N*, by the activity *A* of a sample,

$$S = \frac{N}{A}$$

Scintillation counters have a very high sensitivity compared with a G-M counter, making it feasible to obtain satisfactory counting rates with minute activities of radionuclides; in fact, much smaller than with a G-M counter. Furthermore, it makes possible the use of scintillation counters in automatic scanners.

The *efficiency* of a crystal phosphor depends on a number of factors, various materials being more or less satisfactory as they do or do not possess these qualities. They should be:

1. Good absorbers of the ionizing radiation which they are to detect. This means that a large fraction of the incident radiation will interact with the crystal atoms and, conversely, only a small fraction will escape.

2. Emitters of shorter wavelength visible and ultraviolet photons to increase detectability by the photomultiplier tube.

3. Transparent to the emitted photons. Therefore, phosphors composed of a single large crystal such as anthracene or sodium iodide are superior to zinc sulfide which can be used only in the form of a powder of low transparency.

4. Characterized by minimal phosphorescence (lag or after-glow); that is, the photons should be emitted in an extremely short time interval.

Assuming that we have a phosphor of good quality, we find that its sensitivity is influenced by its *volume*. Thus, the thicker the crystal and the larger its cross-sectional area, the more counts per minute it will detect per μCi of radionuclide. The reason is obvious—as the volume of the crystal is increased, more of the incident radiation will be absorbed and more photons will therefore be emitted. For instance, at a distance of 20 cm, a crystal 3.8 cm in diameter by 3.8 cm thick will yield approximately 2,000 counts per min when exposed to 1 μCi of ^{131}I. If the crystal thickness is doubled, the count is increased to about 2,800 per min. A crystal 2.5 cm in diameter by 2.5 cm thick will produce only 1,000 counts per min under the same conditions. However, it must be borne in mind that although the larger crystals are more efficient, they also require bulkier photomultiplier tubes and, because of the higher background count, heavier lead shielding.

DEVICES FOR COUNTING DETECTOR PULSES

It is impossible to count the G-M or scintillation detector pulses without resorting to special devices which receive, amplify, and register the pulses, thereby permitting comparative counting rates of radioactive samples. We shall describe the two main types of equipment widely used for this purpose: *scalers* and *count rate meters.* It must be emphasized that they do not detect radiation, but merely count the electrical pulses generated by ionizing radiation in the G-M or scintillation detector. However, a source of high voltage is also incorporated in the scaler or rate meter for the operation of the pulse detector.

Scaler. A scaler is essentially a compact unit, including an electronic counting circuit, a mechanical register, a timer, and usually a high voltage source, the latter energizing the G-M tube or scintillation detector. Each electrical pulse is conducted from the detector to the electronic circuit which registers its arrival by means of a flashing signal light on a control panel. Since these pulses arrive too rapidly for individual detection by any type of mechanical register, a scaling circuit must be included to indicate the pulses in groups of 10, 10^2, and 10^3, as in the decade scaler. When operated on a *scale of 1,000,* readings may be made directly from the panel as shown in Figure 14.08. The right vertical column represents units, from 1 to 9. The center column represents tens, from 10 to 90. The left column indicates hundreds, from 100 to 900. After 999 counts have been received, as shown by the top lights in the three columns, the next count will register 1 on the mechanical register at the left of the panel and all of the flashing lights will go out. Continued counting repeats the same sequence until the 2 shows on the register, indicating 2,000 counts.

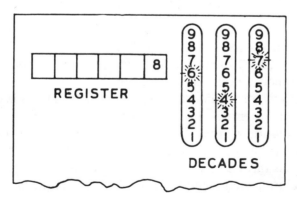

FIGURE 14.08. Arrangement of lights and register in a decade scaler.

Referring again to Figure 14.08, we see 8 on the register, indicating 8,000 counts. To this must be added the signal lights in the vertical columns:

$$8,000 + 600 + 40 + 7 = 8,647 \text{ counts}$$

Thus, by simply reading the number on the register and following it by the lighted numbers in the vertical columns in order from left to right, we can see the total count at a glance.

Besides the scaling circuits and registers themselves, modern scalers incorporate the high voltage supply to operate the radiation detector, and an audio system with audible detection of counts for manual scanning. A timer must also be provided. It is most often used as a *preset timer*, being set for a desired interval of time. When the selected time has elapsed, the timer automatically opens the scaling circuit and the total count is read. The count rate is then obtained by dividing the total count by the time interval. For example, if the total count is 7,985 and the timer was set for 5 minutes, then

$$\frac{7,985}{5} = 1,597 \text{ counts per min (c/min)}$$

Another more elaborate system is one arranged for *preset counting*. Here the timing device is set for a certain predetermined number of counts. As soon as the desired total number of counts has been recorded, the scaling process ceases automatically. The total number of counts divided by the elapsed time equals the number of counts per unit time.

Count Rate Meter. Another method of registering the counts detected by a G-M tube or scintillation probe is embodied in the count rate meter, designed to indicate the number of counts per minute directly on a meter scale (see Fig. 14.09). This is in contrast to the scaler which simply indicates the total number of counts, requiring division by the elapsed time to determine the count rate per minute. In the count rate meter, the electrical pulses from the detector pass through an electronic circuit and build up a charge on a capacitor having a shunt resistor. The greater the rate at which the pulses reach the capacitor (i.e. the higher the count rate), the

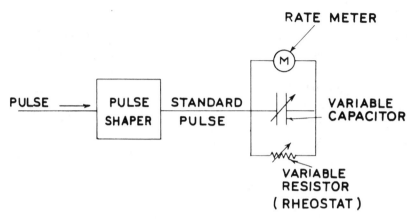

FIGURE 14.09. Simplified diagram of a rate meter circuit. The pulses arriving from the detector (G-M or scintillation) must be shaped and made uniform before they enter the meter circuit. Shaping is more important in scintillation than in G-M counting.

higher the resulting voltage. A circuit from the capacitor to a meter shows the instantaneous voltage fluctuations corresponding to the instantaneous variations in count rate. However, the meter is calibrated to read directly in counts/min.

The function of the capacitor and resistor in parallel is to permit a charge to build up on the capacitor according to the rapidity of the incoming pulses, and at the same time allow the charge to leak across the resistor. When these two opposing tendencies become equalized, the voltage across the circuit is proportional to the average count rate, the rate meter having been so calibrated.

The time required for the capacitor to discharge to about 37 percent of the total charge is called the *time constant* and is equal to resistance times capacitance (RC). Thus, the greater the resistance in parallel with a given capacitance, the longer the time constant or the time required for it to discharge (or charge). If the time constant is short, that is, equal to or less than the average time between pulses, the meter needle will show rapid, wide fluctuations, making it difficult to obtain accurate readings. On the other hand, if the selected time constant is greater than the average interval between pulses, the meter needle will show more leisurely oscillations, and it will be easier to read. However, response will be sluggish, making it difficult to follow rapid changes in count rate. To obtain the accuracy specified by the manufacturer (2 to 5%) the reading should not be taken until full equilibrium between the charging and discharging of the capacitor has been reached. Equilibrium time is usually 4 times the time constant (4RC). For example, if the time constant is 1 sec, a 4 sec waiting period is required for an accurate reading. If, as is usually the case in counting an organ or specimen at a fixed distance, a 10 sec time constant is used, the reading should be made after 40 sec. Rate meters usually have several time constants, any one of which can be chosen by means of a selector switch.

To increase the accuracy of counting with a rate meter, and to obtain a permanent record of the results, provision is made for connecting a chart recorder—a continuous roll of calibrated paper on which are recorded, in ink, the instantaneous deflections of a lever arm activated by the electrical pulses reaching the rate meter. The deflections over a period of time are averaged to obtain the counts per unit time. The shorter the time constant, the greater will be the fluctuations in the record.

Well Counter. Representing an essential instrument in the nuclear medicine laboratory, the well counter permits the determi-

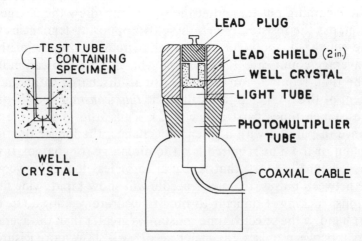

FIGURE 14.10. Well type counter, using a well crystal and scintillation detector. Heavy lead shielding is essential to reduce background.

nation of the activity of a radionuclide in solid or liquid samples. The γ-ray emission of such samples in clinical work, ordinarily body fluids, is so weak that it cannot be counted by conventional G-M or scintillation detectors. In the well counter, a scintillation detector is used with a sodium iodide crystal that is hollowed out to form a well, as shown in Figure 14.10. The radioactive sample is placed in a test tube which is lowered into the well; in effect, the detector surrounds the sample on the sides and bottom. The sensitivity of the well counter is so high that large count rates are obtainable with sources of low activity. In fact, as little as 10^{-5} microcuries (μCi) can be measured. Heavy lead shielding, more than 5 cm in thickness, is ordinarily required to reduce the background count to a sufficiently low level. The greatest field of usefulness of the scintillation well counter in the nuclear medicine laboratory is in the measurement of protein-bound ^{131}I in thyroid investigation; radioactive iodinated serum in the estimation of plasma volume; ^{51}Cr in the determination of red cell survival and red cell mass; ^{60}Co labeled vitamin B_{12} in the diagnosis of pernicious anemia; and ^{59}Fe in studies of red cell production and survival time. The well counter is connected to a scaler to obtain the count rate of a sample.

Radionuclide Scanning. The remarkable sensitivity of the scintillation detector has led to the design of the automatic ***radionuclide scanner*** or ***scintiscanner,*** for the external point-by-point mapping of the distribution of a radionuclide within the body. This has become an extremely important diagnostic tool in nuclear medicine. ***Scans*** or ***scintiscans,*** the visible display of a scanning procedure, are not quantitative but rather indicate pictorially the relative counting rates in different areas of the radionuclide radiation field. The heart of the mechanical scanner is a large scintillation crystal, 7.6 cm (3 in.) or 12.7 cm (5 in.) in diameter. To enable the detector to resolve individual small zones of activity, close ***collimation*** is essential. Special ***multichannel focusing collimators*** are available (see Fig. 14.11) to provide the maximum sensitivity for a given degree of collimation.

The scintillation detector and its collimator move automatically back and forth along parallel lines covering the area of interest, continually recording on X-ray film the light flashes from a small

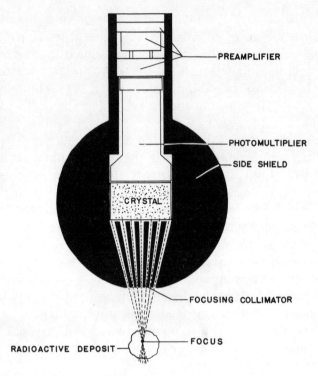

PREAMPLIFIER

PHOTOMULTIPLIER

SIDE SHIELD

CRYSTAL

FOCUSING COLLIMATOR

FOCUS

RADIOACTIVE DEPOSIT

FIGURE 14.11. Diagram of a shielded scintillation detector and focusing collimator used in scanning.

lamp activated by the electric pulses from the detecting system. At the same time this photoscan is being made, a stylus records ink or burn dots on paper as a *dot scan.* The higher the count rate in a particular area, the closer will be the grouping of the dots in both the photoscan and dot scan. An additional system allows the operator to adjust the contrast of the photoscan.

A weakness of the mechanical scanner results from the significant time lapse between the beginning and end of a scan. This makes it difficult or impossible to follow the appearance and disappearance of a radionuclide in an organ; for example, *dynamic processes* such as blood flow through an organ. Stationary devices have been introduced to make possible both *static* and *dynamic scans.* The *Anger Camera* with its large scintillation crystal—28 cm (11 in.) in diameter—can detect and record almost simultaneously the distribution of radioactivity over a relatively large area. Another such device, the ***autofluoroscope,*** consists of a bank of many detector crystals (analogous to the compound eye of an insect) arranged to accomplish the same end. A Polaroid® camera, as well as a 35 mm and a 70 mm rollfilm camera may be used to display the scintiscans produced by both types of gamma cameras. The 70 mm format is preferred because of its convenient size and excellent image definition. A promising new kind of display is embodied in the Microdot® system.

Scanning has become an important method of detecting and localizing primary and metastatic tumors, in addition to the diagnosis of other kinds of lesions. By the use of appropriate radionuclides, abnormalities can be found in the brain, liver, lungs, thyroid gland, pancreas, and kidneys. Of special importance for us is the use of scanning in the localization of metastatic cancer to the liver, brain, and skeletal system.

SOURCES OF ERROR IN COUNTING

Aside from the possibly faulty design of the equipment, or of the procedure itself, there are three main sources of error in counting, all of which must be clearly understood if radionuclide determinations are to be carried out with sufficient precision. They include (1) background, (2) statistical uncertainty, and (3) coincidence loss. Before discussing these, we should point out that the term precision means the reliability or reproducibility of results, provided that the system of measurement is accurate.

Background. If a G-M tube or scintillation detector is operating at the proper voltage with no known source of radiation nearby, counts will be recorded on the scaler or rate meter. These so-called ***background counts*** are due to ***background radiation,*** the sources of which include cosmic rays, natural radioactivity in the earth, and radioactive minerals in the building itself. In addition we have radioactive minerals in the detector and spurious counts resulting from circuitry noise and voltage fluctuation. When a radioactive sample is counted, the total count is the sum of the sample count and the background count. Therefore the background count must be measured separately and subtracted from the total count to obtain the **net sample count.** Then a sample count is run until its total is high enough to satisfy the required precision, and the rate computed. The difference between the sample and background rates is the net count rate of the sample. For example, using a G-M counter,

$$\text{background count} = 420 \text{ in } 10 \text{ min}$$
$$\text{background count rate} = 420/10 = 42 \text{ c/min}$$
$$\text{sample gross count} = 610 \text{ in } 2 \text{ min}$$
$$\text{sample gross count rate} = 610/2 = 305 \text{ c/min}$$
$$\text{gross count rate} - \text{background count rate} = \text{net count rate}$$
$$305 - 42 = 263 \text{ c/min}$$

When the background is very small compared to the sample, it may be neglected without introducing an appreciable error.

As will be shown below, the background count should be reduced to a minimum to improve the accuracy of a counting run. This may be accomplished in part by shielding the detector with lead, leaving only the window unshielded. All radioactive material not being counted should be moved as far as possible from the room where counting is done and should be placed behind lead bricks. It is ordinarily impracticable to shield an entire room against cosmic and γ radiation. Usually a background of 40 c/min for a G-M tube and 250 c/min for a scintillation detector are satisfactory. In general, unless extraordinarily large counts are made, the sample count rate should be at least 9 times that of the background.

Statistical Uncertainty. We may define statistics as the **collection** of a particular set of numerical data and their subsequent **analysis** on the basis of the mathematical **laws of probability** or **chance.** Since radioactive decay is a random process operating in accordance with the laws of probability, statistics plays an important role in radioactive counting. We cannot predict exactly which particular atom in a given sample will undergo nuclear transformation at a given instant in time. Therefore the time intervals between individual transformations vary, and the resulting pulses generated in the detector have a random distribution in time. This is evident from the observation that repeated counting runs of the same radioactive sample yield somewhat different counts despite the existence of a definite statistical rate of decay. For maximum precision, that is, reproducibility of results, an extremely large number of counts must be recorded, from which a nearly ideal average count rate may be calculated. However, it is impracticable to accumulate such large counts routinely, especially with radioactive sources of low activity, and when very high precision is not required.

The precision of a given count is determined by considering its deviation from the ideal average that is obtainable only from an extremely large number of counting runs. By the use of special statistical equations, we can arrive at a statement as to the error that is likely to be present in a particular count. The most useful of these equations gives the **standard deviation,** σ, which is the plus or minus deviation of any count, from the "true" average, that will not be exceeded 68 percent of the time. This will be further clarified after standard deviation has been described in more detail. For our purposes standard deviation is derived from the Poisson Distribution of random and independent events (such as nuclear decay), exemplified by the curves in Figure 14.12. Accordingly, the standard deviation σ is given by

$$\sigma = \pm\sqrt{N} \tag{2}$$

where N is the observed count and is assumed to be the "true" average count. For example, if a given sample count is 6,400, then

$$\sigma = \pm\sqrt{6,400} = \pm 80$$

and the count is stated as $6,400 \pm 80$. According to Figure 14.12, this means that the true average count has a 68 percent chance of lying somewhere between $6,400 - 80$ and $6,400 + 80$, or between 6,320 and 6,480. In other words, there is a 2 to 1 chance that the true average count lies between the values defined by the standard deviation, the **confidence level** being 68 percent.

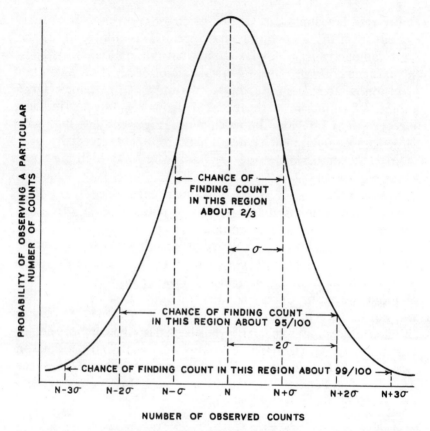

FIGURE 14.12. Normal or "bell-shaped" distribution curve showing probability of variation of an individual count from the mean count N. Note that the probability of finding a particular count within ± 1 standard deviation (σ) from the mean is about 2/3.

The ***percent standard error*** is related to the number of counts as follows:

$$\%S.E. = \pm \frac{\sigma}{N} = \pm \frac{\sqrt{N}}{N} \times 100 \qquad (3)$$

$$\%S.E. = \pm \frac{100}{\sqrt{N}} \qquad (4)$$

In the above example,

$$\%S.E. = \pm \frac{100}{\sqrt{6,400}} = \pm \frac{100}{80} = \pm 1.3\%$$

The count may now be stated as 6,400 ± 1.3 percent. In other words there is a 2 to 1 chance that the error in the count will not exceed 1.3 percent in either direction.

It is obvious from equation (4) that the percent standard error (%S.E.) of a counting run increases as the total number of counts decreases. For example, if the total count is 10,000 then

$$\%S.E. = \pm \frac{100}{\sqrt{10,000}} = \pm \frac{100}{100} = \pm 1\%$$

On the other hand, with a relatively small count such as 400,

$$\%S.E. = \pm \frac{100}{\sqrt{400}} = \pm \frac{100}{20} = \pm 5\%$$

Furthermore, statistical precision depends on the **total count**, and not at all on the counting time.

As already implied, the observer can be 68 percent confident that the "true" count will fall within $\pm 1\sigma$, or the odds are 2:1 that this will be so. Furthermore, he can be 95 percent confident (19:1 odds) that the "true" count will fall within the range of $\pm 2\sigma$. In nuclear medicine enough counts should be accumulated to give a confidence level of 95 percent for a %S.E. of ±2 percent, requiring a total count of 10,000. This can be proved as follows:

$$\sigma = \pm \sqrt{10,000} = \pm 100$$

$$2\sigma = \pm 200 \text{ for } 95\% \text{ confidence with this total count}$$

$$\%S.E. = \frac{\pm 200}{10,000} \times 100 = \pm 2\% \text{ (according to equation [3])}$$

For still higher confidence—99 percent—we must include the range $\pm 3\sigma$, but this exceeds the usual requirements for nuclear medicine.

The above discussion applies to a total count, such as that obtained from a sample and background together. However, in actual practice the net count is obtained by subtracting the background from the total. Since both counts contain statistical errors, the standard deviation of the **net count** must be determined from the standard deviations of the total and background counts. If σ_B applies to the background and σ_T applies to the total count,

$$\sigma = \pm \sqrt{\sigma_B^2 + \sigma_T^2} \tag{5}$$

Since $\sigma = \pm \sqrt{N}$, $\sigma^2 = N$. Substituting in equation (5):

$$\sigma = \pm \sqrt{N_B + N_T}$$

where N_B is the background count and N_T is the total count. The %S.E. is obtained by

$$\%S.E. = \frac{\pm \sqrt{N_B + N_T}}{N_T - N_B} \times 100 \tag{6}$$

Note that (6) is independent of the count rate; we can count as many pulses as necessary in order to obtain the desired precision. The %S.E. derived from equation (6) will then apply to the final calculated count rate. An example will help to clarify this statement. Suppose we are given the following data:

background counted for 10 min—460
gross sample counted for 2 min —7,640

Then from equation (6)

$$\%S.E. = \frac{\pm \sqrt{460 + 7,640}}{7,640 - 460} \times 100 = \frac{\pm \sqrt{8,100}}{7,180} \times 100$$

$$\%S.E. = \pm \frac{90}{7,180} \times 100 = \pm 1.3 \text{ percent}$$

Returning to the original data, we find that

Background count rate is $460/10 = 46$ c/min

Gross sample count rate is $7,640/2 = 3,820$ c/min

Subtracting the two, we obtain 3,774 c/m as the net count rate of the sample itself. Applying the %*S.E.* obtained above, we may state the final rate as $3,774 \pm 1.3\%$. This % *S.E.* is correct for this count rate *only insofar as it is based on the above selected total number of counts.* Furthermore, the higher the background count relative to the sample count, the more total counts must be accumulated. In fact, a background of 40 c/m introduces a negligible error when the total count is of the order of several thousand. On the assumption that the background is so small as to be negligible, relative to the total count (less than 10%), Figure 14.13 shows in graphic form the number of counts required for a given standard error.

Coincidence Loss. In the description of the G-M counter we found that the positive ions released during the avalanche migrate relatively slowly toward the cathode, while the electrons move at

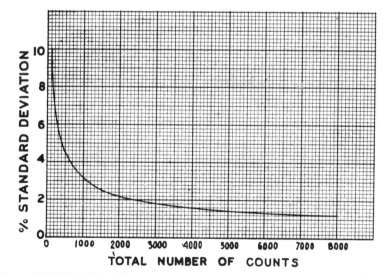

FIGURE 14.13. Variation in percent standard error with the total number of counts in a particular measurement.

a high velocity toward the central wire anode. Because of the lag in movement of the positive ions, the G-M tube is insensitive to further ionizing particles or photons during the time the positive ions are in migration. This period of insensitivity is known variously by the terms **resolving time, recovery time,** or **dead time** of the G-M tube. It may be as short as 2×10^{-4} sec or 0.2 milliseconds. With this resolving time, the counter should record $1/(2 \times 10^{-4}) = 5,000$ evenly spaced ionizing events during each second. However, since the ionizing events are random, due to the random nature of radioactive decay, ionizing particles or photons do not enter the G-M tube at evenly spaced intervals and may even enter during its dead time without being detected. This is more serious at high counting rates, introducing a sizable error in the count. The loss of counts due to ionizing particles or quanta entering the G-M tube too closely spaced to be detected is called **coincidence loss.** It may be computed from the recovery time and the count rate. If the observed count rate is R counts per min and we assume that each count is followed by a resolution or recovery time of t sec or $t/60$ min then the total time in which the counter is insensitive out of each minute is the product of the two:

$$\text{Insensitive time} = \frac{Rt}{60} \text{ min out of each min}$$

Therefore,

$$\frac{Rt}{60} \times 100 = \begin{cases} \% \text{ of time counter is insensitive, or} \\ \% \text{ of counts lost} \end{cases} \quad (8)$$

But the "true" count N_a equals the observed count N plus the number of counts lost, all in the same time interval (e.g. 1 min):

$$N_a = N + (N_a \times \% \text{ lost}) \quad (9)$$

Suppose there is an observed count rate of 20,000 per min and the resolving time is 0.0002 sec. From equation (8):

$$\frac{20,000 \times 0.0002}{60} \times 100 = \% \text{ of counts lost} = 6.7\%$$

Substituting the known values in equation (9):

$$N_a = 20,000 + 0.067\ N_a$$

$$0.933\ N_a = 20,000$$

$$N_a = \frac{20,000}{0.933} = 21,440\ \text{``}true\text{''}\ count$$

Note that the error from coincidence loss alone, at this high counting rate, is more than 5 percent with a G-M counter.

Coincidence loss with scintillation detectors is very small, the dead time being approximately 10 μsec, whereas that for a G-M counter is about 20 times as large.

GENERAL TYPES OF COUNTING

Thus far, we have discussed the types of equipment used in the detection and assay of radionuclides, and mentioned the various sources of error in counting. We must now turn to the methods of counting in nuclear medicine, with a consideration of the two general types: *absolute* and *comparative.*

Absolute Counting. We must emphasize that in counting a radioactive sample, we are not determining directly the decay rate. Figure 14.14 shows how the geometric arrangement prevents

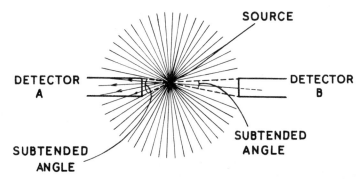

FIGURE 14.14. More particles enter the aperture as the detector is brought closer. Thus, detector *A* would record a higher count rate than detector *B* with the same radioactive sample.

counting all the particles or photons emitted per unit time. Radiation is emitted in every direction in space, passing outward from the source in the form of an increasing spherical surface. However, only a small fraction of the radiation enters the aperture of the counter; the greater the solid angle subtended by the aperture, the greater the *extrinsic efficiency*. If detector A is placed closer to the source as in Figure 14.14, the subtended angle is larger and the efficiency is increased, but at the same time there is a greater error introduced in measuring the *true* distance of the source. Therefore, most workers prefer to use longer distances; for example, in thyroid uptake studies, the distance is usually about 20 to 30 cm. The counting time is increased accordingly to maintain the desired precision.

Of the radiation finally entering the detector, that fraction which the instrument actually detects indicates its *intrinsic efficiency*. As we have already noted, the scintillation counter is considerably more efficient than the G-M tube insofar as γ rays are concerned.

In clinical practice, the *overall efficiency* or *sensitivity* of a detector is more important than the intrinsic or extrinsic efficiency, once the detector has been selected and the geometric setup established. As we have already indicated, the count rate is proportional to the activity of the sample, these two variables being related by a constant called the *sensitivity* or *overall efficiency* of the counter in the geometric arrangement:

$$R = SA \tag{10}$$

where R is the observed count rate, S is the sensitivity, and A is the activity. But R is also proportional to the decay rate D, so

$$R = SD \tag{11}$$

Rearranging,

$$S = R/D$$

If we count a standard having a known decay rate and correct it for background, coincidence loss, and statistical error, we can determine the sensitivity of the counter by using equation (11). In this manner, the detector can be calibrated for actual de-excitations per sec. Standard solutions can be purchased from the

National Bureau of Standards, accompanied by a certificate stating the number of atoms decaying per sec per milliliter (d/s/ml) at a specific time. The d/s/ml can be corrected for decay at some other time by use of the decay curve for that particular radionuclide.

Suppose the standard for ^{131}I has an activity of 10^4 d/s, and at a given distance from the detector we obtain a corrected count of 120/sec. Using equation (11) we find that:

$$S = \frac{120}{10^4} = \frac{120}{10,000}$$

$$S = 0.012 = 1.2\%$$

The sensitivity of the counter under the conditions of measurement is therefore 1.2 percent. If, now, we have an unknown sample of ^{131}I and place it in the same volume of solution at exactly the same distance from the counter as the standard, and obtain 200 c/sec, the number of d/sec can be determined by equation (11):

$$R = SD$$

$$200 = 0.012D$$

$$D = \frac{200}{0.012} = 16,667 \text{ d/s}$$

From the d/s one can readily calculate the activity of the nuclide in curies. Since 1 millicurie $= 3.7 \times 10^7$ d/s,

$$\frac{16,667}{3.7 \times 10^7} = 4.5 \times 10^{-4} \text{ mCi}$$

One mCi $= 1,000$ microcuries (μCi), and, therefore,

$$4.5 \times 10^{-4} \text{ mCi} = 4.5 \times 10^{-4} \times 10^3, \text{ or } 0.45 \ \mu\text{Ci}$$

Comparative Counting. In ordinary tracer studies, absolute counting is seldom required. Since calibrated doses of radionuclides are available commercially, most procedures are based on *comparative counting.* With a given radionuclide the count rate depends on the quantity present, but this is modified by geometric factors: *distance* and *volume* of liquid or tissue containing the nuclide. A third factor is **self-absorption** of radiation in the sample (see page 153). The count rate decreases as the distance of the source from the detector is increased; and, it also decreases as the volume increases. If these geometric factors are maintained constant, the count rate is proportional to the activity of the radionuclide present.

Here is a simple example of comparative counting. Suppose we have a liter of solution containing an unknown activity of a particular radionuclide. We dissolve a known activity of the same radionuclide in 1 liter of water to serve as a standard. We then count the sample and the standard individually under identical conditions, to the desired confidence level. The activity of the sample is obtained by

$$\frac{mCi\ sample}{mCi\ standard} = \frac{c/m\ sample}{c/m\ standard} \qquad (12)$$

PROPERTIES OF RADIONUCLIDES

Since we are primarily concerned with the physics of radiation **therapy,** we shall omit the use of radionuclides in specific diagnostic applications. However, we shall review some of the general characteristics of radioactivity pertinent to the medical use of radionuclides, although the subject has been covered in detail in Chapter 11. Radionuclides are endowed with the property of **radioactivity**—the spontaneous de-excitation or transformation—of nuclei associated with the emission of ionizing radiations. This process is often referred to as decay or, less desirably, as disintegration. The total energy emitted by a nucleus in one de-excitation is called the **transition energy.**

Decay Constant. The rate of decay is constant for a particular radionuclide. Physicists use the term **decay constant** (λ) as the quantitative expression of the **decay rate,** defining it as the fractional amount of a given radionuclide decaying per unit time. The decay constant is **specific** for each radionuclide.

Half-life. Since the decay rate for a given radionuclide is constant, the time required for one-half the original activity of a sample of the radionuclide to decay must also be constant. This specific time is called the **half-life** of that radionuclide. It is readily applicable in nuclear medicine because of its simplicity. The half-life and decay constant of any radionuclide are related as follows:

$$half\text{-}life = \frac{0.693}{\lambda} \qquad (13)$$

It is sometimes convenient to regard the rate of decay in terms of the number of half-lives that have elapsed during a selected time interval. The fractional amount of any radionuclide remaining after n half-lives is equal to $1/2^n$. For example, if we start with 100 mCi of ^{131}I, and we wish to determine the activity remaining after 3 half-lives, the fraction remaining is $(1/2^3) = (1/8)$. Therefore,

$$100 \text{ mCi} \times \frac{1}{8} = 12.5 \text{ mCi}$$

Average Life. Another entity is average life, the average survival time of the atoms of a given radionuclide. It is obtained mathematically as follows:

$$average\ life = \frac{1}{\lambda}$$

Decay Curves. To determine the activity of any radionuclide remaining after a certain length of time, one may employ either tables or graphs. Figures 14.15 and 14.16 are graphs known as **decay curves** for ^{131}I and ^{32}P respectively. But since the decay process is exponential, a straight line is obtained when the data are plotted on semilogarithmic paper, with the **remaining amount** on the vertical axis and the **elapsed time** on the horizontal axis. Therefore, if the half-life of a given radionuclide is known, the decay curve can be obtained simply by plotting two points on a semilog graph. One point must be 100 at zero time, that is, 100 on the vertical axis line. The other point is the coordinate of 50 on the vertical axis, and the time for one half-life. By extending a straight line through these two points, one obtains the complete decay curve, as illustrated in Figures 14.17 and 14.18. Note, for example, in the decay curve of ^{131}I, that at zero time the initial activity as measured along the vertical axis is taken to be 100 percent.

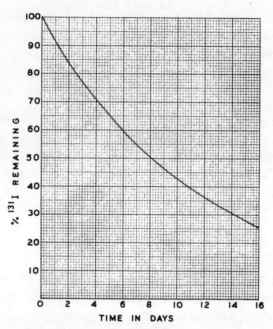

FIGURE 14.15. Decay curve of radioiodine 131 (^{131}I), linear plot.

This is the first point on the straight line curve. The second point is the coordinate of the 50 percent point on the vertical axis, and the 8.1 day point on the horizontal axis since the half-life of ^{131}I is 8.1 days. A straight line drawn through these points, on semilog paper, constitutes the physical decay curve. At 2 half-lives or 16.2 days, for ^{131}I, the curve shows 25 percent activity remaining. This is verified by multiplying

$$100\% \times \frac{1}{2^n} = 100\% \times \frac{1}{2^2} = 100\% \times \frac{1}{4} = 25\%$$

At 3 half-lives or 24 days, the percentage remaining is 12.5. This is verified by :

$$100\% \times \frac{1}{2^3} = 100\% \times \frac{1}{8} = 12.5\%$$

By reversing the above procedure, we can readily find the half-life of an unknown radionuclide. First measure its activity at a recorded time called zero. After a suitable interval of time, measure the sample again. Plot the two points on semilog paper and connect them with a straight line to obtain the decay curve. The time corresponding to 50 percent remaining activity is the half-life.

Units of Activity. The units of *activity* are based on the *curie* (Ci)—the activity of a radionuclide sample undergoing 3.7×10^{10} d/s (37 billion disintegrations per second). The units most often used in nuclear medicine are as follows:

1 millicurie (mCi) $= 3.7 \times 10^7$ d/s, or 10^{-3} curie
1 microcurie (μCi) $= 3.7 \times 10^4$ d/s, or 10^{-6} curie

As we have already pointed out, the activity of a given radioactive sample in mCi or μCi can be determined by comparison with a standard sample of known activity.

Specific Activity. Since a radionuclide decays at a fixed rate, we can say it undergoes a certain number of transformations per second for each gram of sample. This leads to the concept of

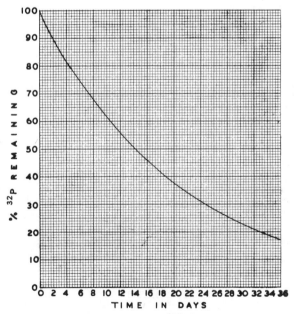

FIGURE 14.16. Decay curve of radiophosphorus 32 (^{32}P), linear plot.

specific activity which is defined as the **number of curies per gram** (Ci/g) of a given radioactive sample. The specific activity may be expressed in the following simple equation:

$$specific\ activity = \frac{curies\ in\ sample}{mass\ of\ sample\ (g)} = Ci/g \qquad (15)$$

It is possible to derive the specific activity of any pure radionuclide in terms of the half-life and atomic weight. The emission rate or number of nuclei de-exciting per second d/s depends on the number of atoms present n and the decay constant λ:

$$d/s = n\lambda \qquad (16)$$

Since $\lambda = 0.693/T$, where T is the half-life, we may substitute this value of λ in equation (16):

$$d/s = \frac{0.693n}{T} \qquad (17)$$

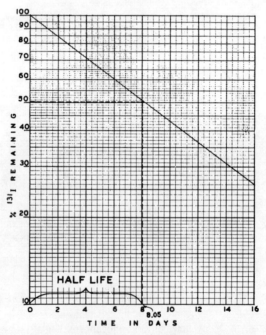

FIGURE 14.17. Decay curve of ^{131}I, semilog plot.

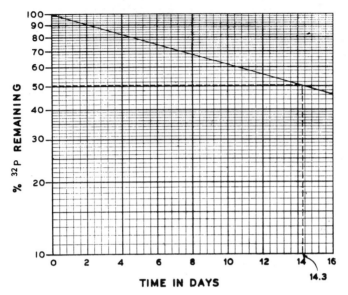

FIGURE 14.18. Decay curve of ^{32}P, semilog plot.

The units of time must be the same throughout the equation, *seconds* in this example. To find the emission rate per gram of pure nuclide, divide both members of the equation by "grams" (g),

$$\frac{d/s}{g} = \frac{0.693n}{Tg} \qquad (18)$$

Since n/g also represents the number of atoms in a gram atomic weight (Avogadro's number 6.02×10^{23}) divided by the atomic weight A of the radionuclide, we may substitute in equation (18), obtaining:

$$\frac{d/s}{g} = \frac{0.693 \times 6.02 \times 10^{23}}{TA} \qquad (19)$$

But 1 Ci represents 3.7×10^{10} d/s, so the right side of equation (19) may be converted to Ci/g by dividing by 3.7×10^{10}.

$$\frac{Ci}{g} = \frac{0.693 \times 6.02 \times 10^{23}}{3.7 \times 10^{10}\, TA}$$

Since Ci/g = specific activity, we may simplify the preceding equation as follows:

$$\frac{specific}{activity} = \frac{1.13 \times 10^{13}}{TA} Ci/g \qquad (20)$$

Thus, if the half-life and the atomic weight (or mass number) of a radionuclide are known, the specific activity of a pure sample can readily be determined by equation (20). For example, ^{131}I has a mass number 131 and a half-life of 8.1 days. First, convert 8.1 days to seconds by multiplying by $24 \times 60 \times 60$. This turns out to be 7.0×10^5 sec. Substituting in equation (20),

$$\frac{specific}{activity} {}^{131}I = \frac{1.13 \times 10^{13}}{7.0 \times 10^5 \times 131} Ci/g$$

$$\frac{specific}{activity} {}^{131}I = 1.23 \times 10^5 \, Ci/g$$

Interestingly enough, a 100 μCi dose of ^{131}I contains only 0.001 μg (i.e. 1 nanogram) of iodine!

Note that specific activity in the above sense refers to the pure radionuclide. If no stable isotope is present in the sample, it is said to be **carrier free.** As we noted earlier, those radionuclides which are produced by artificial transmutation of a different target element (such as ^{32}P from ^{32}S) are readily separated and can, therefore, be obtained carrier free. On the other hand, radionuclides which are produced by neutron irradiation of the stable isotope (such as ^{60}Co from ^{59}Co) are extremely difficult to separate and are therefore contaminated with stable isotopes. (Originally, the term "carrier" referred to the stable isotope that was added to a minute quantity of the radioactive isotope to help precipitate it from a solution.) One may extend the use of the expression "specific activity" to that of a particular sample even though it contains a stable isotope carrier, if it is kept in mind that specific activity then indicates the number of Ci/g of the sample in question.

By taking the reciprocal of equation (20), one can obtain an expression for the number of grams per curie of a pure radionuclide.

$$\frac{g}{Ci} = 8.85 \, TA \times 10^{-14} \qquad (21)$$

Effective Half-life. When a radionuclide is administered internally, its activity in the body decreases progressively as a result of two separate processes. First, there is physical decay—the half-life due to physical decay is called the *physical half-life* of that particular radionuclide. Second, the radionuclide, when it is one that is utilized in metabolism, enters into the physiologic processes of the body. After reaching equilibrium by distribution within the body, it is metabolized and gradually excreted at a nearly constant rate, governed by the *biologic decay constant* λ_b. The half-life due to biologic loss is called the *biologic half-life.*

The *effective decay constant* λ_e is, therefore, a combination of the physical decay constant λ_p and the biologic decay constant λ_b:

$$\lambda_e = \lambda_p + \lambda_b \tag{22}$$

But we showed earlier that the decay constant $\lambda = 0.693/T$ where T is the half-life. Substituting in equation (22):

$$\frac{0.693}{T_e} = \frac{0.693}{T_p} + \frac{0.693}{T_b} \tag{23}$$

Dividing both members of equation (23) by 0.693,

$$\frac{1}{T_e} = \frac{1}{T_p} + \frac{1}{T_b} \tag{24}$$

This equation may be reduced to the more familiar form by simple algebra:

$$T_e = \frac{T_p T_b}{T_p + T_b} \tag{25}$$

or, stated in words:

$$effective\ half\ life = \frac{physical\ half\ life \times biologic\ half\ life}{physical\ half\ life + biologic\ half\ life}$$

In practice, a dose of the desired radionuclide is administered and a series of counts made in an appropriate manner at certain intervals, say daily for two weeks. With *absolute counting,* each daily count will represent the amount of radionuclide remaining in the organ and when plotted as a decay curve, will indicate the progressive loss of radioactivity due to both physical decay and biologic elimination. Therefore, the half-life obtained from such a decay curve will be the **effective half-life** of that particular radionuclide.

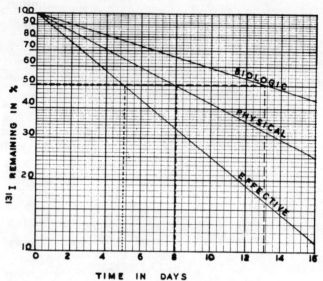

FIGURE 14.19. The three types of decay curves for ^{131}I.

The more common method of **comparative counting,** used in radioiodine uptake studies of thyroid gland function, is carried out at appropriate intervals during the first 24 hours. Comparison of the thyroid counts is made with those of a radioiodine standard having the same activity as the administered dose, and percentage uptake computed.

Biologic Half-life. As mentioned above, **biologic decay** refers to the loss of an administered radionuclide (usually as a tagged compound) resulting from physiologic or pathologic processes only, and neglecting physical decay. This presupposes that biologic decay occurs exponentially, a constant fraction disappearing in unit time. The determination of biologic half-life requires first a series of appropriate absolute counts to derive the **effective half-life.** Published tables give the **physical half-lives** of various radionuclides. The values of T_e and T_p are then substituted in equation (24) rearranged as follows:

$$\frac{1}{T_b} = \frac{1}{T_e} - \frac{1}{T_p} \tag{25a}$$

and T_b computed. For example, suppose the effective half-life of sodium iodide 131 to be 6 days in a particular patient's thyroid gland. Substituting this value as well as that for the physical half-life of ^{131}I (8.1 days) in equation (26),

$$\frac{1}{T_b} = \frac{1}{6} - \frac{1}{8.1}$$

$$= 0.167 - 0.123 = 0.044$$

$$T_b = 1/0.044 = 23 \text{ days}$$

DOSAGE IN SYSTEMIC RADIONUCLIDE THERAPY

The use of radionuclides in therapy is an extension of their application in diagnosis. Doses large enough to cause significant radiation effects in the tissues may be considered to be in the therapeutic range.

Internally administered radionuclides resemble interstitial radium, except that the active foci are submicroscopic in size. The distribution of such nuclides may not be uniform; thus, radiogold is distributed more or less evenly throughout the fluid in a peritoneal or pleural effusion, whereas radioiodine concentrates in the thyroid gland to a significantly higher degree than in other organs. But the nuclide may not be uniformly deposited even in a given organ; for example, in some forms of thyroid disease, radioiodine is fixed in greater concentration in some parts of the gland than in others.

In computing the dosage from internally administered radionuclides, we should record the following data:

1. The description of the treatment in sufficient detail to permit duplication of the technic.

2. The physical and chemical nature of the nuclide, including half-life, and type and energy of radiations emitted.

3. The activity of the nuclide, in millicuries, at the time of administration.

4. The nature and, if possible, the volume (or weight) of both the tissue of interest and the tissue with the maximum concentration of the nuclide.

5. The effective half-life and the pattern of distribution in the target organ and in certain other organs stated as completely as possible.

Absorbed Dose From β^- Emitters. Since the range of β particles in tissues is relatively short (less than 1 cm) most of the radiation effect occurs within the organ in which the nuclide has been deposited. Therefore the calculation of β particle dosage from such internal sources is fairly straightforward. It requires the practical assumption that the radionuclide is uniformly distributed within the organ. If, under these conditions, we achieve a concentration of C μCi of a given β-emitting nuclide per gram of gland, the calculation of absorbed dose would be as follows:

1. The average energy of all the electrons emitted by the radionuclide per disintegration (de-excitation) is called $\bar{E}_\beta$, in units of MeV per de-excitation. This is usually $\frac{1}{3}$ the maximum energy of the β particles if the internal conversion process is not significant. However, for greater reliability, the values for $\bar{E}_\beta$ must be obtained from special tables, such as those of Berger.[4]

2. Certain constants must be used:

    (a) The number of de-excitations/sec per μCi $= 3.7 \times 10^4$ d/s/μCi

    (b) 1 MeV $= 1.6 \times 10^{-6}$ erg

    (c) The energy absorption corresponding to 1 rad $= 100$ ergs/g

First let us apply these values, computing the energy deposited by C μCi in MeV/sec/g:

$$C \; \mu\text{Ci/g} \times 3.7 \times 10^4 \text{ d/s/}\mu\text{Ci} \times \bar{E}_\beta \text{ MeV/d}$$

$$= 3.7 \times 10^4 C\bar{E}_\beta \text{ MeV/s/g}$$

Multiplying by 1.60×10^{-6} erg/MeV to convert MeV to ergs, and dividing by 100 ergs/g to convert to rads,

Energy absorbed in rads/sec

$$= \frac{3.7 \times 10^4 C\bar{E}_\beta \text{ MeV/s/g} \times 1.60 \times 10^{-6} \text{ erg/MeV}}{100 \text{ ergs/g}}$$

$$D_\beta = 5.92 \times 10^{-4} \; C\bar{E}_\beta \text{ rads/sec} \tag{26}$$

where D_β is the absorbed dose contributed by the β^- particles, C is the concentration of radionuclide in μCi/g, and $\bar{E}_\beta$ is the energy per de-excitation in MeV.

To find the energy absorbed during the sojourn to **total decay** of the nuclide in the gland, we must find the average life (effective). If T_e is the effective half-life:

$$average\ life_{eff} = \frac{T_e}{0.693}$$

When T_e is stated in days, it may be applied directly to equation (26) provided the conversion factors to seconds are included. The β^- particle dose D_β to total decay is then:

$$D_\beta = 5.92 \times 10^{-4}\, C\bar{E}_\beta \times \frac{24 \times 60 \times 60}{0.693}\, T_e$$

$$D_\beta = 73.8\, C\bar{E}_\beta T_e\ rads\ to\ total\ decay \tag{27}$$

where C is in μCi/g, $\bar{E}_\beta$ is in MeV, and T_e is in days.

It may be of interest to find the absorbed dose in some time interval, $D_{\beta t}$, other than the total decay time of the radionuclide. This may be done by modifying equation (27) as follows:

$$D_{\beta t} = 73.8\, C\bar{E}_\beta T_e(1 - e^{-(0.693 t/T_e)})\ rads \tag{28}$$

where t is the time interval in days and C is the initial concentration in μCi/g (at beginning of time t).

Equation (28) may be used to find the absorbed dose during three half-lives of the radionuclide, as recommended by the ICRU. In this equation, time t becomes equal to $3T_e$ which may now be substituted:

$$D_\beta = 73.8\, C\bar{E}_\beta T_e(1 - e^{-(0.693 \times 3T_e)/T_e})$$

$$D_\beta = 73.8\, C\bar{E}_\beta T_e(1 - e^{-2.08})\ rads \tag{29}$$

Let us apply the above equations to a hypothetical problem; suppose we wish to determine the total dosage of β^- radiation absorbed by a thyroid gland with an estimated weight of 80 grams, having an uptake of 75 percent, when the administered dose is 5 mCi of ^{131}I. The concentration is then:

$$\frac{5 \text{ mCi} \times 1,000 \times 0.75}{80} = 47 \text{ } \mu\text{Ci/g}$$

From tables, one finds the $\bar{E}_\beta$ for ^{131}I to be 0.182 MeV. The effective half-life in this case is known to be 6 days. According to equation (27),

$$D_\beta = 73.8 \times 47 \text{ } \mu\text{Ci/g} \times 0.182 \text{ MeV} \times 6 \text{ days} = 3790 \text{ rads}$$
$$\text{to total decay}$$

To find the amount of energy absorbed in 3 effective half lives, we may use equation (29):

$$D_\beta = 73.8 \times 47 \times 0.182 \times 6 \, (1 - e^{-2.08})$$

$$= 3790 \, (1 - 0.126)$$

$$D_\beta = 3790 \times 0.874 = 3310 \text{ rads in } 3T_e$$

Note again that the above values of absorbed dose refer only to β^- radiation. The contribution from the γ rays of ^{131}I (mainly 0.364 MeV photons) amounts to about 10 percent of the total dose.

Absorbed Dose From γ-ray Emitters. The determination of the dosage delivered by internally administered γ-ray emitting radionuclides is fraught with many difficulties, mainly because of (1) the long distances traversed by these rays, and (2) the nonuniform distribution of radionuclides in the body.

A series of pamphlets has been issued by the Medical Internal Radiation Dose (MIRD) Committee under the auspices of the Society of Nuclear Medicine. These present, in great detail, the methods of computing β^--particle and γ-ray dosage to various organs from internally deposited radionuclides. Standard sized man and organs have been defined, but these must be inherently subject to error when applied to the individual. Numerous tables are also included. The theory and computations are so complex that they are beyond our scope. Furthermore, the entire subject of internal radiation dosimetry from radionuclides is still in the process of development and, hopefully, simplification at least for practical purposes. Previous methods such as those relying on idealized geometry of the human figure and organs in the shape of spheres or cylinders has proven to be less accurate than the newer methods.

INTERNAL THERAPY WITH RADIONUCLIDES

The first known use of radionuclides in medicine seems to have been the radiophosphorus (^{32}P) treatment of a patient with lymphatic leukemia by John Lawrence in 1937. In fact this antedates by less than one year the diagnostic use of radionuclides, when Saul Hertz performed tracer studies of the thyroid gland with radioiodine (^{131}I). Because of the possibility of depositing organ-specific radionuclides in target organs, it was hoped that a new era of internal radiation therapy was at hand. This idea was reinforced by the first radioiodine treatment of thyrotoxicosis by Hertz and Roberts in 1941. Unfortunately the initial high expectations for radionuclides in internal therapy have not materialized; they have found much greater application in diagnosis and external therapy.

In this section we do not propose to give an exhaustive presentation of internal radionuclide therapy. Instead, we shall focus our attention on ^{131}I, ^{32}P, and ^{198}Au, not only because they are the most widely used, but also because they represent three different forms of internal treatment with radionuclides.

Radioactive Iodine (^{131}I). This nuclide has a physical half-life of 8.1 days, decaying with β^- and γ emission. The β particles have an average energy of 0.182 MeV although the majority (nearly 90 percent) carry a maximum energy of 0.608 MeV. The γ rays have a range of energies, about 82 percent comprising 0.364 MeV. Iodine 131 may be prepared in the nuclear reactor by the irradiation of tellurium with neutrons:

$$^{130}_{52}\text{Te} + ^{1}_{0}\text{n} \longrightarrow \underset{\text{radioactive}}{^{131}_{52}\text{Te}} \longrightarrow \underset{\text{radioactive}}{^{131}_{53}\text{I}} + ^{0}_{-1}\beta + \tilde{\nu}$$

$\underset{\text{stable}}{\phantom{^{130}_{52}\text{Te}}}$

It is also obtainable as a ***fission product*** in the reactor, this now constituting the most abundant source of ^{131}I.

The ^{131}I then decays to stable xenon as follows:

$$^{131}_{53}I \longrightarrow \underset{stable}{^{131}_{54}Xe} + _{-1}^{0}\beta + \gamma + \tilde{v}$$

Before the advent of the nuclear reactor, ^{131}I was obtained by deuterium bombardment of tellurium in the *cyclotron* according to the following reaction:

$$\underset{stable}{^{130}_{52}Te} + {}^{2}_{1}H \longrightarrow \underset{radioactive}{^{132}_{53}I} \quad \text{(half life 2.4 hr)}$$

$$^{132}_{53}I \longrightarrow \underset{radioactive}{^{131}_{53}I} + {}^{1}_{0}n$$

As we have already noted, ^{131}I is readily separated from the target element tellurium by chemical methods so that it can be obtained commercially in relatively pure form; that is, carrier free.

The use of ^{131}I in the therapy of hyperthyroidism depends on the ability of the normal thyroid gland to concentrate inorganic iodine some 25 or more times above the iodine level in the blood. When the thyroid gland functions at an abnormally high level, as in hyperthyroidism, this ratio of thyroid to blood concentration may increase to 500 to 1, or even more.[5] Therefore, assuming that the gland is sensitive to radiation, we can use ^{131}I in therapy by administering it orally or intravenously because it will be selectively absorbed and concentrated in the thyroid gland. The ^{131}I, being rapidly picked up from the circulation (within a few hours), can differentially irradiate the thyroid with a high dose as compared with the dose to the remainder of the body. Since the therapeutic effect of the ^{131}I is due to β particles relative to γ rays by a ratio of about 10 to 1, the energy is dissipated almost entirely within the thyroid. Consequently, the dose delivered to the gland may be several hundred times greater than that to the whole body in a thyrotoxic patient.

Radioiodine therapy has found its widest application in toxic goiter, especially of the *diffuse type*. After the percentage uptake of a tracer dose has been determined (this must *always* precede treatment), we may choose one of several methods to arrive at the therapeutic dose of ^{131}I. First, we must estimate the number of rads to be deposited in the gland. Equation (27) can be used to find C, the number of μCi of ^{131}I per gram of thyroid required to deliver the desired number of rads. Suppose that T_e is known to be 6 days and we wish to deliver a dose of 7,000 rads; substituting these values as well as the known constants in equation (27),

$$D_\beta = 73.8\,C\bar{E}_\beta T_e$$

$$7{,}000 = 73.8 \times C \times 0.182 \times 6$$

$$C = \frac{7{,}000}{73.8 \times 0.182 \times 6} = 87 \ \mu\text{Ci/g}$$

Second, we compute the mCi dose of administered ^{131}I needed to produce this concentration of 87 μCi/g in the thyroid. The following equation may be used:

$$mCi \ given = \frac{100\,W}{\%\ uptake} \times \frac{C}{1{,}000} \tag{30}$$

where W is the estimated weight of the thyroid gland in g and C is the desired concentration of ^{131}I in μCi/g. Suppose the thyroid gland is estimated to weigh 60 g and its uptake is 80 percent. Then,

$$mCi \ given = \frac{60 \text{ g} \times 87 \ \mu\text{Ci/g}}{0.80 \times 1{,}000} = 6.5 \text{ mCi}$$

An approximate expression that is suitable for the β- and γ-ray therapy with ^{131}I has been derived by Quimby:

$$D_{\beta+\gamma} = 90 \times \frac{\mu\text{Ci }^{131}\text{I } in \ gland}{weight \ of \ gland \ (g)} \text{ rads} \tag{31}$$

This equation gives the μCi ^{131}I needed per gram of gland, for the desired dose in rads. From the value of C thus obtained, the administered dose can readily be computed from equation (30).

Despite the apparent accuracy of the above calculations, there are three inherent errors. First, the weight of the thyroid gland *in vivo* is at best an educated guess. Second, the effective half-life of the therapeutic dose may not necessarily be the same as that of the tracer dose. Finally, the assumption that the nuclide is evenly distributed is not entirely valid.

Therefore, in actual practice, most nuclear physicians arbitratily select a predetermined number of microcuries of ^{131}I per gram of gland on an empirical basis, without relating it to the number of rads. There is considerable variation in C, from about 50 to 100 μCi/g, although the tendency at the present time is to use the smaller amount as the initial dose, repeating at the end of several months if necessary. Evidence indicates that of all patients treated with ^{131}I, about 2 percent per year become hypothyroid. In thyrotoxic patients with diffuse involvement of the thyroid gland, the dose is usually 4 to 6 mCi ^{131}I. If sufficient improvement does not occur, the dose may be repeated after about three months. It is inadvisable to repeat therapy sooner than this in order to allow sufficient time for the effect of the first dose to become manifest. It should be pointed out that considerably larger doses, by a factor of 3 or 4, are required in the treatment of *nodular* toxic goiter, although ^{131}I therapy is seldom indicated in this variety of goiter except where surgery is contraindicated.

The second most useful therapeutic application of ^{131}I is in those thyroid cancers which happen to concentrate iodine sufficiently to permit adequate irradiation. Unfortunately, only about 10 to 15 percent of thyroid cancers, especially those with colloid, fall into this category. About 75 percent of follicular carcinomas take up enough radioiodine for effective therapy. Some thyroid cancers, especially those having a glandular structure, take up ^{131}I during the first few hours, only to excrete it promptly within 24 to 36 hours (Corrigan[14]). Unless the biologic half-life is long enough to allow prolonged sojourn of the ^{131}I in the neoplastic tissue, the resulting dose will be inadequate. Complete removal of the carcinomatous thyroid gland before giving the therapeutic dose usually enhances the uptake of ^{131}I by the metastatic deposits. Sometimes this may be further increased by preliminary administration of the thyroid stimulating fraction of the anterior pituitary (TSH) in daily doses of 10 units for about 1 week.

The amount of ^{131}I to be administered in thyroid cancer is even more difficult to estimate than in thyrotoxicosis because of the tremendous variation in uptake by the malignant cells, and the difficulty in judging the volume of thyroid cancer metastasis.

Blahd recommends giving a preliminary test dose of 1 mCi and determining the γ-ray blood dose as well as body retention of ^{131}I. However, treatment is generally *empirical*. The usual therapeutic dose is 100 to 150 mCi ^{131}I, followed by scanning of possible metastatic sites. The dose may then be repeated in a few months, and again uptake sought in possible metastatic sites. Unless there is severe bone marrow depression or other generalized manifestation of radiation damage, the dose may be repeated until the metastases pick up only a small fraction of the administered dose; the smaller the fraction, the longer the intervals between additional doses. When the uptake with a test dose of 1 to 3 mCi falls below 0.01 percent, treatment may be discontinued, then reinstituted if subsequent tracer doses show uptake in the metastatic areas. The patient is maintained in the euthyroid state by exogenous oral thyroid medication which should be discontinued 6 weeks before each therapeutic dose or uptake study (2 weeks if maintained on triiodothyronine) and resumed 2 days thereafter. TSH may be used to enhance the uptake of residual metastatic foci as above. The treatment of complications and sequelae is beyond the scope of this book.

Radiophosphorus (^{32}P) Therapy of Hematologic Diseases. The radioisotope of phosphorus, ^{32}P, is a pure β^- emitter having a half-life of 14.3 days. These β particles have a maximum energy of 1.7 MeV and an average energy of 0.7 MeV. Their maximum range in tissues is 8 mm, although the average is only 2 mm. However, they may travel as far as 4 meters (12 feet) in air.

Radiophosphorus is now produced commercially in the nuclear reactor by the following reaction:

$$^{32}_{16}S + ^{1}_{0}n \longrightarrow ^{32}_{15}P + ^{1}_{1}H$$

The products are easy to separate chemically, so commercially available ^{32}P is carrier free. It is also possible to obtain ^{32}P by slow neutron bombardment of stable ^{31}P, but due to the difficulty in separating the isotopes, the ^{32}P is not carrier free.

Phosphorus 32 can also be manufactured in the cyclotron by firing high energy deuterons at a ^{31}P target, but this is no longer an abundant source of ^{32}P. It will be recalled that ^{32}P can be made by low energy deuteron reaction with ^{31}P by the Oppenheimer-Phillips Mechanism in which the ^{31}P nucleus repels the deuteron's proton, allowing the neutron portion to slip in:

$$^{31}_{15}P + \quad ^{1}_{1}H \cdot ^{1}_{0}n \quad \longrightarrow \quad ^{32}_{15}P + ^{1}_{1}H$$
slow deuteron

Phosphorus has the peculiar ability to concentrate in the **nuclei** of cells because it is incorporated in nucleic acid. Since the nuclei in rapidly proliferating cells, such as those in malignant tumors, tend to have a larger volume than in normal cells, the concentration of phosphorus in malignant cell nuclei may be as high as 3 to 5 times that in normal nuclei. Furthermore, phosphorus is a very important element in the chemical makeup of bone, and it therefore deposits in bone as well as in cells of the reticuloendothelial system. Consequently, it seems rational to employ ^{32}P in the treatment of certain blood dyscrasias in which there is excessive production of red cells (polycythemia vera) and white cells (leukemia), since these cells are irradiated both internally from the ^{32}P fixed in their nuclei, and externally from the ^{32}P fixed in the bone.

When ^{32}P is given by mouth to normal or leukemic patients, as much as 50 percent is lost through the kidneys and intestinal tract in 4 to 6 days, the larger fraction appearing in the feces. About 75 percent of an administered dose is assumed to be absorbed in the gastrointestinal tract, while the remaining 25 percent passes out in the feces. On intravenous administration, 5 to 10 percent is lost in the urine in 24 hours, and about 20 percent in 1 week. There may be more ^{32}P retained by leukemic and polycythemic patients than by normals because of the greater affinity of the rapidly multiplying malignant nuclei for phosphorus. The effective half-life of ^{32}P in the body is about 1 week.

Because of variation in life span of the blood cells, the observed effect of ^{32}P varies. Thus, the granulocytes in chronic myelogenous leukemia have a life span of about 5 days, so at least 1 week will be required to observe the effect of a therapeutic dose. Lymphocytes in chronic lymphatic leukemia have an average life span of about 80 days and erythrocytes about 120 days; therefore, the effect on these cells may require a few months to become manifest.

Using the equation for β-particle dosage to total decay and Lawrence's data on the distribution of ^{32}P in the body, Quimby has calculated the dosimetry of intravenously administered ^{32}P. Her approach to the problem may be illustrated in outline form as follows:

A. Assume an intravenous dose of 3 mCi ^{32}P in a 70 kg patient (that is, 70,000 g).

B. **During first 3 days,** ^{32}P uniformly distributed throughout the body, 12 percent being lost through physical decay. Since

$$D_\beta = 73.8\,C\bar{E}_\beta\,T_e$$

where T_e may be considered equal to the physical half-life during the period of uniform distribution,

$$D_\beta = 73.8 \times \frac{3,000\ \mu\text{Ci}}{70,000\ \text{g}} \times 0.7 \times 14.3\ \text{days} = 31.7\ \text{rads}$$

But only 12 percent has decayed, so that whole body dose during first 3 days is

$$0.12 \times 31 = 3.72\ \text{rads}$$

C. **After third day,** effective half life is 11 days and concentration in "bone" compartment B (bone marrow, spleen, and liver) about 10 times that in remaining soft tissues S. But on third day only 88 percent of initial dose remains:

$$3\ \text{mCi} \times 0.88 = 2.6\ \text{mCi}$$

D. Bone compartment B comprises about 17 percent of total body weight, or 12,000 g, leaving 58,000 g as weight of rest of body. Therefore,

$$concentration\ in\ B = \frac{\mu\text{Ci}\ in\ B}{12,000}$$

$$concentration\ in\ S = \frac{\mu\text{Ci}\ in\ S}{58,000}$$

E. But concentration in bone compartment is about 10 times that in the soft tissues, so that

$$\frac{\mu\text{Ci in B}}{12{,}000} = 10 \times \frac{\mu\text{Ci in S}}{58{,}000}$$

$$\frac{\mu\text{Ci in B}}{\mu\text{Ci in S}} = \frac{12{,}000 \times 10}{58{,}000} = \text{about 2}$$

Thus, ratio of ^{32}P in bone compartment to that in soft tissue is about 2:1, which means that by the fourth day, $\frac{2}{3}$ of the ^{32}P has entered the bone compartment and $\frac{1}{3}$ has entered the soft tissues. In this case,

$$\frac{2}{3} \times 2{,}600 \ \mu\text{Ci} = 1{,}730 \ \mu\text{Ci } in \ B$$

$$\frac{1}{3} \times 2{,}600 \ \mu\text{Ci} = 860 \ \mu\text{Ci } in \ S$$

F. After third day, "bone dose" to total decay is

$$\text{``bone''} \ D_\beta = \frac{1{,}730 \ \mu\text{Ci}}{12{,}000 \ \text{g}} \times \bar{E}_\beta \times T_e \times 73.8$$

$$\text{``bone''} \ D_\beta = \frac{1{,}730 \ \mu\text{Ci}}{12{,}000 \ \text{g}} \times 0.7 \times 11 \times 73.8 = 82 \ \text{rads}$$

The dose to the "soft tissue" compartment is

$$\text{``soft tissue''} \ D = \frac{860}{58{,}000} \times 0.7 \times 11 \times 73.8 = 8.4 \ \text{rads}$$

G. Now add to each the dose delivered during the first 3 days, that is, 3.7 rads:

$$\text{``bone''} \ D_\beta = 3.7 + 82 = 86 \ \text{rads}$$

$$\text{``soft tissue''} \ D_\beta = 3.7 + 8.4 = 12 \ \text{rads}$$

Note that the above calculations omit the factor of excretion which may amount to 25 percent or more during the first three days. In other words, the dose actually delivered is somewhat less than that just derived. According to Osgood,[63] the bone compartment receives a dose of about 10 to 15 rads per mCi ^{32}P.

1. ***Radiophosphorus Therapy of Polycythemia Vera.*** Radio-phosphorus is the treatment of choice in ***polycythemia vera.*** This disease is a manifestation of chronic overactivity of all bone marrow elements, but mainly the red blood cells. The aim of ^{32}P therapy is the inhibition of the manufacture of blood cells by the blood forming (hematopoietic) organs. It does not hasten the destruction of circulating cells. Because of the long average life span of red blood cells, about 120 days, the full effect of a therapeutic dose of ^{32}P is not observed until about 4 months have elapsed; therefore, it should not be repeated at intervals of less than 3 months.

Phosphorus 32 therapy is preferably reserved for those patients who no longer respond satisfactorily to venesection, or who display a very high platelet count of 800,000/ml, or more. However, Osgood's method of therapy of polycythemia ***without*** preliminary venesection is based on the premise that bleeding stimulates the bone marrow to further activity and may favor thrombosis. Dosage of ^{32}P is governed by body weight, as follows:

less than 125 lb—3 mCi intravenously
125 to 175 lb—4 mCi
over 175 lb—5 mCi

The patients return regularly every 12 weeks, but if symptoms are severe, they should be seen as often as every 4 weeks. Followup examination includes a complete blood count and blood volume study. If the RBC, hemoglobin, or blood volume increases by at least 20 percent, the dose is repeated even if the patient has no symptoms. It is rarely necessary to retreat a patient before 1 to 3 years after the initial dose.

According to the National Institutes of Health Polycythemia Study Group, the initial dose should be 2.3 mCi/m^2 of body surface. However, some prefer to use an empirical dose of 3 mCi for all patients.

The results of therapy with ^{32}P are extremely encouraging, with remissions lasting from about 6 months to a year or more. Often the simple repetition of the initial dose after relapse again induces a satisfactory remission. With older methods limited to venesection, phenylhydrazine, or X-ray therapy, median survival time

was about 7 years. This has nearly doubled since the advent of
^{32}P therapy. However, there is some indication of a greater incidence of leukemia in polycythemia vera patients after prolonged
survival with ^{32}P therapy. Whether this results from the natural
history of the disease or from irradiation is still a moot question.

2. *Radiophosphorus Therapy of Chronic Leukemia.* The first satisfactory palliation of chronic leukemia was achieved with X-ray
therapy. This was virtually replaced by ^{32}P when it became available in sufficient quantity following the demonstration of its effectiveness in 1937 by J. Lawrence. However, administration dosage
schedules differed widely among various treatment centers, and
some even included supplemental X-ray therapy. In general, 1 to
2 mCi of ^{32}P as sodium phosphate may be given weekly until the
leukocyte count falls to about 20,000. Usually, 4 to 6 injections
will induce satisfactory palliation during a period of a year or
more, but a total dose of more than 15 to 20 mCi in any one year
should be avoided. Supplemental therapy such as X-ray irradiation of the spleen, blood transfusions, and androgens have often
been used.

Since the advent of chemotherapy, irradiation has been virtually
abandoned except for patients whose disease has become drug resistant, or who develop splenomegaly or leukemic masses. Bu-
sulfan (Myleran®) is preferred for chronic myelogenous leukemia,
and chlorambucil (Leukeran®) for chronic lymphocytic leukemia.

Unfortunately, the long-term results of therapy, whether radiation or drug, are very difficult to evaluate. There is, in fact, no
convincing evidence of prolongation of life, average survival in
chronic myelogenous leukemia being about 3 to 4 years. Nevertheless, there is general agreement that the palliation achieved in
most patients makes treatment worthwhile.

Radiophosphorus Therapy of Metastatic Cancer in Bone. The
majority of metastatic lesions in bone have their origin in cancer
of the breast, prostate, lungs, kidneys, and thyroid gland. In most
instances, when palliative irradiation is indicated, megavoltage
radiation is used. However, skeletal metastases from prostatic
cancer often fail to respond, and it may be possible to achieve
some degree of palliation of intractable pain by giving ^{32}P. Unfor-

tunately, this requires prior stimulation of the uptake mechanism of bone for phosphorus, usually with intramuscular androgens.

Tong[84] has published a method of enhancing the deposition of ^{32}P in bone near the metastatic lesions by first administering para-thormone for one week. Upon withdrawal of the hormone, there is a rebound phenomenon beginning within 24 hours, character-ized by an increased deposition of calcium phosphate in bone. If ^{32}P is given at this time, and in decreasing doses for six weeks thereafter, a large fraction will be taken up by bones generally. However, it is questionable whether this is superior to androgen stimulation to enhance osseous uptake of ^{32}P.

Radiogold (^{198}Au) in Treatment of Malignant Pleural and Peritoneal Effusions. Radiogold is a radioisotope prepared in the nuclear reactor by neutron irradiation of ordinary gold:

$$^{197}_{79}Au + ^{1}_{0}n \longrightarrow \underset{\textit{radioactive}}{^{198}_{79}Au} + \gamma$$

^{198}Au de-excites as follows:

$$^{198}_{79}Au \longrightarrow ^{198}_{80}Hg + ^{0}_{-1}\beta + \gamma + \tilde{\nu}$$

Gold 198 has a half-life of 2.7 days, decaying with emission of β^- particles and γ rays. Of the β^- particles, 99 percent have an energy of 0.96 MeV, and of the γ rays, the most energetic are 0.41 MeV. Since more than 90 percent of the biologic effect is due to the β particles, their penetrating ability assumes major importance. This turns out to be a maximum range of nearly 4 mm in tissue, and an average range of less than 1 mm. Therefore, the efficacy of radiogold in body cavities containing effusions due to metastatic cancer is limited to lesions no greater than 1 mm in thickness, although flocculation of the gold particles on the serosal surface by protein may cause fibrosis of the surface, inhibiting the secretion of fluid. There is some evidence, too, that tumor cells floating freely in the fluid may be destroyed. The γ rays are less effective, but permit external counting and at the same time constitute a hazard to personnel.

A simple method of administration has been devised by Abbott Laboratories to minimize the exposure of personnel. The ^{198}Au colloid is supplied in single dose units (usual dose 75 mCi for pleural cavity, 150 mCi for peritoneal cavity), in a heavily shielded container. After thoracentesis or paracentesis with removal of all but a few hundred ml of fluid, the ^{198}Au colloid is transferred to the body cavity by means of a saline infusion through a two-needle system. Details are given in the package insert, and all precautions should be scrupulously observed because of the large radiation hazard.

It should be noted that 100 mCi of ^{198}Au in the patient gives an exposure of 30 mR/hr at 1 meter at the time of administration, and an average of 15 mR/hr during the first week at the same distance. This is about 10 percent of the dose received under similar conditions from a patient undergoing radium therapy of the cervix. With suitable precautions, the average personnel exposure should not exceed 5 to 10 mR per administration. The patient must not be allowed to leave the hospital until the retained ^{198}Au has decayed to less than 30 mCi.

Radioactive Chromic Phosphate (^{32}P) in Malignant Effusions. A colloidal suspension of chromic phosphate incorporating ^{32}P may be used like ^{198}Au, by direct injection into the pleural or peritoneal cavity, to inhibit the accumulation of fluid resulting from cancer metastases. Since ^{32}P is a pure β^- emitter (while ^{198}Au emits also energetic γ rays) it is safer to handle and is less of a hazard to personnel and others in the vicinity of the patient. The usual dose is 5 mCi for the pleural cavity, and 10 mCi for the peritoneal cavity. Following careful thoracentesis or paracentesis, a saline infusion is started through a polyethylene catheter inserted into the body cavity. The selected dose of colloidal chromic phosphate ^{32}P is then injected through the tubing by means of a properly shielded syringe. Lucite shielding is used instead of lead because we are concerned only with β particles.

The result of this form of therapy with either ^{198}Au or chromic phosphate ^{32}P is palliative in about 50 to 70 percent of selected patients, as manifested by a significant decrease in the accumulation of malignant effusion. Recent clinical experience has shown that similar results are obtained more economically and without radiation exposure, by the intrapleural or intraperitoneal injection of nitrogen mustard or other chemotherapeutic drugs, so that the use of radionuclides for this purpose has been largely abandoned.

CHAPTER 15

Radiobiology

THE special branch of radiology which deals with the mode of action and effects of ionizing radiation on living systems is called *radiobiology*. To gain an understanding of this important subject we must first realize that energy is deposited during the passage of ionizing radiation through all matter, whether non-living or living. However, living tissue is unique in that it responds in a variety of rather typical ways to the ensuing injury. In exploring these responses we must know something of the structure, function, and reproduction of living cells; the manner of energy deposition in them; and the sequential chemical and biologic transformations. Thus, radiobiology partakes of three major sciences— biology, physics, and chemistry.

As we shall see in this chapter, despite the real advances made in the field of radiobiology, much still remains undiscovered, our knowledge at present being at best fragmentary.

PHYSICAL BASIS OF RADIOBIOLOGY

Whenever ionizing radiation traverses body tissues (or any other material medium) it transfers energy to them by the processes of *atomic excitation* and *ionization*. The magnitude of the resulting biologic effects depends on *physical* and *biologic* factors. In this section we shall consider only the physical factors which include (1) the quantity of energy deposited by the radiation in a unit mass of tissue at the site of interest—the *absorbed dose,* and (2) the biologic effectiveness of the radiation, determined by the rate of energy loss (locally absorbed) per unit length of path by the ionizing particle—the *linear energy transfer.* The biologic factors, comprising such entities as the nature and physiologic state of the irradiated tissue and the time-dose relationship, will be described in later sections.

Before the physical factors are discussed, it would be well to review briefly the concept of radiation exposure. As we have seen in Chapter 7, the *exposure* in roentgens is based on the quantity of ionization produced by X or γ rays, with energies up to 3 MeV, in a unit mass of air under specified conditions. The exposure with radiation in the indicated energy range parallels fairly closely the actual flow of energy at the point of interest; but it must be emphasized that it states nothing about the amount of energy absorbed, nor the effects on the tissues, nor the ratio of the radiation absorbed to that transmitted.

Since the biologic effects of radiation depend on the amount of energy locally absorbed, the concept of *absorbed dose* has been introduced to specify this energy absorption. A review of the physical processes involved in absorption will show the rational basis of this idea. On traversing a material medium—body tissues in this case—radiation imparts energy to the atoms of the tissues by the processes of *ionization* and *excitation.* (The latter is believed to be important but is of uncertain significance and will therefore be omitted.) With *electromagnetic radiation,* such as X and γ rays, this energy transfer occurs through the *indirect ionization* of atoms by primary electrons (see Fig. 15.01) liberated initially by the familiar interactions: photoelectric, Compton, and pair production. The relative importance of these interactions

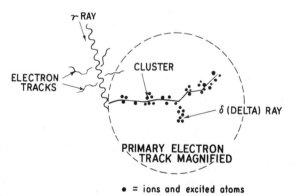

• = ions and excited atoms

FIGURE 15.01. Diagram showing ionization and excitation track of an electron. Ionization and excitation clusters along the primary and delta ray tracks are responsible for producing the radiobiologic lesion, the severity of which depends on linear concentration of the clusters.

depends (in a given medium such as soft tissues) on the energy of the incident radiation, the photoelectric process predominating up to about 50 keV; the Compton interaction with 100 keV to several MeV photons; and pair production in the multimillion volt range. Table 15.01, based on Lea's[50] data, shows the relative

TABLE 15.01
RELATIVE INCIDENCE OF PHOTOELECTRIC AND COMPTON PROCESSES
WHEN PHOTONS WITH VARIOUS ENERGIES INTERACT WITH WATER*

Photon Energy	Wavelength	Percentage of Total Electrons		Percentage of Total Electron Energy	
		Recoil	Photo	Recoil	Photo
keV	Å				
10	1.2	4.5	95.5	0.1	99.9
20	0.6	27.5	72.5	1.4	98.6
50	0.25	85	15	32	68
100	0.12	97	3	85	15
200	0.06	99.6	0.4	98.3	1.7
500	0.02	100	0	100	0
1000	0.01	100	0	100	0

* From Lea, D. E.: *Actions of Radiations on Living Cells,* 1947. Courtesy of The Macmillan Company, Publisher, New York.

importance of the photoelectric and Compton interactions when photons of various energies traverse water; presumably, this parallels their interaction with soft tissues containing a high percentage of water. In the case of *charged particulate radiation* such as α and β particles, ionization is *direct,* by the interaction of their electric fields with those of orbital electrons in the atoms of the tissues being irradiated. With *neutrons* ionization is *indirect* through recoil of atomic nuclei, especially protons. The energy absorbed during these various processes constitutes the *absorbed dose.* In general, the magnitude of a biologic effect produced in a given tissue by a *given type* of radiation depends on the quantity of energy absorbed per unit mass of tissue at the place of interest. The unit of absorbed dose is the *rad* which equals 100 ergs per gram.

The absorbed dose of X or γ rays is proportional to the exposure when the irradiated tissue has a reasonably homogeneous atomic composition and a sufficiently large volume to satisfy the conditions of electronic equilibrium. (Recall that the roentgen as a unit is standardized under conditions of electronic equilibrium.) The constant of proportionality, f, between the absorbed dose (rads) and the exposure (R) depends on the average atomic number of the irradiated medium and the quality of the incident radiation (see pages 217 to 221). Since, in radiotherapy, we deal almost exclusively with soft tissues of water density and with bone, we may justifiably limit our discussion to these two absorbing media. Thus, with X rays having a half value layer (HVL) of 2 mm Cu there is about $1\frac{1}{2}$ times greater energy absorption per roentgen per gram of compact bone than there is per gram of soft tissue such as muscle, because the photoelectric process is still significant in this energy region (about 15% of the liberated energy) and its mass attenuation coefficient is nearly proportional to the cube of the atomic number (Z^3). On the other hand, with 1-MeV radiation the average absorbed dose in equal masses of compact bone and soft tissues is essentially the same because in this energy region interaction is almost exclusively by the Compton process wherein the mass attenuation coefficient is nearly independent of the atomic number of the absorber. This means that with equal exposures in R there may or may not be quantitative differences in the amount of energy absorbed per unit mass of different types of tissues, depending on their average atomic number and the energy of the incident photons.

But the absorbed dose itself does not tell the whole story. The effectiveness of the radiation in producing a stipulated biologic effect in a particular kind of tissue or cell depends also on the **nature** of the radiation—that is, whether it is photonic or particulate—and on its **energy.** In other words, for equal absorbed doses, the magnitude of the biologic effect may differ according to the nature and energy of the radiation.

How can we account for the variation in relative biologic effectiveness of equal absorbed doses of different types of radiation? We know that the distribution, in space and time, of the ions liberated by the radiation along its path, is of fundamental importance in producing biologic effects. The more ions liberated per unit length of path (i.e. the greater the specific ionization) the greater will be the biologic effect. Table 3.03 shows the tremendous differences in the relative ionizing abilities of α and β particles. Alpha particles with dense ionization over a relatively short range may cross only one or a few cells, whereas β particles cross many cells. However, the ion clusters are more closely spaced along α-particle tracks than along primary electron or β-particle tracks, the latter two having ions distributed at relatively long distances, perhaps cells apart. The specific ionization of γ rays depends on the energy of the primary electrons that they set in motion.

A more precise statement than the specific ionization, as far as biologic effect is concerned, is that the greater the **transfer of energy** to the tissues per unit length of path, the greater will be the biologic effect. This concept is embodied in the term **linear energy transfer**—usually called **LET**—defined as the amount of energy lost per unit distance along the track of the primary radiation in a material medium. It includes energy deposition through **both** ionization and excitation. Because of the variation in ion density along the track of an ionizing particle, **increasing as the speed of the particle decreases,** the LET is averaged over the entire path of the particle. LET is an extremely valuable concept. We know, for instance, that the ionization paths of α particles are dense, short, and straight; they display a high rate of energy loss per unit length of path and are characterized by a large average LET. On the other hand, primary electrons and β particles have long, narrow, and irregular ionization paths with an associated smaller rate of energy loss and a smaller average LET than α particles. Furthermore, the LET of heavy particle radiation is generally greater than that of photon radiation, since the latter ionizes through the agency of the electrons which it sets in motion. Some of the typical average values of LET for various kinds of radiation are included in Table 15.02, in which LET is expressed in keV/μ.

In general, the rate of energy loss or LET increases with an increase in the **charge** and/or **mass** of an ionizing particle, but increases with a decrease in the **speed** of the particle. The rate of energy loss of a charged particle is proportional to the square of the charge. Thus, an α particle with a double charge would have a rate of energy loss or LET four times that of an electron or β particle of the same velocity. (Note that only the size of the charge counts, not its sign.) Particle velocity also influences LET; the slower the speed, the more time the particle spends in the vicinity

TABLE 15.02
TYPICAL AVERAGE LINEAR ENERGY TRANSFER (LET) VALUES FOR
VARIOUS KINDS OF RADIATION IN SOFT TISSUES*

Radiation	Energy	LET
		keV/μ
^{60}Co γ rays	1.25 MeV (av.)	0.3
X rays	250 kVp	1.5
Electrons	10 keV	2.3
Electrons	100 keV	0.42
Electrons	1 MeV	0.25
Neutrons	20 MeV	7
Protons	10 MeV	4
Alphas	5 MeV	100
Fission Fragments	Very High	5000

*From Dalrymple, G. V., *et al.*, Eds. *Medical Radiation Biology*, 1973. Courtesy of W. B. Saunders Co., Publisher, Philadelphia.

of an atom and the greater the probability of interaction (ionization and excitation). Heavy particles move more slowly than the much lighter electrons, even when they have the same energy (recall that $K.E. = \frac{1}{2}m_o v^2$). Thus, α *particles* with their large mass, relatively slow speed, and large charge exemplify high-LET radiation.

Fast neutrons also represent high-LET radiation because they ionize indirectly by setting in motion recoil nuclei, mainly *protons*, on interacting with matter. The recoil nuclei have a large mass and, if larger than protons, also a large charge, therefore producing heavy ionization density along their tracks.

It is of interest that for every ion pair produced, the ionizing particle loses about 33.7 eV of energy in soft tissue. With an average of about three ion pairs per cluster along the track of a fast electron this represents an energy deposit of $3 \times 33.7 = 111$ eV in each cluster. However, nearly half the energy of fast electrons is released in tissues by the production of δ (delta) rays, that is, secondary ionization tracks.

Now we must consider the possible existence of biologically significant differences in the LET as between low energy and high energy *photons*. It is known, for example, that the LET of megavoltage radiation is about 85 percent that of orthovoltage. This leads directly to the problem of *energy dependence.* For many years radiobiologists have been concerned with the possible differences in biologic effects produced by identical absorbed doses of X or γ radiation of different wavelengths. Two main difficulties have plagued investigators in their studies on energy dependence; first, the uncertainties involved in administering truly equal absorbed doses with radiation of different qualities; and secondly, the fallacy inherent in transferring experimental results from plants and lower animals to man. It is reasonable to suppose that electrons released by low-energy photons would have relatively lower speed and therefore a higher LET than electrons released by high-energy photons. This has led to the concept of *relative biologic effectiveness—RBE*—which is defined as the ratio of the absorbed dose of a standard type of radiation to that of the radiation in question, to produce the *same degree* of a stipulated biologic effect. The standard radiation is usually 200 to 250 kV X rays. A given type of radiation does not necessarily have a single RBE; the RBE value depends on such diverse factors as the type of cell or tissue, the biologic effect under investigation, the total absorbed dose, and the dose rate. RBE has only limited application in radiation therapy, and is used almost exclusively in experimental radiobiology. (See Fig. 16.01 for relationship between RBE and LET.)

In actual practice, it was found long ago that the γ rays of the radium series require a larger exposure for skin erythema than kilovoltage (orthovoltage) X rays: 1000 R for γ rays, 680 R for 200-kV X rays (HVL 1 mm Cu), and 270 R for 100-kV X rays (HVL 1 mm Al). As already mentioned earlier in this chapter, the generally accepted value of RBE for cobalt 60 γ rays is about 0.85 relative to 200 to 250 kV X rays. Therefore, in radiation therapy the tumor absorbed dose should be increased about 15 percent with a cobalt 60 beam to obtain the same biologic effect (e.g. tumor lethality) as with orthovoltage X rays.

Thus, for the radiation therapist there is a multiplicity of radiobiologic concepts represented by specific units with which he must be conversant, but which have various degrees of clinical applicability. The roentgen is simply a unit of exposure that can be used to determine the absorbed dose with the aid of suitable conversion factors. The two basic processes in radiobiology are (1) the transfer of energy to biologic material in the ionization and excitation processes, represented by the absorbed dose in terms of the energy absorbed per unit mass of tissue at the place of interest—measured in rads; and (2) the average linear energy transfer—$LET_{av.}$—which denotes the average rate of energy loss (locally absorbed) per unit length of path by an ionizing particle. Of the two, the absorbed dose is presently of far greater practical importance in radiotherapy. On the other hand, the LET, although it expresses the ultimate physical basis of radiobiology, is more valuable in research and with newer treatment modalities (e.g. fast neutrons; negative pions) since it furnishes a precise specification of the quality of all types of penetrating radiation. As we have shown previously, the half value layer and tube potential in orthovoltage therapy, and beam energy in megavoltage therapy, serve adequately to specify radiation quality in external beam therapy.

THE CELL

We have learned that the fundamental physical process in radiobiology is energy transfer through ionization and excitation. The ions exert their action on the fundamental biologic units—the *cells* themselves—although the precise mode of action is still uncertain.

Normal Anatomy of the Cell. To understand the changes produced in tissues by ionizing radiations, we must first have a clear concept of the cells which make up the tissues. The *cell* is the fundamental building block of complex living organisms, including man. A typical cell is a microscopic bit of protoplasm consisting of a central *nucleus* surrounded by *cytoplasm* (see Fig. 15.02).

The *nucleus* is the reproductive center of the cell, and also directs and coordinates its activities. It is enclosed by a *nuclear membrane* which is at least intermittently porous to allow interchange of material with the cytoplasm. Within the nucleus are three important constituents: (1) chromatin, (2) one or more nucleoli, and (3) nuclear sap. *Chromatin* (except during mitosis) occurs in the form of thin strands which stain basophilic with appropriate dyes; it is a compound of a simple protein (mainly histone) and *nucleic acid,* that is, a *nucleoprotein.* The main nucleic

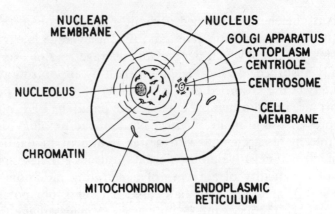

FIGURE 15.02. Schematic representation of the intimate structure of a typical cell.

acid is ***deoxyribonucleic acid (DNA),*** a ***macromolecule*** consisting of two long strands or chains of molecular subunits joined together stepladder fashion by hydrogen bonds. This double strand is coiled into a spiral as shown in Figure 15.03.

Why is DNA so important? Through it the nucleus directs all activities of the cell, both qualitatively and quantitatively; for example, protein and enzyme production, secretion, and antigen-antibody reactions. DNA serves as the storehouse of ***information*** needed for cell activity and survival. This information is in the

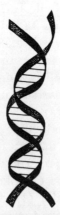

FIGURE 15.03. Double helix structure (Watson-Crick model) of a DNA molecule. The horizontal lines represent the weak chemical (hydrogen) bonds between the nitrogenous bases.

form of a ***code*** which is determined by the sequence of certain molecular subunits—the nitrogenous bases adenine, thymine, cytosine, and guanine—along the DNA chain. Any alteration of their sequence changes the message. Reference to Figure 15.04 will help clarify this discussion. Note that each DNA strand comprises subunits called ***nucleotides*** bonded serially in the chain. Each nucleotide consists of a phosphate group, deoxyribose (a pentose sugar), and a nitrogenous base. The two chains are joined by hydrogen bonding between the bases, but only certain restricted linkages can normally occur between the nitrogenous bases—adenine with thymine, and cytosine with guanine. This, then, is the code—***the sequence of nitrogenous bases along the DNA chain.***

In directing a particular activity such as the manufacture of a specific protein, the DNA in the nucleus transfers its instructions in the form of coded information to ***messenger ribonucleic acid (RNA).*** RNA differs from DNA in its constituents ribose instead of deoxyribose, and uracil instead of thymine. The encoded messenger RNA then leaves the nucleus and moves into the cytoplasm to a ***ribosome*** (a type of particle made up of ribosomal RNA, the function of which is unclear). At the ribosome there is a pool of 20 amino acids, each tagged with ***transfer RNA*** (a product of the nucleus). In accordance with the code carried by the messenger RNA, the transfer RNA bonds the specified amino

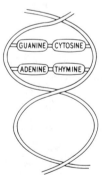

FIGURE 15.04. Chemical linkages of nitrogenous bases in DNA. Linkages can occur only between certain pairs of bases, and the particular sequence of these bases provides specific genetic information, that is, the code for reproduction of specific enzymes and proteins.

acids to form the protein macromolecule programmed by the DNA. The messenger and transfer RNA are believed to "self-destruct" in the process.

All living matter contains DNA and RNA, but species differ in the quantity and sequence of the nucleotides along the chain. Periodically, DNA duplicates itself, or *replicates,* as will be shown later.

The *cytoplasm* does most of the work of the cell such as protein synthesis (including enzymes) under the direction of DNA. Specialized activities such as nerve impulse conduction and muscle contraction are also the function of certain specialized cells. There are several substructures in the cytoplasm, sometimes referred to as *organelles.* As revealed by electron microscopy, they are chiefly membranous structures that include the endoplasmic reticulum, mitochondria, and Golgi apparatus. A triple-layered cover, the *cell membrane.* surrounds the cell.

The *endoplasmic reticulum* is an extensive membranous tubular structure having two forms, rough and smooth, whose function seems to be to channel secretions from the *Golgi apparatus* to the cell surface. The *rough reticulum* has a granular exterior consisting of RNA-rich ribosomes.

Mitochondria are rod-shaped bodies measuring about 0.5 to 1 micron thick and up to 7 micra long, approximately 2000 being scattered throughout the cell cytoplasm. They are really minute chambers lined by a double membrane and are concerned with cell respiration; they contain enzymes required for various metabolic processes (e.g. carbohydrate and lipid metabolism) and also produce *adenosine triphosphate (ATP),* an essential source of energy for such important processes as muscle contraction and nerve discharge.

Cellular Renewal. A cell population continually experiences the death of old cells and the reproduction of new ones of the same kind. Under proper conditions, this should go on indefinitely. In 1912 Alexis Carrell started a culture of cells obtained from the heart of a living chick embryo, and maintained it until 1939 at which time it was still thriving. Naturally, excess cells had to be removed from time to time. It is not surprising, in the light of present knowledge about DNA and RNA, that the cells at the end of the experiment were remarkably like the original ones.

Elementary Genetics. The *chromosomes* are really the seat of activity of the nucleus. They consist of minute particles, called *genes.* lined up in a row in much the same manner as beads on a string. The genes, composed of one or more DNA macromolecules, are the factors which ultimately determine all of the physical, chemical, and physiologic characteristics of the cells and of the individual animal composed of these cells. Their study constitutes the science of *genetics.* In the *body* or *somatic cells,* the chromosomes occur in homologous pairs (except for a nonhomologous pair in the human male); for example every cell in the human body has 23 pairs of chromosomes, each parent having contributed one member of each pair (see below). Therefore, the genes are also paired and all characteristics or traits such as hair type, eye color, and others are determined by a pair of interacting genes derived from the parents. In some instances, each member of the gene pair contributes equally to a given trait. In other cases, one gene completely overshadows its mate and is known as the *dominant* gene as opposed to the other or *recessive* gene. It is obvious that any sort of damage to genes, radiation included, will eventually become manifest as an alteration in some characteristics of the individual or his offspring because of the transmission of chromosomes and their genes by the sex cells. Any such change in the structure of a gene, however induced, is called a *mutation,* and the resulting gene or individual a *mutant.*

Cell Reproduction by Mitosis. The reproduction of most cells occurs by a complicated process known as *mitosis,* initiated spontaneously when the cell has reached a certain size or age, provided it is still capable of reproduction. Just before the onset of mitosis the quantity of nuclear chromatin *doubles* (DNA replication). The chromatin then becomes aggregated in the form of a thread or *spireme.* At the same time a small body, the *centrosome,* lying just outside the nucleus, divides into two parts which begin to separate, building between them a very fine spindle as shown in Figure 15.05. In the meanwhile the chromatin spireme condenses and coils into thicker bodies that become recognizable

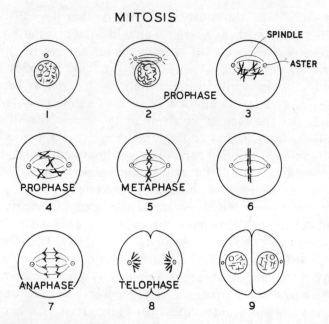

FIGURE 15.05. Cell division by *mitosis*. There has been a doubling of DNA during the synthetic (S) or premitotic phase, resulting in the doubling of the normal somatic chromosome number. During mitosis the normal somatic chromosome number is restored.

as *chromosomes,* the size, number, and shape of which are characteristic of a particular plant or animal species. This is the beginning of the first stage of mitosis known as the *prophase.* The chromosomes at this point actually consist of homologous pairs joined by a tiny body, the *centromere.* Note that the number of chromosomes is *double* the normal number for that species because of prior duplication of chromatin as mentioned above. Prophase is complete when the chromosomes have undergone maximum coiling and the nuclear membrane and nucleoli have disappeared.

Now the *metaphase* starts, the chromosomes arranging themselves in a plane midway between the centrosomes which have by this time reached opposite poles of the cell. The plane of the chromosomes, known as the *equatorial plate,* is perpendicular to the spindle axis. The chromosome pairs, each consisting of two *chromatids,* attach themselves to spindle fibers by their centromere (note: *not* centrosome). The centromeres divide, completing metaphase.

Anaphase starts with the movement of the members (chromatids) of each pair of chromosomes along the spindle to opposite poles.

Finally, during *telophase* all the chromosomes uncoil and revert to a thread-like structure to form the chromatin network, resulting in two complete, resting nuclei. At the same time the nuclear membrane reappears and the cytoplasm divides into two equal portions, each containing one of the daughter nuclei. Note that the original number of chromosomes for that species has been maintained in the daughter cells. The entire mitotic process lasts about one-half to one hour, of which prophase represents the largest fraction.

The "Resting" or Interphase Period. Upon completion of a mitotic cycle, the cell enters the so-called "resting" phase. However, as we shall see, this is not a time of rest but actually a period of intense activity on the molecular level. It is more aptly called the *interphase,* that is, the interval between mitotic cycles. Interphase begins with the G_1 *period* (see Fig. 15.06) in which the cell nucleus contains a fine, lacy network of poorly staining

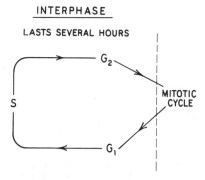

FIGURE 15.06. Diagram of a typical generation cycle of a cell, as proposed by Howard and Pelk (*Heredity, 6:* 261, 1953). There is a general division into two main parts — the synthetic S phase in which DNA is synthesized, and the mitotic phase, M, in which DNA is normally divided equally between two daughter cells. The S and M phases are separated by two gaps, G_1 and G_2, in which other types of cellular activity occur such as synthesis of RNA.

chromatin suspended in the nuclear sap or nucleoplasm. Invisibly, there is an accumulation of nucleotides in preparation for the DNA synthetic or *S period* which is to last several hours. It is during the S period that the DNA replicates, doubling in amount. Duplication of chromosomes (except for the centromere) may also occur during the S period. This is followed by the G_2 *period* which precedes the prophase of the next mitotic cycle; during G_2, proteins and RNA needed in mitosis are synthesized.

Gametogenesis and Meiosis. How are the chromosomes transmitted to the offspring? This occurs during *gametogenesis* or sex cell formation by a modified mitotic process called *meiosis* during which there is a reduction in the number of chromosomes normally present in the somatic or body cells (*diploid* number) to one-half that number (*haploid* number) in the gametes or sex cells. Details are shown in Figure 15.07 in simplified form. In

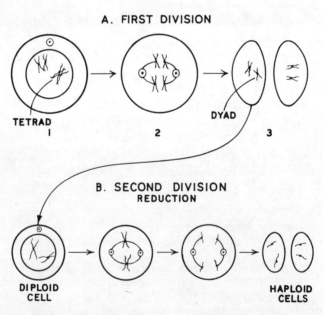

MEIOSIS

A. FIRST DIVISION

TETRAD
I   2   DYAD   3

B. SECOND DIVISION
REDUCTION

DIPLOID CELL   HAPLOID CELLS

FIGURE 15.07. Gametogenesis, the formation of reproductive cells by *meiosis*. In this process the somatic (diploid) chromosome number is reduced by one-half, to the haploid number.

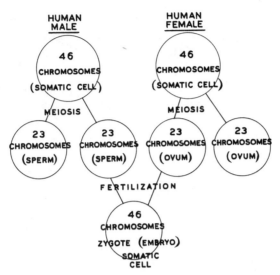

FIGURE 15.08. Genesis of the individual. During meiosis the gametes (sex cells) have each received one-half the number of species-typical somatic cells. Union of two opposite gametes during fertilization restores the full complement of chromosomes in the somatic cells of the embryo.

short, the primordial sex cells in the testes and ovaries reproduce and differentiate by ordinary mitosis until they reach the sperma-tocyte or oocyte stage, respectively. Each cell at this point has the diploid number, 46 chromosomes consisting of 23 homologous pairs *in humans* (except for the male XY pair). Following this, the cells reproduce by meiosis in two cycles. By the time *meiosis I* has started, homologous chromosome pairs, one from each parent, have paired up and come to lie extremely close together, point for point (i.e. gene for gene). They then split longitudinally to form *tetrads* or *bivalents,* each consisting of four strands (a total of 92 strands in humans). During this stage a most important and characteristic event takes place—breaks occur at corre-sponding points in the arms of the homologous chromosomes, apparently at random, and immediately the segments interchange and fuse. This process is called *crossing over.* The tetrads then separate as *dyads* or chromosome pairs on the spindle, one dyad going to each daughter cell as in mitosis. Each daughter cell now has the diploid number (i.e. 23 dyads). Immediately, *meiosis II* starts *without replication of DNA,* the dyads dividing and their constituent chromosomes going to each daughter cell. During this, the *reduction division,* each gamete receives the haploid number of chromosomes—23 in humans.

Fertilization. During *fertilization,* a male and a female gamete unite and their chromosomes intermix, so the full complement of chromosomes is restored in the body cells of the resulting embryo. It is obvious from Figure 15.08 that the offspring inherit one chromosome of each homologous pair from each parent, and therefore both parents determine the characteristics of their descendants by the chromosomes which they transmit through their sex cells.

We should emphasize that crossing over in meiosis I increases the probability of variations occurring in the progeny through increased scrambling of chromosomal fragments including their constituent genes. On the other hand, body cells reproduce by mitosis which virtually assures the identity of the somatic daughter cells with each other and with the parent somatic cells. Biologists are generally agreed that crossing over, in addition to gene mutation, random mixing of paternal and maternal chromosomes during meiosis II, and fertilization, is an important factor in producing intra-species variations that ultimately give rise to new species in the course of biologic evolution.

Malignant Cells. In cancer cells there is derangement of cellular structure characterized mainly by an increase in the amount of chromatin and in the ratio of nuclear material to cytoplasm—*increased nucleocytoplasmic ratio.* However, the actual size of the cell may be unaltered, or may be larger or smaller than its normal counterpart. In fact, highly malignant tumors display a rather marked variation in size and shape of cells called *pleomorphism.* In many malignant tumors, cells lose their ability to stick together, favoring their separation and dissemination. One of the most striking changes observed in malignant cells is an increase in mitotic activity, as well as the occurrence of abnormal mitoses with unequal replication or distribution of chromosomes, and tripolar or multipolar centrosomes with multiple spindles and bizarre mitotic divisions.

MODE OF ACTION OF IONIZING RADIATION

All biologic systems are damaged by ionizing radiation. It is axiomatic that such injury stems from the ionization and excitation induced in the tissues by the absorbed radiation. At the outset, it must be emphasized that no single theory accounts for all the known changes that are brought into play by ionizing radiation as it traverses a tissue. Various aspects of the problem can be explained only by the application of one or more of the prevalent theories. Furthermore, when a cell culture composed of apparently similar cells is irradiated there is a variation in the susceptibility of the cells to the effects of the radiation. If the fraction of surviving cells is plotted as a function of radiation dose, a survival curve is obtained (see Fig. 15.09). Thus, the survival curve is statistical, reflecting the random variation in the response of individuals in a cell culture to irradiation.

Several theories have been proposed to explain the mode of action of ionizing radiation on biologic material. Aside from the generally destructive effects of overwhelming doses of radiation, it is reasonable to suppose that there are sensitive volumes or vital spots, probably essential macromolecules such as DNA and enzymes, in all cells. When such macromolecules are injured by radiation, they cause profound changes in cellular function and reproductive capacity. How this injury may take place will now be described.

1. ***Direct Action.*** According to this concept, an ionizing particle enters a sensitive macromolecule and deposits energy directly within it. Hence it is often referred to as the ***target theory.*** Since the nucleus is the vital center of the cell, the target theory as developed by Lea[50] maintains that ionization in the nucleus occurs in two distinct patterns: (a) ionization within the gene itself (changes in DNA), causing a mutation which may or may not be lethal, and (b) passage of ionization tracks through a chromosome, causing it to break. Such a theory, based on single or multiple hits, presumes an all-or-none effect, the nature of which is still incompletely understood. We do not know as yet the exact identity of the vital target, but there is evidence that it

may be DNA, particularly as the **DNA-protein complex.** Implicit in the target theory is the destruction of individual cells; hence, if recovery takes place at all, it must do so from neighboring undamaged or sublethally damaged cells.

In general, direct action is more likely to occur with heavy charged particles because of their high LET with close spacing of the ion clusters. This increases the probability of (1) hitting a sensitive target and (2) producing multiple hits in a particular target. In other words, we have a "bird-shot" effect.

2. **Indirect Action.** Besides the direct action of ionizing radiation there is an even more important one for radiotherapy, namely, **indirect action.** This is predicated on the formation of substances inside or outside the cell that might in some way interfere with its vital activities, mainly by attacking the sensitive macromolecules through an agency other than direct action. **Free radicals** liberated by the **radiolysis** of water constitute the active agents. However, water molecules probably have to undergo preliminary ionization by irradiation. An electron is stripped from the water molecule leaving it positively charged:

$$H_2O \xrightarrow[radiation]{energy} H_2O^+ + e^-$$

The electron immediately becomes an **aqueous** or **solvated electron** —it is surrounded by water molecules that, because of polarization (oxygen part of molecule slightly negative, hydrogen slightly positive), orient themselves with the hydrogen closer to the electron

$$e^- + H_2O \longrightarrow e^-_{aq}$$

Solvated electrons have an extremely short existence of about 10^{-6} sec. The positively charged water ion is unstable, giving rise to a **free radical** which is believed to result from the presence of an unpaired electron in an outer shell. **Ordinary water** may be represented as follows:

$$H \colon \overset{\cdot\cdot}{\underset{\cdot\cdot}{O}} \colon H$$

Note that there are four pairs of electrons in the outer orbits of the molecule, six of which belong to oxygen and two to hydrogen.

The covalent bonds between hydrogen and oxygen represent electrons which oscillate between the outer orbits of hydrogen and oxygen and are thereby shared.

On the other hand, positively *ionized water* has this configuration

$$H \cdot \overset{\cdot\cdot}{\underset{\cdot}{O}} \cdot H$$

When it dissociates (in 10^{-16} sec), a *free radical* is formed:

$$H_2O^+ \longrightarrow H^+ + OH \cdot$$

where the dot indicates a free radical.

The electron stripped from the water may attach itself to another water molecule, ionizing it negatively

$$H_2O + e^- \longrightarrow H_2O^-$$

which then proceeds to form a free radical

$$H_2O^- \longrightarrow H \cdot + OH^-$$

Water radiolysis is measured in terms of **G-value** which is defined as the number of molecules damaged, or of products formed per 100 eV of energy absorbed. For example, with ^{60}Co γ rays, typical G-values for some of the important radicals at a pH of 3 to 10 are as follows: $H \cdot$ 0.6; H_2O_2 0.7; HO_2^- 0.02; and $OH \cdot$ 2.6. The G-value for e_{aq}^- is 2.6 in acid solution (see Dalrymple).

Why are free radicals so important? There is abundant evidence that they are responsible for the *indirect action* of radiation by transferring energy to other molecules that are vital to living cells. They are extremely reactive, producing their effects within a short life of only 10^{-5} sec, although it has recently been shown that some may have a longer existence. Reactions of free radicals occur in a variety of ways including reactions with each other to produce ordinary water and hydrogen, and, more important, a toxic substance hydrogen peroxide, H_2O_2. They can also react with water to generate other free radicals. *Oxygen* may be involved in reactions with free radicals; this is extremely important because it potentiates the effect of radiation. Finally, they may attack sensitive cellular targets such as *DNA, enzymes,* and *other proteins.* Thus, even though a chromosome or an essential macromolecule may be missed by a direct hit since such events are com-

paratively infrequent, severe damage can still be produced indirectly with greater frequency by free radicals.

Thus, in the theory of indirect action, the radiation transfers
energy first to water molecules resulting in their activation. The
energy is then transferred to certain essential substances which
are decomposed, eventually resulting in cellular injury. In fact,
chromosomal changes are in part due to indirect action by X
and γ rays.

3. *Fluid Flow Theory.* As another type of indirect action,
Failla's theory of fluid flow suggests that ionization causes large
molecules within the cell to break down to smaller molecules
(depolymerization). As a result, the osmotic pressure within the
cell increases so that water enters the cell and causes it to swell.
This may so derange cell metabolism that the cell dies. However,
other workers maintain that the apparent swelling of irradiated
cells is due to a disturbance in their ability to divide, without a
corresponding interference with their growth.

RADIATION-INDUCED INJURIES AT A CELLULAR LEVEL

There are three principal kinds of injuries sustained by cells on
exposure to ionizing radiation: (1) *death,* (2) *mutations,* and (3)
mitotic inhibition. These will be discussed under separate headings.

Cell Death. According to von Borstel[86] there are three ways
in which lethal effects of radiation on cells are expressed: (a) reproductive, (b) genetic, and (c) lytic. Note that these involve
primarily the nucleus.

Reproductive death implies the death of cells through such
profound damage of the reproductive mechanism that the cell
cannot reproduce, or else reproduces once or a few times with
attendant extinction of the cell line. *Genetic death* occurs mainly
as the result of *chromosome breaks, exchanges,* or *deletions* that
are too severe to be repaired, or through *damage to DNA function*
in synthesizing protein. The types of chromosome breaks can be
related to the point of irradiation in the interphase period; thus,
for chromosome damage, G_2 is more sensitive than G_1 or the S
(synthetic) phase. *Dicenters* in which chromosome exchanges have
led to the formation of chromosomes with two centromeres, and

acentrics which are chromosome fragments without a centromere, are lethal to cells. *Lytic* or *immediate death* occurs promptly after irradiation. Its prototype is the lysis of lymphocytes following irradiation. We are still uncertain as to whether this effect is on the nucleus alone or on the whole cell, although there is some evidence for a release of autolytic enzymes which destroy the cell.

Mutations. Radiation is a *mutagen* in that it increases the frequency of mutation beyond the spontaneous frequency. *Mutations* are the sudden, rare, permanent changes that occur at discrete points in a chromosome, that is, in *genes,* and transmitted to offspring. Although the natural mutation rate is about 1 per 100,000 genes in higher animals, not all genes mutate with the same frequency, some being more stable than others. There are other agents such as certain chemicals (e.g. chemotherapeutic agents) that are mutagenic, but radiation is the most potent—an exposure of 40 to 80 R doubles the natural mutation rate. High-LET radiation, because of the closer spacing of ion clusters and the higher concentration of free radicals, is more mutagenic than is low-LET radiation.

Radiation is believed to act on the nitrogenous bases in the DNA macromolecule, causing *base-change* or *base-deletion.* In either event, there is a change or loss, respectively, of genetic information. Some genes are so important to cell survival that mutations in them may result in cell death—they are called *lethal mutations.* In higher animals a gamete may carry a lethally mutated gene which, if dominant, causes death of the embryo. But it must be borne in mind that mutations may vary in the magnitude of their threat to cell survival; for example, some may be mildly detrimental and simply shorten life span without being immediately fatal.

From what has been said, we may surmise that in the vast majority of instances gene mutations are detrimental to individual cells or to the cell line. In fact, gene mutations may be *carcinogenic,* as has been amply observed in humans, and experimentally demonstrated in animals.

Mitotic Inhibition. Even small doses of ionizing radiation inhibit mitosis as shown by *delay* in the start of prophase. (Ultraviolet radiation and chemical mutagens have a similar effect.) However, the manifestation of the effect depends on the position of the cell in the reproductive cycle. Thus, if mitosis is already in progress it may go on to completion. On the other hand, irradiation during interphase delays the onset of prophase, that is, induces *mitotic delay*. In fact, during early prophase the cell may actually return to the interphase status. It has been shown that the length of mitotic delay depends directly on the radiation dose.

As for the apparent inhibition of DNA synthesis, this is now believed to be due to suppression of the number of cells undergoing mitosis. However, individual cells in which mitosis has been delayed continue to synthesize DNA at a normal rate, resulting in the appearance of *giant cells* which are unable to reproduce. In fact the production of giant cells in tumors undergoing irradiation has been used as an index of tumor response.

One of the interesting phenomena associated with mitotic delay is *synchrony*. At the end of the period of mitotic inhibition, the affected cells enter prophase together with the unaffected cells, causing a pronounced increase in the number of mitoses. This is followed by a period in which mitoses disappear. In other words, mitoses appear in waves. These continue to oscillate with decreasing amplitude until the cell population reverts to its preirradiation nonsynchronous status.

ASSESSMENT OF RADIOSENSITIVITY

Following Puck's[71] demonstration that mammalian cells could be cultured artificially in a manner analogous to bacteria, he, as well as others, proceeded to study their response to radiation.[48] A colony of cells produced by a single cell is called a *clone*. If a cell culture with a known number of cells is irradiated and the individual cells explanted to start a new culture, the failure of certain ones to produce a viable clone would be due to lethal injury to these explanted cells. In other words, this would presuppose an all-or-none effect. However, it has been found that a radiation-injured cell may reproduce a few times and often give rise to giant cells which are incapable of further division. Thus, the criteria for cell lethality are not limited to cell death directly, but include also the *loss of sustained reproductive capacity* of the cell. This is, of course, of paramount importance in radiation therapy.

By subjecting a series of identical cell cultures to various doses of radiation and then finding the fraction of cells surviving each dosage level we can obtain an estimate of **radiosensitivity.** When mammalian cells are studied in this way, and the resulting data plotted with the logarithm of the surviving fraction as a function of the dose, the **survival curves** have a typical configuration, an example of which is shown in Figure 15.09. There is an initial **shoulder portion,** followed by a straight line or **exponential portion.** This type of curve fits the theoretical one obtained mathematically on the assumption that the cells contain multiple targets, a certain number of which must be "hit" and inactivated to cause cell death or loss of reproductive capacity. The shoulder suggests that at **least two targets** must be hit to cause loss of cell survival. It indicates that recovery occurs at very low doses. Extrapolation of the exponential portion of the curve to the abscissa gives the **extrapolation number n,** regarded as the average number of dis-

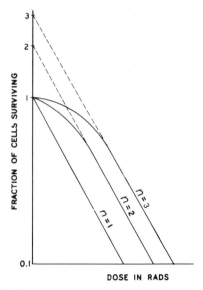

FIGURE 15.09. Typical cell survival curves (cell cultures). When $n = 1$ a single hit of a single target inactivates the cell and no recovery occurs – curve is exponential throughout. When $n = 2$ some cells recover a low dosage as shown by the initial shoulder; extrapolation to the ordinate (vertical axis) indicates an average of 2 targets must be hit for cell inactivation.

crete targets in the cell. Note that with the one-hit model there is no shoulder—lethality results from a single hit.

It is of interest that *in vivo* methods of cell culture (e.g. leukemic cells and skin cells in mice) have also made it possible to study radiation dose-response effects. The resulting survival curves are surprisingly similar to those obtained with *in vitro* cell cultures (see Hall, E. J., in General Bibliography).

An important quantity derived from survival curves is the *mean lethal dose D_o which is the dose increment needed to reduce the surviving cell population to 37 percent of the previous level along the straight line portion of the survival curve.* (Mathematically, it is $1/e$, where e is the natural logarithmic base.) In irradiating a group of cells we deliver inactivating hits not only to unhit cells, but also hit some that have already been inactivated, and even miss some altogether. Hence the *mean lethal dose also represents the dose that gives an average of one hit per cell.*

Another quantity that may be derived for radiation therapy is the *median lethal dose LD_{50}* which kills 50 percent of the cell population. Others may also be derived, such as LD_{90}, LD_{99}, etc.

On the basis of the response of the reproductive capacity of cell cultures to radiation, several definitions of *radiosensitivity* have emerged. One is the *mean lethal dose (D_o)* as was explained above; this has been found to be remarkably constant for *fully oxygenated cell cultures* from a wide variety of normal and malignant mammalian tissues—about 130 rads ± 50 percent. Another measure of radiosensitivity is the *median lethal dose (LD_{50})* which usually applies to whole body irradiation of animals and shows considerable variation among species. In radiation therapy the term radiosensitivity is often used loosely to indicate the speed of response of a tumor or its response to certain dosage ranges, although this may not correlate with radiocurability.

There are no conclusive data regarding the relative importance of direct and indirect action in inactivating mammalian cells. Obviously, a sensitive spot or "target" may be "hit" either by passage of a charged particle or by radicals. It is likely that with X and γ rays the principal mode of action is indirect, whereas, with heavy particles such as protons, deuterons, neutrons, and pions direct action may predominate. In any event, it would seem that the essential targets are DNA and chromosomes, at least insofar as reproductive capacity is concerned.

Survival data indicate that a fraction of X- or γ-irradiated cells does not succumb but somehow manages to recover. A number of factors account for this, including inherent sensitivity, the presence of certain protective substances, the absence of enhancement factors, and the dose rate. For example, we know that mature cells of the central nervous system are less sensitive than those of the hematopoietic system. DNA is capable of repairing itself if not excessively damaged. As will be explained later, *oxygen* potentiates the effects of radiation probably by interplay with free radicals. Certain substances such as the class of antioxidants (glutathione, cysteine, etc.) react with free radicals and thereby diminish their damaging effect on vital targets. Finally, the same radiation dose given over a long time interval may allow the opportunity for repair, whereas the same dose given at once may prevent such restitution.

Although survival experiments have shed much light on some of the fundamental aspects of radiobiology, and have provided us with a better understanding of what takes place during irradiation therapy, they have not yet contributed materially to actual practice.

MODIFICATION OF CELLULAR RESPONSE TO IRRADIATION

Various factors are capable of modifying the response of cells to irradiation, that is, altering their radiosensitivity. However, in too many instances experimental results are contradictory, and even where they are in agreement, there remains the problem of application to medical practice. The more important modifying influences that may bear on radiation therapy will be discussed briefly as follows: (1) fractionation and repair, (2) position of cell in its reproductive cycle, (3) oxygenation, (4) physiologic state, (5) chemical modifiers, and (6) ploidy.

1. *Fractionation and Repair.* According to the multihit or multitarget model (these are *not* exactly alike) the survival curve of a cell culture has an initial shoulder as already described. This represents *intracellular* recovery or repair at low radiation

dosage. Dose fractionation, provided sufficient time elapses between doses, increases the total dose needed for a particular biologic effect. Or, stated differently, multiple small doses require a larger total dose than a single large one to produce the same result. Elkind[21] has shown that if a time interval of at least two hours separates the dose fractions, the survival curve shows the reappearance of the shoulder (see Fig. 15.10). In fact, with multiple fractions, the shoulder reappears each time. This indicates that recovery has taken place after each exposure provided the latter is reasonably small. Thus, treatment of a cell culture in a series of small daily fractions will give a survival or dose-response curve that is *less steep* than that with a single large dose to achieve

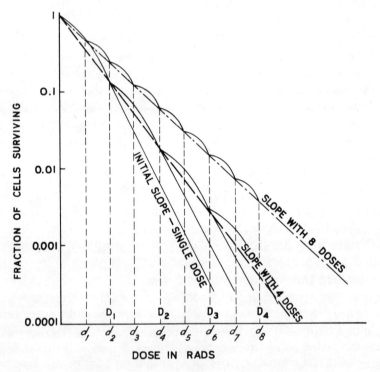

FIGURE 15.10. Modification of cell survival curves by multiple doses of radiation (fractionation). Between doses separated by several hours, partial recovery takes place as indicated by reappearance of the shoulder (called "return of *n*"). This is known as *Elkind or fast recovery*. The larger the total number of fractions for the same total dose, the less steep will be the average curve.

the same end point; in other words, *fractionation decreases radiosensitivity.* Since the letter *n* is often used to symbolize the *extrapolation number* (i.e. the number of hits for inactivation of a cell), the reappearance of the shoulder on fractionation is referred to as *"return of n."* In human normal and tumor tissue the extrapolation number *n* ranges from about 2 to 10 for X and γ rays. With *heavily ionizing particles* such as protons, neutrons, and deuterons—high-LET radiation—*n* approaches 1; consequently, there is a steeper slope of the survival curve (greater RBE), no significant recovery takes place, and fractionation does not decrease radiosensitivity.

How recovery occurs is uncertain. It is undoubtedly a complex process. For example, a single break in a DNA strand is repaired first by enzyme digestion of the separated fragment and second by reconstruction of the missing fragment by the complementary strand. However, if both strands are broken, especially when this occurs in corresponding segments, repair may be incomplete. This may lead to profound changes in cell function and even death of the cell. Multiple breaks are more apt to occur with high-LET radiation and at high dose rates, the former producing closely spaced ion clusters, and the latter not permitting enough time for repair.

Cohen[11] has attempted to draw an interesting analogy between the response of biologic systems and of photographic emulsions to ionizing radiation. Ordinarily, a particular photographic effect may be equated to the product of the radiation intensity and the exposure time. Thus, an increase in one factor must be compensated by a proportionate decrease in the other, as expressed in the *Bunsen and Roscoe Reciprocity Law,*

$$IT = K \qquad (2)$$

where *I* is the intensity, *T* is the time, and *K* is a constant. This resembles the single-hit genetic effects in biologic systems. However, with very low intensity of visible light (not direct action of X rays) on photographic emulsions, the reciprocity law fails and we have, instead, the *Schwarzchild Effect.* Now the photographic effect at low intensity is exceeded at high intensity even if there is proportional reduction in exposure time, indicating that recovery may take place during very prolonged low intensity exposure. This empirical relationship resembles that in tumors or other tissues subjected to ionizing radiation wherein recovery occurs with a fractionated treatment schedule.

2. *Position of Cell in Reproductive Cycle.* Although it is a fact that the radiosensitivity of a cell varies with its position in the reproductive cycle, this is not the same for all kinds of cells. In general, cells are *most sensitive during mitosis.* But there are also peaks and valleys of radiosensitivity during interphase. For example, many kinds of cells exhibit increased sensitivity also during the G_2 phase (postsynthetic), whereas mouse cells and HeLa cells (human epidermoid cancer of cervix in culture) do so during the G_1 phase (presynthetic). Therefore, except for the mitotic phase itself, we cannot generally relate the radiosensitivity of cells to their position in the reproductive cycle, nor can we state at which point within mitosis the cell is most vulnerable although this may well be during prophase. Attempts continue in the direction of producing synchronous cell populations by the use of blocking agents such as colcemide and thymidine, to study the phase sensitivity of cells, but thus far many of the results have been contradictory. One factor that must not be ignored is the possible influence of the blocking agent itself on the radiosensitivity of cells at various points in the reproductive cycle.

3. *Oxygenation.* Experimental evidence is in good agreement on this point: *radiosensitivity of cells increases with an increase in the concentration of molecular oxygen at the instant of irradiation.* This is known as the *oxygen effect.* It occurs predominantly at *low* O_2 partial pressure—less than about 20 mm Hg. As shown in Figure 15.11, the radiosensitivity curve rises steeply as the O_2 pressure increases from zero to about 20 mm Hg, then levels off rapidly. The *O_2 enhancement ratio* (*OER*) is the ratio of the radiation dose under anoxia, to the dose under full oxygenation, for the same biologic effect. Typical OER values are: 2.5 to 3 for X and γ rays, about 1.7 for fast neutrons, and virtually unity for α particles. In other words, this ratio indicates how much more sensitive cells are when fully oxygenated than when they are anoxic. The importance of this phenomenon in radiation therapy is quite obvious and will be discussed later.

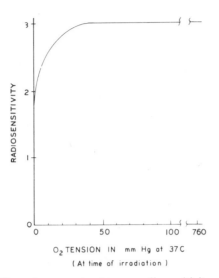

FIGURE 15.11. Effect of oxygen tension on radiosensitivity. Above about 40 mm Hg, a further increase in O_2 tension has no significant additional effect on radiosensitivity. (After L. H. Gray.)

No entirely satisfactory explanation of the oxygen effect has thus far been proposed. As has already been mentioned, one possible mechanism is the interplay of O_2 with free radicals. For example, O_2 may combine with H˙ to form HO_2, or with e_{aq}^- to form O_2^-, products known to be toxic to cells. Support for this explanation of the oxygen effect is adduced from the observation that O_2 provides little or no sensitization of cells to irradiation by heavy particles which cause significant injury by direct action. Another explanation of the oxygen effect postulates the union of O_2 with a macromolecule that has been attacked by a free radical, thereby preventing its repair.

4. *Physiologic State.* In higher animals various physiologic factors may influence radiosensitivity, either of the cells directly, or of the organism as a whole. The *age* of the animal at the time of irradiation is very important—it is well known that embryos are much more radiosensitive than older individuals largely because of their inherently greater cellular radiosensitivity (high mitotic rate, immaturity). For example, in mice the LD_{50} increases nearly in proportion to the logarithm of the age up to about 13

weeks, then levels off and finally decreases during old age (Kohn and Kallman).[48] Furthermore, it has been found that the *life-shortening* effect of radiation increases, the earlier in life the animals are irradiated. *Endocrine status* may influence radiosensitivity; thus, hyperthyroid individuals are more sensitive than normals. Another example is lower radiosensitivity of female than male mice, probably because of circulating estrogens. *Low temperature* decreases radiosensitivity, probably by inducing a hypometabolic state (reverse of thyrotoxicosis). Cooling the skin was found years ago to decrease its sensitivity to irradiation with X rays. Finally, *nutritional state* is a factor in that well-nourished animals exhibit increased tolerance to radiation.

5. *Chemical Modifiers.* Because of its outstanding importance, oxygen, a chemical modifier, has been discussed above under a separate heading. There are a number of compounds that modify radiosensitivity, either enhancing or inhibiting it. An example of a *chemical sensitizer* is 5-bromouracil (5-BU) prepared by the substitution of bromine for a methyl group in thymidine. Such a thymidine analog is readily incorporated in the DNA chain in cells cultured, for example, from human bone marrow or epidermoid carcinoma, and increases their radiosensitivity. Other halogenated thymidine analogs have a similar action. Unfortunately, radiosensitizers have not yet become practicable in radiation therapy.

The opposite type of modifier—*chemical protector*—includes first the *sulfhydryl compounds* exemplified by glutathione and cysteine. Protection is relative, not absolute. To be effective, these compounds must be present at the time of irradiation, just as in the case of O_2. They inhibit radiation effects on cultures of bacteria, plants, bone marrow cells, and certain human cancer cells. Unfortunately, their toxicity for higher animals prevents their use in averting radiation injury. Several possible mechanisms have been invoked to explain the protective action of sulfhydryl compounds: (a) they may block the oxygen effect either by reacting with O_2, or by increasing the utilization of O_2 by the target macromolecules; (b) they may capture free radicals, for they are more effective against indirect action; and (c) they may transfer hydrogen to a radiation-damaged macromolecule and thereby aid its repair. Another compound that has been found to give a measure of protection in experimental animals is colchicine which causes metaphase arrest of mitosis. This, too, has not yet proved to be practicable in higher animals.

6. *Ploidy.* Radiosensitivity of haploid cells (1 set of chromosomes) is greater than that of diploid cells (2 sets of chromosomes). This is evidenced by the 1-hit type survival curves (no shoulder) with haploid cells, and multihit type curves (shoulder) for diploid and polyploid cells. It is obvious that a damaged gene in a haploid cell does not have a complementary gene or *allele* to cover for it, as occurs in a diploid cell where a normal gene is present on the other member of the chromosome pair. At the same time, radiosensitivity increases with chromosomal mass; in fact, D_o is nearly proportional to the square root of the nuclear DNA mass.

RADIATION EFFECTS ON CYTOPLASM

Although we have emphasized that the effects of radiation predominate in the nucleus, the cytoplasm is by no means spared. *Cytoplasmic injury* may be structural, functional, or both. When irradiated cells are studied at a magnification of a few thousand times, cytoplasmic changes may appear before nuclear damage is apparent. One possible mechanism is the entrance of water into the cell, causing liquefaction and death (fluid flow theory). Certain important structures in the cytoplasm are also injured. For example, the *mitochondria* may be so altered by swelling and by dissolution of their membranes that the secretions of certain cells may be impaired. Swelling of the *endoplasmic reticulum* also occurs. These changes may be produced by doses ranging from about 2000 to 5000 rads. Injury of the *Golgi apparatus* may interfere with the transfer of secretions to the surface of the cell. One-celled animals, as well as the sperm of mammals, may lose their motility, although very large doses of radiation are required. Changes in enzymes, and proteins generally, may profoundly affect cellular metabolism. Radiation may damage *lysozymes*— enzyme-containing vesicles—with release of enzymes; these may be sufficient in amount to destroy the cell. Finally, even low doses of radiation can so *alter the permeability of the cell membrane* that the exchange of important substances between the cell and its environment is seriously impaired. Increased permeability of the cell membrane may enhance the flow of water into the cell until it is destroyed.

Irradiation of resting cells produces two results. Some cells may rapidly degenerate and die, while other cells suffer mitotic inhibition and therefore differentiate to a more mature type. Tumors which are capable of differentiating do so when irradiated. For example, Glucksmann[34] found that some carcinomas of the cervix, following irradiation, exhibit decreased mitosis and increased differentiation to mature squamous cells. Such a change indicates a good prognosis because it heralds cell death through differentiation.

THE RESPONSE OF TUMORS TO IONIZING RADIATION

Let us now apply the basic data from the preceding sections to the radiotherapy of malignant tumors. Their response is governed by a number of factors, some known and others unknown, roughly paralleling the response of cell cultures. We must emphasize that rapid shrinkage of a tumor—often regarded as an index of clinical radiosensitivity—does not necessarily correlate with radiocurability. The more important factors contributing to a favorable tumor response will now be discussed.

Cellular Radiosensitivity. We may define radiosensitivity as the vulnerability of cells to lethal injury by ionizing radiation. However, we should distinguish between *reproductive death* in which cells may still reproduce one or more times or form giant cells, and *interphase death* in which cells die promptly, within a few hours. As measured experimentally, the mean lethal dose D_o is an index of radiosensitivity based mainly on reproductive death (lethally injured cells are unable to produce viable colonies or giant cells). As noted before, D_o is nearly constant for all mammalian cells in *tissues culture*—about 130 rads ± 50 percent. On the other hand, there is a wide variation in radiosensitivity of cells undergoing interphase (prompt or lytic) death. This may be the main reason for differences in the *inherent* radiosensitivity of various kinds of mammalian tumors *in vivo*. In general there is a spectrum of tumor radiosensitivity according to cell lineage. Table 15.03 shows the relative susceptibility of various tissues to irradiation, with cell death as the endpoint. However, in actual practice the speed of tumor regression does not necessarily correlate with radiocurability. Thus, while the primary tumor may be readily controlled, it may have already metastasized widely, thereby precluding radiotherapeutic cure.

In 1904, following extensive research on the effect of X rays on the normal rat testis, Bergonié and Tribondeau formulated the following law: *The radiation effect is greatest in cells having the highest mitotic rate, the least differentiation of structure and function, and the longest mitotic phase* (although cells do not have to be in mitosis to be injured by radiation). In other words those cells which are most active in reproduction and most poorly differentiated are the most sensitive to radiation. Although this law is based on the behavior of normal cells, an attempt has been made to apply it also to malignant cells—insofar as radiobiology is concerned, there is no specific effect of radiation on tumor cells; they should obey the law in the same manner as normal cells. Thus, the more undifferentiated the neoplasm and the greater

TABLE 15.03
DECREASING ORDER OF RADIOSENSITIVITY OF MAMMALIAN CELLS
WITH LETHALITY AS THE ENDPOINT*

1. Lymphocytes
2. Erythroblasts
3. Myeloblasts
4. Megakaryocytes
5. Spermatogonia
6. Oogonia
7. Cells of small intestinal crypts
8. Basal cells of skin and its appendages
9. Cells of lens of eye
10. Cartilage cells
11. Osteoblasts
12. Endothelial cells of blood vessels
13. Glandular epithelium
14. Liver cells
15. Renal tubular cells
16. Glia cells
17. Nerve cells
18. Pulmonary alveolar cells
19. Muscle cells
20. Osteocytes
21. Connective tissue cells

* From Errera, M., and Forssberg, A.: *Mechanisms in Radiobiology,* 1960, 1961. Courtesy of Academic Press, Publisher, New York.

its mitotic activity, the more radiosensitive it should be. In general, malignant cells exhibit radiosensitivity that is roughly parallel to that of the normal cells from which they are derived.

It should be stressed that the Law of Bergonié and Tribondeau must be applied with caution to malignant tumors. An apparent contradiction is the marked radioresistance of certain anaplastic tumors. This may be explained on the assumption that such tumors are not really undifferentiated, but are rather ***dedifferentiated.*** In other words, arising from differentiated cells which have regressed in the process of becoming malignant, they are just as resistant as the normal parent cells. Although they appear undifferentiated, they are not so biologically and hence are not radiosensitive. However, there are exceptions to the law that cannot be explained in this manner; for example, the greater degree of radiosensitivity of mature lymphocytes in contrast to the immature cells from which they originate. It simply means that the radiation effects in tumors are extremely complex and cannot be explained by a formal rule of thumb.

At this juncture, another misconception must be pointed out— the confusion between ***radiosensitivity*** and ***radiocurability.*** Just because a tumor responds rapidly to irradiation, we must not assume that it is readily curable. For example, lymphoblastic lymphosarcoma is radiosensitive, but is rarely, if ever, radiocurable because it is almost always generalized by the time therapy is instituted. On the other hand, epidermoid carcinoma of the cervix requires relatively high dosage but is often curable. Here, the factor of maturation of tumor cells as the result of inhibition of mitosis favors a high degree of curability, at least in the more localized stages.

Also important is the fact that despite the variation in radiosensitivity of different tumors of the same species—for example, epidermoid carcinoma—they should all receive essentially the same dose in radiotherapy. Therefore, histologic grading of tumors does not aid the radiotherapist, and may actually mislead him if he is not aware of the importance of complete therapy according to the tumor species. On the same basis, the rate of regression must not be used as a yardstick for radiation dosage; a rapidly regressing tumor must receive just as complete treatment as more slowly regressing tumors of the same species.

A recurrent tumor is usually less responsive than the primary, owing at least in part to regrowth from a more radioresistant cell population. Another factor, as we shall soon find, may well be hypoxia associated with a poorer blood supply engendered by previous irradiation.

The Oxygen Effect. As noted earlier, radiosensitivity is enhanced by molecular oxygen (O_2) *if it is present at the time of irradiation,* and is manifested at low partial pressures ranging from 0 to 20 mm Hg. The *oxygen enhancement ratio* (*OER*) has already been defined as follows:

$$OER = \frac{dose\ (anoxia)}{dose\ (full\ oxygenation)}\ for\ same\ biologic\ effect$$

or, alternatively,

$$OER = \frac{D_0\ (anoxia)}{D_0\ (full\ oxygenation)}\ for\ same\ biologic\ effect$$

In a typical mammalian tumor *in vivo* there is a progressively enlarging necrotic center surrounded by a zone of viable cells (see Fig. 15.12). It has been known for a number of years that the maximum diffusion distance for O_2 in tissues is about 150 microns $(150 \times 10^{-3}\ mm)$. Furthermore, the thickness of the viable cell layer is surprisingly constant for most tumors, about 160 to 180 microns. Thus, if the dying center of the tumor is more than this critical range from the capillaries, it will contain hypoxic and anoxic cells which are more radioresistant by a factor of 2.5 to 3, and regrowth of the tumor can occur from these cells if their

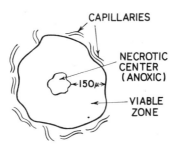

FIGURE 15.12. Oxygen can diffuse over a distance of about 150 μ from a capillary. Beyond this distance, anoxia supervenes. This may explain the loss of radiosensitivity of the central regions of tumor cords or masses.

TABLE 15.04

DIAMETERS (CM) OF TUMORS FOR 90 PERCENT PROBABILITY OF CURE
AT THE INDICATED EXPOSURE LEVEL*

^{60}Co γ rays—exposure in R

Degree of Oxygenation	2,000	2,500	3,000	3,500	4,000	4,500	5,000	5,500	6,000	6,500	7,000	7,500	8,000	8,500	9,000	9,500	10,000
Cells Fully Oxygenated	0.07	2	5	13	36	75											
1% of Cells Oxygenated				1.3	2.1	3.2	5.0	7.9	13	20.4	32	50	75				
All Cells Anoxic							1.0	1.6	2.4	3.8	5.9	9.0	14	21	32	50	75

*Adapted from Fowler, J. F., Morgan, R. L., and Wood, C. A. P., *Brit. J. Radiol. 36:77*, 1963; based on data of H. B. Hewitt. Courtesy of The British Journal of Radiology.

anoxic state is ignored in radiotherapy. In fact, radio*in*curable tumors may well be those which contain significant numbers of anoxic cells.

We may summarize the problem of tumor oxygenation by stating that it is a function of four factors: (a) the distance between the capillary and the farthest tumor cell, as described in the preceding paragraph, (b) the O_2 tension in the capillary blood, (c) the rate of utilization of O_2 by the intervening viable cells, and (d) the rate of O_2 diffusion into the tumor mass.

In a series of ingenious experiments Powers and Tolmach[68] found that a particular murine lymphosarcoma consists of a mixed population of 1 percent radioresistant ($D_o = 260$ rads) and 99 percent radiosensitive ($D_o = 110$ rads) cells. This difference in sensitivity to X rays is related to the state of oxygenation, as indicated by the response of cells irradiated *in vitro* (well oxygenated), and as transplants rendered anoxic by killing the host animals. Interestingly enough, the ratio of the survival curve slopes of the two components is $260/110 = 2.3$, the factor by which the radiosensitivity of oxygenated cells usually exceeds that of anoxic cells exposed to low-LET radiation. It has been estimated that even if only 1 percent of the cells in a tumor are anoxic, the curative dose approaches that needed for a wholly anoxic population!

The same authors[68] have quoted from the literature the 90 percent curative dose for tumors of various sizes under different degrees of oxygenation. Table 15.04 and Figure 15.13 show how an increase in tumor size and/or a decrease in oxygenation increases the dose needed for 90 percent "cure." It is at least theoretically possible that deficient oxygenation may occur in human tumors as the result of such factors as large size, torsion, or scarring.

Unfortunately, direct clinical application of this principle by deliberately increasing the O_2 tension of tumors is still in the experimental stage. Although O_2 tension can be increased by placing the patient in a hyperbaric chamber during irradiation, the method is fraught with technical problems and the results are thus far equivocal. Another approach has been to have the patient breath pure O_2 but this, too, is still under investigation. The use of intra-arterial hydrogen perioxide to perfuse the tumor

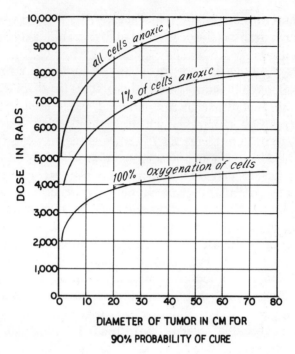

FIGURE 15.13. Dose required for 90 percent probability of cure, related to the diameter of the tumor and its state of oxygenation. Based on same data as Table 15.03. Note that the "curative" dose increases with the size of the tumor, and with the degree of anoxia.

volume at first offered considerable promise, but further clinical experience has not confirmed initial optimism. Another approach has been to reduce local oxygenation in an effort to decrease the radiosensitivity of the normal tissues and here, too, the results are inconclusive. Finally, hypothermia which is known to induce local hypoxia is being tried as a means of enhancing the difference in radiosensitivity of the tumor and the normal tissues.

Radiation Quality At present the mainstay of radiation therapy is ^{60}Co γ rays (1.25 MeV), now being challenged by megavoltage linac X rays (4 to 8 MV). Although these have effected an improvement in dosage distribution, with skin and bone sparing, their dissipation of energy is still via the release of energetic electrons which are in the low-LET region, just as are those produced by 250-kV X rays. In fact, megavoltage radiation has a relative biologic effectiveness (RBE) 15 to 20 percent less than that of orthovoltage X rays. (Recall that the LET of a charged particle increases with its charge and decreases with its velocity.)

Low-LET radiation (fast electrons released by X or γ rays) produces sublethal injury of tumor cells with possible recovery, multiple hits being needed for lethality. More highly lethal are ***intermediate-LET radiation*** such as cyclotron fast neutrons (see pages 610 to 612), and ***high-LET radiation*** such as fission spectrum fast neutrons, and cyclotron negative pions (π^-) as described on pages 612 to 615. The fast neutrons deposit energy by releasing recoil nuclei, especially protons; whereas, the π^- pions, upon capture, cause star formation with the release of α particles, protons, neutrons, and nuclear fragments. These are highly ionizing, and the ion clusters are closely spaced; a single hit as the charged particle crosses a cell nucleus usually suffices to kill the cell. There is virtually no recovery from sublethal injury, in contrast to the situation with megavoltage photon radiation.

The discussion of radiation quality would be incomplete without reference to the ***oxygen effect.*** With low-LET radiation there is a significant oxygen effect, the oxygen enhancement ratio (OER) decreasing from a maximum to a minimum in the LET range of 10 to 100 keV/micron, while the RBE increases inversely (see Fig. 16.01). On the other hand, with intermediate and high-LET radiation, the OER approaches unity, and cell anoxia is no longer a determining factor in complete tumor control. The radiobiologic properties of high-LET radiation with its potential application in radiotherapy will be taken up in greater detail in the next chapter.

Volume Effect. The irradiated volume should include the entire tumor and a "safe" margin of apparently normal tissue. However, this so-called ***volume of interest*** should be kept as small as possible for at least two reasons. ***First,*** the tolerance of normal tissues (i.e. recuperative ability) varies inversely with the irradiated volume. This is a complex function of such factors as the release of toxic products, the number of normal cells inactivated with resulting interference in ***repopulation*** of the normal tissues, injury to the vascular components of the stroma, and host immunologic response. Because a large volume of normal tissue must necessarily be included in the radiation field of a large tumor, there is a greater risk of irreparable damage than with a small tumor treated to the same total dose. On the other hand, larger tumors require a larger curative dose of radiation because of the inverse relationship of sensitivity to tumor volume. This is explained mainly by the *oxygen effect.* Obviously, the larger the tumor the more likely it is to have zones of poor vascularization containing hypoxic and anoxic cells which, as we have seen, are radioresistant. As an example, Von Essen[87] found in treating epidermoid carcinoma of the skin that single curative exposures ranged from 2700 R for field areas measuring less than 10 cm^2, to more than 3700 R for field areas of 100 cm^2.

Second, the integral dose increases with an increase in the irradiated volume. This is manifested by a corresponding decrease in whole body tolerance.

Since current methods of radiotherapy are relatively ineffective in destroying all anoxic cells at least to a critical level of about 30 cells, especially in bulky tumors, other approaches are under investigation. As noted in the preceding section, these include methods of inducing increased tumor oxygenation and hypothermia, high-LET radiation, and radiosensitizers.

Abscopal Effect (Effect at a Distance). On less certain grounds is the clinical observation that exposure of certain tumors to radiation may result in regression of similar tumor deposits located remote from the treatment site. For example, it is a common observation that in patients with Hodgkin's disease, radiation therapy of a group of nodes in the neck may cause shrinkage of untreated nodes elsewhere in the body. It is not known whether this is due to the liberation of certain substances in the irradiated area that are toxic to the same tumor elsewhere, or to a rallying of the natural body defenses against the same tumor type generally by a sort of immune reaction, or to some other mechanism as yet unidentified. This type of response is not limited to irradiation therapy, but may occur after an infection, transfusion reaction, or rarely after a biopsy of one of the lesions.

Time-Dose Relationship and Tissue Recovery. The aim of clinical radiation therapy is to deliver a *lethal dose* to virtually every tumor cell in a localized lesion, without irreparable injury to the adjoining normal tissues. This requires information about the differential radiosensitivity of the two types of tissue in question. However, this is only one side of the coin. The other side is concerned with the difference in the recovery rates between neoplastic and normal tissue. Both these factors, *differential sensitivity* and *differential recovery* are of paramount importance in tumor control by radiation therapy. In radiotherapy this relationship is embodied in the concept of the *therapeutic ratio* (see pages 591 to 593).

It is generally recognized that normal cells have a greater degree of recuperative power *in vivo* than do *sensitive* tumor cells. There are several possible explanations for this behavior. First, normal tissues harboring tumors usually display less reproductive activity and are therefore not so vulnerable to ionizing radiation. Second, normal cells possess better vascular and nerve supplies which aid in their recovery. Finally, even when normal cells, (mainly connective tissue) suffer nuclear damage, there seems to be a greater tendency to recovery, probably in large part due to replacement from undamaged cells nearby.

The *rate* of recovery of normal cells is also greater than that of certain tumor cells with the usual clinical doses of radiation. *Intracellular recovery* occurs during the first few hours and is more pronounced in normal cells, corresponding to the shoulder of the survival curve with X or γ radiation.

Full advantage should be taken of the differential sensitivity and recovery rates between the tumor and its surrounding normal tissues. Any factor which enhances this difference is bound to improve the results of radiotherapy. It had been known since 1918 that more total radiation could be given safely if the dose were divided into daily *fractions,* than could be given in a single massive dose. Coutard[15] (1932) recognized this in his extensive clinical experience with carcinoma of the head and neck, laying the groundwork for modern radiotherapy by placing the *principle of fractionation* on a firm clinical basis. He ascribed the marked improvement in results with fractionated treatment to these factors:

1. Improved recovery of normal tissues as compared with cancer (enhanced differential recovery), that is, improved therapeutic ratio.

2. Greater opportunity of irradiating tumor cells during periods of heightened sensitivity, that is, during mitosis.

3. Cyclic changes in sensitivity of tumor cells on the thirteenth and twenty-sixth days, lasting three or four days. Coutard discovered that with fractionation he could deliver larger total doses with impunity. For example, with a 75 cm^2 field, the following exposures could safely be given to an undifferentiated carcinoma:

700 R daily for 5 days   3,500 R total
450 R daily for 10 days   4,500 R total
350 R daily for 13 days   4,550 R total

He observed an epithelial reaction (*epithelite*) on the thirteenth day and epidermal reaction (*epidermite*) on the twenty-sixth day.

With differentiated carcinoma Coutard advised 160 R daily for 40 days, for a total of 6,400 R. Because of the cyclic increase in sensitivity mentioned above, he suggested a larger dose, 500 to 600 R, a few days before the thirteenth and twenty-sixth days of the treatment course.

In 1933 Reisner[74] published data on the effect of fractionation of X rays on the exposure required to produce **skin erythema.** His results, summarized in Table 15.05, indicate that with daily

TABLE 15.05
FRACTIONAL DAILY EXPOSURES REQUIRED TO PRODUCE SKIN
ERYTHEMA (2 × 2 CM^2 AREA), ACCORDING TO REISNER[74]

No. of Daily Exposures	R Per Exposure	R Total	% Total Exposure
1	1000	1000	100
2	650	1300	130
3	500	1500	150
4	400	1600	160
7	300	2100	210
12	200	2400	240
27	100	2700	270

fractionation over one week, the total exposure needed for the same skin effect is double that in a single exposure. If fractionation is carried to four weeks, the total exposure is nearly tripled. Furthermore, the greatest recovery rate occurs in the early days of the treatment course as shown graphically in Figure 15.14. Presumably, there is cumulative damage to the tumor bed as treatment progresses, gradually decreasing the recovery rate.

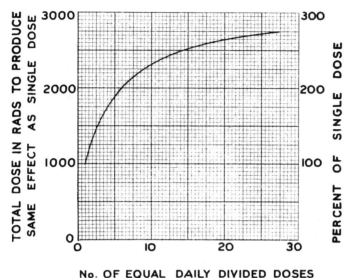

No. OF EQUAL DAILY DIVIDED DOSES

FIGURE 15.14. Effect of fractionation of kilovoltage X rays on the total dose needed for a particular effect, such as erythema. (From A. Reisner.[74])

In 1934, Duffy, Arneson, and Voke[18] investigated skin recovery by first determining the single exposure of 200-kV (1 mm Cu HVL) radiation required to produce skin erythema. This turned out to be 660 R including backscatter. They next attempted to produce an erythema with two equal fractions separated by a period of 24 hours, and found that two exposures of 500 R each, or a total of 1,000 R was required, using the same quality of radiation. This was an increase of 150 percent over the single erythema exposure, or 2 × 75 percent. Therefore, they reasoned that the skin behaved as though the second increment of 75 percent was added to 25 percent remaining from the first exposure to give a 100 percent erythema exposure; in other words, 25/75 or one-third of the first exposure remained in the skin, representing a recovery of about two-thirds during the first 24 hours. Later, Quimby and McComb[73] calculated a recovery ranging from 31 percent for day 2, to 5 percent for day 21. Here again as therapy is prolonged the daily recovery rate diminishes probably because of cumulative injury of the supporting tissues of the skin. The total exposure of 200-kV X rays required in four weeks is nearly three times the single exposure.

Some authorities have warned that the results of Reisner and of Quimby are experimental, are based on increments of only 100 R per day for one month, and are concerned with a mild erythema. The same degree of recovery cannot be assumed to hold for a schedule of 250 R per day, carried to the severe skin reaction that is often required with orthovoltage radiation. However, the skin tolerance is of about the same order of magnitude, despite these differences. Table 15.06, based on Paterson's[66] ex-

TABLE 15.06

MAXIMUM TOLERATED SKIN EXPOSURES * WITH VARIOUS DEGREES OF FRACTIONATION AND WITH VARIOUS FIELD AREAS. THE QUALITY OF THE RADIATION IS 1.5 MM CU HVL.

No. of Daily Exposures	Field Size in Cm^2				
	20–40	40–60	75–125	150–200	300–400
1	2100	1900	1700	1500	—
4	3700	3400	2900	2500	—
8	4700	4300	3800	3300	2700
10 **	5100	4700	4100	3600	3000
15 **	5500	5100	4500	4000	3400
25 **	6300	5900	5300	4800	4300

* From Paterson, R.: *The Treatment of Malignant Disease by Radium and X-rays,* 1963. Courtesy of Edward Arnold, Publisher, London.
** Saturdays and Sundays excluded.

perience, shows the variation in skin tolerance for various areas in terms of the total exposure administered over various total periods of time. It can readily be seen from this empirical table that with any given field size the skin tolerance, when therapy is fractionated over one month, is about 3 times the single exposure tolerance. This is in surprisingly close agreement with the observations of Reisner, and of Quimby and McComb, considering the biological nature of the experiments.

A classic in clinical research is Strandqvist's[80] report on the treatment of skin cancer, published in 1944. He studied a large series of patients who had been treated for assorted cancers of the skin, varying in size from about 5 to 30 cm^2, and determined the optimal total exposure relative to the degree of fractionation, midway between overdosage and underdosage (necrosis and recurrence, respectively). In summary, the optimal single exposure for lesions this size is 2,000 R, and if treatment is fractionated over a period of 7 days, the total exposure must be increased to

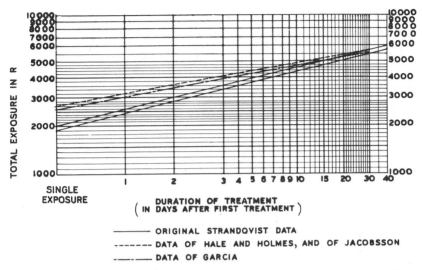

SINGLE EXPOSURE

DURATION OF TREATMENT
(IN DAYS AFTER FIRST TREATMENT)

——————— ORIGINAL STRANDQVIST DATA

------- DATA OF HALE AND HOLMES, AND OF JACOBSSON

—·—·— DATA OF GARCIA

FIGURE 15.15. Comparison of recovery curves obtained by various authors. Note that the curves are all straight lines on a log-log plot of the data. (Compiled from M. Strandqvist;[80] C. H. Hale and G. W. Holmes;[37] F. Jacobsson;[42] and M. Garcia.[32])

3,800 R. Two-week fractionation requires 4,500 R. It cannot be too strongly emphasized that the **treatment area** is an important factor in the time-dose relationship; as already noted, although a larger exposure is required for a larger lesion, the tolerance is at the same time reduced. Figure 15.15 is a graph based on Strandqvist's data. The data of other investigators are included for comparison, and it is interesting to note the similarity in the curves. Paterson's[66] data for lethal doses in epidermoid cancer are comparable to those of Strandqvist, as shown in Table 15.07.

TABLE 15.07
MINIMAL TUMOR LETHAL EXPOSURES OF X RAY, ACCORDING TO
PATERSON[66] AND STRANDQVIST,[80] FOR VARIOUS DEGREES OF
FRACTIONATION; AND FOR VARIOUS TYPES OF SKIN CANCER

Fractionation (No. of Daily Exposures)	Paterson (Epidermoid Cancer)	Strandqvist (Skin Cancer)
1	2000	2000
4	4000	3600
8	5000	4200
18	5500	4800
32	6000	5500

Strandqvist found that when he plotted the various total exposures against the corresponding overall treatment times on log-log paper, he obtained virtually a straight line curve. He explained this on the basis of the following parabolic function which best fits the time-dose relationship:

$$D = kt^n \qquad (1)$$

where D is the total dose required for a specific effect in a given tissue, k is a constant under the conditions specified for D, t is the total time during which daily fractionation is carried out, and n is a constant (positive fraction) known as the *recovery exponent* (*not* the same as extrapolation number n in cell survival curves). Equation (1) represents a parabola, characterized by a straight line curve or *time-dose regression line* on a double log plot.

The meaning of the constants k and n requires clarification. If a specific effect, such as a tumor lethal dose, is to be produced in a single irradiation, $t = 1$ day and $t^n = 1$ regardless of the value of n. In this case, $D = k$ and we may therefore define k as that single dose of radiation which will produce the desired effect. If the treatment is to be fractionated, the value of the total dose D will be greater than k and can be found by equation (1). The constant n is the slope of the time-dose curve on a double log plot; the greater the value of n, that is, the steeper the slope of the curve, the greater the recovery rate of the tissue in question. In general, if n is less for a given tumor than it is for the normal tissues, it indicates a favorable differential recovery rate, and fractionation is advantageous. Any factor or factors which steepen the slope of the curve for normal tissues, or lower that of the tumor, improve differential recovery in favor of destruction of the tumor by fractionation. According to Strandqvist, the values of the constants in equation (1) are $k = 2,000$ R and $n = 0.22$ for skin cancer.

In a study of 60 patients with carcinoma of the breast, Cohen[12,13] found the time-dose relationship to follow the same equation as the Strandqvist data, but with a different set of constants. Thus, $k = 1,270$ R and $n = 0.35$ for the median lethal dose in carcinoma of the breast, indicating greater sensitivity and faster recovery than with epidermoid carcinoma. Since n for normal skin is about 0.32, nearly the same as that of breast carcinoma, prolonged fractionation should be of no particular value with this type of tumor.

Garcia[32] in 1955 published the results of radiation therapy in a large series of patients with epidermoid carcinoma of the cervix and found the time-dose relationship to follow a regression line similar to the plots obtained previously with equation (1). In other words, a similar time-dose relationship was found by Garcia in epidermoid carcinoma of the cervix to that of Strandqvist in carcinoma of the skin, Paterson in epidermoid skin cancer, and Cohen in carcinoma of the breast. Garcia's constants were $k = 2,575$ R and $n = 0.23$ for the median effective dose. The similarity between Garcia's constants, and those for epidermoid carcinoma of the skin ($k = 2,750$ R and $n = 0.23$ according to Andrews and Moody[1]) are quite striking. Finally, the values of these constants for moist desquamation of the skin, as pointed out by Andrews and Moody,[1] are $k = 1,500$ R and $n = 0.32$.

The application of equation (1) to various types of tissue with the appropriate constants may be summarized as follows:

$D = 1,500\ t^{0.32}$ for moist desquamation of skin

$D = 2,000\ t^{0.22}$ for regression of skin cancer (Strandqvist)

$D = 2,575\ t^{0.23}$ for median effective dose in epidermoid carcinoma of the cervix

$D = 2,750\ t^{0.23}$ for regression of skin epidermoid carcinoma

$D = 1,270\ t^{0.35}$ for median lethal dose in carcinoma of the breast

According to these equations, 2,750 R in a single irradiation should cause regression of epidermoid cancer of the skin. If the treatment is fractionated over a total time t, then the total exposure would have to be increased to a value determined by the appropriate equation. The constant in Strandqvist's equation is 2,000 because of the manner in which he plotted his data; as modified by Andrews and Moody, the constant becomes 2,750. Since the recovery exponent is less than that for normal skin, there is an indication for fractionation which takes advantage of the differential recovery rate.

Mention should also be made of the possible influence of *dose rate* on radiobiologic response. Under ordinary conditions, in the range of about 100 to a few hundred rads per min, there is no conclusive evidence for a dose rate effect. Only with extremely high dose rates of thousands of rads per sec, and in microsecond pulsed exposures, is there an intensification of biologic effects. On the other hand, with very low dose rates, such as exist in the case of low intensity radium needles, there is suggestive evidence for an improved therapeutic ratio (see Hall, E. J., in General Bibliography).

Radiation Dose Fractionation. Since the goal of radiotherapy is to deliver a lethal dose to virtually every cell in a particular tumor without causing irreparable injury to the neighboring normal cells, we must know about the differential response of the two kinds of tissue in question. Obviously, the greater the damage to tumor cells relative to normal cells, the higher will be the probability of tumor control by irradiation. In radiotherapy, this relationship is embodied in the concept *therapeutic ratio*, to be discussed on pages 591 to 593.

We have already seen that fractionation therapy regimens have been established on more or less empirical grounds as being generally far superior to single dose therapy. We also know, at least from radiobiologic experiments, that all mammalian cells (i.e. when fully oxygenated) exhibit practically the same degree of inherent radiosensitivity. What then is the scientific basis for fractionation? Experiments *in vitro* and *in vivo* have revealed the operation, to varying degrees, of four major radiobiologic factors which can be represented by the acronym ROMP, standing for

(1) Repair of sublethal injury (fast recovery)
(2) Oxygenation
(3) Mitotic cycle
(4) Proliferation (slow recovery)

These will now be discussed individually.

1. *Repair of Sublethal Injury.* This is manifested experimentally by the reappearance of the shoulder in cell survival curves within a few hours after each dose fraction. First published by Elkind,[21,22] this is called *fast* or *Elkind type recovery*. As the number of fractions in a given overall treatment time are increased, the expo-

nential (straight line) portion of the survival curve assumes a smaller slope indicating lessened radiosensitivity, as shown in Figure 15.10. However, if this effect of diminished sensitivity through fractionation were the same in both tumor and normal cells, there would be no advantage in fractionated over single dose radiotherapy schedules. Fortunately, normal cells generally have a greater proclivity to repair sublethal radiation injury than do most kinds of tumor cells, and so fractionation enhances the therapeutic ratio. At the same time, it must be borne in mind that there is evidence for a significantly greater influence of the number of fractions than of the overall treatment time on producing a given radiobiologic effect.

2. *Oxygenation.* The relation of cellular response to fractionated doses of radiation, as determined by the availability of oxygen, has been observed in experiments with cell cultures. As we know, anoxic cells are about one-third as radiosensitive as fully oxygenated cells when exposed to X or γ radiation. Since tumors are likely to have zones of hypoxia while normal cells are ordinarily well-oxygenated, additional oxygen should have a relatively greater sensitizing effect on tumor cells than on normal cells. Thus, oxygen may be said to improve the therapeutic ratio. To carry this a step farther, we may assume that fractionation of doses permits the degree of oxygenation to improve as the tumor shrinks; again the oxygen effect will be relatively greater on tumor cells than on normal cells, and so the therapeutic ratio should improve as a result of fractionation. Hall* has shown that in cell cultures *in vitro* no repair of sublethal injury occurs between dose fractions under **hypoxic** conditions, although repair does occur if oxygen is supplied during the radiation-free intervals. Therefore, on the assumption that such experimental results hold true in radiotherapy, fractionation improves the therapeutic ratio by (a) increasing the differential radiosensitivity of tumor cells through re-oxygenation between fractions, and (b) counteracting the protective effect of hypoxia by impairing the recovery of tumor cells from sublethal damage.

---

*Hall, E. J., Lehnert, S., and Roizin-Towle, L.: Split dose experiments with hypoxic cells. *Radiol. 112:*425, 1974.

3. *Mitotic Cycle.* As noted earlier, the radiosensitivity of cells depends on their respective positions in the mitotic cycle, being a maximum during the mitotic and G_2 phases in many cell systems. Irradiation of an asynchronous population of cells (i.e. cells in various phases of the cycle at any particular instant) will, for the most part, cause the greatest inhibition in the most sensitive phases, with a resulting tendency for the cell population to become synchronous. However, synchrony lasts for a relatively short time and there is no firm evidence as yet as to how much this factor influences the improved therapeutic results obtained by dose fractionation. It is possible that in the future we may be able to enhance the therapeutic ratio by inducing synchrony through the use of appropriate drugs in conjunction with radiation.

4. *Population Kinetics.* While rapid recovery of sublethal injury occurs within a few hours after radiation exposure, repopulation by reproduction of surviving cells is more a function of the overall treatment time than of the number of fractions. Since normal cells retain their reproductive capacity better than tumor cells following irradiation, a fractionated therapy program with a reasonably long overall treatment time should improve the therapeutic ratio. At the present time our knowledge of recovery from radiation injury in humans is based chiefly on normal skin and on epidermoid carcinoma. To transpose these data to other types of tumors without further research may be erroneous. One must not assume that the same fractionation will produce similar results in all kinds of tumors. Yet, that is precisely what is being assumed in present day clinical therapy, mainly because there is inadequate information to guide us in modifying fractionation for various types of tumors in different locations. Furthermore, the subject is considerably more complex than one would guess from equation (1). For example, a great deal of uncertainty still surrounds the selection of the number of fractions with respect to the overall treatment time for a particular variety of tumor. Equation (1) simply relates total dosage to overall treatment time and states nothing about the number of fractions, although the data underlying the equation are based on daily treatment fractions.

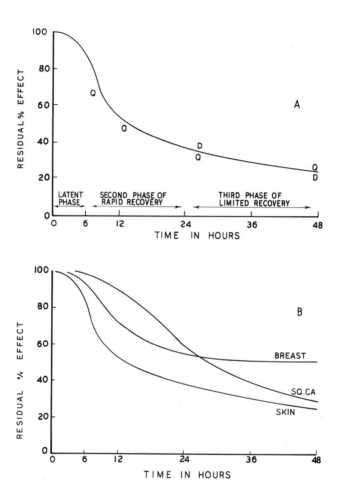

FIGURE 15.16. In *A* is shown a composite recovery curve as a function of time after a single radiation exposure of human skin, based on the data of E. H. Quimby and W. S. McComb[73] (Q), and of J. J. Duffy, A. N. Arneson, and F. L. Voke[18] (D).

In *B* are three hypothetical variations in the shapes of the recovery curves to explain the clinical observations on two types of cancer as compared with normal skin, following a single dose of radiation. Note that the maximum differential recovery between breast carcinoma and normal skin occurs at about 48 hr, whereas that between squamous cell cancer and normal skin occurs at about 12 hr. (Courtesy of N. G. DeMoor, D. Durbach, J. Levin, and L. Cohen[16] and *Radiology.*)

As an interesting example of differential radiation response of normal and of tumor cells, Duffy and others[19] have obtained suggestive evidence that maximum differential recovery of skin versus epidermoid carcinoma occurs at 12 hours after irradiation, but according to Cohen[12] this occurs at 48 hours for mammary adenocarcinoma (see Fig. 15.16). On this basis, we should adopt a twice-daily or at least daily schedule for treatment of skin epidermoid carcinoma, and an alternate-day schedule for mammary adenocarcinoma.

Obviously, there is urgent need of further investigations along these lines before radiotherapy of the great multiplicity of neoplasms can be established on a firm scientific foundation. In fact it is not unreasonable to suppose that a change in the method of fractionation in the right direction may be of much greater importance than the quality of the radiation employed. The lack of adequate flexibility of fractionation in various neoplasms may account, at least in part, for the failure of ^{60}Co and megavoltage X-ray therapy to yield spectacular improvement in the long-term curability of most varieties of cancer.

NOMINAL STANDARD DOSE AND THE RET

As we have just learned, modern radiation therapy is based on the delivery of a series of dose fractions over a designated period of time. There has long been a need for a unit that could provide a basis of comparison between various dosage schedules and also permit variation in them while retaining the same biologic effect.

In 1965 Ellis[24] first proposed such a unit which he called the *ret* (radiation equivalent therapy), the biologic dose being the *nominal standard dose (NSD)*. To arrive at its formulation, he made certain assumptions based on data acquired from radiobiologic research and from clinical experience. These include the following:

1. Normal and malignant cells respond *similarly* to radiation injury insofar as lethality, loss of reproductive capacity, and intracellular repair of sublethal injury are concerned. This is borne out by the similarity of survival curves of various cell cultures.

2. Only **normal cells** can recover by the intervention of extra-cellular or homeostatic factors (e.g. healing of tissues by fibro-blasts, capillaries, immune factors). **Malignant cells** are **not** subject to such extracellular repair, this being a major difference between the response of malignant and normal cells.

3. Intracellular repair is **rapid** (Elkind type), occurring well within 24 hours, whereas extracellular repair is **slow**, requiring days or weeks. Hence, intracellular recovery depends on the number of fractions, but extracellular recovery depends on the overall treatment time.

On the basis of such considerations Ellis separated the fraction-ation factor which is related to fast recovery, from the total treat-ment time in days which is related to slow recovery. Since the re-sponse of skin cancer is presumably subject only to intracellular recovery (if repair occurs) and the slope of the time-dose regression curve is 0.22 as shown in Figure 15.17, he adopted this value as the exponent for rapid recovery (fractionation factor), correcting it to 0.24 for 5-day per week treatment. Recall that this type of recovery is characterized by reappearance of the shoulder in the survival curve after each fraction. On the other hand, the time-dose regression curve for normal skin contains two components—one for rapid recovery and the other for slow recovery. The time-dose regression curve for normal skin has a slope of 0.33. The difference between the exponents $0.33 - 0.22 = 0.11$ represents the exponent for slow recovery related to the overall treatment time in days.

From the above hypothesis came the following relation:

$$D = NSD \times N^{0.24} \times T^{0.11} \text{ rads} \qquad (3)$$

where D is the total dose in rads (for ^{60}Co γ rays), NSD is the nominal standard dose in **rets**, N is the number of fractions, and T is the total treatment time in days between the first and last treatment. Ellis emphasizes that the fractions must be separated by at least 16 hours and must be evenly spaced (5-day per week schedule permissible); and T must be in the range 3 to 100 days.

The NSD is a dose representing a biologic effect related to normal connective tissue tolerance. Thus, it is the real limiting factor in radiation therapy. Furthermore, it is incorrect to regard it as a single dose because then the factor of slow recovery would not have time to come into play and equation (3) would not be valid.

Although Ellis uses 1800 rets as the maximum normal connective tissue tolerance he recommends that each radiotherapy center establish its own value depending on the experience of its therapists as to the tolerable connective tissue dose. In the case of radiosensitive tumors such as Hodgkin's disease in the treatment of which there is little likelihood of reaching normal tissue tolerance, only $N^{0.24}$ need be considered, and we can obtain a *tumor standard dose* (*TSD*) in rets from the following equation:

$$D = TSD \cdot N^{0.24} \qquad (4)$$

Ellis warns that in applying equation (3) to a portion of a treatment course the dosage in rets is based on the portion of the fractions given. For example, if the total contemplated *NSD* is 1800 rets in 30 fractions and only 15 fractions are given, then the given *NSD* is $15/30 \times 1800 = 900$ rets.

There has been wide divergence in the opinion of radiotherapists and physicists as to the validity of the *NSD* concept. While it is not a substitute for careful radiotherapy planning, it does succeed in furnishing an approximate common denominator for intercomparison of treatment schedules and for introducing a degree of flexibility in varying dosage schedules. For example, as an approximate generalization, 400 rads twice weekly has about the same radiobiologic effect as 200 rads 5 times weekly.

The NSD apparently has a sufficient factor of safety to avoid excessive irradiation of normal tissue, but still should be used with caution.

Moving-strip Technic. As an example of the application of the time-dose relationship, the moving-strip technic (M.D. Anderson Hospital and Tumor Institute modification for ^{60}Co therapy, of Manchester method for orthovoltage X-ray therapy) permits the irradiation of large body cavities without intolerable regional or systemic reactions in most patients. In ovarian carcinoma with its all too frequent peritoneal implants, and in extensive pleural neoplasia, large field therapy of the abdomen or hemithorax is poorly tolerated when carried to significant dosage.

In moving-strip therapy of the abdomen we lay off directly opposed anterior and posterior strips measuring 2.5 cm high and covering the width of the abdomen. These strips are numbered sequentially from the symphysis upward, corresponding anterior and posterior strips being treated on alternate days. Strip number 1 is treated anteriorly on the first day, and posteriorly on the second day. Then strips number 1 and 2 are combined and treated anteriorly on the third day, and posteriorly on the fourth. The addition of strips one at a time continues in this manner until four (10 cm high) are treated anteriorly and posteriorly on alternate days. Next, the 10-cm port is moved up 2.5 cm every

TABLE 15.08
MOVING-STRIP TECHNIC* FOR ABDOMINAL IRRADIATION.
IN THIS HYPOTHETICAL CASE, THE ABDOMEN MEASURES 30 CM IN
HEIGHT, REQUIRING 12 STRIPS 2.5 CM IN HEIGHT

	Strips Treated		
Day	Anterior	Height of Treated Port in cm	Posterior
1	1	2.5	
2		2.5	1
3	1 + 2	5	
4		5	1 + 2
5	1 + 2 + 3	7.5	
6		7.5	1 + 2 + 3
7	1 + 2 + 3 + 4	10	
8		10	1 + 2 + 3 + 4
9	2 + 3 + 4 + 5	10	
10		10	2 + 3 + 4 + 5
11	3 + 4 + 5 + 6	10	
12		10	3 + 4 + 5 + 6
*		10	*
*		10	*
23	9 + 10 + 11 + 12	10	
24		10	9 + 10 + 11 + 12
25	10 + 11 + 12	7.5	
26		7.5	10 + 11 + 12
27	11 + 12	5	
28		5	11 + 12
29	12	2.5	
30		2.5	12

* Described by Delclos, L., Braun, E. J., Herrera, J. R., Jr., Sampiere, V. A., and van Roosenbeek, E.: *Radiology 81:* 632, 1963.
** Sequence continued on days 13 through 22, uppermost strip being reached on day 23.

other day (in effect, one strip removed from bottom and one added at the top) until the topmost strip has been reached, after which the height is reduced by successively removing a lower strip every other day until the last 2.5-cm strip has been treated posteriorly on the last day. The kidneys must be shielded **posteriorly** with 2 HVL of lead to avoid radiation nephritis. The dose to the liver must not exceed 2000 rads. Table 15.08 shows the treatment schedule in detail.

Although the planned midline total dose is 2500 to 3000 rads in an overall treatment time of 6 weeks, the actual treatment time for each strip is 16 days (each strip receives direct radiation 8 times, and penumbra 4 times except the top and bottom strips which receive penumbra twice) including the weekends on a 5-day per week schedule. For the same total dose we should anticipate a greater radiobiologic effect in this curtailed treatment time relative to that with large field irradiation over a 6-week period.

Let us see how a midline dose of 3000 rads by the moving-strip method compares with the same dose by conventional large-field therapy on the basis of the *NSD*. Rearranging equation (3) in terms of *NSD*:

$$NSD = dose \times N^{-0.24} \times T^{-0.11} \text{ rets} \qquad (4)$$

Moving-strip Method

> $dose = 3000$ rads
> $N = 12$ fractions
> $T = 16$ days

$$NSD = 3000 \times (12)^{-0.24} \times (16)^{-0.11}$$

$$= 1218 \text{ rets}$$

Large-field Method

> $dose = 3000$ rads
> $N = 28$ fractions
> $T = 40$ days

$$NSD = 3000 \times (28)^{-0.24} \times (40)^{-0.11}$$

$$= 898 \text{ rets}$$

Despite the larger biologically effective dose with moving-strip therapy, patient tolerance is usually superior to that with large-field therapy. For example, with the latter a dose of 4065 rads in 6 weeks gives the same NSD—1218 rets—as 3000 rads with the moving strip in $2\frac{1}{2}$ weeks, but causes significantly greater regional and systemic reactions. This difference is probably due to the comparatively smaller volume treated on any one day by the moving-strip method.

THERAPEUTIC RATIO

First introduced by Paterson,[66] the *therapeutic ratio* is one possible index of the local radiocurability of a tumor. It is based on the concept that the smaller the cancericidal dose for a particular tumor relative to the necrotizing dose of the associated normal tissue, the better the chance of achieving local control of the tumor. Thus,

$$therapeutic\ ratio = \frac{normal\ tolerance\ dose}{tumor\ lethal\ dose}$$

Obviously, any factor which augments the numerator or diminishes the denominator improves the therapeutic ratio. The factors we have discussed pertaining to tumor response should affect the therapeutic ratio; they are presented in the following outline, where ↑ indicates enhancement of the therapeutic ratio, and ↓ the opposite.

The therapeutic ratio may be expressed alternatively as the ratio of the t^n from equation (1), for normal tissue and for a particular tumor. Thus, the therapeutic ratio (T.R.) for skin cancer (see pages 580 and 581) may be obtained as follows:

$$T.R. = \frac{t^{0.32}}{t^{0.22}} = t^{0.10}$$

Therapeutic ratio influenced by:
1. Tumor Radiosensitivity
   a. Intrinsic—cell variety less differentiated ↑
   b. Extrinsic
      1) location in adequate vascular bed ↑

    2) oxygen tension high ↑

    3) tumor volume small ↑

  c. Acquired radioresistance (e.g. previous irradiation, probably from reduced oxygen supply) ↓

2. Normal Tissue Tolerance

  a. Cell type radioresistant ↑

  b. Vascularity adequate ↑

  c. Systemic tolerance

    1) Age—young ↑

    2) Infection ↓

    3) General state of health—good ↑

    4) Host resistance (immunity) ↑

  d. Volume—small ↑

3. Fractionation (with low-LET radiation) ↑

4. Overall treatment time long (within limits) ↑

5. Relative biologic effectiveness (if greater for tumor than for normal cells) ↑

Note that the therapeutic ratio is useful only as a guide in therapy and does not have absolute significance because no absolute values can be assigned to the factors which govern it. Furthermore, normal tissue tolerance is a relative term. For example, in attempting radical irradiation of a potentially curable lesion a 2 percent incidence of necrosis of normal tissue may be acceptable. But patients must be individualized; thus, in an elderly patient whose malignant tumor has a natural history longer than life expectancy, the dose may be arbitrarily reduced about 10 to 20 percent to reduce the danger of serious necrosis.

It must be borne in mind that there is no single dose that is lethal for every case of a particular type of neoplasm, as has been amply observed experimentally and clinically. In general, as the absorbed dose is increased, the probability of tumor control increases. The curve representing percent tumor lethality as a function of absorbed dose is sigmoid shaped (see Fig. 15.17). Similarly, the incidence of necrosis as a function of absorbed dose follows a sigmoid curve. Obviously, any factor that separates these curves, moving the tumor-response curve to the left, and the necrosis-incidence curve to the right, increases the therapeutic ratio. This important concept should be kept in mind by the therapist as he plans a course of radiation therapy.

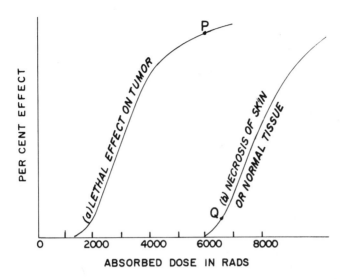

FIGURE 15.17. Typical sigmoid dose-response curves showing per-cent effect produced by various doses of radiation. Beyond some point *P* on curve (*a*) virtually all tumors are killed; thus, *P* may be called the *tumor lethal dose*. At some point *Q* on curve (**b**) there is a steep rise in the incidence of necrosis with increasing dose. The ratio of dose *Q* to dose *P* is the *therapeutic ratio*, which increases as the separation between the curves increases. (After R. Paterson.[64])

TISSUE AND ORGAN REACTIONS IN RADIOTHERAPY

In this section we shall describe various postirradiation changes in normal tissues and in radiosensitive tumors. With orthovoltage therapy of malignant tumors a radiation reaction is usually necessary, but overdosage with its attendant delayed or absent healing must be avoided. However, tissue reactions also occur with megavoltage and particle therapy carried to high dosage. In Table 15.09 are shown tolerance doses for a number of important organs. Note particularly the low tolerance of the liver, kidney, bone marrow, lens, and whole lung, and also the fact that many organs have a tolerance close to the therapeutic dose of tumors they may habor.

During a course of intensive X-ray therapy in the kilovoltage energy range of *200 to 250 kV,* the skin exhibits a sequence of reactions following a general pattern:

1. *Latent Period.* During the first 1 to 2 weeks, no visible change

TABLE 15.09

RADIATION TOLERANCE DOSES OF VARIOUS ORGANS, RANGING FROM MINIMAL ($TD_{5/5}$) TO MAXIMAL ($TD_{50/5}$). BASED ON STANDARD TREATMENT SCHEDULE OF 1000 RADS/WK, 2 DAYS' REST/WK, PHOTON RADIATION ENERGY 1 TO 6 MeV.*

Organ	Injury at 5 years	1–5% $TD_{5/5}$**	25–50% $TD_{50/5}$***	Volume or Length
Skin	Ulcer, severe fibrosis	5500	7000	100 cm³
Oral mucosa	Ulcer, severe fibrosis	6000	7500	50 cm³
Esophagus	Ulcer, stricture	6000	7500	75 cm³
Stomach	Ulcer, perforation	4500	5000	100 cm³
Intestine (small and large)	Ulcer, stricture	4500	6500	100 cm³
Rectum	Ulcer, stricture	5500	8000	100 cm³
Salivary glands	Xerostomia	5000	7000	50 cm³
Liver	Liver failure, ascites	3500†	4500†	Whole
Kidney	Nephrosclerosis	2300	2800	Whole
Bladder	Ulcer, contracture	6000	8000	Whole
Testes	Permanent sterilization	500–1500	2000	Whole
Ovaries	Permanent sterilization	200– 300	625–1200	Whole
Vagina	Ulcer, fistula	9000	>10,000	5 cm³
Breast (child)	No development	1000	1500	5 cm³
Breast (adult)	Atrophy and necrosis	>5000	>10,000	Whole
Lung	Pneumonitis, fibrosis	4000	6000	Lobe
			2500	Whole
Heart	Pericarditis, pancarditis	4000	>10,000	Whole
Bone (child)	Arrested growth	2000	3000	10 cm³
Bone (adult)	Necrosis, fracture	6000	15,000	10 cm³
Cartilage (child)	Arrested growth	1000	3000	Whole
Cartilage (adult)	Necrosis	6000	10,000	Whole
Muscle (child)	No development	2000–3000	4000–5000	Whole
Brain	Necrosis	5000	>6000	Whole
Spinal cord	Necrosis, transection	5000	>6000	5 cm³
Eye	Panophthalmitis, hemorrhage	5500	10,000	Whole
Lens	Cataract	250– 500	1200	Whole
Ear (inner)	Deafness	>6000	—	Whole
Thyroid gland	Hypothyroidism	4500	15,000	Whole
Adrenal glands	Hypoadrenalism	>6000	—	Whole
Pituitary gland	Hypopituitarism	4500	25,000	Whole
Bone marrow	Hypoplasia	200	550	Whole
		2000	4000–5000	Localized
Lymph nodes	Atrophy	4500	>7000	—
Fetus	Death	200	400	—

* Data from Dalrymple, G. V., *et al., Medical Radiation Biology.* Courtesy of the author and Publisher, W. B. Saunders, Philadelphia, 1973.

** $TD_{5/5}$ is dose that, under these conditions, results in no more than 5% severe complication rate in 5 years.

*** $TD_{50/5}$ is dose that, under these conditions, results in a 50% severe complication rate in 5 years.

† These values may be too high especially with moving strip technique wherein doses of 2,450 to 2,920 rads in 2½ weeks caused a high incidence of fatal radiation hepatitis. (J. T. Wharton, *et al., Am. J. Roentgenol.* 117:73, 1973.)

occurs. Presumably, there is cumulative damage to the skin which soon reaches a visible threshold by a:

2. *First Degree Reaction.* A moderate dose produces erythema

in the treatment field, often accompanied by mild itching or burning. If the radiation dosage is high enough, dry, bran-like scaling of the skin occurs, followed by tanning which may persist for several months. Rarely, the treated skin may be bleached. Still higher doses, particularly in sensitive moist areas such as the axillas, groins, and perineum lead to:

3. *Second Degree Reaction.* This follows the erythema (without intermediate tanning), appearing at the end of the third or fourth week after the start of therapy. It consists of blistering, with moist desquamation and denudation of the epithelium, followed by repeated crust formation with bleeding when the crusts are removed. Healing by regeneration of the epidermis from the edges of the denuded zone requires several weeks, although it may be delayed several months if the maximum tolerance dose of radiation has been reached. In late sequelae after fractionated radiation, that is, years after healing, the skin may show various degrees of atrophy, telangiectasia, and hyper- or depigmentation. If excessive doses are not used initially, later radiation-induced skin cancer rarely if ever occurs.

With gross overdosage, the skin reaction passes from the second degree reaction into the:

4. *Third Degree Reaction.* Regeneration is absent or incomplete. A deep ulcer forms, characterized by a sharp hard margin and a leathery gray base. It may heal slowly or become chronic, causing marked pain and discomfort to the patient. This is known as a *radiation ulcer.* In some instances, it may not appear for some years after therapy, arising as the result of trauma or infection in an area of atrophic, poorly vascularized skin. Therefore, any patient who has been subjected to intensive radiation therapy should be warned about the low resistance of the treated tissues to trauma, infection, or sunlight. Areas of the body which should probably never be given cancericidal doses of X ray for skin cancer include the back of the hand, pretibial area, dorsum of the foot, sacrum, and back of the neck. These areas show poor healing and if they do recover, are quite prone to ulceration upon minor traumatization.

The hair follicles are very susceptible to radiation damage, epilation occurring with doses smaller than those required to produce erythema. Minimal epilating doses cause temporary loss of hair, with regrowth in about one month. The new hair may be similar to the normal hair, or may differ in color and/or texture. Desquamating doses may induce permanent epilation.

Reactions of normal **mucous membranes** resemble those in the skin, but appear earlier. Erythema is mild and of short duration, being quickly followed by complete denudation of epithelium accompanied by a white, fibrinous membrane—the so-called **diphtheroid membrane.** Recovery takes place by regeneration from the margin just as in the skin. Overdosage may result in chronic ulceration and delayed or nonhealing.

In radiation therapy of the head and neck, the salivary glands may be profoundly altered in their function. The secretion becomes thick and ropy, interfering with mastication of food. If the dose is less than 1,000 rads recovery may occur in about one month. With larger doses, the damage to the salivary glands may be permanent as manifested by complete loss of secretion. In addition, teeth in the radiation field are often seriously damaged at the dento-enamel junction. Injury to the salivary glands and teeth is just as probable with megavoltage as with orthovoltage radiation for equal absorbed doses.

Edema of the subcutaneous tissues is very prone to occur in the upper part of the neck and lower part of the face. This may last many months, or even become permanent. With large doses, especially with megavoltage radiation, the subcutaneous tissues may eventually become fibrotic, this process even extending into the muscles.

Bone and cartilage are often damaged by radiation in the 200 to 250 kV range if the increased energy deposit in these structures relative to soft tissues is not kept in mind. Whenever bone or cartilage lies within the irradiated volume, care must be taken not to exceed their tolerance while attention is focused on skin tolerance. Megavoltage radiation does not remove the danger of osteoradionecrosis, despite the fact that absorption of energy is about equal per unit mass of bone and soft tissue. Bone destroyed by radiation forms a dead sequestrum which eventually ulcerates through the skin. Only when the sequestrum is known to be complete should it be removed. Cartilage necrosis is most apt to occur in the outer ear, the larynx, and the nose. Surgical removal may be necessary. With ordinary cancericidal doses cartilage necrosis is more likely to occur if the tumor has invaded the cartilage prior to therapy. In any case, if radiation therapy is selected for treatment of skin cancer on the ear or nose, the fields must be generous because cancer does not readily penetrate cartilage. Instead, it grows down to the cartilage and then spreads peripherally along the surface beyond the reaches of the visible portion of the lesion.

Many radiotherapists, the author included, insist on complete dental extraction in all patients with head and neck cancer requiring radiotherapy through the jaws. Experience has shown, all too often, that following such irradiation, dental extraction results in a very high incidence of osteoradionecrosis.

The reaction of tumor cells to irradiation has already been described. Clinically, a deep-seated tumor reacts by shrinking in volume as treatment progresses. The rate of shrinkage depends on the radiosensitivity of the tumor. Lymphosarcoma and Hodgkin's disease may show beginning regression after only 400 to 600 rads, although 3600 to 4000 rads in $3\frac{1}{2}$ to 4 weeks are required for complete disappearance. Usually, malignant tumors require 6 to 8 weeks for complete involution. Superficial carcinomas, as in the skin, gradually disappear, being replaced by moist desquamation. This heals by ingrowth of normal cells from the margin. Unless the original lesion has penetrated deeply beneath the surface, there is usually no permanent defect. In the treatment of cancer of a mucous membrane, there is an epithelitis with denudation similar to that in the normal skin, followed by regeneration from the margin of the treated area.

ACUTE RADIATION SYNDROMES

Thus far, we have been concerned only with the biologic effects engendered in tissues by ionizing radiation administered through limited ports during therapy. We shall now take up the radiobiology of whole body exposure to *single* massive amounts of radiation, resulting from the explosion of atomic weapons or from industrial accidents. As will be seen later, such exposure induces profound and often fatal effects due mainly to neutrons and γ rays. The damage resulting from the mechanical aspects of the explosion—the so-called blast—will not be included.

In general, whole body irradiation *shortens life,* the degree of shortening being *dose dependent up to about 1,000 R.* Between 1,000 and 10,000 R, survival time in experimental animals is no longer dose dependent, but becomes so again above 10,000 R. Survival times of individuals in an irradiated population have a random distribution at any particular dosage level.

Ordinarily the lethal effect of radiation is designated by the median lethal dose LD_{50}, the dose that causes 50 percent of the irradiated population to die within a specified period of time. In the case of small mammals, lethality usually becomes manifest within 30 days; therefore, the corresponding 50 percent lethal dose is expressed by $LD_{50/30}$. On the other hand, survival in humans may be as long as 60 days with low or moderate doses and we use the expression $LD_{50/60}$. It is customary to regard a radiation dose as being *immediately lethal* if its effect occurs within 30 days for small mammals, and 60 days for humans.

For the purpose of this discussion, we shall use exposure in R to express radiation quantity because of the difficulty of estimating absorbed doses in many of the published studies. In any case, the stated quantities are at best approximate.

The lethal exposure of whole body radiation varies with different animal species. The LD_{50} in man has been derived from the A-bombing experience in Hiroshima and Nagasaki. According to the United States Public Health Service, the following LD_{50} doses are representative of species variation:

Guinea Pig	175–250 R
Dog	325
Goat	350
MAN	360
Mouse	530
Rabbit	800
Rat	850
Bacteria	20,000–50,000
Virus	50,000–1,000,000

It is interesting to note that in man the LD_{50} is about 360 R when administered to the whole body, although much larger exposures may be given deliberately to localized areas in radio-therapy. As is well known, small doses of X rays have been applied to the whole body in the treatment of chronic leukemia and generalized lymphoma. It is estimated that in man a whole body exposure of 200 R will give a lethal probability of 1 to 3 percent, and an exposure of 600 R, 95 percent, within 60 days. Obviously, whole body exposures in lethal quantities would be likely to result only from accidental exposure in atomic energy plants, or in atomic warfare.

The sum total of the radiobiologic effects in the individual following whole body exposure to a lethal or near-lethal dose of ionizing radiation is called the *acute radiation syndrome.* This comprises a definite chain of events, the severity of which depends on the nature of the ionizing radiation, and more specifically, on the relative biologically effective dose (rems). Furthermore, the sequence of events is remarkably similar in various animals.

As the *whole body* dose to a reasonably homogeneous population is increased, the following symptoms appear in increasing numbers: nausea, vomiting, depilation, anorexia, malaise, pharyngitis, petechiae, diarrhea, weight loss, and death.

The three main pathologic processes resulting from *heavy* total body exposure include the following:

1. *Necrosis* or cell death. The most sensitive cells are obviously destroyed first. Chief among these, in descending order of sensitivity, are (a) lymph nodes; (b) blood-forming (hematopoietic) organs; (c) gonads, the testes being more susceptible than the ovaries; (d) gastrointestinal tract epithelium; and (e) skin.

2. *Hemorrhages* distributed widely throughout the body: skin, gastrointestinal tract, respiratory tract, and other internal organs. The reason for the onset of hemorrhage is, above all, the suppression of platelets (thrombocytopenia), interfering with the clotting of blood. A second factor is the damage to capillaries resulting in increased permeability. In addition, especially with large doses, inflammation occurs in and about small blood vessels.

3. *Infection* supervenes due to depletion of the body's defenses: loss of leukocytes, general debility, death of cells, hemorrhage, anemia.

There are at present three (or possibly four) main subsyndromes of the acute radiation syndrome: (1) **hematopoietic or bone marrow,** (2) **gastrointestinal,** and (3) **vascular.** A fourth type has been recognized in animal experiments and is known as the **central nervous system syndrome;** this has not been observed in man except as a manifestation of the vascular syndrome.

Hematopoietic or Bone Marrow Syndrome. When the whole body single exposure range is 200 to 600 R, death occurs mainly in the second to third week after exposure, but may be delayed as long as two months. During the **prodromal period** lasting about two days, the individual experiences nausea with or without vomiting, and indigestion. (If these symptoms appear within one or two hours, the exposure was probably about 1,000 R). A **latent period** follows during which the victim seems to be normal, but there is actually rapid cellular depletion of the bone marrow. Following the latent period the individual becomes severely ill, with ulcerative stomatitis, bloody diarrhea, hemorrhage into tissues, infection, anemia, and fluid and electrolyte imbalance. Circulating blood elements—lymphocytes, platelets, and granulocytes—are depleted. Depilation, weight loss, and depression of oogenesis and spermatogenesis also occur. However, the cause of death in this subsyndrome is basically **hematologic.** It should be noted that there is a sharp increase in mortality in the range of 200 to 800 R. Survivors of less exposure may enter a chronic stage characterized by ulcerating lesions and severe, refractory anemia.

Gastrointestinal Syndrome. With a whole body exposure ranging from about 600 to 1,000 R death in at least 95 percent of individuals occurs on or near the sixth day as the result of **failure of the lining cells of the small intestine,** accompanied by hematopoietic failure. There is rapid depletion of bone marrow causing agranulocytosis within three days. However, the main manifestation of the gastrointestinal syndrome is **denudation and failure of regeneration of the small intestinal epithelium** from the crypts, although abortive attempts at regeneration may occur. Hemal concentration occurs due to the profound anorexia, leakage of fluids into the small bowel, failure to absorb liquids, diarrhea, and electrolyte imbalance. Because bile salts cannot be absorbed in the distal ileum they pass into the colon, irritating it and intensifying the diarrhea. Small bowel denudation also favors ingress of bacteria resulting in *sepsis*. Thus, even though there is damage to the bone marrow and other susceptible organs, death results primarily from the severe damage to the lining of the small intestine.

Vascular Radiation Syndrome. Very large doses of penetrating radiation, about 4,000 R or more to the whole body, cause generalized vascular and perivascular inflammation associated with cardiovascular collapse. In two similar but unrelated accidents (one reported by Shipman and associates,[77] the other by Fanger and Lushbaugh[25]) a male employee was engaged in processing fissionable wastes, plutonium in one instance and uranium 235 in the other. The material was poured into a large tank containing a liquid with which it did not readily mix, and an electric stirring paddle was activated. Immediately, the fissionable material was drawn into the vortex resulting in *supercriticality:* that is, *nuclear excursion*—and a chain reaction. The extremely high intensity γ and neutron radiation delivered a whole body exposure of approximately 4,500 R to one victim, and 8,800 R to the other, with death occurring at 35 and 49 hours, respectively. There were extensive inflammatory vascular damage, interstitial edema, body cavity effusions, myocardial and meningeal vascular injury, and pancreatitis. Although the first of these patients experienced rapid onset of ataxia, mental incapacity, and mania, the authors thought that the central nervous system changes were secondary to vascular injury, no direct evidence of radiation-induced lesions being found in the neural tissues. Although propulsive watery diarrhea and bone marrow depletion also occurred, these did not have an opportunity to contribute significantly to the fatal outcome, death resulting primarily from cardiovascular collapse.

In experimental animals a dose above about 5,000 rads produces severe central nervous system symptoms such as disorientation, disequilibrium, ataxia, and convulsions. In addition, vomiting and diarrhea appear early. Damage is found mainly in certain cerebellar cells. However, there are also severe vascular changes resembling those found in the human cases just described, so that the *central nervous system syndrome* may actually be a manifestation of the vascular radiation syndrome.

A **sublethal dose** (i.e. less than LD_{50}) of approximately 100 to 300 R to the whole body gives rise to a **pancytopenic** form of the acute radiation syndrome from which a majority of individuals will recover. There may or may not be mild initial nausea, vomiting, and malaise, with a very short course of 12 to 24 hours. Initial mild erythema of the skin may also occur; this may fade and then return, going on to blistering and ulceration if the exposure approaches 500 R. About 3 to 5 weeks after exposure, epilation occurs with subsequent restoration of hair. Along with epilation, there may be mild pharyngitis, weakness, and malaise. In addition to leukopenia, progressive anemia supervenes, occasionally resulting in death in 2 to 4 months after exposure. Cataracts occur in a high percentage of survivors in 2 to 6 years. Some victims do not recover fully, but enter the chronic stage, remaining feeble, emaciated, and anemic for months. Statistically, there is an increased incidence of leukemia in the survivors—estimated at 9 times the incidence in the general, unexposed population.

MODIFICATION OF RADIATION INJURY

By far, the bulk of the data on the modification of tissue response to penetrating radiation is based on the experimental induction of the acute radiation syndrome or death in animals. The usual criterion is the $LD_{50/30}$ dose, namely, that whole body dose that causes the death of 50 percent of exposed animals in 30 days. The ratio of $LD_{50/30}$ with the protective agent, to the $LD_{50/30}$ without it, is the **dose reduction factor**. A number of such **modifying factors** have been found to influence the mortality of animals subjected to massive doses of radiation. These factors have been classified by Ellinger[23] as (1) physical, (2) chemical, and (3) physiologic. The relationship of the time of application of the factor to the time of irradiation is important.

1. **Physical Factors.** The most significant of these is the lead shielding of certain organs such as spleen, liver, or hind leg of mice during whole body irradiation. Shielding in this manner reduces the mortality in animals, as compared with unshielded controls. Two explanations for this effect have been proposed:

a. Certain organs, when shielded, in some manner enhance the recovery of blood forming organs.

b. Even a small amount of protected bone marrow aids in the regeneration of blood. This has been proved by a very ingenious experiment. Tails of rats normally contain no red marrow, and if shielded during whole body irradiation, there is no effect on mortality. If red marrow production is first induced in rats' tails, and the tails are then shielded during whole body irradiation, there is a significant drop in mortality.

2. *Chemical Factors.* A great variety of hormones and other chemicals has been found to affect the mortality resulting from whole body exposure; thus, desoxycorticosterone (DOCA), estradiol, epinephrine, and histamine decrease mortality, if given before the exposure. Cortisone increases the mortality, probably because it enhances susceptibility to infection. Of the chemicals, those containing the $-SH$ (sulfhydryl) group are most effective in protecting against radiation damage. Examples of such compounds are glutathione and cysteine. They apparently protect certain oxidation-reduction enzyme systems in the tissues. More recently, the class of amino-alkyl thiols, the simplest being aminoethyl-phosphorothioate (MEAP) has been found to yield the sulfhydryl group on hydrolysis, with less toxicity than glutathione or cysteine. It is possible that they act through the induction of tissue anoxia which is known to decrease radiosensitivity. Antibiotics, especially streptomycin and aureomycin, are valuable in combatting the infection occurring in the acute radiation syndrome. Saline solutions administered intravenously offer protection, probably in a manner similar to DOCA.

3. *Physiologic Factors.* As the result of experiments with parabiotic twins, an indirect effect has been demonstrated, probably humoral in nature, as well as a direct effect on the gastrointestinal tract. Transfusion of whole blood has not proved very successful, but transfusions of homogenates of spleen or *bone marrow* are definitely protective. These do not require the presence of cells. Transplants of certain organs, such as the spleen, into irradiated animals decrease mortality.

There is evidence that bone marrow transfusions may prove

beneficial in humans. In 4 of 5 persons accidentally receiving large exposures to the whole body, Mathé[54] found that injection of homologous bone marrow 30 days after the incident caused partial repopulation of the recipients' marrow. The donor cells gradually disappeared as the recipients' hematopoietic systems recovered.

In summary, then, a number of agents can be called upon to reduce the mortality in total body irradiation, but unfortunately the vast majority must be administered before the exposure. Most of them act either by enhancing bone marrow regeneration, by inducing tissue anoxia, by regulating salt and water balance, or by combatting infection. Unfortunately, the improvement in recovery which they evoke may be just as pronounced in malignant tumors as in normal tissues, so that their use in radiotherapy is contraindicated. However, in time, research along the lines of such modifying agents may evolve more effective treatment of the acute radiation syndrome.

CHAPTER 16

Radiotherapy with Heavy Particles

IN the last few years there has been a resurgence of interest in the use of heavy particles—*high-LET radiation*—in radiation therapy. This is not surprising in view of the general impression among radiotherapists that we have pushed the radiocurability of tumors as far as possible with megavoltage beams, and there still remain a significant number of malignant lesions which are uncontrollable with low-LET radiation.

As we have seen in Chapter 15, X and γ rays liberate primary electrons which cause sparse ionization along their tracks. Typical LET values for this kind of radiation range from about 3 keV/μ for kilovoltage X rays to about 0.35 keV/μ for ^{60}Co γ rays. By way of contrast, the LET for intermediate neutrons ranges from about 8 to 50 keV/μ; the ion clusters being closely spaced, we should anticipate greater damage to cells.

In the next section we shall discuss some of the pertinent radiobiologic characteristics of high-LET radiation as exemplified by fast (really intermediate) neutrons, and include a few discordant notes that have appeared in the literature regarding its efficacy in the control of human neoplasia.

RADIOBIOLOGY OF HIGH-LET RADIATION

1. *Oxygen Effect.* In Chapter 15 (pages 569 to 572) we pointed out that fully oxygenated (oxic) cells are more sensitive to X and γ rays than are hypoxic cells by a factor of nearly 3, at least experimentally. Thus, hypoxia seems to have a protective effect against low-LET radiation. Since most solid tumors contain regions of low oxygen tension, we might suppose that a dose of low-LET radiation capable of destroying oxic cells may fail to eliminate hypoxic cells which may therefore remain clonogenic, that is, go on to reproduce and cause tumor recurrence.

It has been found that high-LET radiation such as *fast neutrons* and *negative pi mesons* (*pions*) show less discrimination than low-

605

LET radiation between oxic and hypoxic cells. Furthermore, the killing ability of high-LET radiation is not greatly enhanced by oxygenation at the time of irradiation.[6,27,38,47] Thus, the *oxygen enhancement ratio (OER)*—defined as the ratio of the dose in the absence of oxygen, to the dose in its presence, to achieve the same effect—of high-LET radiation such as fast neutrons and pions is about 1.5 to 2.0, in contrast to a value of about 2.5 to 3 for X or γ rays, provided that the oxygen is present during the irradiation. Barendsen[3] has shown that the RBE increases from 1 for low-LET radiation (X and γ rays) to a peak value of about 8 for high-LET radiation (heavy ions) beyond 100 keV/μ. At the same time, the OER falls from about 2.6 for low-LET radiation to a value of 1 for high-LET radiation of 100 keV/μ (see Fig. 16.01).

As a result of the oxygen effect, it would be anticipated that the use of heavy particles such as neutrons and pions might augment the probability of local control of various tumors, provided we could have a beam with adequate output and suitable distri-

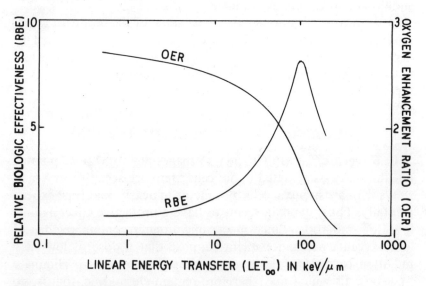

FIGURE 16.01. Relationship of OER (oxygen enhancement ratio) and RBE (relative biologic effectiveness) to the LET (linear energy transfer averaged over the entire track of the ionizing particle). Note that with low-LET radiation, which has a low RBE, the presence of oxygen greatly enhances radiosensitivity. The OER is much less for high-LET (high RBE) radiation. (After Barendsen.[3])

bution in the tumor. However, Withers[90] has challenged the dogmatic concept that hypoxia is a limiting factor in the radio-curability of all human tumors, especially when they are treated by a fractionated dosage schedule. For example, many human tumors are cured locally by low doses of fractionated X or γ rays, equivalent to a single dose of 1800 to 2000 rads. This raises a serious question as to the percentage of hypoxic cells in most human tumors; on the other hand, if there is a significant fraction of hypoxic cells, their influence on tumor control might be less than would be anticipated from studies on cell cultures.

Favorable response under these conditions may depend on two factors: (1) reoxygenation of surviving hypoxic cells between dose fractions, possibly due to decreased competition for available oxygen as the oxic cells are killed, and (2) death of hypoxic cells between fractions. In fact, even if 10 percent of cells are hypoxic, a mammalian cell cultures displays no appreciable difference in response to low- and high-LET radiation at the usual therapeutic dose level of about 200 rads. According to Withers,[90] if dose fractionation is so designed as to keep at least 90 percent of the surviving cells oxygenated, response to subsequent doses of 200 rads should be unaffected by the hypoxic cells. Perhaps, at least in theory, most small human tumors respond in this manner.

In the case of bulky tumors, the hypoxic component may be large enough to lessen curability with low-LET radiation, all the more so if invasion of avascular tissue such as cartilage, fat, or myxomatous connective tissue has occurred. Under such conditions, irradiation with high-LET radiation should produce a significant therapeutic gain over low-LET radiation.

2. *Mitotic Phase.* The position of the tumor cells in the mitotic cycle may also play a role in their response to high-LET radiation. A number of workers have found that the radiosensitivity of cells to X or γ rays varies with their position in the reproductive cycle, as noted on page 562. In contrast, such cyclic variation in radio-sensitivity is less pronounced with high-LET radiation such as neutrons. Obviously, a tumor containing a larger fraction of resistant cells than the associated normal tissue would succumb more readily to injury by neutrons than by X rays. In other words, the RBE (relative biologic effectiveness) for the tumor would ex-

ceed that for the normal cells. On the other hand, if the normal tissue contained a higher percentage of cells in a resistant stage of the cycle, conditions would be reversed, the RBE being greater for the normal tissue; now therapy with neutrons would be detrimental, as compared with X or γ rays. Withers has suggested that these cyclic variations in radiation response may be more significant than the variation in the state of oxygenation in radiotherapy.

3. *Survival Curves.* It has been found that the survival curves of mammalian cell cultures exposed to neutrons are steeper than those for X rays, but the RBE depends on the dose.[38] For example, the RBE for neutrons may range from about 25 for a dose of 5 rads, to about 1.5 for 800 rads, with a value of 3 for a typical therapy dose of 200 rads (see Fig. 16.02). Furthermore, as shown in Figure 16.03 as the number of fractions in a particular overall treatment time is increased in the case of low-LET radiation the survival curve becomes less steep on account of the reappearance of the shoulder between fractions.[11] Recall that this represents

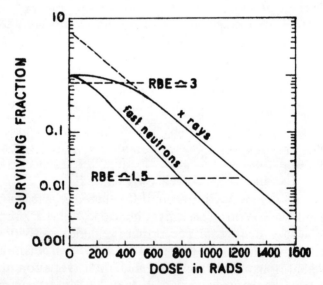

FIGURE 16.02. Comparison of survival curves of cultured mammalian cells irradiated with X rays and with neutrons. Inasmuch as neutrons cause much denser ionization (high LET), they produce a survival curve having a steeper slope. Furthermore, the RBE of neutrons decreases with increasing dose because of the "waste" of neutrons at high dosage. (Courtesy of E. J. Hall[38] and *Radiology.*)

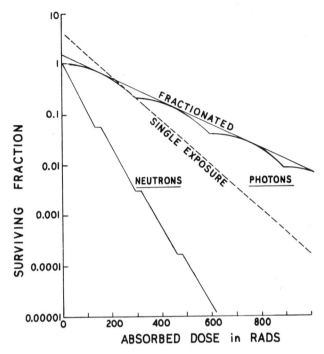

FIGURE 16.03. Comparison of the effect of fractionated irradiation of mammalian cells by photons and neutrons on the corresponding survival curves. Note how fractionation reduces the slope of the curve in the case of photon radiation, indicating diminished radiosensitivity. By way of contrast, the steepness of the survival curve with neutrons is independent of fractionation because of the absence of Elkind or fast recovery. (From L. Cohen, "Radiation Response and Recovery," in E. E. Schwartz, ed., *The Biological Basis of Radiation Therapy* [Philadelphia, J. B. Lippincott Company, 1966], pp. 266–267.)

Elkind or fast recovery (intracellular) between fractions. On the other hand, with neutron therapy, the recoil of nuclei, principally protons, causes dense ionization tracks which so severely injure cells that they cannot recover. In other words, there is virtually no sublethal injury from high-LET radiation. Therefore the survival curve with neutrons has almost no shoulder and remains exponential throughout. Since the survival curve for low-LET radiation becomes less steep as the number of fractions is increased (the size of each fraction decreased correspondingly), and that for neutrons remains essentially unchanged, it is obvious that the resulting RBE of neutrons increases with a larger number of fractions, and with smaller doses. Because of this phenomenon, experience with X- and γ-ray therapy cannot be transferred directly to therapy with high-LET radiation. In fact, this probably accounts in large part for the disastrous results in many patients treated with neutrons in the early days.[76] In any event, unless it can be shown that the steepness of the survival curve for neutron therapy is greater for neoplastic tissue than for the normal relevant tissues, we should not expect a therapeutic gain from the use of neutrons.

NEUTRON BEAM THERAPY

A number of years ago neutron beam therapy was abandoned because of intolerable reactions in normal tissues resulting from failure to recognize the large exit dose, and from inability of normal tissues to recover between fractions as with photon radiation.[76] With renewed interest in neutron therapy and the availability of equipment for the production of suitable neutron beams, various treatment plans are now being tried, taking into account the inherent differences between low- and high-LET radiation with regard to radiobiologic effects. The fast neutrons under investigation have energies ranging from about 6 to 50 MeV; these are really intermediate in energy. Slow neutrons do not have adequate penetrating ability, whereas very fast neutrons have low LET. Treatment distances range from about 50 to 125 cm, the former providing a depth dose distribution similar to ^{137}Cs, and the latter more nearly that of ^{60}Co. Skin reactions with 1440 rads given in fractions three times weekly over a period of 25 days resemble those with about 4100 rads of kilovoltage X rays.[10] Skin sparing is of about the same degree as with ^{60}Co γ rays.

Because of the high probability of interaction with protons, that is, with hydrogen nuclei, there is relatively more absorption in fat than in muscle; therefore the possibility of fat necrosis must not be overlooked, especially in areas where there is a large amount of subcutaneous fat. On the other hand, bone contains significantly less hydrogen than muscle and hence absorbs neutrons to a smaller degree, so fast neutrons are bone sparing.

Equipment is still far from ideal. One type uses the ***deuterium-tritium reaction***[20,29] in which deuterium ions are fired at a tritium target in a sealed tube with production of 14-MeV neutrons. Depth doses with beams of this energy are slightly better than those with ^{60}Co γ rays. However, tube life and radiation output are limited. A typical output is 6 rads/min at a treatment distance of 75 cm, requiring a treatment time of 10 to 20 min.[29] Figure 16.04 shows isodose distributions with 14-MeV neutrons.[57]

Another important type of neutron generator utilizes deuterons accelerated in a cyclotron. At present the M. D. Anderson Hospital and Tumor Institute is using the variable energy cyclotron at Texas A & M University. This provides a high neutron output, long target life, and large depth dose, but lacks the flexibility of more conventional γ-ray beams. A neutron beam generated by 50-MeV deuterons is being used in the treatment of deeply situated tumors, but a 16-MeV beam is available for selected superficial lesions. Thus far, the most responsive cancers have been those of the head and neck, and breast.

Collimation must be carefully designed. It utilizes a steel shield for absorption of fast neutrons, surrounded by a boron shield that is usually incorporated in plastic to absorb slow neutrons.

It is still too early to predict the position of fast neutron therapy

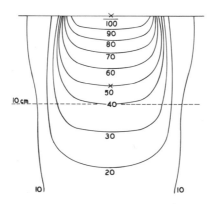

FIGURE 16.04. Isodose distribution for a 10×10 cm^2 14-MeV neutron beam at SSD 75 cm. (Courtesy of W. J. Meredith, and J. B. Massey, *Fundamental Physics of Radiology* [Baltimore, Williams and Wilkins, 1972].)

in the future. However, careful investigation may reveal its potentiality in the control of certain lesions that are now resistant to megavoltage photon radiation.

NEGATIVE PI MESON (PION) THERAPY

Another completely different kind of high-LET radiation is under investigation,[6,27,47] namely, that produced by interactions of *negative pions* (π^-) at the end of their range in tissues. Bombardment of matter with high energy protons in a cyclotron, or extremely high energy electrons in a linac, yields, among other nuclear particles, a sufficient number of π^- pions for radiotherapy, at least on an experimental basis.

Negative pions are unstable singly-charged particles having a mass 273 times that of a resting electron, and 15 percent that of a proton. A π^- decays in a vacuum in 2.6×10^{-6} sec, producing a muon and a neutrino. However, in matter it dissipates its kinetic energy in ionizing atoms much like an electron of similar energy. But the π^-, as it slows down at the end of its range, has the unique property of entering an atomic orbit to form a pi-mesic atom. This process occurs especially in oxygen and carbon, and to a much smaller degree in nitrogen. In about 10^{-13} sec the π^- falls to a lower atomic energy level and is captured by the nucleus which disintegrates with a burst of energy called *star formation.* Extremely high-LET radiation is released, consisting mainly of α particles, protons, neutrons, and nuclear fragments. On the average, each star yields one α particle, one proton, and 2 to 3 neutrons. In the capture of a π^- by an oxygen atom, about 140 MeV of energy is released, of which 96 MeV is carried by the heavy particles, and the remainder as de-excitation γ rays and nuclear binding energy.

Typical of the energy distribution by the π^- beam is a plateau followed by a peak as shown in Figure 16.05. Peculiar to this peak is the fact that it consists of (1) a primary *Bragg peak* representing the augmented ionization due to the slowing of the pions (just as with other ionizing particles), on which is superimposed (2) a still higher ionization peak due to star formation.

While the plateau portion comprises low-LET π^- pions (be-

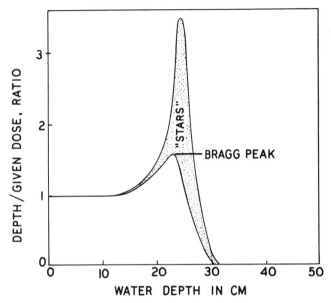

FIGURE 16.05. Ratio of depth dose to given dose for a negative pion beam. Note the lower Bragg peak due to increased ionization as the pions slow down, and the higher peak due to star formation. It is obviously desirable to have this peak region encompassing the tumor volume. (Courtesy of V. P. Bond[6] and *The American Journal of Roentgenology*.)

having much like fast electrons), the star region contains high-LET heavy particles (α particles, protons, neutrons). Because of this, the absorbed dose in the peak region is about 3 to 4 times greater than the entrance dose (plateau region), and the dose equivalent in the peak region exceeds that in the plateau by a factor of about 10. Obviously, it would be desirable for the plateau to fall in the normal tissues outside the tumor, and the peak entirely within the tumor.

Typical values of the high-LET radiation are as follows:[6]

1. **RBE** (relative biologic effectiveness) ranges from 2 for a single large exposure, to 4 or more for fractionated exposures.

2. **OER** (oxygen enhancement ratio) ranges from about 1.35 to 1.8.* As we found earlier in this chapter, high-LET radiation

* Data of Raju and Richman, quoted in H. S. Kaplan, et. al., "A Hospital-based Superconducting Accelerator Facility for Negative Pi-Meson Beam Radiotherapy," *Radiology*, Vol. 108 (1973), p. 159.

is more effective than megavoltage photon radiation in engendering cell damage (high RBE) and, at the same time, is more effective in killing anoxic cells (low OER). Furthermore, cells that have been injured sublethally by high LET radiation show virtually no recovery. But it should be pointed out that the OER of the particles in the pion star is no better than that of neutrons, and may even be inferior.

Clinical, as well as experimental, studies show that fractionated dosage schedules with low-LET radiation allow recovery between fractions, but such recovery does not occur to any significant degree with high-LET radiation (see pages 561 and 609). Thus, fractionation with a π^- beam should permit recovery in the plateau region (normal tissues), while preventing recovery in the star region (tumor), provided the geometric configuration of the beam can be suitably designed.

The π^- beam has a number of interesting features. It can be sharply collimated by the use of electromagnets. Although skin sparing is less than with megavoltage photons, the skin dose is about one fourth the tumor dose at a 10 cm depth. There is no exit dose. Because of the possibility, at least theoretically, of tailoring the beam so as to provide maximum energy release within the tumor itself, a large dose can be delivered into the tumor while sparing the surrounding normal tissues; hence, a **high therapeutic ratio**. Isodose curves from a π^- beam are shown in Figure 16.06.

Despite the theoretical advantages of π^- beam therapy, the high cost of production and the narrow dose peak with present equipment makes it unlikely that it will become widely used in the near future. However, an elaborate hospital-based facility is being planned for the Stanford University Medical Center,[47] but this is an extremely costly project. It is a 500-MV superconducting linac in which electrons will strike a titanium or titanium carbide target. Electron contamination of the beam amounts to about 10 percent. Imaging of the star region can be achieved by using one or more of the secondary radiations produced at various stages of π^- capture in the tissues. These include characteristic X rays emitted by pi-mesic atoms, and γ rays emitted during subsequent de-excitation. A method must be found to delineate precisely the

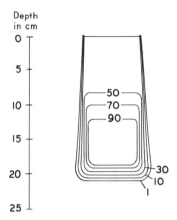

FIGURE 16.06. Isodose curves for pure negative pions stopped in tissue, beam having been shaped by a trapezoidal collimator. (After A. Thiessen.[82])

tumor volume so that the star region may be tailored to encompass it. Finally, an adequate computer system must be designed to control the foregoing parameters as well as the radiotherapy process itself, including beam intensity and patient position. All in all, this is a formidable undertaking whose progress should be watched with interest by all those concerned with radiation therapy.

CHAPTER 17

Protection in Radiotherapy:
Health Physics

RADIOTHERAPY has proved to be a great boon to mankind in the control of certain diseases, a number of which are amenable to no other form of treatment. However, in common with other therapeutic agents, radiation produces a number of undesirable side effects. These are unique in the case of radiation in that they are not limited to the patient alone, but may also jeopardize the attending personnel. Such undesirable exposure of personnel may arise from X rays, radium, artificial radionuclides, or other sources of ionizing radiation. Incidentally, this hazard may also involve individuals other than personnel who happen to be in the radiation field.

Health physics deals with the protection of individuals from unnecessary exposure to ionizing radiation, whether it involves the patient, the radiotherapy personnel, or the general public. In this chapter we shall survey the field of health physics as it pertains to irradiation therapy.

BACKGROUND RADIATION

Before discussing the exposure of individuals to radiotherapeutic devices or agents, we must call attention to the fact that man is continuously being exposed to ionizing radiation arising in the natural environment. This is called **natural background radiation** and includes not only external sources but also radioactive material in the body.

What are the sources of natural background radiation? These may be classified as *external* and *internal.*

1. *External sources* include, first, *cosmic rays* which are of two kinds, primary and secondary. *Primary cosmic rays* originate in outer space and consist mainly of high energy protons (energy exceeding 2.5 billion electron volts), but also include α particles,

atomic nuclei, and high energy electrons and photons. When these interact with the earth's atmosphere they produce *secondary cosmic* rays which consist mainly of mesons, electrons, and γ rays. (Mesons are subatomic particles having masses several hundred times that of the resting electron, positive or negative charge, and extremely short average lives of the order of 10^{-6} sec or less.) Most cosmic rays detected at the earth's surface are of the secondary type; they are so penetrating that they can pass through lead (Pb) several meters thick.

A second source of background radiation is the naturally radioactive minerals in the earth itself. These occur in various amounts everywhere, but in large concentration in deposits of uranium, thorium, and actinium. Because of the wide distribution of such radioactive minerals, they are present in at least minute amounts in building materials. It is of interest that terrestrial background radiation varies widely from place; thus, in Kerala, India, it is about ten times greater than the average in the United States.

2. *Internal sources* include naturally radioactive nuclides incorporated in the body tissues and in the materials of which the radiation detector itself is constructed. The main radionuclides comprising the internal sources are potassium 40 and carbon 14.

To natural background radiation must be added *artificial background radiation* from the following sources: medical and dental X rays, occupation (for example, X-ray, radium, and radionuclide technology), environs of atomic energy plants, and atomic bomb fallout. Whereas natural background radiation is unavoidable, man can exercise at least some measure of control over artificial background radiation.

Table 17.01 summarizes the average background exposure of the general population of the United States on an annual basis, and also includes the accumulated dose per individual from conception to age 30 years. This age span is selected because about 80 percent of children have been born by the time the parents have reached age 30. Obviously we are concerned here with the genetic effects rather than with any possible damage to the individual, although this may not be negligible. Because the tabulated values are approximate they should not be applied with any semblance of precision to the individual.

TABLE 17.01
AVERAGE RADIATION EXPOSURE PER PERSON DUE TO NATURAL
AND ARTIFICIAL BACKGROUND*
(NOT TO BE APPLIED CRITICALLY TO THE INDIVIDUAL)

| | Whole Body Dose | |
Source	rems/year/person (based on entire population)	rems conception to age 30 (in procreative segment of population only)
Natural—total	0.1	3.0
Cosmic	0.03	0.9
Earth and Housing	0.05	1.5
Internal	0.025	0.75
Artificial—total	0.17–0.33	1.5–4.8
Medical and Dental	0.15–0.3	1.0–4.0
Occupational	0.005	0.15
Plant Environs	0.005	0.15
Fallout	0.01–0.015	0.3–0.45
TOTAL—all sources	0.3–0.4	4.5–7.8

* Data from American College of Radiology.

MAXIMUM PERMISSIBLE DOSE EQUIVALENT

The original "tolerance" dose to the whole body of an occupationally exposed person was based strictly on *empirical* data accumulated in large radiation therapy centers. As more experience was gained, and as protective measures improved, the tolerance dose was gradually decreased. Furthermore, the term "tolerance" was abandoned and replaced by the term *maximum permissible dose equivalent (MPD),* because there is no certainty that doses of even this small order of magnitude are entirely harmless. For example, experimental evidence indicates that there is no threshold dose for the induction of gene mutations or the inception of leukemia. On the other hand, we can never completely escape exposure to ionizing radiation because there is no method of avoiding background radiation. In other words, the problem of protection in radiology involves the radiation exposure incurred by personnel over and above background.

The *permissible* or *acceptable dose* for an individual is that dose, accumulated over a long period of time or received in a single exposure, which carries a negligible risk of significant somatic or genetic damage in the light of present knowledge. The International Commission on Radiation Protection (ICRP) has specified a maximum permissible dose on the basis of a balance of the risks versus the benefits of radiation exposure.

In 1971 the National Council on Radiation Protection and Measurements (NCRP), in *Report No. 39*, while acknowledging the need to keep radiation exposure to the lowest possible level, made a number of dose-limiting recommendations. These may be summarized as follows:

1. *Accumulated Dose* (Radiation Workers):

a. *External exposure to critical organs:* The *maximum permissible dose equivalent (MPD) for radiation workers* is *based on* the cumulative dose over the *entire lifetime* of the individual. Thus, the *occupational MPD to the whole body and to certain radiosensitive organs*—gonads, hematopoietic organs, lens of eye, head, and trunk—*from all sources, shall not exceed*

$$\text{cumulative MPD} = 5(N - 18) \text{ rems} \qquad (1)$$

where N is the age in years and is greater than 18. The dose in any 13-week period shall not exceed 3 rems. This recommendation applies to any radiation that is sufficiently penetrating to affect a significant fraction of the critical tissues.

b. *External exposure to other organs:*

Skin (unlimited area, except lens of eye): for electrons and low energy photons, 15 rems in any one year.

Hands: 75 rems in any one year, but not more than 25 rems in any one quarter. If possible, try to keep at level recommended for skin.

Forearms: 30 rems in any one year, but not more than 10 rems in any one quarter. If possible, try to keep at level recommended for skin.

Other organs (except those under 1a): 15 rems in any one year.

Fertile women: 0.5 rems *during entire gestation period*

c. *Internal Exposure:*

Permissible levels shall be consistent with the age-proration scheme described in 1a, by limiting the body burden (concentration) of radionuclides. The maximum permissible concentration of radionuclides specifies an annual dose of 15 rems for most individuals organs including the thyroid or skin, and 5 rems for the gonads. Figure 17.01 shows the occupational MPD for the whole body and for various critical organs.

2. ***Emergency Exposure*** (Radiation Workers):

An accidental dose of 25 rems to the whole body once in a lifetime need not be included in the radiation exposure status of the individual.

3. ***Medical Exposure*** (Radiation Workers):

Radiation exposures required for medical or dental procedures are not included in the radiation exposure status of the person concerned.

4. ***Exposure of Persons Outside Controlled Areas:***

When normal operations are in progress in a controlled area (one under radiologic supervision) persons outside the controlled

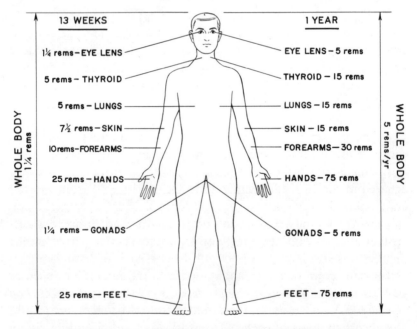

FIGURE 17.01. Maximum permissible dose equivalent (MPD) to various organs and the whole body of radiation workers, for 13 weeks (left column) and for 1 year (right column).

area shall receive no more than *0.5 rem* in any one year. This smaller MPD is to minimize the genetic dose to the general population. The maximum permissible body burden shall not exceed that for radiation workers.

Certain interesting features of the rules proposed by the NCRP will now be pointed out:

1. Summation of exposure over a lifetime beginning with age 18 permits a smaller total MPD up to age 40 than from age 40 onward. It is assumed that a very small fraction of the lifetime exposure (occupational) would be incurred before the age of 18 years. Thus, up to age 40, the MPD is $5(40 - 18) = 110$ rems as compared with an accumulated MPD in the next 40 years of $5 \times 40 = 200$ rems. Since the total MPD for an 80-year lifetime is $5(80 - 18) = 310$ rems, the fraction allowed during the first 40 years would be about $\frac{1}{3}$ of the total, and during the second 40 years about $\frac{2}{3}$ of the total.

2. The emphasis on a lower accumulated MPD during the first 40 years implies recognition of the danger of genetic injury and possible delayed carcinogenic effects from chronic exposure of the whole body to small amounts of ionizing radiation.

3. The rules recognize the increased sensitivity of certain critical organs.

4. Consideration is given to persons outside controlled areas.

Monitor film badges should be worn for *at least 4 weeks* to enhance the accuracy of the dosage reading.

At this point we should explain the meaning of the unit *rem* designated in the MPD formula. With X-, γ-, or β-radiation the rad may be used as the unit of dosage because equal absorbed doses of these three types of radiation produce virtually the same effects in tissues. However, to engender a particular effect in tissues, a smaller dose (rads) is required with heavy particles such as α particles, deuterons, or neutrons than with X or γ rays. Thus, *one rad of α particles or fast neutrons produces a greater tissue effect than one rad of X or γ rays*, and it would therefore be incorrect to add the absorbed doses of such different kinds of radiation in arriving at the total MPD. In order to be able to express on a common scale, for *protection purposes only*, the irradiation incurred by exposed persons for all types of radiation, the quantity **dose equivalent (DE)** has been introduced by the ICRU. By definition, the *DE* is the product of the absorbed dose and appropriate modifying factors which depend on the particular radiation hazard involved. In this regard the **quality factor (QF)** suffices for our purpose. Thus,

$$\text{dose equivalent} = \text{absorbed dose} \times \text{quality factor} \qquad (2)$$
$$DE = \text{absorbed dose} \times QF$$
$$rems = \qquad\qquad rads \times QF$$

The unit of *DE* is the **rem,** and the value of *QF* varies with the type of radiation. For kilovoltage and megavoltage photons, and for β particles, *QF* has been arbitrarily assigned the value 1. Therefore,

$$DE = \text{absorbed dose} \times 1$$
$$= 1 \text{ rad} \times 1 = 1 \text{ rem}$$

or, 1 rad = 1 rem *for X, beta, and gamma rays*

(The **millirem,** abbreviated mrem, is 0.001 rem.)

On the other hand, the *QF* for the cataractogenic effect of fast neutrons is 10 (e.g. 1 rad of fast neutrons is 10 times as effective as 1 rad of X rays in producing cataract); hence,

$$DE = \text{absorbed dose} \times 10$$
$$= 1 \text{ rad} \times 10 = 10 \text{ rems}$$
or, 1 rad = 10 rems *for fast neutrons*

This means that with fast neutrons, 1 rad gives a *DE* of 10 rems insofar as cataract induction is concerned. The *QF* for α particles is 20, so that 1 rad of this radiation gives a *DE* of 20 rems. It must be emphasized that the rems of different kinds of radiation, insofar as a particular biologic effect is concerned, are equivalent (*DE*) and can be added. For example, if an individual were exposed to a mixture of radiations and received 1 rad from X rays, 1 rad from fast neutrons, and 1 rad from α particles, the total absorbed dose would be 3 rads. However, this would seriously underestimate the radiation hazard. By converting these doses to **dose equivalents**, we would obtain:

X rays	$1 \text{ rad} \times 1 = 1$ rem
fast neutrons	$1 \text{ rad} \times 10 = 10$ rems
α particles	$1 \text{ rad} \times 20 = 20$ rems

31 rems *total DE*

Thus, the dose equivalent in rems provides a more realistic measure of the radiation hazard when the quality factor is different from 1. However, in the average hospital Radiology Department exposure is usually limited to radiation with a quality factor of 1 so that the MPD under these conditions may be stated in rads, or even in R.

MEASUREMENT OF WHOLE BODY EXPOSURE

Before discussing the various methods of reducing the exposure of personnel to ionizing radiation in the therapy department, we shall describe the procedures used in measuring the whole body exposure level. These are included under the general heading of **radiation surveying** and **monitoring.** A protection survey to evaluate radiation hazards includes first a physical survey of the arrangement and use of equipment, and second, the measurement of exposure rates under anticipated conditions of use.

Two types of surveying and monitoring for radiation levels are ordinarily available: (1) monitoring of personnel and (2) surveying of various areas to determine the existence of hazardous conditions.

Personnel Monitoring. The most widely used method of ascertaining individual whole body exposure to radiation is the **film badge** service provided commercially by a number of laboratories. A typical film badge consists of a dental film covered by a thin copper stepped-wedge filter to permit the detection of radiation of various qualities. The film is backed by lead foil to absorb back-scattered radiation. The film badge is worn on the clothing in a position subjected to the prevailing radiation, initially for a period of one week. The commercial laboratory furnishes a fresh supply each week, to be used the following week and returned to the laboratory. There the films are processed and compared densitometrically with standard films exposed to known quantities of radiation. In this manner, the dose received by the wearer's film badge is obtained and is reported to the radiology department where it must be filed permanently. With dosage levels well below the weekly MPD (0.1 rad) the film badge may be worn and returned *monthly*, especially if the type and volume of radiologic procedures remain reasonably constant. The one-month period is preferable because of greater convenience and more precise calibration.

For workers in the vicinity of nuclear reactors, the *neutron badge* containing a special type of film is used to evaluate personnel exposure to neutrons. The dosage with the neutron badge is not recorded in rads or rems, but rather in terms of the number of proton recoil tracks per unit area as determined under a microscope.

Another procedure in personnel monitoring utilizes the *self-reading pocket dosimeter,* which resembles a fountain pen externally, but consists of: (1) an ionization chamber, and (2) a built-in electrometer for reading the radiation dosage (see Fig. 17.02). This device operates on the same principle as a Victoreen R-meter. Some dosimeters have a built-in charger, but others require an auxiliary charger. The dosimeter records the number of milliroentgens, usually up to a full scale reading of 200 mR received in a given period of time. For example, in conducting an experiment with radioactive material, we can determine when the maximum permissible exposure is being approached, and either discon-

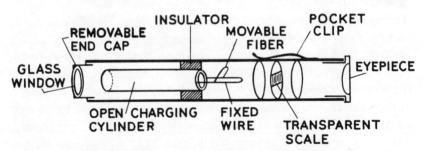

FIGURE 17.02. Diagram of a self-reading pocket dosimeter.

tinue the experiment or increase the shielding. In routine monitoring, the dosimeter should be worn for a specified period of time; the observer then reads the accumulated exposure by looking through the end of the dosimeter at a source of light. Pocket dosimeters are also available with full scale ranges of 5 or 10 R for civil defense and emergency purposes.

Pocket chambers, another variety of dosimeters, also resemble a fountain pen but consist of an ionization chamber only. They require an auxiliary charging and reading device, much the same as a Victoreen R-meter. It should be mentioned that pocket dosimeters and chambers are neither so convenient nor so suitable as film badges for continuous personnel monitoring. Furthermore, they do not provide a permanent record, as does the commercial film badge laboratory. Therefore, whenever pocket chambers or dosimeters are used, a film badge should also be worn.

A new kind of personnel monitor, still in the developmental stages, is the ***thermoluminescent dosimeter*** (TLD). This depends on the unique ability of certain crystalline materials to store energy on exposure to radiation, because of the trapping of valence electrons in crystal lattice defects. Upon being heated under strictly controlled conditions, the electrons return to their normal state, releasing the stored energy in the form of light. Measurement of the light by a photomultiplier device gives a measure of the initial radiation exposure, since the two are very nearly proportional. The dosimeters can be returned to a commercial laboratory for readout if desired. Lithium fluoride (LiF) seems at present to be the most suitable material for TLD. There are many advantages of TLD over film badge monitoring: (1) low cost and small size of detector—for example, 1 mm × 6 mm—which can be sealed in Teflon to avoid mechanical damage; (2) direct reading possible at any time; (3) response to radiation proportional up to about 1000 R; (4) response almost independent of radiation energy (film badge is not); (5) response very similar to that of human tissues; (6) wide exposure range detectable—10 mR to 100,000 R; (7) accuracy about ±5 percent (film badge varies from ±10 to 50 percent); (8) can be incorporated in jewelry to make it unobtrusive. For these reasons, it is very likely that TLD will eventually become the method of choice in personnel monitoring.

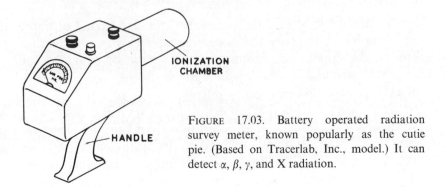

IONIZATION
CHAMBER

HANDLE

FIGURE 17.03. Battery operated radiation survey meter, known popularly as the cutie pie. (Based on Tracerlab, Inc., model.) It can detect α, β, γ, and X radiation.

Laboratory Survey. When radionuclides, natural or artificial, are used in the Radiology Department, special instruments must be available to determine the presence of hazardous conditions. This holds especially for radionuclides which may be accidentally spilled or may otherwise contaminate glassware and other laboratory apparatus. A very useful radiation survey meter, known popularly as the ***cutie pie***. appears in Figure 17.03. It is a battery operated ionization-type instrument, light in weight and suitable for surveying the safety of protective barriers and determining the radiation hazard of various experimental radionuclide procedures. It may also be used to survey a patient's abdomen or chest following the injection of radiogold for effusions, to ascertain the uniformity of distribution and the dosage levels at various distances from the patient. The exposure rate of γ rays from 7 keV to 2 MeV can be measured with this device. There are 4 full scale ranges (25; 250; 2,500; and 25,000 R/hr) with a precision of about ± 10 percent of the full scale reading. It must be emphasized that this survey meter, though adequate for protection problems, should not be used in the calibration of therapy equipment. In ordinary use, for detection of X or γ rays, a bakelite shield is placed over the window at the end of the chamber. Removal of this shield admits low energy β particles (above 70 keV) into the chamber so that they can be measured.

A simple ***rate meter*** provided with a G-M counter and an audio circuit to permit hearing the counts, can be used as a laboratory monitor both to explore areas suspected of contamination, and to provide steady monitoring of the background level. It also detects contamination of the hands, clothing, glassware, or apparatus. The meter of this type of instrument indicates the counts per minute. Because of the audible "clicking," any increase in count rate becomes obvious to the personnel occupying the area.

A battery operated ***portable rate meter*** is useful in conducting radiation surveys both in the laboratory and in the field (see Fig. 17.04). Its application resembles that of the laboratory rate meter just described. The portable meter detects both β and γ radiation and, when provided with a special G-M counter, to α particles as well. It is calibrated in counts per minute (up to 50,000), and in mR per hour in three ranges of 0.25, 2.5, and 25; or 1, 10, and 100. Headphones are available for audible detection.

Careful monitoring virtually obviates the likelihood of incurring radiation injury. When, under ***unusual*** circumstances, there is evidence of damage to the blood-forming organs, corrective steps should be taken immediately. First, the affected individual should be removed until he has recovered completely. Second, a radiation physicist should survey the Radiology Department and recommend the best means of eliminating the hazardous condi-

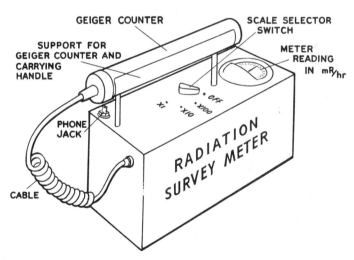

FIGURE 17.04. Portable rate meter with G-M counter, battery operated, used as a radiation survey meter. A phone jack is included for audible detection. (Based on Nuclear-Chicago model.)

tions. However, it must be emphasized here that safety rules must be continually obeyed by all personnel, and enforced by the Radiation Safety Officer.

X- AND GAMMA-RAY PROTECTION UP TO 10 MeV

The subject of protection is covered in great detail in the National Council on Radiation Protection and Measurements (NCRP) *Report No. 33*. When specific problems arise, this publication should be referred to, preferably in consultation with a radiation physicist. We shall limit our discussion to basic principles.

First we shall define the origin of radiation with which we are concerned:

1. *Useful beam* is the radiation passing through the aperture, cone, or collimator of the source housing.
2. *Leakage radiation* includes all radiation coming from within the source housing, other than the useful beam.
3. *Scattered radiation* is radiation that has undergone a change of direction during passage through matter. It may also have decreased in energy. (Strictly speaking, *secondary radiation* is radiation that is emitted by irradiated matter.)
4. *Stray radiation* is the sum of leakage and scattered radiation.

It is obvious that exposure to any of the foregoing sources of radiation may be hazardous to personnel so the total exposure should not exceed the MPD of 0.1 R per week. (In radiotherapy with photons we ordinarily use R instead of rads in protection computations because they are nearly equal numerically.) No one besides the patient should remain in the therapy room while treatment is in progress.

Radiation Sources. All *X-ray tubes* must be of rayproof type; that is, the manufacturer must enclose the tubes in a metal housing that reduces leakage radiation to a prescribed safe level. The specifications for such protective enclosures are given in *NCRP Report No. 33*. With **orthovoltage X-ray therapy tubes** (150 to 500 kV), the exposure rate from leakage radiation shall not exceed 1 R/hr at 1 meter. ("Shall" denotes a *necessary* condition, whereas "should" indicates an *advisable* condition, to meet currently acceptable protection standards.) In addition to protective housing, specifications are prescribed in the same report governing collimation, exposure timers, filter systems, shielding of the patient, and other factors.

Radioactive *sources* used in *teletherapy*—cobalt 60 and cesium 137—shall be doubly sealed in stainless steel and tested for leakage by the manufacturer who shall provide a certificate attesting to the absence of leakage. In addition, leakage tests shall be conducted every six months by the user (this also includes semiannual leakage tests for sealed radium sources such as needles and tubes, and for strontium 90 eye applicators). A leakage test for radioactive sources is performed by carefully wiping the collimator leaves and the edges of the final collimator aperture with a long-handled cotton applicator moistened with dilute detergent solution. The swab can either be sent in a special container to a commercial laboratory or it can be tested by the method of Rose—the cotton is held near the unshielded window of a G-M survey meter (30 mg/cm^2 window). Any increase over background counting rate with earphones indicates a minimum leak of 10^{-9} Ci. A leak only ten times as great (i.e. 10^{-8} Ci) will give thousands of counts per min and kick the indicator needle off the scale. When this occurs, the equipment shall be promptly checked by a radiation physicist or other qualified person. Radium needles and tubes as well as strontium 90 applicators can be tested in this way. In addition, radium needles and tubes should be placed in a stoppered test tube together with activated charcoal for 24 hours, and then the charcoal is tested as above. Leaking needles shall be sent promptly in a suitable container to the supplier for repair.

Wall Protective Barriers. Personnel outside the therapy room must be protected from radiation that might pass through the walls. Protection must also be afforded the general public. This requires the use of built-in protective barriers that reduce transmitted radiation to the appropriate MPD. These barriers are defined as follows:

1. *Primary protective barrier* is one that is sufficient in atomic number and thickness to attenuate the *useful beam* to the required degree.

2. **Secondary protective barrier** is one that is sufficient in atomic number and thickness to attenuate **stray radiation** to the required degree.

The significance of these two types of barriers becomes apparent when it is realized that only those areas of the therapy room wall which may be struck by the useful beam require a primary protective barrier. Other areas of the wall need only a secondary protective barrier.

Wall protection should be planned in advance by a radiation physicist qualified in this field, to avoid expensive alteration after the building has been completed. On the other hand, poor planning may result in excessive wall protection which becomes unnecessarily expensive. An important basic principle in permanent barriers is that joints and holes must be occluded by the same or equivalent protective barrier as the wall. Proper wall protection varies with the **energy of the radiation** modified by certain factors described in *NCRP Report No. 34.*

There are two kinds of occupied areas in the vicinity of a therapy room—"controlled" and "uncontrolled." A **controlled area** is under the supervision of the Radiation Safety Officer and concerns **radiological personnel.** On the other hand, an **uncontrolled area** is not under supervision and involves nonradiological personnel. In accordance with the previously stated radiation limits, the MPD is now 100 mR per week for all controlled areas, and 10 mR for an uncontrolled area. It is of interest that Braestrup and Wyckoff[7] have recently suggested that the limits should be reduced to 10 mR per week for all controlled areas insofar as shielding only is concerned (not the MPD in general) to achieve the lowest practicable exposure level, without unreasonable increase in construction costs. For example, they estimate an added expense of only 1000 dollars to change the design limits from 100 to 10 mR per week for a 4-MV installation.

Several **basic principles** in the arrangement of protective barriers should aid in understanding the more detailed data in *NCRP Report No. 34.* Thorough comprehension of these principles should guarantee adequate protection with minimum shielding, thereby holding down the cost of construction.

1. *Application of Inverse Square Law.* Because of the rapid attenuation of beam intensity with increasing distance from the source, distance itself assumes considerable importance in protection requirements. This principle may be applied in two ways:

(a) *Location of Main Protective Barrier as Close as Possible to the Source or Tube.* The barrier decreases in area the closer it is to the source, according to the inverse square law. Hence a smaller total mass of lead barrier is required if it encloses the tube or source (except at the aperture) then if it is placed at some distance away. Note, however, that the required lead *thickness* is not reduced by being placed closer to the source. Due to the relatively large amount of scattered radiation emerging from the patient, leakage radiation need not be reduced to less than 10 percent of the scattered radiation. The incorporation of the main protective barrier in the housing restricts the patient's exposure to the useful beam, at the same time affording protection from leakage radiation.

(b) *Location of the Therapy Room.* The farther removed the therapy room from occupied areas, the less will be the barrier requirements for the walls, ceilings, and floors. However, in selecting an outside or corner room we must not fail to take into account the distance of outside occupied areas or neighboring buildings in planning the wall protective barriers. Furthermore the roof of a one-story structure housing a therapy installation must have an adequate barrier since megavoltage radiation passing through the roof is scattered downward toward the environs by *aerial* or *atmospheric scatter.*

2. *Restriction in the Directions of the Useful Beam.* Significant economy in construction costs may be effected by limiting beam direction with suitable stops, provided this does not unduly impair the flexibility of the equipment. Only the limited area of the wall exposed to the useful beam and an adequate margin (usually 30 cm [1 ft]) are treated as a primary protective barrier. Further reduction in wall protection is possible if the useful beam can be restricted to an unoccupied area.

3. *Attenuation of Radiation by Scattering.* When radiation of any energy is scattered by the patient or nearby objects, the exposure rate of the 90-degree scattered radiation at 1 meter is 1/1,000

that of the incident radiation at that point. Furthermore, the same degree of attenuation occurs with each subsequent scattering. This explains why the secondary protective barrier requirement is less than the primary.

4. **Computation of Shielding for a Full Eight-Hour Day.** It is poor economy to plan the barrier thickness exactly for present patient load. In the first place, the trend is almost universally toward increasing patient loads, so that future therapy volume must be considered in the planning of a department. Secondly, a reduction in the number of working hours per day does not reduce the barrier thickness by the same fraction. Thus, the thickness of wall barrier is very little less for a 4-hour day than for an 8-hour day, whereas construction costs are almost the same in both cases.

5. **Work Load (W).** This represents the degree of utilization of an X-ray or γ-ray source. W is ordinarily expressed in milliampere-minutes per week for X-ray equipment operating below 2 MV, and in roentgens per week at 1 meter for the useful beam of γ-ray treatment sources and for X-ray equipment operating at or above 2 MV. Note the use of the unit **R** because it is numerically close enough to the absorbed dose for protection purposes. Values of W for typical installations and a treatment load of 32 patients a day are 20,000 mA-min/week for orthovoltage (200 to 300 kV) therapy, and 40,000 R/week at 1 meter for a ^{60}Co unit at a source-skin distance of 80 cm.

6. **Use Factor (U).** Also known as the beam direction factor, this refers to the fraction of the work load during which the beam under consideration is pointed to a particular barrier. For example, the usual value of U is 1 for the floor, $\frac{1}{4}$ for the walls, and not more than $\frac{1}{4}$ for the ceiling. However, this would have to be determined for a particular installation.

7. **Occupancy Factor (T).** Considerable saving in protective barrier may be effected by application of the so-called occupancy factor, defined as the factor by which the work load is multiplied to correct for the degree or type of occupancy of the area in question. According to *NCRP Report No. 34,* there are three degrees of occupancy:

(a) *Full Occupancy.* Control space, wards, office workrooms, corridors and waiting space large enough to hold desks; rest rooms used by the radiologic staff and others routinely exposed to radiation; play areas; and occupied rooms in adjacent rooms or buildings. The occupancy factor is 1.

(b) *Partial Occupancy.* Corridors in Radiology Department too narrow for future desk space, rest rooms not used by radiologic personnel, unattended parking lots, and utility rooms. The occupancy factor is $\frac{1}{4}$.

(c) *Occasional Occupancy.* Stairways, automatic elevators, outside areas used only for pedestrians and vehicular traffic, closets too small for future workrooms, and toilets not used by radiologic personnel. The occupancy factor is $\frac{1}{16}$.

One should exercise the utmost caution in estimating the occupancy factors in various parts of the Radiology Department, because areas with initially low occupancy may later acquire increased occupancy and then be found to have inadequate shielding.

8. *Use of the Most Efficient Material in Protective Barriers.* Only approximate thicknesses of the appropriate shielding material will now be given. Later, an example of the general principles in the planning of a ^{60}Co installation will be presented.

a. *Orthovoltage X-ray Therapy*—about 150 to 300 kV. Here the primary protective barrier is about $\frac{3}{8}$ in. Pb extending $7\frac{1}{3}$ ft. up from the floor. The secondary barrier of $\frac{1}{8}$ in. Pb should overlap the primary barrier about $\frac{1}{2}$ in. and extend to the ceiling. Overlap at seams should be as wide as the lead is thick.

Protection of the floor and ceiling depends strongly on beam energy and other factors and must be determined in advance by a qualified expert.

The leaded glass observation port should have the same lead equivalent as the adjacent wall and should be overlapped about $\frac{1}{2}$ in. by the lead in the wall. Leaded glass ordinarily requires about four times the thickness of sheet lead for equivalent protection; for example, 1 in. leaded glass is equivalent to $\frac{1}{4}$ in. sheet lead.

In wall construction the laminated lead concrete block serves as an economical building material. Another, possibly less expensive, method is to nail sheet lead with lead-headed nails between double studs placed flatwise. Lead barriers $\frac{1}{8}$ in. or more in thickness are much easier and cheaper to apply in multiple layers of $\frac{1}{16}$ in. because this thickness can be cut with suitable shears and can be lifted more readily. One-eighth inch lead must be chiseled and is difficult to lift because of its weight. Furthermore, $\frac{1}{16}$-in. lead can be overlapped more easily at seams and joints.

b. *Megavoltage therapy*—0.5 to 10 MeV range (cobalt 60 and megavoltage X ray in energy region). Concrete of density 2.35 g/cc (147 lb/cu ft) is most economical for wall material here because it provides both adequate protection and structural strength. Only approximate values of thickness will be given—accurate advance planning by a qualified expert is imperative. In the average cobalt 60 installation, about 3 ft or more of concrete of the above density is required for the primary barrier, and about 2 ft for the secondary barrier. This will vary, of course, with the energy of the beam, size of the source, and other protective factors. The primary barrier may be significantly decreased in thickness if the beam direction is restricted or if, as with ^{60}Co, an isocontour shield is used (see Fig. 17.11). This is a heavy lead shield located diametrically opposite the source on the far side of the patient, whose purpose is to receive and attenuate the transmitted beam. The shield is affixed to the source housing by a rigid arm to keep it always opposite the source regardless of the treatment position. *Leakage radiation* is an important item, since the housing for ^{60}Co provides only relative protection and the source radiates continuously. The exposure rate from leakage radiation must be added to that from scattered radiation (the two together comprise *stray radiation*) in calculating wall thickness for the secondary barrier. Radiation that has scattered twice is usually reduced to a safe level by a barrier of $\frac{1}{4}$ in. Pb, but this must be verified. An observation port of leaded glass must be about 12 in. thick for the average ^{60}Co teletherapy room. A less expensive and far more satisfactory method uses closed circuit television to monitor the patient, with an auxiliary system of mirrors for viewing the patient in the event of failure of the television system.

Care must be taken to design and shield properly all apertures in any barrier, such as those needed for plumbing, electrical wiring, air conditioning vents, and door pulls.

9. *Allowance of a Safety Factor.* It has not been sufficiently stressed that, in view of the gradual reduction of the MPD over the years, there is some likelihood that this trend may continue. Therefore, in computing barrier thickness and therapy room location, we should take cognizance of this trend and allow a reasonable safety factor. While it is uneconomical to plan too far ahead, barrier thickness should, if possible, be adjusted for possible future requirements. (See page 630 for recent suggestion of Braestrup and Wyckoff concerning the desirability of increasing shielding requirements to reduce the limits from 100 to 10 mR per week for controlled areas.)

Computation of Protective Barriers for a ^{60}Co Teletherapy Room. It goes without saying that a qualified radiation physicist should plan the protective barriers for a radiology department, especially when it includes high energy equipment. However, this does not absolve the radiotherapist from the responsibility of participating in the computation and planning of the required protective barriers. Although the published equations may seem formidable, they are actually derived from rather simple principles, involving mainly the inverse square law and arithemetic. To illustrate these principles we shall describe how a typical ^{60}Co teletherapy room may be designed to meet the established requirements for radiation protection.

Figure 17.05 is a layout of such a room. Beam direction is to be so restricted that it can be angled *only* toward wall A; otherwise it must be aimed straight down. In other words, the useful beam cannot strike any other wall than A. Thus, a passerby in the parking lot (uncontrolled area) at point I would have to be protected from exposure to the useful beam, whereas a person at the control desk (controlled area) at point II would need protection from scattered and leakage radiation as defined above. Now the problem is fundamentally that of finding the barrier thickness needed to reduce the weekly exposure anywhere outside the room to the MPD applicable to that particular area. We shall use concrete (density 2.35 g/cm^3 or 147 lb/ft.^{3}) for three reasons: (1) gram for gram it is just as efficient an absorber of high energy γ rays as is lead because absorption is predominantly by Compton interaction which is independent of the atomic number of the absorber;

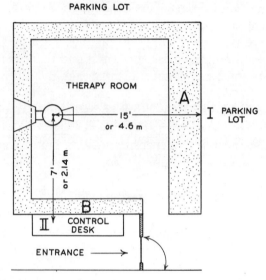

FIGURE 17.05. Sample floor plan for a cobalt 60 therapy room, to serve as a basis for calculating protective barriers. (See text.)

(2) concrete is much cheaper than lead, gram for gram; and (3) concrete is structurally strong. Since we are only exemplifying the computation of barrier thickness we shall consider only walls A and B which require primary and secondary barriers, respectively.

In this particular installation we are to plan for a patient load of 40 per day and an average exposure of 400 R per patient at a treatment distance (SSD) of 100 cm (1 m). For a 5-day week this gives a workload W of about $40 \times 400 \times 5 = 80,000$ R/wk at 1 m. Now we may proceed with the calculation of the barrier thicknesses.

1. **Primary Barrier Computation.** If no barrier were used and the useful beam were directed toward a person at position I in Figure 17.05, the exposure X would be

$$X = \frac{W}{D^2} \quad R/wk \qquad (3)$$

where W is the workload and D is the distance between the source and point I. However, X is further decreased by the *fraction* of the time the beam is directed toward I (use factor U) and by the *fraction* of the time that I is occupied by someone (occupancy factor T), so the exposure at I becomes

$$X = \frac{WUT}{D^2} \quad R/wk \tag{4}$$

But we must reduce this exposure to the weekly MPD which, for an uncontrolled area such as a parking lot, is 0.01 R/wk. To achieve this we must insert a concrete barrier between the source and the point of interest, the barrier being of such thickness that the fraction of radiation it transmits does not exceed the weekly MPD. This fraction is the **transmission factor B.** Equation (4) then becomes

$$0.01 = \frac{BWUT}{D^2} \quad R/wk \tag{5}$$

All terms in equation (5) are known except B which can be related to the required thickness of concrete by the use of appropriate published curves (see Fig. 17.06). Rearranging equation (5),

$$B = \frac{0.01\, D^2}{WUT} \tag{6}$$

From Figure 17.05, $D = 15$ ft or $15/3.28 = 4.6$ m. The workload W has been estimated to be 80,000 R/wk at 1 m. If the beam is directed horizontally at I about $\frac{1}{4}$ W, $U = \frac{1}{4}$. If I is occupied about 1/16 the time, $T = 1/16$. Substituting these values in equation (6),

$$B = \frac{0.01 \times 4.6 \times 4.6}{80{,}000 \times 1/4 \times 1/16}$$

$$B = 0.00017$$

Referring to the ^{60}Co curve in Figure 16.06, we locate 0.00017 on the ordinate, read over to the curve and then down to the abscissa where the thickness of concrete is found to be 33 in. (84 cm). This thickness of concrete will decrease the exposure by a factor of 0.00017 to the MPD of 0.01 R/wk.

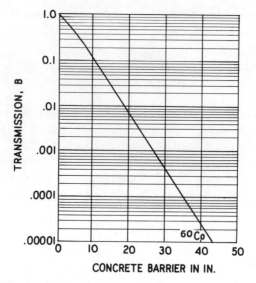

FIGURE 17.06. ^{60}Co γ-ray transmission B through concrete (density 2.35 g/cm^3 or 147 lb/ft^3). Adapted from NCRP *Report No. 34*, data of F. S. Kirn, R. J. Kennedy, and H. O. Wyckoff, *Radiology*, Vol. 63, [1954], p. 94.)

It should be pointed out that for an SSD other than 1 m, conversion to 1 m must be made according to the inverse square law. For example, if the SSD is 80 cm and the exposure per patient is 400 R, then the exposure at 1 m is

$$\frac{0.8 \times 0.8}{1 \times 1} \times 400 = 256 \text{ R}$$

and the workload W becomes

$$256 \ R/pt \times 40 \ pt/day \times 5 \ days/wk = 51{,}000 \ R/wk$$

2. *Secondary Barrier Computation.* Let us turn now to the barrier required to protect a technologist at position II from scattered and leakage radiation (as already postulated, the useful beam is restricted so that it cannot be aimed at position II). The treatment of scattered and of leakage radiation is different, and they will therefore be discussed separately.

a. *Barrier thickness for scattered radiation* is obtained by reasoning similar to that used in deriving the equation for the primary barrier. However, the fraction of the useful beam scattered in a particular direction depends on the scattering angle (Compton effect), so it must enter the equation. *NCRP Report No. 34* (Table B-2) gives the fraction of the radiation scattered at various angles at the position of the patient. Suppose we consider only the radiation scattered at 90°, for which the fraction is found to be 9×10^{-4}. The work load is multiplied by this factor and the MPD is changed to 0.1 R/wk for this controlled area. The new equation is

$$B_s = \frac{0.1 D^2}{9 \times 10^{-4} \, WUT} \tag{7}$$

In this case U and T are both unity. D according to Figure 17.05 is 7 ft. or $7/3.28 = 2.13$ m. Substituting the appropriate values in equation (7),

$$B_s = \frac{0.1 \times 2.13 \times 2.13}{9 \times 10^{-4} \times 80,000} = 0.0063$$

According to Figure 17.07, for 90° scattering this value of B_s requires a concrete barrier 13 in. (33 cm) thick. Note that the HVL

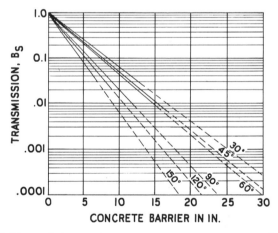

FIGURE 17.07. Transmission B_s through concrete (density 2.35 g/cm³ or 147 lb/ft³) of ⁶⁰Co scattered radiation, at various angles, from a cylindrical Masonite phantom, 20 cm field at 1 meter from the source. Adapted from NCRP *Report No. 34*, data of R. T. Mooney, and C. B. Braestrup, AEC *Report NYO 2165* (1957).

of the scattered radiation (softer than that in the useful beam) is about 1.82 in. concrete, increasing as the scattering angle is decreased. Note how this contrasts with an HVL of 2.45 in. concrete for the useful beam.

It should be pointed out that SSD's other than 1 m must be normalized to 1 m by means of the inverse square law. This is done by introducing the $\overline{SSD}^2$ as a factor in the numerator of equation (7)

$$B_s = \frac{0.1\, D^2\, \overline{SSD}^2}{9 \times 10^{-4}\, WUT} \tag{8}$$

b. **Barrier thickness for leakage radiation** is based on *NCRP Report No. 33* that the maximum permissible leakage shall not exceed 0.1 percent of the useful beam at 1 m from the source in the **"on"** position. The maximum permissible leakage in the **"off"** position shall not exceed, on the average, 2 mR/hr. Obviously, the hazard from leakage radiation is limited to that with the unit in the "on" position. Furthermore, the more protection incorporated in the source housing, the less will be needed in the walls, with resulting economy in construction. For the sake of this discussion, suppose that we have the maximum allowable leakage—$0.1\%\,W$ or $0.001\,W$ at 1 m. The values of U and T are again unity. Hence the exposure at I without a barrier would be $0.001\,W$ R/wk. This must be decreased to the MPD of 0.1 R/wk (controlled area) by the **leakage transmission factor B_L** and is further decreased according to the inverse square law applied to the distance 7 ft = 2.13 m. We then have equation

$$0.1 = \frac{0.001\, W B_L}{D^2}\, \text{R/wk} \tag{9}$$

Rearranging,

$$B_L = \frac{0.1\, D^2}{0.001\, W} \tag{10}$$

Substituting the known values and solving,

$$B_L = \frac{0.1 \times 2.13 \times 2.13}{0.001 \times 80{,}000} = 0.0063$$

Since leakage radiation has the same energy as the useful beam, we use the same transmission curves as shown in Figure 17.06. For a B_L of 0.0063 the required thickness of concrete is found to be 20 in. (51 cm).

Leakage radiation should actually be measured by the physicist so that full advantage can be taken of all protection incorporated in the source housing.

We must now find the thickness of the secondary barrier for **both leakage and scattered radiation.** In this example, 13 in. of concrete are needed for scattered radiation, and 20 in. for leakage. According to NCRP recommendations in *Report No. 34,* when the barrier thicknesses for scattered and leakage radiation differ by *less* than 3 HVL's, we simply add 1 HVL to the larger thickness. Therefore, our secondary barrier should have a thickness of

$$20 \text{ in.} + 2.45 \text{ in.} = 22.45 \text{ in.}$$

This may be rounded to 22 in.

In the event that the barriers for the two types of radiation differ by *more* than 3 HVL's, the thicker of the two will suffice.

RADIUM PROTECTION

In this section, protective measures will be discussed only as they pertain to *sealed radium sources.* Just as with other kinds of radiation sources, the problem of inadvertent exposure of personnel includes: (1) whole body or systemic irradiation and (2) local irradiation.

Protection Against Whole Body Exposure. Before the advent of radionuclide therapy, relatively little consideration was given to whole body exposure of personnel to Ra, especially when it concerned the Ra sources within a patient. Most emphasis was placed on local exposure of the hands. Now there is much greater awareness of the large doses that can be accumulated by radiological and nursing personnel attending patients who are undergoing interstitial or intracavitary Ra (or Ra-substitute) therapy. In general, whole body exposure to the γ rays of Ra may be incurred in four ways: proximity to stored Ra, manipulation of Ra applicators, proximity to patients undergoing Ra therapy, and transportation of Ra.

1. ***Storage of Radium.*** The best protection from stored Ra includes a suitable ***lead barrier*** and ***distance.*** The latter is of great importance because of the inverse square law. We can easily compute the thickness of lead and the distance for any given quantity of stored Ra,. or for that matter, any γ ray emitter. The minimal distance from such a source, at which dosage does not exceed the MPD, may be designated as the ***shortest permissible distance*** (SPD). It depends on the specific γ-ray constant Γ and the inverse square law. Recall that the specific γ-ray constant is defined as the γ-ray exposure rate in R/hr at 1 cm from a 1-mCi point source of any radionuclide. Γ values for various radionuclides are given in Table 17.02. Note that a 0.5 mm Pt filter is specified for radium.

TABLE 17.02
MEAN GAMMA-RAY ENERGY AND SPECIFIC GAMMA-RAY CONSTANT (Γ)
OF VARIOUS RADIONUCLIDES

Element	Radionuclide	Mean γ-ray Energy	Γ
		MeV	R/mCi-hr at 1 cm
Gold	^{198}Au	0.41	2.3
Iodine	^{131}I	0.40	2.18
Cesium	^{137}Cs	0.66	3.3
Radium (*0.5 mm Pt filter*)	^{226}Ra	0.83	8.25
Cobalt	^{60}Co	1.25	13.0

Since Γ is in R/mCi-hr at 1 cm, we must find the SPD at which the exposure will be reduced to the MPD (occupational) of 0.0025 R/hr for a 40-hr week. Applying the inverse square law,

$$\frac{d^2}{1^2} = \frac{\Gamma A}{0.0025}$$

where d is the SPD in cm, A is the radionuclide activity in mCi, and 0.0025 is the occupational whole body MPD in R/hr. Therefore

$$d = \sqrt{\frac{\Gamma A}{0.0025}} \text{ cm}$$

$$d = 20\sqrt{\Gamma A} \text{ cm} \tag{11}$$

The SPD d_{Ra} for Ra may be found by substituting its Γ in general equation (11):

$$d_{Ra} = 20\sqrt{8.25A} \text{ cm}$$

$$d_{Ra} = 57\sqrt{A} \text{ cm} \tag{12}$$

For example, if the Ra source is 100 mg ($= 100$ mCi):

$$d_{Ra} = 57\sqrt{100}$$

$$d_{Ra} = 57 \times 10 = 570 \text{ cm}$$

Thus, at 570 cm from a 100-mg Ra source, the maximum permissible exposure of 2.5 mR/hr (100 mR/wk) will not be exceeded even in the absence of protective shielding.

The SPD may be reduced by *shielding* a γ-ray emitter with an appropriate barrier. If the half value layer (HVL) of the γ rays in any material is known, then the required barrier thickness for a given SPD can be calculated. Table 17.03 shows the HVL's in lead and in concrete for the more commonly used γ emitters. Equation (12) may be combined with the data for HVL to find the various combinations of lead barrier thickness and distance needed to store "safely" any given quantity of Ra. At a given distance each added HVL of barrier material reduces the γ-ray exposure rate by one-half. For example, if 100 mg Ra is stored at

TABLE 17.03
HALF VALUE LAYERS OF SOME COMMONLY USED γ-RAY EMITTERS.
THE HVL IS GIVEN IN CM FOR LEAD, AND
IN INCHES FOR CONCRETE*

Element	Radionuclide	Half Value Layer	
		cm Pb	*in. Concrete*
Iodine	^{131}I	0.3	—
Gold	^{198}Au	0.33	
Cesium	^{137}Cs	0.65	1.9
Cobalt	^{60}Co	1.2	2.5
Radium	^{226}Ra	1.4	2.7

*NCRP *Report No. 40*.

a certain distance and is surrounded by a lead barrier 1.4 cm thick (1 HVL) the exposure rate decreases 50 percent at that same distance. An additional barrier of 1.4 cm lead further reduces the exposure rate 50 percent, that is, to one-fourth the initial value $[(\frac{1}{2})^2 = \frac{1}{4}]$. The next HVL will reduce it to $(\frac{1}{2})^3$ or $\frac{1}{8}$. Therefore, we can introduce the expression 2^n into the right member of equation (12), n representing the number of HVL's of a particular barrier. The new equation assumes the form:

$$d_{Ra} = 57 \sqrt{\frac{mg\,Ra}{2^n}} \text{ cm} \tag{13}$$

(It should be emphasized that 57 is a constant applicable only to Ra, as derived above.) If no protective barrier is used, $n = 0$ and $2^0 = 1$, so that equation (13) reverts to equation (12).

Let us now apply equation (13) to an actual Ra storage problem. Suppose we have 100 mg Ra that is to be stored at 100 cm (1 meter) from an occupied area. What thickness of lead container is needed to decrease the exposure rate to the MPD of 2.5 mR/hr? Substituting these values in equation (13):

$$100 = 57 \sqrt{\frac{100}{2^n}}$$

$$100 = \frac{57 \times 10}{\sqrt{2^n}}$$

$$\sqrt{2^n} = \frac{57 \times 10}{100} = 5.7$$

Squaring both sides:

$$2^n = 5.7 \times 5.7 = 32.5$$

The next step requires the use of logarithms:

$$n \log 2 = \log 32.5$$

$$0.301n = 1.5119$$

$$n = 5 \text{ HVL}$$

Thus, 5 HVL's of protective barrier are needed to store 100 mg of Ra at a distance of 100 cm. Since, from Table 17.03 the HVL of Ra γ rays in lead is 1.4 cm,

$$5 \times 1.4 \text{ cm} = 7.0 \text{ cm lead}$$

For those not familiar with logarithms, Figure 17.08 is a graph showing the protective barriers required for various quantities of Ra at 1, 2, and 3 meters, in HVL. To find the actual thickness of a particular barrier material, simply multiply the indicated number of HVL's by the appropriate HVL in the given material, as shown above.

Because of the essentially monochromatic γ radiation emitted by Ra filtered by 0.5 mm Pt, the relationship of mgRa/d^2 to the required number of HVL's follows a straight line curve when plotted on semilog paper, as in Figure 17.09. This provides a con-

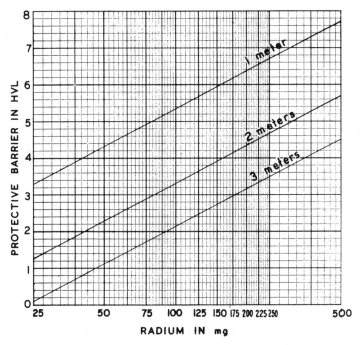

FIGURE 17.08. Graph showing protective barrier of any material in half value layers for a given quantity of radium stored at 1, 2, or 3 meters. Based on a 40-hour work week.

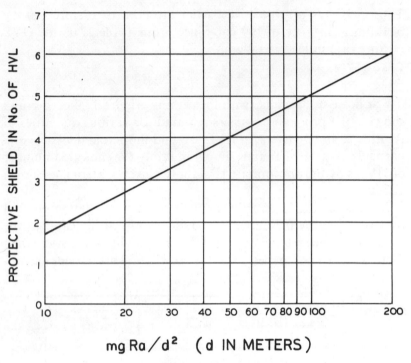

mg Ra/d² (d IN METERS)

FIGURE 17.09. Graph for determining the protective shield in HVL for radium of various quantities stored at various distances. The graph is simplified by combining Ra in mg, and distance in meters, as mg/d² on the horizontal axis. Based on a 40-hr week.

venient method of summarizing protective barrier data for various quantities of Ra and their corresponding danger ranges, as related to HVL. As an example of the use of this graph, suppose we wish to determine the thickness of lead barrier needed for 50 mg Ra at a distance of 1.5 m. The value of mgRa/d^2 at this distance is:

$$\frac{\text{mgRa}}{d^2} = \frac{50}{1.5 \times 1.5} = \frac{50}{2.25} = 22.2 \text{ mgRa/m}^2$$

Looking up this value on the ordinate of the graph, we find that it intersects the curve at 2.8 HVL, so that 2.8 × 1.4 = 3.9 cm of lead is required to furnish adequate protection (based on a 40-hr working week).

The shielding of Ra can be accomplished satisfactorily by the use of concrete of proper specific gravity (2.35 g cm³ or 147 lb/ft³). According to Figure 17.09 the thicknesses of concrete barrier (HVL 6.6 cm or 2.6 in.) for 100 mg Ra at various shortest permissible distances are as follows:

1 meter —100 mg Ra— 5 HVL—33 cm (13 in.) concrete
2 meters—100 mg Ra— 3 HVL—20 cm (8 in.)   concrete
3 meters—100 mg Ra—1.8 HVL—12 cm (4.7 in.) concrete

Values for other combinations may be readily obtained from the graph.

It must be emphasized that the indicated lead or concrete shielding of Ra will attenuate the γ radiation to the permissible level at the corresponding distance during a 40-hour working week, from Ra alone. If personnel should be exposed to other sources in addition, the exposure to Ra must be decreased accordingly so that the total will not exceed 100 mR/wk. This may necessitate the storage of Ra at a greater distance from occupied areas, and/or the use of additional protective barriers.

2. *Manipulation of Radium* in loading or unloading applicators, and the application of Ra to the patient, should be done with the greatest possible speed at the longest possible distance, using forceps at least 25 cm (10 in.) long. An L-shaped lead block at least 5 cm (2 in.) thick should always be used (see Fig. 17.10), the thickness depending on the work load. It should measure about 40 cm (16 in.) wide, 50 cm (20 in.) high, and 35 cm (14 in.) deep.

3. *Hazards From Patients Containing Radium.* Personnel should remain as far as possible from patients receiving Ra therapy. Nursing procedures must be carried out as rapidly as is consistent with the patient's welfare, and nurses should be rotated on duty. Visiting of Ra patients by youngsters and pregnant women shall be prohibited, and by adults under 45 avoided or reduced to a minimum. Radiology personnel should also avoid frequent and prolonged visiting of patients, unless it is absolutely necessary. The exposure rate should be measured and calculated at 1 m from the source itself, and recorded on the patient's chart.

Transportation of Radium. This requires long-handled containers lined with sufficient lead. For example, 100 mg Ra should be carried in a container having a 2-cm lead wall, suspended by a handle 45 cm long. Transportation should be as rapid as possible, and should preferably be intrusted to responsible persons not ordinarily exposed to ionizing radiation.

Film badge monitoring will readily indicate excessive accumulation of whole body radiation from external sources. If the MPD is exceeded, immediate steps must be taken to modify handling technics or to rotate personnel so that satisfactory dosage levels may be attained.

Protection Against Local Exposure. Here *speed* and *distance* give the best protection. Forceps at least 25 cm long should always be used; under no circumstances should Ra be picked up directly with the fingers. Lead-lined gloves do not contain sufficient lead to be of any practical value in protection and would even increase the exposure because of lead characteristic radiation. Exposure of the radiologist's hands during the introduction of Ra into the patient is sometimes unavoidable, but should be kept to a minimum. Local injury by Ra or its substitutes may take many years to manifest itself, so one should not be lulled into a false sense of security. However, limitation of exposure to the present maximum permissible weekly 1,500 mR to the hands should produce no untoward sequelae. If a finger badge monitor

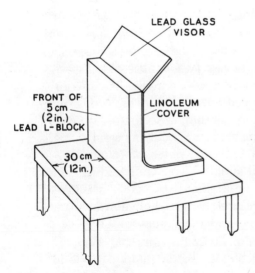

FIGURE 17.10. Lead protective L-black for loading and unloading radium applicators. The required thickness must be verified by appropriate radiation survey for the individual department.

of the thermoluminescent type indicates that this exposure is regularly being exceeded, rotation of personnel in the handling of the Ra should be instituted. *Afterloading technics* bring about significant reduction in personnel exposure.

The *gonads* (testes and ovaries) may also receive significant local exposure. As already noted, there is no threshold for genetic effects, but the mutation rate is roughly proportional to the accumulated dose. The mutation doubling rate approximates 40–80 R. On the basis of 5 R per year, the maximum permissible weekly gonadal exposure is 100 mR. To reduce the gonadal exposure, especially when large amounts of Ra are handled, a thick lead L-block should be used (see Fig. 17.10). Depending on the amount of Ra being handled, the front and bottom of the L should measure at least 5 cm in thickness. The front of the L-block should be about 30 cm behind the front edge of the table. Almost as important as lead shielding is *speed* in loading and unloading of applicators. Speed can best be acquired by practicing with dummy Ra sources. Only when maximum dexterity has been attained, should real Ra sources replace the dummies.

HAZARDS IN THE USE OF RADIONUCLIDES IN TELETHERAPY

The same principles governing X-ray and radium protection also apply to radionuclides. When used in *teletherapy*, ^{60}Co and ^{137}Cs require primary and secondary protective barriers (see pages 629 to 630). Radionuclides used in *nuclear medicine* for tracer studies and therapy require protective measures similar to discrete radium sources. However, there are the additional problems of accidental spill of radionuclides in solution, and of waste disposal. Health physics related to nuclear medicine will be discussed later. Here we shall take up the hazards arising in teletherapy with radionuclides.

Since we are concerned with γ radiation from telecurie sources, particularly ^{60}Co, the MPD applicable to the whole body, extremities, blood-forming organs, eyes, and other anatomic regions is the same as for X rays.

The housing for the ^{60}Co teletherapy source must contain sufficient shielding (lead, tungsten, or an alloy of lead-tungsten-spent uranium) to accord adequate protection to both patient and personnel with respect to leakage radiation. The protective housing must reduce leakage radiation to the levels prescribed in NCRP *Report No. 33;* that is, a maximum of 10 mR/hr and an average of 2 mR/hr at a distance of 1 m in the "off" position, and a maximum of 0.1 percent of the useful beam at a distance of 1 m in the "on" position.

The collimating device shall reduce the intensity outside the edge of the useful beam to 5 percent (or less) of the useful beam intensity at that level. The mechanism which puts the beam in the "off" and "on" position (that is, the shutter or the source transfer mechanism) shall have both automatic and manual controls. In the event of failure of the automatic closing device, the manual control can then be brought into play. However, it must be so arranged that it can be operated with minimum exposure to personnel. The automatic control shall be so designed that in the event of breakdown, the closing device promptly returns to the "off" position. Signal lights on the control panel shall indicate whether the beam is "on" or "off" A preset timer serves to terminate the exposure and engage the control device which then automatically returns to the "off" position.

Primary and secondary barriers are required for the walls of the teletherapy room and have been discussed in detail above (see pages 629 to 641). Although ^{60}Co teletherapy is in the megavoltage region, the scattered radiation from the patient is considerably softer than the useful beam, so that different absorption curves may be used in computing the two types of barriers. The primary protective barrier must be provided for any area that can possibly receive the useful beam, and it must extend at least 30 cm beyond the useful beam. An *isocontour shield* (see Fig. 17.11) reduces the thickness of protective barrier needed in the walls. Areas subjected to scattered and leakage radiation require a secondary protective barrier.

No one but the patient should remain inside the therapy room while treatment with telecurie ^{60}Co or ^{137}Cs is in progress. (The same applies to any form of ortho- or megavoltage therapy.) Furthermore, the lead-protected entrance door shall be so inter-

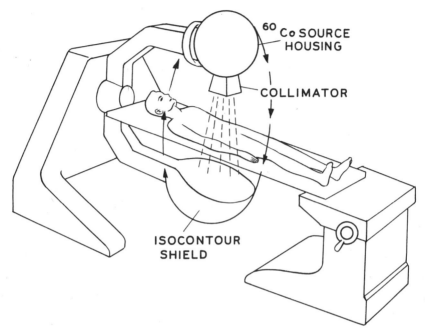

FIGURE 17.11. Diagram of a ^{60}Co teletherapy unit with a protective isocontour shield. (Based on Picker ^{60}Co Unit.)

locked electrically with the control mechanism that when the door is opened the source immediately returns to the "off" position. Personnel shall not enter the room while the source is in the "on" position due to the deliberate inactivation of the door interlock during an emergency, unless a suitable protective assembly is used to prevent dangerous whole body exposure.

PERSONNEL HAZARDS IN NUCLEAR MEDICINE

Since World War II, the nuclear reactor has provided an abundance of radionuclides for use in medicine and industry. As a result of their rapidly increasing application in medicine, ***personnel exposure*** has become sufficiently important to require protective measures, many of which simply extend the principles of protection from X-ray and γ-ray therapy. However, the internal administration of radionuclides entails the further hazard of exposure to

radioactive solutions and dusts, necessitating certain special precautions. In this section we shall consider the general principles
of radionuclide protection of personnel entrusted with the handling of these materials. The excellent *NCRP Report No. 37* deals
with precautions in managing patients who have received therapeutic amounts of radionuclides.

Because ordinary medical radionuclides emit either β or γ rays,
or both, protection should be considered with relation to these
two types of radiation.

What are the hazards to personnel in handling radionuclides?
These include:

1. External Radiation Hazards
    a. To the whole body
        1) β particles
        2) γ rays
    b. To local anatomic regions
        1) β particles
        2) γ rays
2. Internal Radiation Hazards
    a. Ingestion
    b. Inhalation
    c. Absorption through intact skin
    d. Absorption through broken skin

These radiation dangers will now be discussed separately.

External Radionuclide Hazards to Personnel

Gamma Radiation. Whole body exposure to γ radiation may
result from contaminated laboratory equipment, from stored radionuclides, or from patients receiving therapeutic doses. As already
emphasized, the continuous *occupational* whole body exposure to
γ rays must not exceed 100 mR/wk and, in fact, should be well
below this level.

There are four principal methods of reducing personnel exposure: (1) distance, (2) shielding, (3) time of exposure, and (4) limitation of the quantity of radionuclides on hand.

1. *Distance.* Since γ rays are photons having tremendous penetrating ability, they cannot be completely absorbed by any type

of practical barrier. Protection follows the same rules as those given for Ra. **Distance** is a very important safety factor. According to the familiar inverse square law, the exposure rate falls rapidly with increasing distance from the source. Since our aim is to reduce the exposure rate to the MPD of 100 mR/wk, we may conveniently express the "safe distance" from a given quantity of a particular radionuclide as the shortest permissible distance (SPD), in the same manner as with Ra. For example, 10 mCi of ^{131}I may be stored without shielding at a minimal distance of about 3 feet. Such information derives from the general equation

$$d = 20\sqrt{\Gamma A} \text{ cm}$$

where d is the SPD in cm, Γ is the specific γ-ray constant of a given γ emitter, and A is the activity in mCi of the radionuclide under consideration. The value of Γ for ^{131}I being 2.18 R/hr at 1 cm, the SPD for 10 mCi of unshielded ^{131}I is:

$$d = 20\sqrt{2.18 \times 10}$$

$$d = 93 \text{ cm or 3 ft}$$

The inverse square law holds not only for the storage but also for the handling of γ-emitting radionuclides. This is accomplished by the use of long-handled forceps or tongs; an unshielded source should never be picked up directly. Obviously, rubber gloves offer no protection against γ rays, although they should be worn to protect the hands from contamination by radioactive solutions.

2. **Shielding.** Another important means of minimizing γ-ray hazard is **lead shielding** of appropriate thickness. This, too, relates to the MPD of 100 mR/wk. From the equation for SPD, an expression for the protective barrier may be derived, as has already been done in the section on Ra protection:

$$d = 20\sqrt{\frac{\Gamma A}{2^n}} \text{ cm}$$

where n is the number of HVL's of barrier material, and the other terms have the same meaning as above.

Let us find the thickness of lead barrier required for 100 mCi

^{131}I at a distance of 1 foot. Here, d is 1 ft or 32 cm and Γ is 2.18 R/mCi-hr at 1 cm. Therefore,

$$32 = 20\sqrt{\frac{2.18 \times 100}{2^n}}$$

Squaring both sides:

$$32 \times 32 = 20 \times 20 \times 218/2^n$$

$$2^n = \frac{20 \times 20 \times 218}{32 \times 32} = 85$$

$$n \log 2 = \log 85$$

$$n \times 0.301 = 1.9294$$

$$n = 6.4 \text{ HVL}$$

Since the HVL of the γ radiation from ^{131}I is 0.3 cm lead, 6.4 HVL would be $6.4 \times 0.3 = 1.9$ cm lead, this being about $\frac{3}{4}$ in. Figure 17.12 shows the relationship of mCi/d^2 to the required HVL for ^{131}I.

In actual practice, a γ-emitting radionuclide is shielded by storage in its lead shipping container. Additional protection may be afforded by 5-cm (2-in.) lead bricks around the radioactive sample on those sides which constitute an exposure hazard. A radiation survey meter should be used to test the adequacy of this protective barrier.

Personnel exposure to parenterally administered γ-emitting nuclides, even in tracer amounts, should be minimized by a **lead shield** fitted to the syringe. Such shields are available commercially in a variety of sizes. Therapeutic quantities of γ-emitting nuclides of high activity such as ^{131}I in thyroid cancer and ^{198}Au in effusions require special remote systems of administration to reduce exposure to a tolerable level.

3. *Time of Exposure.* Another factor in the control of γ-ray exposure, previously mentioned, is *speed*. The less time spent with various radionuclide procedures, the smaller will be the exposure.

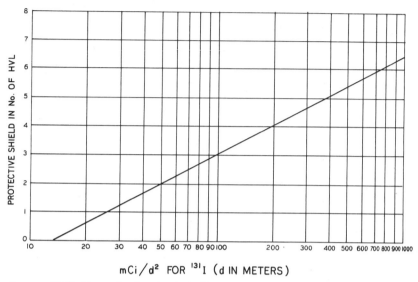

y-axis: PROTECTIVE SHIELD IN No. OF HVL

x-axis: mCi/d² FOR ¹³¹I (d IN METERS)

FIGURE 17.12. Protective barrier in half value layers required for the storage of various quantities of ^{131}I at various distances. The amount of ^{131}I in mCi and the distance in meters have been combined in the form mCi/d² to simplify the graph. Based on a 40-hr week.

4. *Limitation of Stored Quantities.* Limiting the quantities of radionuclides on hand to the minimum needed for a reasonable length of time will obviously reduce protective barrier requirements.

Beta Radiation. Just as with other kinds of radiation, the key factors in protection from external sources of β radiation are time, distance, and shielding. Time must be kept to a minimum, and distance to a maximum, commensurate with the requirements of a particular procedure. In general, the range of β particles in any medium depends on their energy; as an approximation, the range in cm of air is numerically equal to one-half their energy in MeV. Thus, the β particles of ^{32}P ($E_{max} = 1.7$ MeV) and of ^{90}Sr-^{90}Y ($E_{max} = 2.18$ MeV) are very penetrating; in fact, they may reach a depth of 8 to 10 mm within the body. Therefore special shielding is required. Plastics (e.g. polystyrene or lucite) or aluminum are superior shielding materials because their low atomic number makes them poor emitters of brems radiation while, at the same time, providing satisfactory absorption of β particles. About 7 mm ($\frac{1}{4}$ in.) plastic is sufficient for ^{32}P, and 10 mm ($\frac{3}{8}$ in.) for ^{90}Sr-^{90}Y. Air also contributes to the protective barrier. Thus, the handling of these β emitters does not pose a serious radiation hazard in the presence of a sufficient thickness and area of plastic barrier.

Exposure of Hands or Other Noncritical Areas to Beta or Gamma Radiation. In general, the occupational MPD for all parts of the body, other than the hands, is identical to that of the whole body, 100 mrem per week. However, the MPD to the hands is 1,500 mR per week or 75 R per year for both β and γ rays, since they both have similar biologic effectiveness.

Contamination of the hands by radioactive solutions can be avoided by the use of disposable plastic gloves. If spill should occur the gloves can be peeled carefully from the hands inside out and stored in the decay chamber to a safe radiation level. When ^{32}P is to be injected the hands should be protected by a plastic shield designed to fit the syringe, as well as by plastic gloves. A lead-shielded syringe should be used with low activity, therapeutic quantities of γ emitters such as ^{131}I; remote systems must be used for doses of high activity.

It must be pointed out that when exposure involves more than one of the above hazards, the total must not exceed the MPD. In other words, if the total body exposure in a given week is 60 mR of γ rays, any additional exposure to radionuclides or other sources of ionizing radiation must not exceed 40 mrem, the total from both sources being limited to 100 mrem.

Internal Radionuclide Hazards to Personnel

In performing laboratory procedures involving radionuclides, personnel is subjected not only to the hazards of external radiation, as already described, but also to the dangers of internal radiation from nuclides accidentally entering the body. Such internal contamination may be due to carelessness on the part of the worker, or to unsuspected radioactive fumes or dust in a poorly controlled laboratory. The principal routes of entry of radionuclides include ingestion, inhalation, and absorption through the skin. The fate of a radionuclide, once it has entered the body, depends on its decay rate, its physical and chemical properties, its mode of entry, its localization within the body, and its rate of excretion. Thus, the problem of determining the internal hazard of any particular nuclide is unique, and is much more difficult to solve than the problem of external exposure. Furthermore, as we shall see later, the peril of internal contamination may greatly exceed that of external contamination.

Ingestion may occur as the result of carelessness, such as allowing contaminated hands to convey food or cigarettes to the mouth. Radioactive solutions should never be pipetted by mouth because only a minute volume of solution accidentally swallowed may exceed the daily MPD. The ingested radionuclide may then be absorbed from the gastrointestinal tract, enter the blood stream, and be deposited in various tissues. The rate of excretion may be slow or rapid, depending on the nature of the compound. Obviously, a radionuclide having a long effective half-life (long physical half-life and slow rate of excretion) constitutes a more serious radiation hazard than one with a short effective half-life.

Inhalation may result from the presence of radioactive dust, fumes, or gas. For example, ^{131}I in solution in an open container readily vaporizes to contaminate the laboratory air. Furthermore, ^{131}I vaporizes almost immediately upon contact with ordinary city tap water due to the presence of chlorine. The inhaled material may remain in the lungs or may be absorbed in the blood stream to be deposited in various parts of the body; or it may be coughed up and swallowed.

Absorption of radionuclides in significant amounts may occur either through the intact or broken skin. The absorbed nuclide then enters the circulation and is deposited in various organs. To avoid absorption, disposable plastic or rubber gloves should always be worn when therapeutic amounts of radioactive solutions are handled. The gloves do not offer protection against the radiation itself, but do guard against absorption that might follow accidental spill. With tracer quantities the hands should be washed thoroughly after each procedure.

Why do radionuclides which gain access to the internal organs of personnel constitute such a grave hazard? First of all, their sojourn in the body depends on their effective half-life, determined by the biologic half-life (excretion) and physical half-life (radioactive decay). A radionuclide of long effective half-life would act as a source of internal radiation hazard for a longer time than one of short effective half-life. In many cases, excretion is slow and there may be no way to hasten it.

In the second place, radionuclides which emit β particles do not ordinarily present a serious external radiation hazard because of the simplicity of shielding. However, once a β particle emitter such as ^{32}P enters the body, its ionizing particles are absorbed in the tissues. Obviously, there is no way of erecting a barrier against the radiation from such internally deposited emitters.

Finally, internal radionuclides in most instances are not deposited uniformly. For example, ^{90}Sr concentrates almost entirely in the bones, ^{131}I in the thyroid, and ^{32}P in the bones and in rapidly multiplying cells. Because of this uneven distribution, the laboratory worker accidentally absorbing radionuclides may suffer damage to those organs receiving the greatest concentration. Unfortunately, the problem is too complex to permit accurate localization and dosage determination. Besides, there is an element of uncertainty as to how much has entered the body in the first place during accidental contamination.

What is the maximum permissible concentration of the commonly used medical radionuclides in water, in air, and in the body? The old U.S. Bureau of Standards *Handbook 52* contained such data, and also showed the necessary calculations for deriving similar data for these and other nuclides, but we have revised them on the basis of more recent data. Table 17.04 includes the revised maximum permissible concentrations of ^{131}I and ^{32}P. The maximum permissible concentration in the total body is also called the **total body burden** of a given radionuclide. Only minute amounts are allowable in air or water. For example, if one consumes 2 quarts of water a day, equivalent to 2 liters or 2,000 milliliters (ml), then according to Table 17.04, the maximum permissible amount of ^{32}P contamination would be

$$2{,}000 \text{ ml} \times 2 \times 10^{-5} \ \mu\text{Ci/ml} = 0.04 \ \mu\text{Ci}$$

Thus, 0.04 μCi ^{32}P is the maximum permissible daily activity of this nuclide alone, assuming there is no additional radiation ex-

TABLE 17.04
MAXIMUM PERMISSIBLE CONCENTRATIONS OF ^{131}I AND ^{32}P
IN THE BODY, IN WATER, AND IN AIR*

Radioisotope	Organ	μCi in Whole Body	μCi Per ml Water	μCi Per ml Air
^{131}I	Thyroid	0.1	2×10^{-6}	3×10^{-6}
^{32}P	Bone	0.6	2×10^{-5}	2×10^{-9}

*Based on data in J. Shapiro: *Radiation Protection. A Guide for Scientists and Physicians* (Table 2.9), 1972. Courtesy of the Publisher, Harvard University Press, Cambridge, Mass.

posure. If we have a solution of ^{32}P containing 1 mCi/ml (1×10^3 μCi/ml) it would take only:

$$\frac{0.04 \ \mu Ci}{1 \times 10^3 \ \mu Ci/ml} = 4 \times 10^{-5} \ ml$$

that is, four one hundred-thousandths of an ml per day to carry the maximum permissible amount of this radionuclide. It is no wonder, therefore, that every effort must be made to prevent the entrance of radionuclides into the body except in known quantities for specific medical reasons.

It may be pointed out that in small departments relying mainly on precalibrated doses in capsule form, there is virtually no danger of internal contamination of personnel. This danger exists only when solutions are used, especially those containing large quantities of radioactive material. However, the same degree of technical care must be exercised with all radioactive liquids, in view of the minute quantities that are capable of exceeding the maximum permissible body burden.

LABORATORY DESIGN AND FACILITIES

Although the size and arrangement of the Nuclear Medicine Department may vary with the number and types of procedures, careful planning should obviate serious external and internal radiation hazards to personnel, as well as to patients. A discussion of the detailed layout will not be attempted. However, the more important general principles of laboratory design and protective devices will be presented.

Arrangement and Location. Optimum efficiency demands at least two rooms—one for receiving, preparing, and storing the radionuclides and the other for measuring samples and patients. Adequate shielding of stored material is essential as already noted. In larger departments where nuclides are received "raw" without precalibration a separate radiochemistry room facilitates proper safeguards against exposure or accidental contamination. On the other hand, for the small laboratory relying on precalibrated doses, especially in capsule form, personnel protection is greatly simplified.

The Nuclear Medicine Department should be separate from a high level nuclear research installation to avoid accidental interchange of nonmedical with medical nuclides. The same applies to large differences in levels of activity that may exist between the two facilities.

Surface Material. When liquid solutions are used, whether precalibrated or not, additional precautions must be taken against accidental spill, whereupon proper decontamination procedures must be instituted immediately. These are facilitated by having all exposed areas of floors, walls, and laboratory tables covered with nonporous material. Stainless steel or plastic trays lined with absorbent paper on which bottles containing radioactive solutions may be placed, will help to confine any spilled material.

Shielding. It is neither feasible nor necessary to provide shielding in the walls of a Nuclear Medicine Department. A more practical method is to shield the radioactive samples themselves, first with the lead shipping container. Stacked lead bricks provide additional shielding on all exposed sides. Lead is more efficient for γ-ray protection, but steel bricks fit more closely and retain their shape better than lead. The arrangement of the bricks can readily be changed as required, making for a very flexible type of barrier. Beta emitters are sufficiently shielded by their glass containers, but if they are handled at a short distance, plastic shields may be required for sufficient protection as described earlier in this chapter. The *adequacy of shielding must be checked at frequent intervals* with a survey meter. Lead-shielded syringes should be used for the injection of γ-ray emitters, and remote control methods with nuclides of high level activity, such as ^{131}I and ^{198}Au. With ^{32}P, lucite shields 7 mm ($\frac{1}{4}$ in.) thick are obtainable for various size syringes.

Decay Chamber. Since there is danger of causing further contamination in attempting to clean gloves, clothing, linens, shoes, or other materials which may have been soiled with radioactive material, they are best stored until activity has declined to a safe level. With the short half-life radionuclides used in medicine, decay for about 7 half lives, or 1 to 2 months, usually suffices. In any case, the location of the decay chamber should permit adequate shielding on all exposed sides. Before anything is removed from storage, it should be checked with a survey meter. Contaminated sponges in which radioactivity has dropped to a permissible level may then be incinerated. Glassware may be placed in the decay chamber, but if one is careful and the level of activity is low to begin with, ^{131}I may be removed by the use of an alkaline solution. ^{32}P may be removed simply by prolonged rinsing with hot water. ^{198}Au has such a short half-life that contaminated glassware should be placed in storage for a few weeks or longer depending on the activity of the material.

Oral solutions of ^{131}I or ^{32}P are most conveniently given with a drinking straw. The container is then filled several times with water, the patient drinking each refill. Both the straw and container are then stored in the decay chamber as long as necessary.

Laboratory Monitoring. Despite all precautions in handling radionuclides, the only certain method of determining whether or not accidental or incidental contamination has occurred is to survey the area with one of the instruments described earlier in this chapter. When radionuclides are used in solution, a portable survey meter serves to check the floors, bench tops, clothing, shoes, and hands. It is a good idea to place an audible G-M unit just outside the door of a high level laboratory to determine if any of the personnel accidentally harbors excessive quantities of radionuclides on the skin or clothing. If the outside surface of a container housing a radioactive sample is thought to be contaminated, or if there is any possibility of loose radioactive material on the floor or bench, a wipe test shall be done. This consists in rubbing a forceps-held piece of filter paper over the suspected area and then checking the paper with a survey meter. Such a procedure is essential in a high level (or so-called "hot") laboratory where the high background prevents instrumentation; the filter paper can be carried to the measuring room for counting with a survey meter.

All personnel shall wear an approved type of personnel monitor, usually a film badge, while on duty. Although this is quite satisfactory for whole body exposure, it is inadequate for the control of hand exposure or internal contamination. Special thermoluminescent dosimeters are available as finger rings. However, the hands should also be checked with a survey meter at least once daily, and more often in the event of suspected contamination.

DISPOSAL OF RADIOACTIVE WASTES

In the Nuclear Medicine Department we are faced with the problem of disposing of a number of radioactive waste products. These include such items as unused stocks of radionuclides, contaminated disposable materials coming into contact with the patient, cleanup rags and papers, and patients' excretions and vomitus. Fortunately, there are no longer any restrictions on the disposal of patients' excreta; these can be discharged directly into the public sewage system regardless of the dose of radionuclide the patient has received. There remains the problem of disposing of the other kinds of radioactive wastes.

1. *Sewage disposal* of unused radionuclides must not exceed the limits set by federal and state regulations for each particular nuclide, or combinations in various proportions. To be released in the public sewage system the radioactive material must be water soluble and shall not exceed the maximum permissible concentration when diluted by the effluent. For example, with ^{131}I the diluted effluent shall contain no more than 6×10^{-5} μCi/ml/day. Suppose this applied to a 200-bed hospital with an estimated average sewage flow of 200,000 liters or 2×10^8 ml/day. Then the maximum allowable sewage disposal for this institution would be

$$2 \times 10^8 \times 6 \times 10^{-5} = 12,000 \ \mu\text{Ci or 12 mCi/day}$$

In any case, the gross activity of all radionuclides released per year shall not exceed 1 Ci. As already noted, radionuclides discharged in patients' excreta are exempt from this limitation.

2. *Incineration* is covered by very strict regulations because of

atmospheric contamination. It shall not be used without specific approval by the responsible state agency. Under most circumstances in nuclear medicine it is preferable to allow contaminated materials to remain in the decay chamber until activity reaches the permissible level.

DECONTAMINATION

Any medical facility using therapeutic quantities of radioactive nuclides shall have a Radiation Safety Officer who not only sets out the proper procedures for the department, but also takes charge in the event of an accident. If necessary, he should seek consultation with the proper authorities. Because of the wide variability in the types of radionuclide procedures and the variation in the levels of activity from one department to another, routines should be established for each individual department, best suited to its needs. All that can be done here is to point out general principles which can be modified as required.

Skin contamination may be avoided by the wearing of disposable plastic or rubber gloves. However, contaminated skin should be washed with copious amounts of water and detergent until a monitor check shows no significant residual activity. Special detergents facilitate removal of various radionuclides, and should be close at hand for immediate cleansing. As a general rule, contaiminated skin should be cleansed until an end window G-M tube placed in contact indicates no more than about 100 counts/min. Contaminated open wounds should be washed thoroughly in running water, and bleeding encouraged, to aid in flushing out the radioactive material.

Contaminated clothing and linens are best handled, as already suggested, by storage in the decay chamber until a survey indicates a permissible level of radiation. Usually, 7 half-lives suffice. The count at contact with a G-M tube should not exceed about 100/min before linens are sent to the laundry. Shoes may be impossible to decontaminate, and probably can best be handled by storage or deep burial.

In any case, whenever an accident occurs, the Radiation Safety Officer should be notified immediately so that he may supervise cleanup. Each State Health Department now has experts designated on a regional basis for consultation in any type of radionuclide accident. The Radiation Safety Officer should have the phone number and address of the designated consultant posted in a conspicuous place.

RECOMMENDATIONS FOR NURSING PROCEDURES

Whenever therapeutic amounts of radionuclides are administered, the nursing personnel, whether in the hospital or in the patient's home, should be given specific instructions by the physician-in-charge, for the care of such patients, their excreta, and their linens. Obviously, such instructions are unnecessary with tracer doses.

The external hazard to nursing personnel is usually controllable, just as with laboratory personnel. It is advisable that nurses and other attendants follow the same procedures as the personnel in the Nuclear Medicine Department. Disposable plastic or rubber gloves shall be worn when significant contamination hazard is present in bed linens, bedpans, vomitus, urine, feces, or other potentially soiled articles. In addition, the nurse shall wear gloves in bathing patients who have received large doses of radionuclides. The gloves should be washed while on the hands, peeled off the hands inside out, and placed in a plastic bag to be monitored for residual activity by a qualified person. If contamination of nurses' hands is suspected, they shall be washed and receive a monitor survey. All contaminated linens must be placed in specially marked plastic bag to be saved for monitoring. All linens shall be checked before laundering.

Special Nursing Instructions With Radioiodine (^{131}I). No special instructions are required for tracer doses. However, with ^{131}I in the treatment of **hyperthyroidism**, only a few recommendations are necessary. Visiting need not be restricted, and there is no danger to patients in adjacent beds. If the patient is ambulatory, he should use the bathroom. Otherwise, for the first 3 days, the nurse shall handle the bedpan with disposable plastic or rubber gloves and take the precautions described above. If the patient is incontinent of urine, the linens shall be saved in a disposable plastic bag for monitor survey by a responsible member of the Nuclear Medicine Department. Contaminated linens shall be handled only with gloves as above. The same precautions apply to vomitus. No special precautions are required for feces.

When ^{131}I is given in large doses in the treatment of *thyroid carcinoma* or for inhibition of the thyroid gland in *heart disease*, that is, 25 mCi or more, the urine is heavily loaded with excreted radionuclide for the first few days. All nursing personnel in charge of the patient should wear film badges or equivalent monitoring devices. The same nursing precautions are to be taken as in treatment of hyperthyroidism with ^{131}I: gloves must be worn in attending the patient and in handling urinals, bedpans, linens, catheters, and emesis basins. No baths shall be given during the first 2 days following the administration of ^{131}I at this activity level. Ordinarily, the external radiation hazard poses no significant problem, but this should be checked by some responsible member of the Nuclear Medicine Department. We can determine the shortest permissible distance by the use of equation (11):

$$d = 20\sqrt{\Gamma\ mCi}\ \text{cm}$$

For example, a patient receives 150 mCi of ^{131}I. What is the minimum working distance for nursing personnel during the first day? Table 17.02 shows Γ for ^{131}I to be 2.18. Substituting these values in the equation,

$$d = 20\sqrt{2.18 \times 150}$$

$$d = 20\sqrt{327}$$

$$d = 360\ \text{cm or 140 in. or 12 ft}$$

This means that at a distance of 12 feet, the hourly maximum permissible whole body exposure of a nurse attending the patient will not be exceeded, during an 8-hour working day. Approximately the same results are obtained with ^{198}Au because the Γ is nearly the same for both radionuclides. If the nurse works closer to the patient, say at a 30-cm (1-ft) distance, the hourly exposure will be 12^2 or 144 times as great, and therefore it will be permissible to work only 1/144 as long or 8/144 hr or about 3 min out of a total 8-hour working day. At a 60-cm (2-ft.) working distance the hourly exposure will be $\frac{1}{4}$ as great as at 1 ft. and it will be permissible to work at the 2 ft. distance for a period of 12 min. out of each 8-hour day. Table 17.05 shows the approximate permissible exposure of nursing personnel at various distances from patients receiving ^{131}I or ^{198}Au therapy. The corresponding figures for radium are also shown for comparison. It should be emphasized that the exposure of nursing personnel to patients undergoing internal radium therapy is even more serious than with ^{131}I or ^{198}Au. For example, 50 mg of radium presents about the same external radiation hazard to nurses as does 150 mCi of ^{131}I or ^{198}Au. This external hazard may be minimized by spending the least possible amount of time in the vicinity of the patient, compatible with adequate patient care. Nurses should be trained to plan carefully every step of a procedure which they are about to carry out, before approaching the patient, so that it can be completed efficiently in the shortest possible time. Rotation of nursing personnel will aid in maintaining exposure within permissible limits.

Special Nursing Instructions With Radiophosphorus (^{32}P). Since ^{32}P is a pure β emitter, it does not pose a significant external hazard. Furthermore, no precautions are necessary other than plastic gloves if the patient is incontinent or vomits during the first 24 hours, but contaminated linens shall be placed in a plastic bag and a responsible member of the Nuclear Medicine

TOTAL 17.05
MINIMUM PERMISSIBLE WORKING DISTANCES AND DAILY EXPOSURE
TIMES FOR PERSONNEL ATTENDING PATIENTS RECEIVING
VARIOUS DOSES OF RADIONUCLIDES

^{131}I or ^{198}Au (first 2 days)	Ra or Rn	Maximum Permissible Daily Exposure Times in Minutes for Various Distances			
mCi	mCi	30 cm (1 ft)	60 cm (2 ft)	1 m (3 ft)	2 m (6 ft)
25	—	20	90	200	800
50	—	10	45	100	400
150	50	3	15	35	140
200	—	2½	12	25	100
300	100	1½	7½	17	70

Department notified about the incident. No special precautions are required for colloidal ^{32}P, except for possible leakage from the puncture wound. Dressings should be changed only when directed by the physician in charge. All dressings shall be saved in a plastic bag and monitored as already described. If dressings become stained, wet, or bloody, a responsible member of the Nuclear Medicine Department must be notified immediately.

Special Nursing Instructions With Radiogold (^{198}Au). It is assumed that the ^{198}Au has been introduced into the pleural or abdominal cavity under direct supervision of the physician in charge of radionuclide procedures, or some responsible person designated by him. The nurses then caring for the patient should be carefully monitored for several days. Since ^{198}Au is a γ as well as a β emitter, the handling of the patient and all other items such as linens, urinals, and bedpans should follow the same rules as with patients receiving ^{131}I for cancer. Plastic or rubber gloves must always be worn, of course. These precautions shall be taken during the first 48 hrs. Dressings from paracentesis or thoracentesis wounds shall be placed only in waterproof containers, clearly labeled, and sent to the Nuclear Medicine Department. The handling of the equipment used in administering the ^{198}Au shall be under direct supervision of qualified personnel. Because of the short half-life of ^{198}Au, contaminated articles can most readily be taken care of by storage in the decay chamber. The external hazards are about the same as those with equal doses of ^{131}I, as shown in Table 17.05.

UNSAFE PRACTICES IN HANDLING RADIONUCLIDES

The Atomic Energy Commission found, in the course of conducting periodic surveys, that certain improper procedures, from the standpoint of radiation safety, were frequently encountered. They suggest the corrective steps for each of these unsafe practices, the most prevalent of which will now be listed.

1. *Inadequate Planning of Procedures.* All procedures involving radionuclides, especially new and untried ones, should be carefully planned in advance. Trial runs with inactive dummy samples will increase the speed of operation, thereby reducing exposure.

2. *Improper Monitoring.* The safety monitoring instruments should be carefully selected, and the operator should thoroughly familiarize himself with their operation. Ionization chambers are best for quantitative work, such as accurate calibration of samples. G-M tubes may be used for qualitative work, to detect dangerous levels of contamination. Personnel monitoring instruments or film badges should be selected, depending on the type and amount of radiation, and type of procedure being used.

3. *Inadequate Shielding.* The proper shielding materials, adequate in thickness, should be selected as barriers against primary and scattered radiation.

4. *Inadequate Use of Trays and Paper Covering.* All work surfaces should be covered with absorbent paper which can be taken up in the event of spill. Trays should be used under all apparatus and equipment to confine accidental spill.

5. *Pipetting by Mouth.* Of all improper procedures, this is one of the most pernicious and should never be allowed. A hand-operated, remote control pipetting device should always be used.

6. *Poor Work Habits.* These often develop along with familiarity with certain procedures. Familiarity should never breed contempt for radiation safety.

7. *Inadequate Use of Protective Clothing.* Plastic or rubber gloves should be worn whenever solutions of radionuclides in more than tracer amounts, or contaminated articles, are handled. In certain high level operations, such as one may encounter in research facilities, special clothing may be required.

8. *Improper Disposal.* The disposal of radioactive wastes should always be preceded by careful study of the available facilities, and the proper methods planned in advance.

9. *Improper Fume Hoods.* These are unnecessary in the vast majority of clinical departments. However, when required for high level activity, the hood should be properly designed for air intake and exhaust, without excess turbulence.

10. *Changing Types or Levels of Activity and Procedures* without reorientation as to procedures and equipment may jeopardize personnel safety.

11. *Failure to Maintain Detailed Radiation Safety Records.* Complete records shall be kept in the Nuclear Medicine Depart-

ment covering surveys, waste disposal, and personnel exposure. The latter shall include film badge reports and/or dosimeter readings with the corresponding dates. Accidents shall also be recorded, as well as the decontamination procedures employed.

12. *Failure to Post Signs.* Approved signs shall be posted to mark work, storage, and disposal areas, and on all doors leading into rooms that contain an actual or potential radiation hazard.

References

1. Andrews, J.R., and Moody, J.M.: The dose-time relationship in radiotherapy. *Am J Roentgenol, 75:*590, 1956.
2. Attix, F.H., and Ritz, V.H.: A determination of the gamma-ray emission of radium. *J Res NBS, 59:*293, 1957.
3. Barendsen, G.W.: Responses of cultured cells, tumors, and normal tissues to radiations of different linear energy transfer. In Ebert, M., and Howard, A. (Eds.): *Current Topics in Radiation Research.* Amsterdam, North Holland Publishing Co., 1968, vol. IV.
4. Berger, M.J.: MIRD pamphlet No. 7. *J Nucl Med* (Suppl. 5), *12:* 1971.
5. Blahd, W.H.: *Nuclear Medicine.* New York, McGraw, 1971.
6. Bond, V.P.: Negative pions: Their possible use in radiotherapy. *Am J Roentgenol, 111:*9, 1971.
7. Braestrup, C.B., and Wyckoff, H.O.: Shielding designs for radiology departments. *Radiology, 107:*445, 1973.
8. British Hospital Physicists' Association: Depth dose tables for use in radiotherapy. *Br J Radiol,* Suppl. 10. 1961.
9. Case, J.T.: The early history of radium therapy and the American Radium Society. *Am J Roentgenol, 82:*574, 1959.
10. Catterall, M., Rogers, C., Thomlinson, R.H., and Field, S.B.: Investigation into the clinical effects of fast neutrons: methods and early observations. *Br J Radiol, 44:*603, 1971.
11. Cohen, L.: Radiation response and recovery. In Schwartz, E.E. (Ed.): *The Biological Basis of Radiation Therapy.* Philadelphia, Lippincott, 1966, pp. 266–267.
12. Cohen, L.: Radiotherapy in breast cancer. *Br J Radiol 25:*636. 1952.
13. Cohen, L., and Shapiro, M.P.: Practical applications. *Br J Radiol, 25:*643, 1952.
14. Corrigan, K.E., and Hayden, H.S.: Diagnostic studies with radioactive isotope tracers. *Radiology, 59:*1, 1952.
15. Coutard, H.: Roentgenotherapy of epitheliomas of the tonsillar region, hypopharynx, and larynx from 1920–1926. *Am J Roentgenol, 28:*313, 1932.
16. DeMoor, N.G., Durbach, D., Levin, J., and Cohen, L.: Radiation therapy in breast cancer; optimal combination of technical factors; analysis of five-year results. *Radiology, 77:*35, 1961.
17. Demy, N.G.: Beam localization and depth dose determination. *Radiology, 51:* 89, 1948.
18. Duffy, J.J., Arneson, A.N., and Voke, F.L.: The rate of recuperation of human skin following irradiation. *Radiology, 33:*486, 1934.
19. Duffy, J.J., McNattin, R.F., Copeland, M., and Quimby, E.H.: The relative effects produced by 200 kV roentgen rays, 700 kV roentgen rays, and gamma

rays. V. Comparison based on the production of erythema in the human skin. *Am J Roentgenol, 29:*343, 1933.

20. Duncan, W., Green, D., and Meredith, W.J.: Consideration of the uses of 14-MeV fast neutrons for radiotherapy. *Br J Radiol, 44:*713, 1971.

21. Elkind, M.M.: Cellular aspects of tumor therapy. *Radiology, 74:*529, 1960.

22. Elkind, M.M., Sutton, H., and Moses, W.B.: Postirradiation survival kinetics of mammalian cells grown in culture. *J Cell Physiol, 58:*113, 1961.

23. Ellinger, F.: *Medical Radiation Biology.* Springfield, Thomas, 1957.

24. Ellis, F.: Dose, time, and fractionation: a clinical hypothesis. *Clin Radiol, 20:* 1, 1969.

25. Fanger, H., and Lushbaugh, C.C.: Radiation death from cardiovascular shock following a criticality accident. *Arch Pathol, 83:*446, 1967.

26. Fedoruk, S.O., and Johns, H.E.: Transmission dose measurements for cobalt 60 radiation with special reference to rotation therapy. *Br J Radiol, 30:*190, 1957.

27. Feola, J., and Marayuma, Y.: Radiobiologic considerations of pions in radio-therapy. *Oncology, 25:*536, 1971.

28. Fields, T., and Seed, L.: *Clinical Use of Radioisotopes.* Chicago, Year Bk, 1961.

29. Fowler, J.F.: High-LET radiation: clinical facilities available with neutron beams. *Radiology, 108:*139, 1973.

30. Friedell, H.L., Thomas, C.I., and Krohmer, J.S.: An evaluation of the clinical use of a strontium 90 beta ray applicator with a review of the underlying principles. *Am J Roentgenol, 71:*25, 1954.

31. Friedman, M., Southard, M.E., and Ellet, W.: Supervoltage (2 MeV) rotation irradiation of carcinoma of the head and neck. *Am J Roentgenol, 81:*402, 1959.

32. Garcia, M.: Further observations on tissue dosage in cancer of the cervix uteri. *Am J Roentgenol, 73:*35, 1955.

33. Glasser, O., et al.: *Physical Foundations of Radiology.* New York, Hoeber, 1959.

34. Glucksmann, A.: Response of human tissues to radiation with special reference to differentiation. *Br J Radiol, 25:*38, 1952.

35. Goodwin, P.N., Quimby, E.H., and Morgan, R.H.: *Physical Foundations of Radiology.* New York, Har-Row, 1970.

36. Greenfield, M.A., Tichman, M., and Norman, A.: Dosage tables for linear radium sources filtered by 0.5 and 1.0 mm of platinum. *Radiology, 73:*418, 1959.

37. Hale, C.H., and Holmes, G.W.: Carcinoma of skin: influence of dosage on success of treatment. *Radiology, 48:*563, 1947.

38. Hall, E.J.: Radiobiology of heavy particle radiation therapy. Cellular studies. *Radiology, 108:*119, 1973.

39. Hall, E.J., Rossi, H.H., and Roizin, L.A.: Low dose rate irradiation of mam-malian cells with radium and 252-californium: comparison of effects on actively proliferating cell population. *Radiology, 99:*445, 1971.

40. Hendee, W.R.: *Medical Radiation Physics.* Chicago, Year Bk, 1970.

41. Hewitt, H.B., and Wilson, C.W.: Survival curves of tumor cells irradiated *in vitro. Ann NY Acad Sci, 95:*818, 1961.
42. Jacobsson, F.: Carcinoma of hypopharynx, clinical study of 322 cases, treated at Radiumhemmet, from 1939 to 1947. *Acta Radiol, 35:*1, 1951.
43. Johns, H.E.: Physical aspects of rotation therapy. *Am J Roentgenol, 79:*373, 1958.
44. Johns, H.E., and Cunningham, J.R.: *The Physics of Radiology.* Springfield, Thomas, 1969.
45. Jolles, B.: *X-ray Sieve (Grid) Therapy in Cancer: A Connective Tissue Problem.* Boston, Little, 1953.
46. Jones, C.H., and Dermentzoglu, F.: Practical aspects of ^{90}Sr ophthalmic applicator dosimetry. *Br J Radiol, 44:*203, 1971.
47. Kaplan, H.S., Schwettman, H.A., Fairbank, W.M., Boyd, D., and Bagshaw, M.A.: A hospital-based superconducting accelerator facility for negative pi-meson beam radiotherapy. *Radiology, 108:*159, 1973.
48. Kohn, H.I., and Kallman, R.F.: Age, growth, and the LD_{50} of X Rays. *Science, 124:*1078, 1956.
49. Krishnaswamy, V.: Dose distributions about ^{137}Cs sources in tissue. *Radiology, 105:*181, 1972.
50. Lea, D.E.: *Actions of Radiations on Living Cells.* New York, Macmillan, 1947.
51. Lidén, K.: SI units in radiology and radiation measurement. *Radiology, 107:*463, 1973.
52. Martin, C.L., and Martin, J.A.: *Low Intensity Radium Therapy.* Boston, Little, 1959.
53. Massey, J.B.: *Manual of Dosimetry in Radiotherapy,* Technical Reports Series 110, Vienna, International Atomic Energy Agency, 1970.
54. Mathé, G., Jammet, H., and Pendic, B.: Transfusions et greffes de moelle osseuse homologue chez des humains irradiés a haute dose accidentellement. *Rev Eur Étud Clin Biol, 4:*226, 1959.
55. Mayneord, W.V., and Lamerton, L.F.: A survey of depth dose data. *Br J Radiol, 14:*255, 1941.
56. Meredith, W.J.: *Radium Dosage. The Manchester System.* Edinburgh, 2nd ed., Baltimore, Williams & Wilkins, 1963.
57. Meredith, W.J., and Massey, J.B.: *Fundamental Physics of Radiology.* Baltimore, Williams & Wilkins, 1972.
58. Meredith, W.J., and Stephenson, S.K.: Calculation of dosage and an additional distribution rule for cylindric "volume" implantation with radium. *Br J Radiol, 18:*45, 1945.
59. Neary, G.J.: Dose measurements with radium beta ray applicators. *Br J Radiol, 19:*357, 1946.
60. Nuttall, J.R., and Spiers, F.W.: Dosage control in interstitial radium therapy. *Br J Radiol, 19:*135, 1946.
61. Oddie, T.H.: A method of routine preparation of radon. *Br J Radiol, 10:*348, 1937.
62. Oddie, T.H.: A note on dosage data for radium therapy. *Br J Radiol, 13:*389, 1940.

63. Osgood, E.E.: The relative dosage required of total body X ray vs. intravenous ^{32}P for equal effectiveness against leukemic cells of the lymphatic series or granulocyte series in chronic leukemia. *J Nucl Med, 6:*421, 1965.

64. Paterson, R., and Parker, H.M.: A dosage system for gamma-ray therapy. *Br J Radiol, 7:*592, 1934.

65. Paterson, R., Parker, H.M., and Spiers, F.W.: A system of dosage for cylindrical distributions of radium. *Br J Radiol, 9:*487, 1936.

66. Paterson, R.: *The Treatment of Malignant Disease by Radium and X Rays.* London, Arnold. 2nd edition, 1963.

67. Paterson, R., and Parker, H.M.: A dosage system for interstitial radium therapy. *Br J Radiol, 11:*252 and 313, 1938.

68. Powers, W.E., and Tolmach, I.J.: Demonstration of an anoxic component in a mouse tumor cell population by *in vivo* assay of survival following irradiation. *Radiology, 83:*328, 1964.

69. Proctor, B., Lofstrom, J.E., and Nurnberger, C.E.: The use of contact therapy in the treatment of carcinoma of the larynx. *Laryngoscope, 58:*000, 1948.

70. Puck, T.T., and Marcus, P.I.: Action of X rays on mammalian cells. *J Exp Med, 103:*653, 1956.

71. Puck, T.T., Marcus, P.I., and Cieciura, S.J.: Clonal growth of mammalian cells *in vitro*. *J Exp Med, 103:*272, 1956..

72. Quimby, E.H., and Laurence, G.C.: The radiological society of North America standardization committee, Technical Bulletin No. 1. *Radiology, 35:*138, 1940.

73. Quimby, E.H., and McComb, W.S.: Further studies on the rate of recovery of human skin from the effects of roentgen or gamma-ray irradiation. *Radiology, 29:*305, 1937.

74. Reisner, A.: Hauterythem und Röntgenstrahlen. *Ergebn Med Strahlenforsch, 6:*1, 1933.

75. Rogers, A.W.: *Technique of Autoradiography.* New York, Elseviere, 1967.

76. Sheline, G.E., Phillips, T.E., Field, S.B., Brennan, J.T., and Raventos, A.: Effects of fast neutrons on human skin. *Am J Roentgenol, 111:*31, 1971.

77. Shipman, T.L., Lushbaugh, C.C., Petersen, D.F., Langhans, W.H., Harris, P.S., and Lawrence, J.N.P.: Acute radiation death resulting from accidental nuclear excursion. *J Occup Med, 3:*145, 1961.

78. Sinclair, W.K., and Blackwell, L.H. in *Radiation Biology in Cancer.* Austin, U. of Tex. Pr., 1958.

79. Sinclair, W.K., and Blondal, H.: ^{32}P beta sources for superficial therapy. *Br J Radiol, 25:*360, 1952.

80. Strandqvist, M.: Studien über die kumulative Wirkung der Röntgenstrahlen bei der Fractioneerung. *Acta Radiol.* (Suppl. 55), 1944.

81. Suit, H.D.: Radiation biology: a basis for radiotherapy. In Fletcher, G.H. (Ed.): *Textbook of Radiotherapy.* Philadelphia, Lea & Febiger, 1966, p. 93.

82. Thiessen, A.: Design study of π^- beams for biomedical applications at LAMPF. *Los Alamos Scientific Laboratory Document LA-DC 9789,* 1968.

83. Tod, M.C., and Meredith, W.J.: A dosage system for use in the treatment of cancer of the uterine cervix. *Br J Radiol, 11:*809, 1938.

84. Tong, E.C.K.: Parathormone and ^{32}P therapy in prostatic cancer with bone metastases. *Radiology, 98:*343, 1971.
85. Trump, J.G., Wright, K.A., Evans, W.W., Anson, J.H., Hare, H.E., Fromer, J.L., Jacque, G., and Horne, K.: High energy electrons for the treatment of extensive superficial malignant lesions. *Am J Roentgenol, 69:*623, 1953.
86. Von Borstel, R.C.: Effects of radiation on cells. In Schwartz, E.E. (Ed.): *The Biological Basis of Radiation Therapy.* Philadelphia, Lippincott, 1966, p. 79.
87. von Essen, C.F.: Roentgen therapy of skin and lip carcinoma: factors influencing success and failure. *Am J Roentgenol, 83:*556, 1960.
88. Wachsmann, F.: Neue Gesichtpunkte fur Ermittlung der Dosis bei der Bestrahlung tiefliegender Herde. *Strahlentherapie, 87:*253, 1952.
89. White, T.N., Marinelli, L.D., and Failla, G.: Measurement of gamma radiation in roentgens. *Am J Roentgenol, 44:*889, 1940.
90. Withers, H.R.: Biologic basis for high-LET radiotherapy. *Radiology, 108:* 131, 1973.
91. Wright, C.N., Boulogne, A.R., Reinig, W.C., and Evans, A.G.: Implantable californium 252 neutron sources for radiotherapy. *Radiology, 89:*337, 1967.

General Bibliography

Cloutier, R.J., Edwards, C.L., and Snyder, W.S.: *Medical Radionuclides: Radiation Dose and Effects*. United States Atomic Energy Commission, 1970.

Conference on Radiobiology and Radiotherapy, *Natl Cancer Inst Monogr (No. 24)*. Washington, U.S. Department of Health, Education and Welfare, 1967.

Dalrymple, G.V., Gaulden, M.E., Kollmorgen, G.M., and Vogel, H.H., Jr.: *Medical Radiation Biology*. Philadelphia, Saunders, 1973.

Early, P.J., Razzak, M.A., and Sodee, D.B.: *Textbook of Nuclear Medicine Technology*. St. Louis, Mosby, 1969.

Fields, T., and Seed, L.: *Clinical Use of Radioisotopes*. Chicago, Year Bk, 1961.

Fletcher, G.H.: *Textbook of Radiotherapy*. Philadelphia, Lea & Febiger, 1973.

Goodwin, P., Quimby, E.H., and Morgan, R.H.: *Physical Foundations of Radiology*. New York, Har-Row, 1970.

Hall, E.J.: *Radiobiology for the Radiologist*. New York, Har-Row, 1973.

Hendee, W.R.: *Medical Radiation Physics*. Chicago, Year Bk Med, 1970.

International Commission on Radiologic Units and Measurements (ICRU): *Handbook, 87, Clinical Dosimetry*. 1963.

International Commission on Radiation Units and Measurements (ICRU): *Report 20*. 1971.

Jackson, H.L.: *Basic Nuclear Physics for Medical Personnel*. Springfield, Thomas, 1973.

Johns, H.E., and Cunningham, J.R.: *The Physics of Radiology*. Springfield, Thomas, 1969.

Lea, D.E.: *Action of Radiation on Living Cells*. New York, Macmillan, 1947.

Meredith, W.J., and Massey, J.B.: *Fundamental Physics of Radiology*. Baltimore, Williams & Wilkins, 1972.

Moss, W.T., Brand, N.W., and Battifora, H.: *Therapeutic Radiology. Rationale, Technique, Results*. St. Louis, Mosby, 1973.

Murphy, W.T.: *Radiation Therapy*. Philadelphia, Saunders, 1967.

National Council on Radiation Protection and Measurements (NCRP): Reports, NCRP P.O. Box 4867, Washington, D.C., 20008.

24. *Protection Against Radiations from Sealed Gamma Sources* (1960).
30. *Safe Handling of Radioactive Materials* (1964).
33. *Medical X-ray and Gamma-ray Protection for Energies up to 10 MeV—Equipment Design and Use* (1968).
34. *Medical X-ray and Gamma-ray Protection for Energies up to 10 MeV—Structural Shielding Design and Evaluation* (1970).
37. *Precautions in the Management of Patients Who Have Received Therapeutic Amounts of Radionuclides* (1970).
39. *Basic Radiation Protection Criteria* (1971).
40. *Protection Against Radiation from Brachytherapy Sources* (1972).

675

Pizzarello, D.J., and Witcofski, R.L.: *Basic Radiation Biology*. Philadelphia, Lea & Febiger, 1967.

Purdom, C.E.: *Genetic Effects of Radiation*. New York, Acad Pr, 1963.

Schwartz, E.E.: *The Biological Basis of Radiation Therapy*. Philadelphia, Lippincott, 1966.

Shapiro, J.: *Radiation Protection. A Guide for Scientists and Physicians*. Cambridge, Harvard U Pr, 1972.

Stanton, L.: *Basic Medical Radiation Physics*. New York, Appleton, 1969.

Van Cleave, C.D.: *Late Somatic Effects of Ionizing Radiation*. United States Atomic Energy Commission. 1968.

Appendix

Tables A-1 through A-6 are adapted from Johns, H. E., and Cunningham, J.R.: *The Physics of Radiology*, 1969. Courtesy of Charles C Thomas, Publisher, Springfield.

Tables A-7 through A-9 are from Supplement 10. Courtesy of British Journal of Radiology.

TABLE A-1
CENTRAL AXIS PERCENTAGE DEPTH DOSES FOR SQUARE FIELDS

HVL 1.0 mm Cu   TSD 50 cm

Depth in cm	0	16	25	36	50	64	81	100	225	400	Depth in cm
*	100.0	118.0	121.1	125.2	127.9	131.1	133.3	135.7	143.0	148.7	*
0	100.0	100.0	100.0	100.0	100.0	100.0	100.0	100.0	100.0	100.0	0
1	79.0	92.0	94.7	96.9	97.9	99.1	99.8	100.6	102.6	103.0	1
2	63.0	81.3	84.3	87.9	89.6	91.6	92.8	94.0	97.0	98.4	2
3	50.5	70.3	73.5	77.4	79.8	82.5	84.2	86.1	90.9	93.4	3
4	40.5	60.0	63.2	67.2	69.7	72.6	74.5	76.6	82.8	86.1	4
5	32.5	50.7	53.8	57.7	60.2	63.2	65.2	67.3	74.0	77.8	5
6	26.3	42.7	45.5	49.2	51.6	54.6	56.6	58.8	65.6	69.7	6
7	21.3	35.8	38.3	41.7	44.1	46.9	48.9	51.1	57.9	62.2	7
8	17.3	29.9	32.2	35.3	37.6	40.2	42.1	44.2	50.9	55.3	8
9	14.0	25.0	27.1	29.9	32.0	34.4	36.2	38.2	44.6	49.1	9
10	11.3	20.9	22.8	25.3	27.2	29.4	31.1	32.9	39.0	43.4	10
11	9.1	17.4	19.2	21.4	23.1	25.1	26.6	28.3	34.0	38.2	11
12	7.4	14.6	16.2	18.1	19.6	21.4	22.7	24.3	29.6	33.5	12
13	5.9	12.2	13.6	15.3	16.6	18.3	19.4	20.8	25.8	29.3	13
14	4.8	10.2	11.4	12.9	14.1	15.6	16.6	17.8	22.4	25.7	14
15	3.9	8.6	9.6	10.9	12.0	13.2	14.2	15.3	19.4	22.5	15
16	3.2	7.2	8.1	9.2	10.2	11.2	12.1	13.1	16.9	19.7	16
17	2.6	6.0	6.8	7.8	8.6	9.5	10.3	11.2	14.7	17.2	17
18	2.1	5.0	5.7	6.6	7.3	8.1	8.8	9.6	12.7	15.1	18
19	1.7	4.2	4.8	5.6	6.2	7.0	7.6	8.3	11.0	13.2	19
20	1.4	3.5	4.0	4.7	5.3	6.0	6.5	7.1	9.5	11.5	20

* This line gives the dose (including backscatter) to a small mass of tissue at the surface, for 100 rads of primary radiation (without backscatter) to the same mass of tissue. Division by 100 gives the backscatter factor.

677

TABLE A-2
CENTRAL AXIS PERCENTAGE DEPTH DOSES FOR SQUARE FIELDS

HVL 2.0 mm Cu   TSD 50 cm

Depth in cm	0	16	25	36	50	64	81	100	225	400	Depth in cm
			Field area in cm² (open-ended applicator)								
*	100.0	114.4	116.9	120.1	122.2	124.8	126.5	128.6	135.8	141.5	*
0	100.0	100.0	100.0	100.0	100.0	100.0	100.0	100.0	100.0	100.0	0
1	81.4	93.8	95.2	96.8	97.7	98.6	99.3	99.9	101.7	102.4	1
2	66.5	83.9	85.9	88.4	89.8	91.4	92.5	93.6	96.9	98.9	2
3	54.0	72.5	75.2	78.6	80.6	83.0	84.5	86.1	90.9	93.6	3
4	44.2	62.1	65.0	68.7	71.0	73.6	75.4	77.4	83.4	86.8	4
5	36.2	52.9	55.7	59.5	61.9	64.7	66.6	68.7	75.1	79.1	5
6	29.6	44.9	47.6	51.3	53.7	56.5	58.5	60.6	67.3	71.6	6
7	24.3	38.0	40.6	44.1	46.4	49.2	51.1	53.2	60.1	64.6	7
8	19.9	32.1	34.6	37.8	40.1	42.7	44.5	46.6	53.5	58.1	8
9	16.4	27.1	29.4	32.4	34.5	37.0	38.7	40.7	47.5	52.1	9
10	13.4	22.9	25.0	27.7	29.7	32.0	33.6	35.5	42.0	46.5	10
11	11.1	19.4	21.3	23.6	25.5	27.6	29.1	30.9	37.1	41.4	11
12	9.1	16.5	18.1	20.2	21.9	23.8	25.2	26.9	32.7	36.7	12
13	7.5	14.0	15.4	17.3	18.8	20.5	21.8	23.4	28.7	32.5	13
14	6.2	11.9	13.1	14.8	16.1	17.6	18.9	20.3	25.2	28.7	14
15	5.1	10.1	11.2	12.7	13.8	15.2	16.3	17.6	22.2	25.4	15
16	4.2	8.5	9.5	10.9	11.8	13.1	14.1	15.2	19.5	22.5	16
17	3.5	7.2	8.1	9.3	10.1	11.3	12.2	13.2	17.2	19.9	17
18	2.9	6.1	6.9	7.9	8.7	9.8	10.5	11.5	15.2	17.6	18
19	2.4	5.2	5.9	6.7	7.5	8.4	9.1	10.0	13.4	15.6	19
20	2.0	4.4	4.9	5.7	6.4	7.2	7.9	8.7	11.7	13.7	20

*This line gives the dose (including backscatter) to a small mass of tissue at the surface, for 100 rads of primary radiation (without backscatter) to the same mass of tissue. Division by 100 gives the backscatter factor.

TABLE A-3
CENTRAL AXIS PERCENTAGE DEPTH DOSES FOR SQUARE FIELDS

HVL 3.0 mm Cu   TSD 50 cm

Depth in cm	0	16	25	36	50	64	81	100	225	400	Depth in cm
*	100.0	111.6	113.7	116.4	118.2	120.4	121.9	123.7	129.6	133.7	*
0	100.0	100.0	100.0	100.0	100.0	100.0	100.0	100.0	100.0	100.0	0
1	82.3	93.9	95.1	96.5	97.1	97.9	98.3	98.9	100.6	101.4	1
2	68.0	84.6	86.2	88.3	89.4	90.7	91.6	92.6	95.6	96.8	2
3	56.2	73.7	76.0	78.8	80.5	82.4	83.7	85.1	89.5	92.3	3
4	46.4	63.1	65.8	69.0	71.0	73.4	74.9	76.7	82.1	85.7	4
5	38.6	54.2	56.7	60.1	62.2	64.8	66.5	68.4	74.5	78.3	5
6	32.0	46.3	48.7	52.0	54.2	56.8	58.6	60.6	67.0	71.3	6
7	26.5	39.3	41.7	44.9	47.1	49.7	51.5	53.6	60.1	64.2	7
8	22.0	33.4	35.7	38.7	40.9	43.4	45.2	47.2	53.7	57.9	8
9	18.4	28.5	30.6	33.4	35.4	37.8	39.6	41.5	47.9	52.0	9
10	15.4	24.3	26.2	28.7	30.6	32.8	34.5	36.3	42.6	46.7	10
11	12.8	20.7	22.4	24.7	26.4	28.5	30.0	31.7	37.7	41.7	11
12	10.7	17.6	19.1	21.2	22.8	24.8	26.1	27.7	33.3	37.2	12
13	9.0	15.1	16.3	18.2	19.7	21.5	22.7	24.2	29.4	33.1	13
14	7.5	12.9	14.0	15.7	17.0	18.6	19.7	21.1	25.9	29.4	14
15	6.3	11.0	12.0	13.5	14.6	16.1	17.1	18.4	22.9	26.2	15
16	5.3	9.4	10.3	11.6	12.6	13.9	14.9	16.0	20.2	23.2	16
17	4.5	8.0	8.8	10.0	10.9	12.0	13.0	13.9	17.8	20.7	17
18	3.7	6.8	7.5	8.6	9.4	10.4	11.3	12.2	15.7	18.5	18
19	3.1	5.8	6.4	7.4	8.1	9.0	9.8	10.7	13.9	16.4	19
20	2.6	4.9	5.5	6.3	7.0	7.8	8.5	9.3	12.3	14.5	20

*This line gives the dose (including backscatter) to a small mass of tissue at the surface, for 100 rads of primary radiation (without backscatter) to the same mass of tissue. Division by 100 gives the backscatter factor.

The Basic Physics of Radiation Therapy

TABLE A-4
CENTRAL AXIS PERCENTAGE DEPTH DOSES FOR SQUARE FIELDS

Cobalt 60				*Open-ended applicator*					60 cm SSD	
Depth in cm				Field area in cm^2						Depth in cm
	0	16	25	36	49	64	81	100	225	400	
*	100.0	101.5	101.8	102.2	102.5	102.9	103.2	103.5	105.1	106.3	*
0				Surface dose 30 to 50% depending upon collimator							0
0.5	100.0	100.0	100.0	100.0	100.0	100.0	100.0	100.0	100.0	100.0	0.5
1	95.0	96.5	96.7	97.0	97.2	97.4	97.5	97.7	98.0	98.1	1
2	86.0	98.7	90.2	90.8	91.2	91.7	91.9	92.1	92.7	93.0	2
3	77.9	83.2	83.9	84.8	85.3	86.0	86.3	86.6	87.5	88.0	3
4	70.7	77.0	77.8	78.9	79.6	80.3	80.7	81.2	82.4	83.1	4
5	64.2	71.0	71.9	73.2	74.0	74.8	75.3	75.9	77.4	78.3	5
6	58.3	65.4	66.4	67.7	68.6	69.5	70.0	70.7	72.5	73.7	6
7	53.0	60.1	61.2	62.5	63.4	64.4	64.9	65.6	67.8	69.2	7
8	48.2	55.1	56.2	57.6	58.4	59.5	60.1	60.8	63.3	64.9	8
9	43.9	50.4	51.5	53.0	53.8	54.9	55.6	56.3	59.0	60.9	9
10	39.9	46.1	47.2	48.7	49.5	50.6	51.3	52.1	54.9	57.0	10
11	36.3	42.2	43.3	44.8	45.6	46.7	47.4	48.2	51.1	53.4	11
12	33.1	38.7	39.8	41.2	42.0	43.1	43.8	44.6	47.6	50.0	12
13	30.2	35.5	36.5	37.9	38.7	39.8	40.5	41.3	44.4	46.9	13
14	27.5	32.5	33.5	34.8	35.7	36.7	37.5	38.2	41.4	43.9	14
15	25.1	29.8	30.8	32.0	32.9	33.9	34.6	35.4	38.6	41.1	15
16	22.9	27.4	28.3	29.4	30.3	31.3	32.0	32.8	36.0	38.5	16
17	20.9	25.2	26.1	27.1	28.0	28.9	29.6	30.4	33.6	36.1	17
18	19.1	23.2	24.0	25.0	25.8	26.7	27.4	28.2	31.4	33.9	18
19	17.4	21.3	22.1	23.0	23.8	24.7	25.4	26.2	29.3	31.8	19
20	15.9	19.5	20.3	21.1	21.9	22.8	23.4	24.2	27.3	29.8	20

*This line gives the dose at maximum (5 mm depth), for 100 rads to a small mass of tissue (equilibrium thickness) at the same location in "free space." Division by 100 gives the backscatter factor.

TABLE A-5
CENTRAL AXIS PERCENTAGE DEPTH DOSES FOR SQUARE FIELDS

Cobalt 60				Open ended applicator						80 cm SSD
Depth in cm				Field area in cm²						Depth in cm
	0	16	25	36	49	64	81	100	225	400	
*	100.0	101.5	101.8	102.2	102.5	102.9	103.2	103.5	105.1	106.3	*
0	Surface dose 30 to 50% depending upon collimator										0
0.5	100.0	100.0	100.0	100.0	100.0	100.0	100.0	100.0	100.0	100.0	0.5
1	95.4	96.8	97.0	97.4	97.6	97.8	98.0	98.2	98.4	98.4	1
2	87.1	90.6	91.2	91.9	92.2	92.7	93.0	93.3	93.9	94.0	2
3	79.5	84.7	85.5	86.5	86.9	87.6	87.9	88.3	89.3	89.6	3
4	72.7	79.0	79.9	81.1	81.7	82.5	82.9	83.4	84.7	85.2	4
5	66.5	73.5	74.5	75.9	76.6	77.4	77.9	78.5	80.1	80.8	5
6	60.8	68.1	69.2	70.7	71.5	72.4	73.0	73.6	75.4	76.4	6
7	55.6	62.9	64.1	65.7	66.5	67.5	68.1	68.8	70.8	72.1	7
8	50.9	58.0	59.2	60.8	61.7	62.7	63.4	64.1	66.5	68.0	8
9	46.6	53.5	54.7	56.2	57.1	58.2	58.9	59.7	62.3	64.0	9
10	42.7	49.3	50.5	52.0	52.9	54.0	54.8	55.6	58.4	60.2	10
11	39.2	45.5	46.6	48.1	49.0	50.1	50.9	51.7	54.7	56.6	11
12	35.9	41.9	43.0	44.5	45.4	46.5	47.3	48.1	51.2	53.2	12
13	32.9	38.6	39.7	41.1	42.0	43.2	44.0	44.8	47.9	50.0	13
14	30.2	35.6	36.6	38.0	38.9	40.1	40.9	41.8	44.9	47.0	14
15	27.7	32.9	33.8	35.2	36.1	37.2	38.0	38.9	42.0	44.2	15
16	25.4	30.4	31.3	32.6	33.5	34.5	35.3	36.2	39.3	41.5	16
17	23.3	28.1	29.0	30.2	31.1	32.1	32.8	33.7	36.8	39.0	17
18	21.4	26.0	26.9	28.0	28.8	29.8	30.5	31.4	34.5	36.7	18
19	19.6	24.0	24.9	26.0	26.7	27.7	28.4	29.2	32.3	34.6	19
20	18.0	22.1	22.9	24.0	24.8	25.7	26.4	27.2	30.3	32.6	20

*This line gives the dose at maximum (5 mm depth), for 100 rads to a small mass of tissue (equilibrium thickness) at the same location in "free space." Division by 100 gives the backscatter factor.

TABLE A-6
CENTRAL AXIS PERCENTAGE DEPTH DOSES FOR SQUARE FIELDS

Cobalt 60				Open ended applicator						100 cm SSD
Depth in cm				Field area in cm^2						Depth in cm
	0	16	25	36	49	64	81	100	225	400	
*	100.0	101.5	101.8	102.2	102.5	102.9	103.2	103.5	105.1	106.3	*
0				Surface dose 30 to 50% depending upon collimator							0
0.5	100.0	100.0	100.0	100.0	100.0	100.0	100.0	100.0	100.0	100.0	0.5
1	95.9	97.1	97.3	97.7	97.9	98.1	98.3	98.6	99.0	98.9	1
2	87.9	91.4	91.9	92.6	92.9	93.3	93.6	93.9	94.6	94.7	2
3	80.7	85.8	86.5	87.5	87.9	88.5	88.9	89.3	90.2	90.5	3
4	73.8	80.2	81.2	82.4	83.0	83.7	84.2	84.7	85.9	86.3	4
5	67.8	74.8	76.0	77.3	78.1	78.9	79.6	80.1	81.6	82.2	5
6	62.3	69.7	70.9	72.4	73.2	74.2	74.9	75.5	77.3	78.1	6
7	57.3	64.8	66.0	67.6	68.4	69.5	70.2	70.9	73.0	74.0	7
8	52.7	60.1	61.3	62.9	63.8	64.9	65.6	66.4	68.7	70.0	8
9	48.5	55.7	56.9	58.4	59.4	60.5	61.2	62.0	64.5	66.1	9
10	44.7	51.5	52.7	54.2	55.2	56.3	57.0	57.8	60.6	62.3	10
11	41.2	47.7	48.8	50.3	51.3	52.4	53.1	53.9	56.9	58.7	11
12	38.0	44.1	45.2	46.7	47.7	48.7	49.5	50.3	53.4	55.3	12
13	35.0	40.8	41.9	43.3	44.3	45.4	46.1	47.0	50.2	52.1	13
14	32.2	37.8	38.9	40.2	41.2	42.3	43.0	43.9	47.1	49.1	14
15	29.6	35.0	36.1	37.4	38.3	39.4	40.1	41.0	44.2	46.2	15
16	27.2	32.5	33.5	34.8	35.6	36.7	37.4	38.3	41.5	43.5	16
17	25.0	30.1	31.1	32.3	33.1	34.2	34.9	35.8	39.0	41.0	17
18	23.0	27.9	28.8	30.0	30.8	31.9	32.6	33.5	36.7	38.6	18
19	21.2	25.8	26.7	27.9	28.7	29.7	30.5	31.3	34.5	36.4	19
20	19.5	23.8	24.7	25.9	26.7	27.7	28.5	29.3	32.4	34.4	20

*This line gives the dose at maximum (5 mm depth), for 100 rads to a small mass of tissue (equilibrium thickness) at the same location in "free space." Division by 100 gives the backscatter factor.

TABLE A-7
CENTRAL AXIS PERCENTAGE DEPTH DOSES FOR SQUARE FIELDS

4 MV Linear Accelerator SD 100 cm
Field area in cm² (open-ended applicator)

Depth in cm	4 × 4	5 × 5	6 × 6	7 × 7	8 × 8	10 × 10	12 × 12	15 × 15	20 × 20	Depth in cm
1	100.0	100.0	100.0	100.0	100.0	100.0	100.0	100.0	100.0	1
2	96.5	96.8	97.2	97.4	97.5	97.6	97.7	97.9	98.2	2
3	91.3	92.0	92.5	92.9	93.0	93.3	93.5	93.7	94.3	3
4	85.9	86.8	87.4	88.2	88.2	88.7	89.2	89.7	90.5	4
5	80.4	81.3	82.2	82.9	83.4	84.0	84.4	84.9	85.7	5
6	74.9	76.1	77.0	77.9	78.6	79.5	80.1	80.7	81.5	6
7	69.9	71.3	72.2	73.2	74.0	75.0	75.8	76.4	77.3	7
8	65.6	66.9	68.0	69.1	69.8	71.0	71.7	72.3	73.4	8
9	61.2	62.8	63.7	64.7	65.5	66.6	67.7	68.5	69.8	9
10	57.2	58.5	59.8	60.8	61.7	62.7	63.7	64.7	66.2	10
11	53.4	54.9	56.0	57.0	57.8	59.0	60.0	61.4	62.7	11
12	49.8	51.1	52.3	53.4	54.3	55.7	56.8	58.1	59.5	12
13	46.6	47.8	49.0	50.0	51.0	52.4	53.5	54.9	56.3	13
14	43.5	44.7	45.8	46.9	47.8	49.3	50.3	51.7	53.4	14
15	40.7	41.9	43.0	44.0	45.0	46.4	47.5	48.8	50.3	15
16	37.9	39.2	40.3	41.3	42.1	43.6	44.7	46.0	47.8	16
17	35.4	36.6	37.8	38.7	39.5	40.9	42.0	43.4	45.0	17
18	33.0	34.2	35.2	36.2	37.0	38.5	39.6	40.9	42.6	18
19	30.9	32.0	32.9	34.0	34.8	36.0	37.2	38.5	40.1	19
20	28.9	29.9	30.8	31.8	32.7	34.0	35.1	36.3	38.1	20
22	25.3	26.2	27.1	27.9	28.7	30.0	31.0	32.4	34.2	21
24	22.1	23.0	23.9	24.6	25.4	26.5	27.6	28.9	30.6	22
26	(19.4)	(20.2)	(20.9)	(21.6)	(22.3)	(23.5)	(24.5)	(25.8)	(27.4)	23
28	(16.9)	(17.7)	(18.3)	(19.0)	(19.7)	(20.7)	(21.7)	(22.9)	(24.6)	24
30	(14.9)	(15.5)	(16.1)	(16.8)	(17.4)	(18.4)	(19.4)	(20.4)	(21.9)	25

TABLE A-8
BETATRON X RAYS—CENTRAL AXIS PERCENTAGE DEPTH DOSES

Depth cm	15 MV, TSD 100 cm Field area (cm²)			22 MV, TSD 100 cm	31 MV, TSD 100 cm
	25	100	200–400	Field sizes larger than 50 cm²	
0.5	61.5	64.5	68.0	50.0	
1	81.0	82.0	86.5	70.0	
2	98.5	98.0	98.5	90.1	83.5
3	100.0	100.0	100.0	98.0	94.0
4	98.0	98.0	97.5	100.0	99.5
5	94.5	94.5	94.0	99.5	100.0
6	90.5	91.0	90.5	96.6	99.0
7	86.5	87.0	87.5	93.0	96.0
8	83.0	84.0	84.0	89.1	93.0
10	76.0	77.0	77.5	81.9	88.0
12	69.0	71.0	71.5	75.5	82.0
14	62.5	64.5	65.5	69.6	76.5
16	57.0	59.0	60.0	64.2	71.5
18	52.0	54.0	55.5	59.1	66.0
20	47.5	50.0	51.0	54.5	62.0

TABLE A-9
HIGH ENERGY ELECTRONS—DEPTH IN CM FOR INDICATED PERCENTAGE DEPTH DOSE

Percentage Depth Dose	15-MeV Electrons Field area (cm²)				20-MeV Electrons Field area (cm²)				30-MeV Electrons Field area (cm²)			
	2 × 2	4 × 4	6 × 6	10 × 10	4 × 4	6 × 6	10 × 10	15 × 15	4 × 4	6 × 6	10 × 10	15 × 15
100	1.0	1.6	1.7	1.8	1.8	1.9	2.1	2.1	2.3	2.4	2.6	2.7
95	1.9	2.7	2.9	3.1	3.1	3.5	4.0	4.0	3.8	4.5	5.5	5.7
90	2.3	3.5	3.7	4.0	4.0	4.4	4.9	5.0	5.1	5.9	6.8	7.0
80	2.9	4.0	4.3	4.6	4.8	5.5	5.8	5.9	6.3	7.5	8.3	8.7
70	3.4	4.5	4.9	5.2	5.4	6.2	6.6	6.7	7.5	8.7	9.5	9.9
60	4.0	4.9	5.3	5.5	6.1	6.9	7.2	7.3	8.5	9.8	10.5	11.0
50	4.5	5.4	5.7	6.0	6.7	7.4	7.8	7.9	9.4	10.8	11.3	11.8
40	4.9	5.8	6.1	6.3	7.3	8.0	8.3	8.4	10.4	11.6	12.2	12.6
30	5.4	6.2	6.4	6.7	7.8	8.4	8.7	8.8	11.3	12.5	13.0	13.4
20	5.9	6.5	6.9	7.1	8.3	8.7	9.0	9.0	12.5	13.3	13.7	14.1
10	6.3	7.3	7.4	7.5	9.7	9.8	9.8	9.8	14.2	14.5	14.9	15.0

TABLE A-10
USEFUL PHYSICAL DATA

alpha-particle mass (m_a) = 6.65×10^{-24} g

1 ampere (amp) = 3×10^9 esu of charge/sec
                = 6.25×10^{18} electrons/sec

1 angstrom (Å) = 10^{-8} cm

1 atomic mass unit (amu) = 1.66×10^{-24} g
                         = 931.2 MeV

Avogadro's number = 6.023×10^{23} atoms/gram-atomic weight

1 calorie (cal) = 4.185×10^7 erg/g

1 curie (Ci)——3.7×10^{10} de-excitations/sec
   1 millicurie (mCi)——3.7×10^7 d/s
   1 microcurie (μCi)——3.7×10^4 d/s

diameter of lighter atoms = about 3×10^{-8} cm (3 Å)

electron charge (e) = 4.803×10^{-10} esu
                    = 1.602×10^{-19} coulomb

electron rest mass (m_e) = 0.000549 amu
                           = 9.108×10^{-28} g
                           = 0.511 MeV

1 electron volt (ev) = 1.602×10^{-12} erg
   10^3 electron volts (keV) = 1.602×10^{-9} erg
   10^6 electron volts (MeV) = 1.602×10^{-6} erg

1 electrostatic unit of charge (esu) = 2.083×10^9 electrons

1 erg = 6.24×10^5 MeV

1 gram (g) = 6.024×10^{23} amu
           = 5.61×10^{26} MeV

neutron rest mass (m_n) = 1.00866 amu
                          = 1.675×10^{-24} g
                          = 939.5 MeV

Planck's constant (h) = 6.625×10^{-27} erg-sec

proton rest mass (m_p) = 1.00727 amu
                         = 1.672×10^{-24} g
                         = 938.2 MeV

1 roentgen (R) produces ionization :
   = 1 esu/cc standard air
   = 2.083×10^9 ion pairs/cc standard air
   = 1.61×10^{12} ion pairs/g air
   = 7.01×10^4 MeV/cc standard air
   = 5.42×10^7 MeV/g air
   = 87 ergs/g air
   = about 96 ergs/g soft tissue

TABLE A-10 (*continued*)

velocity of electromagnetic radiation = 2.998×10^{10} cm/sec in vacuum or air

$W = 33.7$ eV/ion pair, average for radiations in the usual therapy range (X and γ rays with energy above 20 keV)

TABLE A-11
USEFUL EQUATIONS

Kinetic Energy: $K.E. = \frac{1}{2}mv^2$
   where $K.E.$ is energy in ergs, m is mass in g, and v is velocity of body in cm/sec.

Mass-energy: $E = mc^2$
   where E is energy in ergs, m is mass in g, and c is velocity of light in cm/sec.

$$\text{Relativistic Mass:} \quad m = \frac{m_o}{\sqrt{1 - \dfrac{v^2}{c^2}}}$$

where m is mass at velocity v cm/sec, m_o is rest mass, and c is velocity of light in cm/sec.

Photon Energy: $E = hv$
   where E is energy in ergs, h is Planck's constant, and v is frequency of electromagnetic wave.

Wavelength-frequency Relationship: $c = v\lambda$
   where c is velocity of electromagnetic wave *in vacuo* (constant) in cm/sec, is frequency, λ is wavelength in cm.

Minimum Wavelength: $\lambda_{min} = \dfrac{12.4}{kVp}$ Å

where λ_{min} is minimum wavelength in Å, and kVp is peak kilovoltage. If photon energy is known in keV, the equation gives the wavelength of the electromagnetic wave.

Inverse Square Law: $ID^2 = \text{constant}$
   where I is the exposure and D the distance.

Photoelectric Equation: $hv = W + E_e$
   where hv is energy of incident photon, W is energy needed to remove electron from shell, and E_e is kinetic energy of photoelectron.

Compton Effect: $\Delta\lambda = 0.024(1 - \cos\phi)$ Å
   where $\Delta\lambda$ is lengthening of wavelength and ϕ is scattering angle (photon).

Pair Production: $hv = e^- + e^+ + \text{kinetic energy}$
   where hv is energy of photon (minimum 1.02 MeV), e^- is negatron, and e^+ is positron.

Attenuation of X or γ rays:

$$I = I_o e^{-\mu d}$$

where I is intensity of monoenergetic radiation transmitted radiation through layer of thickness d, I_o is initial intensity, e is base of natural logarithms, and μ is linear attenuation coefficient.

TABLE A-11 (*continued*)

Mass Attenuation Coefficient: $\mu_m = \tau_m + \sigma_m + \pi_m$
  where μ_m is total mass attenuation coefficient, τ_m is photoelectric mass attenuation coefficient, σ_m is Compton mass attenuation coefficient, and π_m is pair production mass attenuation coefficient.

Bragg-Gray Relation: $E_m = J_a \rho W$
  where E_m is energy/g absorbed in solid, J_a number of ion pairs/g formed in gas cavity, ρ is ratio of stopping powers for secondary particles in solid to that in gas, and W is average energy to form 1 ion pair in gas.

Half Value Layer: $\text{HVL} = \dfrac{0.693}{\mu_l}$

  where μ_l is linear attenuation coefficient.

Homogeneity Coefficient: $\text{H.C.} = \dfrac{\text{HVL}_1}{\text{HVL}_2}$

Integral Dose (approximate): $I = 1.44 A D_0 d_{1/2} \left\{ 1 + \dfrac{2.88 d_{1/2}}{f} \right\}$

  where A is area of beam, D_0 is surface dose, $d_{1/2}$ is depth of 50% central axis depth dose, and f is the source to skin distance.

Radioactive Decay: $A = A_o e^{\lambda t}$
  where A is activity of radionuclide remaining at time t, A_o is activity of radionuclide at time zero, e is base of natural logarithms, and λ is decay or transformation constant.

Half-life: $T = \dfrac{0.693}{\lambda}$

  where T is half-life and λ is decay constant.

Average Life: $t_a = \dfrac{1}{\lambda}$

  where t_a is average life and λ is decay constant.

Specific Activity of a Radionuclide $= \dfrac{1.13 \times 10^{13}}{TA}$ curies/g

  where T is half-life and A is atomic weight.

Effective Half-life of a Radionuclide:

$$T_e = \frac{T_b T_p}{T_b + T_p}$$

where T_e is effective half-life, T_b is biologic half-life, and T_p is physical half-life.

TABLE A-11 (*continued*)

Beta Dosage of Internal Radionuclide:

$$D_\beta = 5.92 \times 10^{-4} C \bar{E}_\beta \text{ rad/sec}$$

$$D_\beta = 73.8 C \bar{E}_\beta T_e \text{ rads to total decay}$$

where D_β is dosage due to β particles, C is concentration of radionuclide in μCi/g, E_β is average energy of β particles in MeV, and T_e is effective half-life in days.

Standard Deviation in Counting Technics: $\sigma = \pm \sqrt{N}$
where σ is standard deviation and N is number of observed counts.

Percent Standard Error: $\%S.E. = \pm \dfrac{100}{\sqrt{N}}$

where N is number of observed counts.

Resolving Time of Counter: $t = \dfrac{N_1 + N_2 - N_{12}}{2N_1 N_2}$

where N_1 is net count rate of first sample, N_2 second sample, and N_{12} both samples.

Correction for Coincidence Loss: $N_\alpha = \dfrac{N}{1 - (Nt/60)}$

where N_α is corrected count rate, N is observed count rate, each in counts/min; t is resolving time in sec.

Accumulated Maximum Permissible Dose Equivalent for Occupational Exposure:

$$MPD = 5(N - 18) \text{ rems}$$

where MPD is maximum permisslbe whole body dose equivalent in rems, N is age in years and is greater than 18.

Dose Equivalent = Absorbed Dose × Quality Factor
  rems = rads × QF

Shortest Permissible Distance from External γ-ray Emitters (40-hr week):

General Form: $d = 20 \sqrt{\dfrac{\Gamma A}{2^n}} \text{ cm}$

Radium Source: $d = 57 \sqrt{\dfrac{mg\ Ra}{2^n}} \text{ cm}$

where d is shortest permissible distance in cm, Γ is specific γ-ray constant in R/mCi-hr at 1 cm, A is the activity of the radionuclide in mCi, $mg\ Ra$ is number of milligrams of radium in source, and n is number of half value layers of protective shield.

TABLE A-12
THE GREEK ALPHABET

Small	Large	Name
α	A	alpha
β	B	beta
γ	Γ	gamma
δ	Δ	delta
ε	E	epsilon
ζ	Z	zeta
η	H	eta
θ	Θ	theta
ι	I	iota
κ	K	kappa
λ	Λ	lambda
μ	M	mu
ν	N	nu
ξ	Ξ	xi
ο	O	omicron
π	Π	pi
ρ	P	rho
σ	Σ	sigma
τ	T	tau
υ	Υ	upsilon
φ	Φ	phi
χ	X	chi
ψ	Ψ	psi
ω	Ω	omega

ATLAS OF ISODOSE CURVES FOR THE ERNST APPLICATOR

The isodose curves in Figures A-1 to A-12 were calculated by Robert J. Shalek by means of the RADCOMP III computer program,* at the M.D. Anderson Hospital and Tumor Institute.

Factors used in the calculations for the various radium loadings are:

Active length	12.0 mm
Physical length	20.0 mm
Nominal filter thickness	0.5 mm Pt
Effective filter thickness	0.541 mm Pt
Filter absorption coefficient	0.170^{-1}
Exposure rate at 1 cm for 1 mg Ra (unfiltered)	9.09 R/hr
Rad/roentgen	0.957

Distribution of Ra in mg is shown in each figure. The values indicated on the individual curves represent dose rates in rads/hr with the designated Ra distribution. Allowance has been made for attenuation in tissues.

Isodose distributions in rads per hour about a variety of useful radium loadings of the Ernst expanding cervicouterine applicator. The curves were generated by the computer at the University of Texas M.D. Anderson Hospital.

Original point-by-point manual measurement and plotting of exposures in R per hour were published some years ago in booklet form (now out of print) by Ansco (GAF) under the title *Dosage Measurements in Radium Therapy,* by Edwin C. Ernst, Sr. When these data are corrected for the latest value of Γ_{Ra} and converted to rads per hour, the results are in reasonably good agreement with the isodose curves, at least at certain critical points. However, the curves provide a much better conception of the dosage distribution about the applicator.

Note that Tod's points A and B have been shown in each figure. These continue to be useful points of reference, provided their limitations are kept in mind. These limitations are less relevant with the Ernst applicator because the lesion is usually adapted geographically to the applicator.

The Ernst device continues to be widely used on account of its flexibility and adaptability to the great majority of cervicouterine lesions. One of its outstanding advantages is the known relationship of all the radium sources to each other and to the lesion, making it possible to use a standard set of isodose curves for dosage determination.

*Details of method of calculation are given in a series of three papers by R. J. Shalek and M. Stovall, and by G. Batten, Jr., under the general title: The M. D. Anderson Method for the computation of isodose curves around interstitial and intracavitary radiation sources. *Am. J. Roentgenol., 102*:662, 1968.

FRONT VIEW

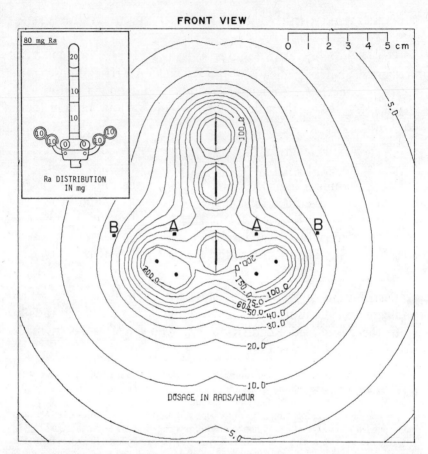

FIGURE A-1. Radium loading of Ernst expanding applicator for *carcinoma of the cervix* with adequate depth (7 cm) of the cervicouterine canal, and average width (6 cm) of the vaginal vault.

SIDE VIEW

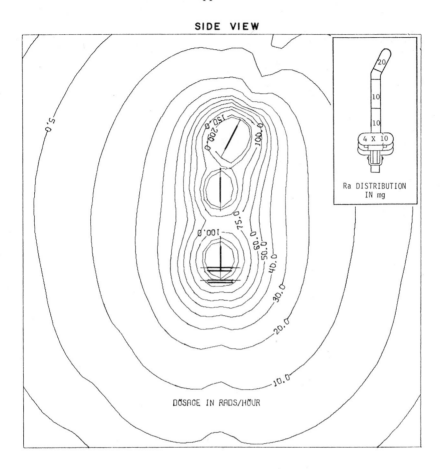

DOSAGE IN RADS/HOUR

Ra DISTRIBUTION
IN mg

FRONT VIEW

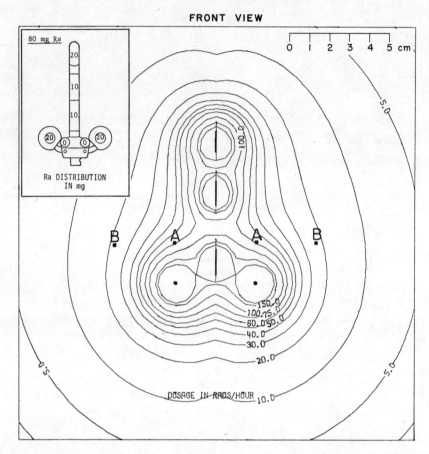

FIGURE A-2. Radium loading of Ernst expanding applicator provided with *plastic ovoids* in the vaginal portion (the lateralmost colpostats have been removed), for *carcinoma of the cervix*. The vaginal vault and cervicouterine canal are of average dimensions as in Figure A-1.

SIDE VIEW

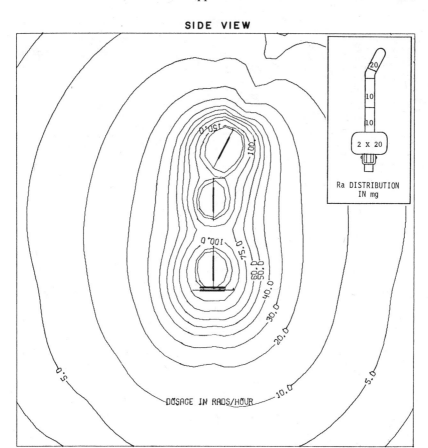

FRONT VIEW

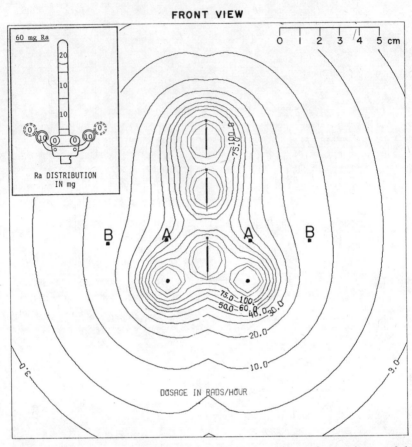

FIGURE A-3. Radium loading of Ernst expanding applicator for *carcinoma of the cervix* with adequate depth (7 cm) of the cervicouterine canal, but with a narrow vaginal vault (5 cm). The lateralmost colpostats have been detached.

SIDE VIEW

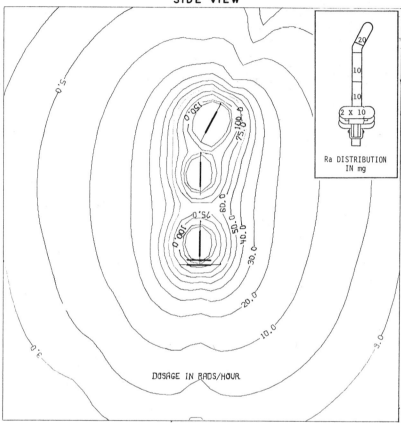

DOSAGE IN RADS/HOUR

Ra DISTRIBUTION
IN mg

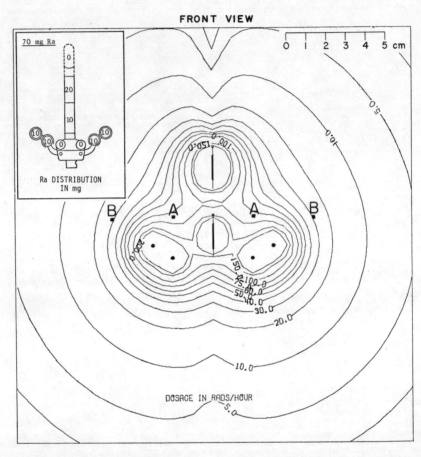

FIGURE A-4. Radium loading of Ernst expanding applicator for *carcinoma of the cervix* when the cervicouterine canal is shallow (5 cm deep), but the vaginal vault is adequate (6 cm). Only two segments of the tandem can be accommodated.

SIDE VIEW

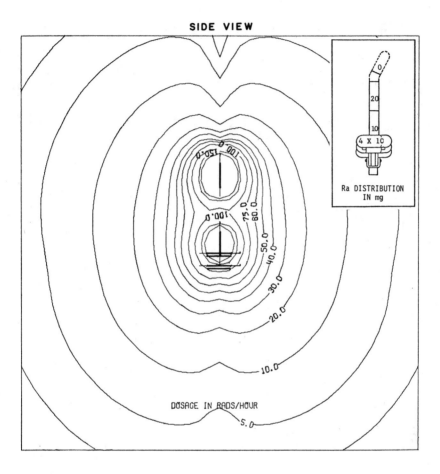

DOSAGE IN RADS/HOUR

Ra DISTRIBUTION IN mg

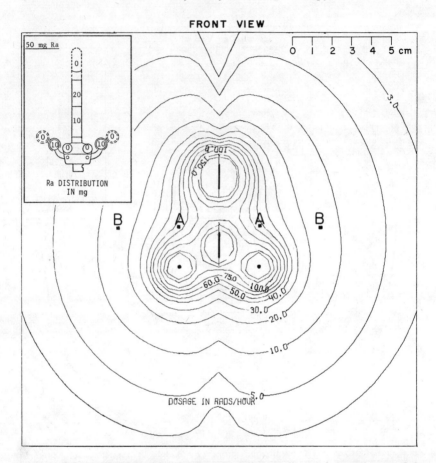

FRONT VIEW

FIGURE A-5. Radium loading of Ernst expanding applicator for ***carcinoma of the cervix*** when the cervicouterine canal is shallow (5 cm) and the vaginal vault is narrow (5 cm). Only two tandem segments can be accommodated, and the lateralmost colpostats have been detached.

SIDE VIEW

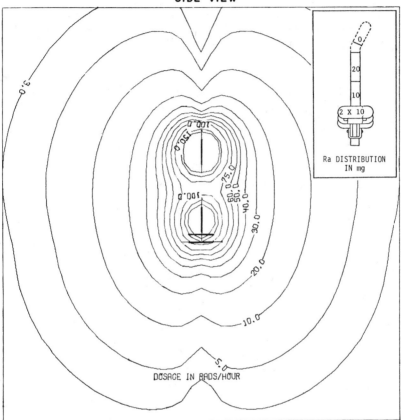

Ra DISTRIBUTION
IN mg

DOSAGE IN RADS/HOUR

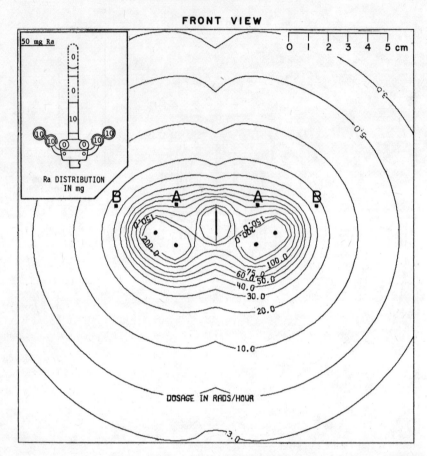

FIGURE A-6. Radium loading of Ernst expanding applicator for ***advanced carcinoma of the cervix,*** or ***carcinoma of the cervical stump.*** Only one tandem can be accommodated because the cervicouterine canal is only 2 cm deep. However, the vaginal vault is normal in width (6 cm). Sometimes, in advanced cervical carcinoma the canal may become patent after the first application, and a second one with better distribution of radium becomes possible.

SIDE VIEW

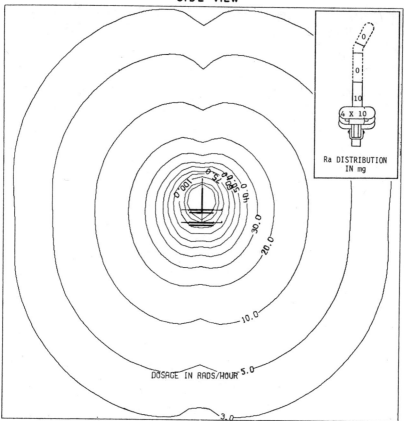

FRONT VIEW

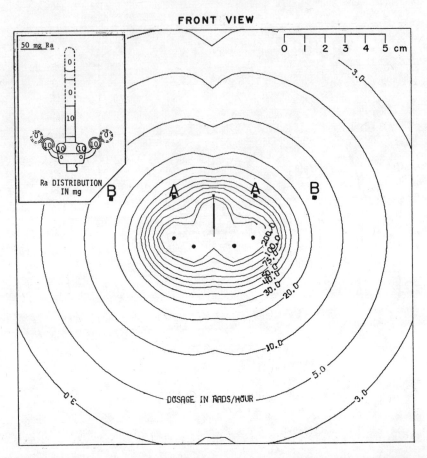

FIGURE A-7. Radium loading of Ernst expanding applicator for ***advanced carcinoma of the cervix,*** or ***carcinoma of the cervical stump,*** when the cervicouterine canal is only 2 cm deep, and the vaginal vault is narrow. The lateralmost colpostats are removed and the remaining four colpostats loaded.

SIDE VIEW

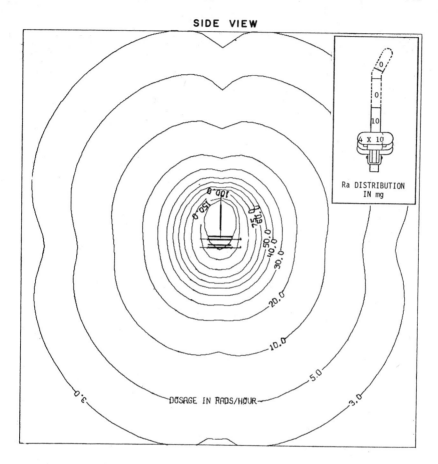

Ra DISTRIBUTION IN mg

DOSAGE IN RADS/HOUR

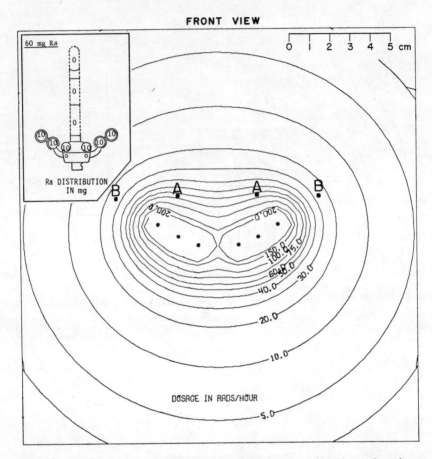

FIGURE A-8. Radium loading of Ernst expanding applicator for ***advanced carcinoma of the cervix,*** or ***carcinoma of the cervical stump,*** when the cervicouterine canal is completely obliterated, but the vaginal vault is still normal in width (6 cm). In advanced carcinoma the canal may open after the first application, and a second one with better distribution of radium may become possible.

SIDE VIEW

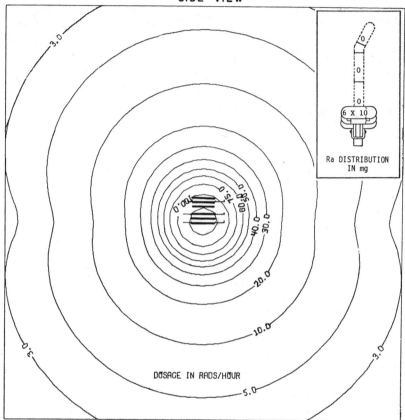

Ra DISTRIBUTION
IN mg

DOSAGE IN RADS/HOUR

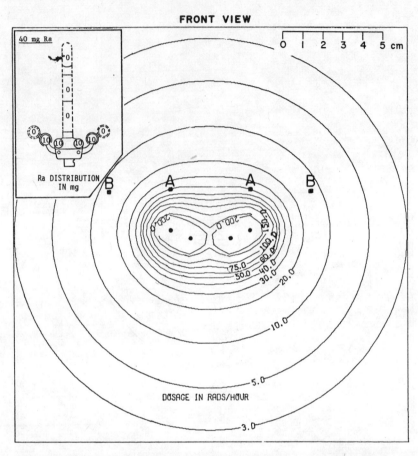

FRONT VIEW

FIGURE A-9. Radium loading of Ernst expanding applicator for *advanced carcinoma of the cervix,* or *carcinoma of the cervical stump,* when the vaginal vault is narrow and the cervicouterine canal obliterated. The canal may become patent after the first application, making possible a second one with better distribution of radium.

SIDE VIEW

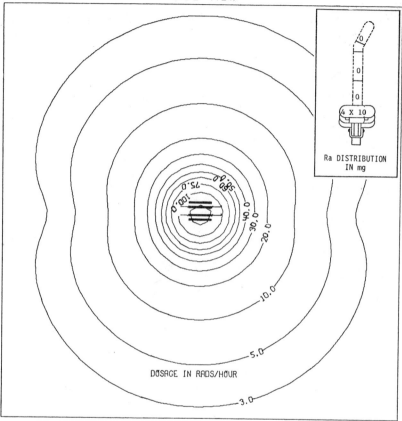

DOSAGE IN RADS/HOUR

Ra DISTRIBUTION IN mg

FRONT VIEW

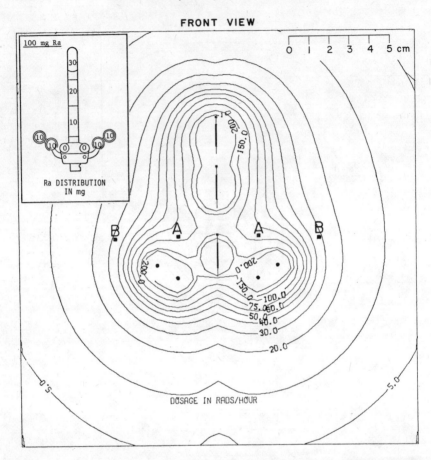

FIGURE A-10. Radium loading of Ernst expanding applicator for *carcinoma of the corpus uteri.* Caution must be used to avoid overirradiation of the normal tissues in the paracervical triangle (Point A). This form of therapy should be limited to the uterus with a normal size cavity; otherwise, the packing technic of Heyman, either alone or in combination with the Ernst method, is preferable.

SIDE VIEW

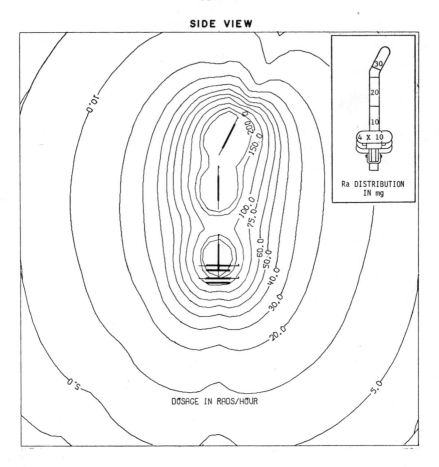

DOSAGE IN RADS/HOUR

Ra DISTRIBUTION IN mg

FRONT VIEW

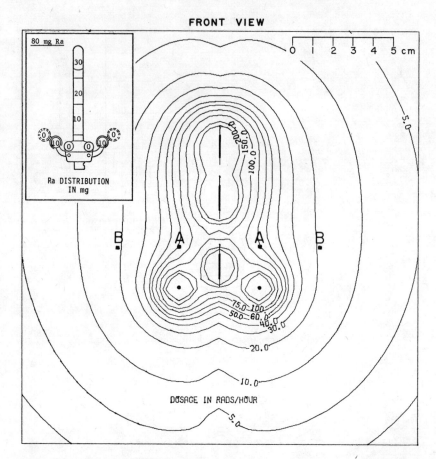

FIGURE A-11. Radium loading of Ernst expanding applicator for *carcinoma of the corpus uteri* when the vaginal vault is narrow. The lateralmost colpostats have been removed. This form of therapy should be limited to the uterus with a small cavity; otherwise, the packing technic of Heyman, either alone or in combination with the Ernst method, is preferable.

SIDE VIEW

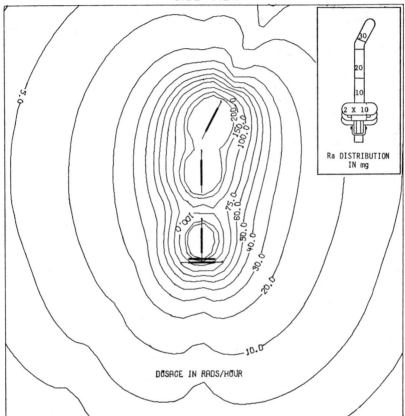

DOSAGE IN RADS/HOUR

Ra DISTRIBUTION
IN mg

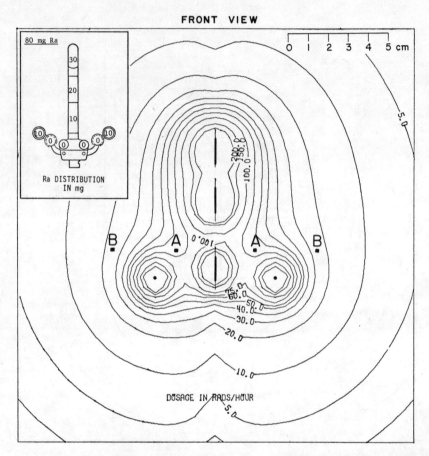

FRONT VIEW

FIGURE A-12. Radium loading of Ernst expanding applicator for *carcinoma of the corpus uteri* when the vaginal vault is normal in width (6 cm) and only the lateral-most colpostats are loaded. Note the smaller dose rate in the cervical and para-cervical regions with this radium distribution, as compared with the one in Figure A-10.

SIDE VIEW

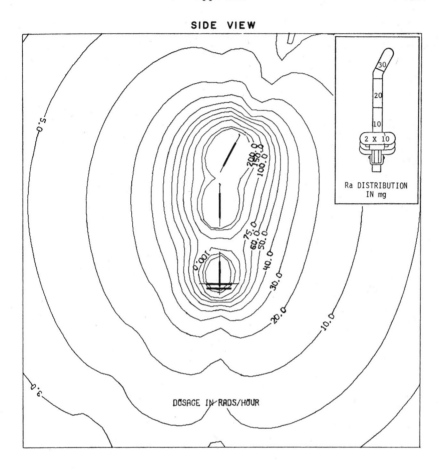

DOSAGE IN RADS/HOUR

Ra DISTRIBUTION
IN mg

Index